Diabetes: From Basic Science to Clinical Practice

Diabetes: From Basic Science to Clinical Practice

Edited by Edwina Orion

hayle
medical

New York

Hayle Medical,
750 Third Avenue, 9th Floor,
New York, NY 10017, USA

Visit us on the World Wide Web at:
www.haylemedical.com

ISBN: 978-1-63241-597-4

Cataloging-in-Publication Data

Diabetes : from basic science to clinical practice / edited by Edwina Orion.
   p. cm.
Includes bibliographical references and index.
ISBN 978-1-63241-597-4
1. Diabetes. 2. Carbohydrate intolerance. 3. Endocrine glands--Diseases.
4. Diabetes clinics. I. Orion, Edwina.
RC660 .D53 2019
616.4--dc23

Table of Contents

Permissions

List of Contributors

Index

Preface

The condition in which high blood sugar levels persist over prolonged periods of time in the human body is known as diabetes or diabetes mellitus (DM). Some of its symptoms are increased thirst and hunger, unintended weight loss and frequent urination. These symptoms may vary for Type 1 and Type 2 DM. Headache, blurred vision, fatigue and itchy skin may also occur. Diabetic emergencies can arise in cases of severe drops in blood sugar levels, diabetic ketoacidosis and hyperosmolar hyperglycemic state. DM can also result in long-term complications, such as damage to the eyes, nerves and kidneys, diabetes-related foot problems, cardiovascular diseases, stroke, etc. This book is a valuable compilation of topics, ranging from basic science to clinical practice in the field of diabetes. From theories to research, case studies related to all medical aspects of relevance have been included herein. It will prove to be immensely beneficial to students and researchers in this field.

Various studies have approached the subject by analyzing it with a single perspective, but the present book provides diverse methodologies and techniques to address this field. This book contains theories and applications needed for understanding the subject from different perspectives. The aim is to keep the readers informed about the progresses in the field; therefore, the contributions were carefully examined to compile novel researches by specialists from across the globe.

Indeed, the job of the editor is the most crucial and challenging in compiling all chapters into a single book. In the end, I would extend my sincere thanks to the chapter authors for their profound work. I am also thankful for the support provided by my family and colleagues during the compilation of this book.

Editor

Driving and diabetes: problems, licensing restrictions and recommendations for safe driving

Alex J. Graveling[1]* and Brian M. Frier[2]

Abstract

Driving is a complex process that places considerable demands on cognitive and physical functions. Many complications of diabetes can potentially impair driving performance, including those affecting vision, cognition and peripheral neural function. Hypoglycemia is a common side-effect of insulin and sulfonylurea therapy, impairing many cognitive domains necessary for safe driving performance. Driving simulator studies have demonstrated how driving performance deteriorates during hypoglycemia. Driving behavior that may predispose to hypoglycemia while driving is examined. Studies examining the risk of road traffic accidents in people with insulin-treated diabetes have produced conflicting results, but the potential risk of hypoglycemia-related road traffic accidents has led to many countries imposing restrictions on the type and duration of driving licenses that can be issued to drivers with diabetes. Guidance that promotes safe driving practice has been provided for drivers with insulin-treated diabetes, which is the group principally addressed in this review.

Keywords: Diabetes, Type 1 diabetes, Type 2 diabetes, Insulin therapy, Hypoglycemia, Automobile driving, Driving performance, Driving license, Road traffic accident, Motor vehicle accident

Introduction
Background

Driving has important business and recreational roles for transport in most countries, allowing people to travel to and from work, pursue their employment, and undertake multiple social and domestic activities. Most people regard driving to be a fundamental part of daily life; especially those with limited access to public transport [1]. Safe driving requires complex psychomotor skills, rapid information processing, vigilance and sound judgment [2]. Driving is classified as a light physical activity [3] but has considerable metabolic demands as has been demonstrated by driving simulator studies, which have shown high glucose consumption (predominantly cerebral) while driving [4].

Many of the microvascular and macrovascular complications of diabetes as well as some associated conditions (e.g., sleep apnea) can interfere with driving performance. Most of the cognitive functions required for driving are impaired by hypoglycemia [5, 6]. For many years diabetes, and in particular hypoglycemia, has been reported anecdotally to

impair driving performance; this can lead to driving mishaps and cause road traffic accidents. Drivers have reported incidents such as driving the wrong way along motorways and injudicious parking during hypoglycemia [7].

The majority of driving licensing authorities in developed countries make a distinction between people with diabetes who require insulin therapy to treat their diabetes and those who do not. This is principally related to the risk of hypoglycemia associated with insulin therapy. Other glucose-lowering agents, particularly the insulin secretagogues, the sulfonylureas and glinides, can also cause hypoglycemia, although are seldom reviewed in relation to driving performance. Recognition that the level of accident risk depends on factors other than insulin treatment has encouraged licensing authorities to assess insulin-treated drivers individually. In some countries this has influenced changes in driving regulations to allow insulin-treated drivers who are free of complications and able to demonstrate management practises that promote driving safety (such as regular blood glucose monitoring), to be licensed to drive large commercial vehicles from which they were previously debarred. The present review focuses mainly on drivers who require insulin treatment for their diabetes.

* Correspondence: alex.graveling@nhs.net
[1]JJR Macleod Centre for Diabetes & Endocrinology, Aberdeen Royal Infirmary, Foresterhill, Aberdeen AB25 2ZP, UK
Full list of author information is available at the end of the article

Literature search

A MEDLINE search (1946–2015) was conducted in January 2015 by combining the following subject terms: diabetes mellitus, diabetes mellitus type 1, diabetes mellitus type 2, automobile driving, traffic accidents, automobiles, whiplash injuries, motor vehicles and automobile driver examination. Limits of 'human' and 'English language' were imposed; the citations were then considered for relevance. Papers from the authors' personal files were included, and lists of published references were checked to identify any other relevant material.

Review
Diabetes & driving performance

How can diabetes affect driving performance? The considerable impact of hypoglycemia on driving performance is discussed below. Other complications of diabetes such as peripheral neuropathy, visual impairment and cerebrovascular disease leading to cognitive impairment may also affect driving performance. Peripheral vascular disease is not discussed but a lower limb amputation may impair the ability of the individual to operate the foot pedals. Adaptation of the vehicle to use hand-operated controls is a possible solution. Disorders associated with type 2 diabetes (T2DM), such as sleep apnea, can have an adverse impact on driving performance.

How does hypoglycemia affect driving performance? Hypoglycemia is a common side effect of insulin therapy for diabetes for people with type 1 and type 2 diabetes [8]. Experimental laboratory studies have demonstrated that cognitive functions critical to driving (such as attention, reaction times and hand-eye coordination) are impaired during hypoglycemia [5, 9]. The changes in visual information processing that occur during hypoglycemia could affect visual perception under conditions of limited perceptual time and low visual contrast (poor light); this would also have a significant effect on driving performance [10]. Studies using a sophisticated driving simulator have shown that driving performance is affected adversely by moderate hypoglycemia, causing problems such as inappropriate speeding or braking, ignoring road signs and traffic lights and not keeping to traffic lanes [11, 12]. During simulation studies, driving *per se* required higher dextrose infusion rates to maintain normoglycemia compared to passively watching a driving video; this increased metabolic demand in drivers may risk promoting hypoglycemia, particularly if their blood glucose is <5.0 mmol/l (90 mg/dl) [4].

Does hyperglycemia affect driving performance? The effect of hyperglycemia on driving performance has received very little attention and depends on how hyperglycemia is defined. A questionnaire-based study reported that hyperglycemia disrupted driving activities; 8 % of participants with T1DM reported at least one episode of disrupted driving associated with hyperglycemia over 1 year compared with 40 % of participants with insulin-treated type 2 diabetes [13]. No studies have examined the effect on driving performance but hyperglycemia does affect some measures of cognitive function and mood in people with T1DM and T2DM [14, 15].

How does peripheral neuropathy affect driving performance? When reduced sensation and impaired proprioception affect the lower limbs of people with diabetes they may find it more difficult to gauge pressure on the accelerator, brake or clutch pedals. In addition many of the agents used for neuropathic pain such as gabapentin or amitriptyline can have a sedative effect, although a recent driving simulator study in people without diabetes did not show any effect of pregabalin on driving performance [16]. To our knowledge, no studies to ascertain the potential effects of peripheral neuropathy on driving performance have been performed [17].

How does visual impairment affect driving performance? It is self-evident that vision is essential to safe driving performance and any impairment therefore has the potential to impair driving performance. Diabetes increases the risk of developing several eye disorders that can impair eyesight, such as cataract. Both proliferative, severe non-proliferative retinopathy and maculopathy can result in reduced visual acuity and affect visual fields. In the UK diabetes is no longer the commonest cause of blindness in working age people, but it remains a significant cause of visual impairment [18]. Because of the potential risk of visual impairment occurring through diabetic eye disease, in most westernized countries applicants for a driving license must be able to demonstrate an adequate level of vision. The assessment of people who have had photocoagulation for proliferative retinopathy usually includes the assessment of visual fields using perimetry.

How does cognitive impairment affect driving performance? People with diabetes may experience cognitive impairment from various causes, including cerebrovascular disease in the older person. Despite resolution of hypoglycemic symptoms and counter regulatory hormonal responses after hypoglycemia is treated, recovery of cognitive function has been shown to lag behind the restoration of normoglycemia (between 20 to 75 min) [5, 19]. Cognitive impairment has been shown to impair driving performance both in simulator studies and in "real-world" assessments of driving performance [20].

How does sleep apnea affect driving performance?
Sleep apnea is associated with obesity and type 2 diabetes. With the increased prevalence of obesity in many countries people are at increased risk of developing sleep apnea. Poor sleep quality overnight leads to daytime somnolence. Performance in driving simulator studies is worse in people with sleep apnea than in those without [21, 22]. A systematic review demonstrated that the risk of road traffic accidents was three-fold higher in people with sleep apnea; treatment of sleep apnea with continuous positive airway pressure improves driving performance and reduces accident risk [23, 24].

Diabetes and the risk of road traffic accidents (RTAs)
This has been reviewed previously in detail for drivers with insulin-treated diabetes [25]. Some studies have reported that RTA rates appear to be no higher in drivers with diabetes [26–28] whereas other studies have reported an increased risk [29, 30]. The differences may result from the considerable heterogeneity in the design of these studies. One reason why many studies failed to show a significant difference in RTA rates at a population level between people at risk of hypoglycemia (mainly those with insulin-treated diabetes) and the general population with driving licenses is that many countries impose restrictions on drivers with insulin-treated diabetes and remove those who are at high risk of having an accident. Drivers with diabetes who have problems such as deteriorating eyesight or impaired awareness of hypoglycemia may voluntarily restrict or cease their driving activities to avoid putting themselves and others at risk. However, a RTA is likely to have multifactorial causation and it may be difficult to control for concomitant fatigue, adverse weather or road conditions, mechanical failure of the vehicle, or to the use of drugs or alcohol.

A British study suggested that drivers with insulin-treated diabetes were not at increased risk [31], but one confounding factor was that the percentages holding a driving license in populations with and without diabetes were not determined [32]. Drivers with non-insulin treated diabetes have received less scrutiny despite the fact that the risk of severe hypoglycemia with sulfonylurea therapy is similar to that of people with T2DM who have been treated with insulin for less than two years [8]. Analysis of a claims database showed that the risk of road traffic accidents was significantly increased (hazard ratio 1.8) in people with a history of requiring medical attention to treat a hypoglycemic episode; the anti-diabetes medications being used were not reported (Fig. 1) [33].

In Canada, the province of Ontario has mandatory physician reporting of drivers with medical disorders who may be unfit to drive, including people with diabetes. By providing a financial incentive for physicians to report drivers at risk (which increased the incidence of

reporting) the RTA rate was lowered in those drivers who received warnings [34]. The Canadian National Population Health Survey (a large, representative longitudinal study) used self-reporting of diabetes status, insulin treatment and frequency of RTAs. The proportion of those with diabetes and/or treatment with insulin was not significantly higher in those who self-reported a history of RTAs in the preceding 12 months [35].

The largest study that examined RTA risk in drivers with diabetes analyzed data from the entire adult Norwegian population (3.1 million) for slightly over 2 years; just over 170,000 were taking anti-diabetes medications [36]. People with insulin-treated diabetes had a modestly increased risk of RTAs compared with the population as a whole, with an odds ratio of 1.4 (1.2–1.6). Those taking medication for peptic ulcers or gastro-esophageal reflux (neither of which are thought to influence driving performance) had a similar elevation in risk with an odds ratio of 1.3 (1.2–1.4). A meta-analysis of data from all these studies failed to show a significantly higher accident rate, with a non-significant risk ratio of 1.26 [37].

Can high-risk drivers with diabetes be identified?
Hypoglycemia is recognized to be the cause of some RTAs. When 452 people with T1DM who possessed current driving licenses were followed prospectively for 12 months with monthly reporting, 52 % reported at least one hypoglycemia-related mishap with 5 % recording as many as six or more [38]. People with a history of road traffic accidents exhibited poorer working memory during hypoglycemia compared with no history of accidents [39]. Adolescent drivers are well known to have an increased risk of accidents; parents of adolescent drivers with T1DM reported that 31 % of them had experienced a collision in the preceding year that had been attributed to hypoglycemia [40].

The factor that has most consistently been identified to be associated with an increased risk of RTAs in people with diabetes is previous exposure to severe hypoglycemia; a history of severe hypoglycemia in the preceding two years was associated with a four-fold higher risk of accidents [38, 41]. Driving problems included a variety of incidents including disruptive hypoglycemia occurring while driving and another passenger having to take over driving because of the driver's incapacity. When adjusted for annual mileage, severe hypoglycemia, experience of hypoglycemia while driving and a previous history of a RTA within the previous two years were all associated with an increased risk of a driving mishap [38]. Stricter glycemic control (HbA1c of 7.4 % (59 mmol/mol) versus 7.9 % (63 mmol/mol)) has been reported to be associated with a higher risk of RTAs [38]. The type of diabetes was not stated in this very small study but as the mean age at diagnosis was 31.6 years and 80 % were receiving insulin therapy, most

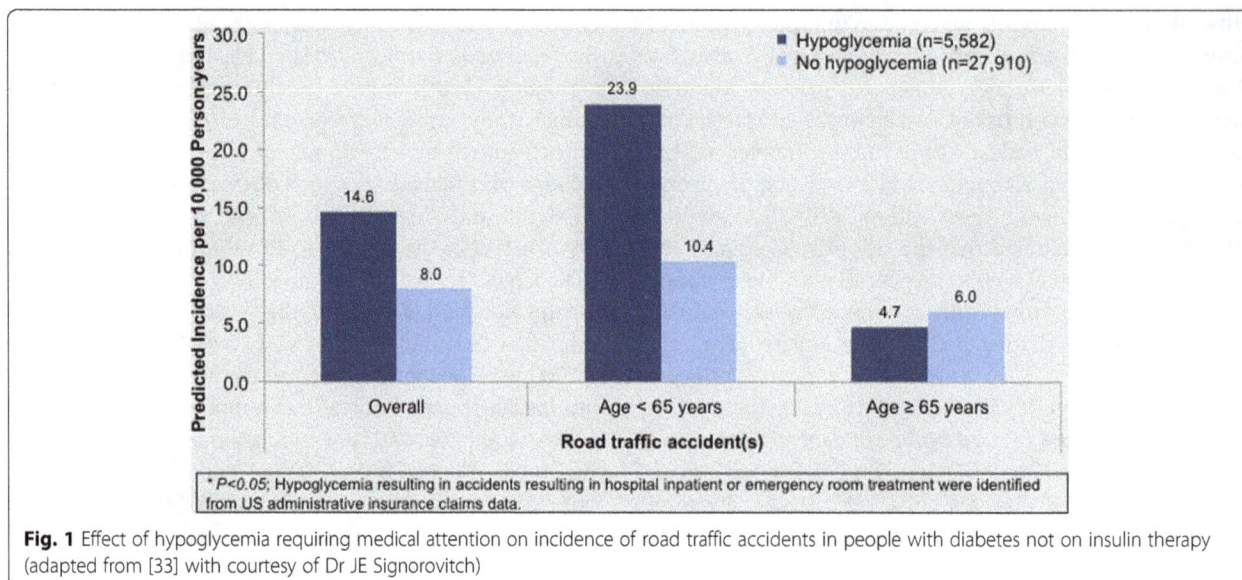

Fig. 1 Effect of hypoglycemia requiring medical attention on incidence of road traffic accidents in people with diabetes not on insulin therapy (adapted from [33] with courtesy of Dr JE Signorovitch)

drivers presumably had T1DM [41]. However, in people with T2DM on glucose-lowering therapies, the risk of severe hypoglycemia is similar across all levels of glycemic control except in those with near-normal or very poor glycemic control, so HbA1c is unlikely to be a useful index of risk for severe hypoglycemic events and resulting RTAs [42].

Drivers with type 1 diabetes (T1DM) who had a history of driving mishaps in the previous 12 months were compared to those with those with no such history [43, 44]. Other than a greater risk of severe hypoglycemia in the later study, the groups were well matched in terms of duration of diabetes, age and glycemic control. The driving performance of those with a history of driving mishaps deteriorated to a greater extent during hypoglycemia, thus perhaps identifying a subset of drivers who are more vulnerable to hypoglycemia affecting their driving performance adversely. An 11-item questionnaire attempted to identify the "at risk" drivers with diabetes [45]. Those scoring in the upper quartile reported more driving mishaps than those in the lower quartile. The most discriminating questions regarding accident risk were those that quantified annual mileage, identified a history of hypoglycemia-related RTAs, elicited poor self-management of hypoglycemic episodes and screened for the presence of lower limb neuropathy. An internet-based management programme undertaken by drivers with T1DM reduced the frequency of driving mishaps in high-risk drivers [46].

Hypoglycemia while driving; recognition and management

Experience of hypoglycemia while driving Previous experience of hypoglycemia while driving has been reported by between 15–66 % of drivers in surveys in the United Kingdom and New Zealand [47–49]; experience of hypoglycemia while driving in the preceding year was reported by 13–29 % [26, 50]. A prospective survey in the USA observed that over a 12-month period, 41 % of drivers reported experienced "disruptive" hypoglycemia while driving; the median number of hypoglycemia episodes reported by each driver was 2.7 (range of 1–26) [38]. This would suggest that a subset of drivers experience hypoglycemia more frequently than others while driving. A small study in eastern Europe that used blinded continuous glucose monitoring showed that many drivers with T1DM develop hypoglycemia while driving, including many asymptomatic episodes [51]. In-vehicle monitoring has been suggested as a possible solution using technologies, such as continuous glucose monitoring, which are linked to the car's dashboard display system [52].

The decision to drive including testing blood glucose levels before and during driving A driver with insulin-treated diabetes needs to have accurate knowledge of their blood glucose, and appreciate the minimum level compatible with safe driving. Subjective estimates of blood glucose based on symptoms are unreliable [53–55]; this has been clearly demonstrated in drivers with T1DM before driving [47, 48]. The ability of deciding when it is safe to drive may also be unreliable or absent, particularly in those with impaired awareness of hypoglycemia. During a driving simulator study only 4 % of those with normal hypoglycemia awareness stated that they would drive while hypoglycemic compared to 43 % with impaired awareness of hypoglycemia [56]. In a laboratory study [57], 38 % of subjects felt able to drive safely when their blood glucose was 2.8 mmol/L (50 mg/dl), and in a driving simulator study three quarters of subjects neither recognized the impairment of their driving performance, nor the presence of hypoglycemia, at blood glucose levels as low as 2.8 mmol/l (50 mg/dl) [12]. It is therefore preferable that the individual's decision to drive should be based on an actual measurement of blood glucose, though this is not enforceable in drivers with ordinary (European Group 1) driving licenses. Similar findings were observed in a prospective study when drivers with insulin-treated diabetes reported that they felt safe to drive on around 25 % of occasions when they had already ascertained that their capillary blood glucose was low (below 2.2 mmol/l (40 mg/dl)), suggesting that errors of judgment can arise from misperceptions about the safety of driving with a low blood glucose [58]. Abnormal behavior with pronounced cognitive impairment associated with hypoglycemia (becoming disorientated, getting lost or arriving at their destination with no memory of how they got there) was reported by 18 % of drivers [38], a state described in legal parlance as "automatism".

Questionnaire-based surveys have shown that 75–91 % of drivers are able to proffer an appropriate level for the minimum blood glucose for safe driving, i.e., 4.0 mmol/l (72 mg/dl) or higher. However, it is disconcerting that almost 40–60 % of drivers with insulin-treated diabetes reported that they never test blood glucose before driving, or test only if they feel hypoglycemic [47, 50, 59]. Although testing before driving was more common in participants with impaired hypoglycemia awareness, only a small minority in this high-risk group reported regular testing. Most participants (77 %) reported never testing during journeys of any length, indicating a lack of vigilance even when the risk of hypoglycemia is not negligible [50]. This is particularly relevant in view of the metabolic demands of driving [4].

Failure to measure blood glucose could have major medico-legal consequences. In a previous prosecution within the Scottish jurisdiction, a driver with T1DM, was found guilty of causing death by dangerous driving while hypoglycemic, and was strongly criticized because he had not measured his blood glucose before driving. In passing judgment, the Sheriff highlighted the risk associated with diabetes and driving, and stated that the privilege of a driving license carries a responsibility to ensure safety by measuring blood glucose. It is important that health care professionals ensure that the potential legal consequences of not testing blood glucose in relation to driving are communicated to their patients.

Treatment of hypoglycemia that occurs while driving
Appropriate treatment of hypoglycemia while driving is vital. Most drivers (83–88 %) have reported that they carry carbohydrate with them in their vehicles, but very few wait for more than 30 min after self-treatment before resuming driving, although cognitive function may

not have recovered fully until 45 min after restoration of normoglycemia [47, 50, 59–62]. The exact time required for recovery of sufficient cognitive function for driving has not yet been determined and drivers should be advised to err on the side of caution.

Although the definition of safe practice is debatable, any of the following omissions is unsatisfactory: not measuring blood glucose before driving; not carrying carbohydrate when driving; not stopping the vehicle when driving to self-treat hypoglycemia; and believing that a blood glucose level below 3.0 mmol/l (54 mg/dl) is compatible with safe driving. Almost half of the participants in an Edinburgh-based study failed to meet one or more of these basic standards [50]; a similar study in New Zealand reported that 33 % of drivers failed to meet one or more of these criteria [47].

Driving regulations for drivers with insulin-treated diabetes
It is beyond the scope of this review to describe the regulations for drivers with insulin-treated diabetes in every country or continent, and in many parts of the world no such driving regulations exist. Many developed countries place restrictions on those with diabetes; the principal concern is the development of hypoglycemia while driving that may cause a RTA.

Driving regulations for drivers with insulin-treated diabetes in the European Union (EU)
Many European countries previously imposed a blanket ban on most drivers with insulin-treated diabetes, particularly to drive large goods vehicles or passenger carrying vehicles. This rather draconian approach failed to acknowledge that the distribution of severe hypoglycemia is skewed, with many drivers seldom or never experiencing hypoglycemia [63]. In 2006 the European Union issued its 3rd Directive on driving that addressed several medical conditions and licensing for driving, which included diabetes and aimed to harmonize the driving regulations applied by member states [64, 65]. The European regulations were also an attempt to individualize the risk associated with driving and allow some people with insulin-treated diabetes to drive Group 2 vehicles (large goods vehicles), provided they met strict criteria and could demonstrate safe driving practices.

In the EU, driving licenses are issued as a Group 1 license (an ordinary driving license for a car, light van or motorcycle) and as a Group 2 license (a vocational driving license for a large goods vehicle (LGV) or a passenger carrying vehicle (PCV)). In the United Kingdom (UK), where 40 million people hold a driving license, approximately 575,000 are held by people with diabetes, with 13 % of these being Group 2 licenses [66]. Licensing is processed by the Driver and Vehicle Licensing Agency (DVLA).

Following the issue of the 3rd EU Directive on Driving, the regulations for driving licenses have been changed throughout Europe. Medical fitness to drive has to be reviewed at least every 5 years for renewal of the driving license. In addition the requirement was introduced that any driver with diabetes holding a Group 1 driving license who experienced more than one episode of severe hypoglycemia in any 12 month period must inform their national licensing authority and the driving license revoked until this problem was addressed and the annual frequency of severe events had declined to one per year [25]. In the context of hypoglycemia risk, this change in legislation would have meant that 44 % of the intensively treated group and 17 % of the conventionally treated group in the Diabetes Control and Complications Trial (DCCT) would have lost their driving licenses at some time during the trial period [67]. A recent study in Denmark has shown that following implementation of this legislation self-reported rates of severe hypoglycemia have fallen by 55 %, suggesting that the licensing change will encourage concealment of severe hypoglycemia [68]. People with impaired awareness of hypoglycemia have also to be debarred from driving, but this condition was not defined and how this is identified and managed has been left to individual countries.

By contrast, the regulations for Group 2 licenses have been relaxed for insulin-treated drivers, who previously had been debarred from driving LGVs and PCVs. Insulin-treated drivers are now able to apply for a Group 2 license although the medical fitness requirements are stringent; they must report any severe hypoglycemic episode, must have no evidence of impaired awareness of hypoglycemia and must test their blood glucose regularly at times relevant to driving and provide an accurate diary record.

Current guidelines for drivers with insulin-treated diabetes in the USA and Canada

The American Diabetes Association (ADA) recommends that "people with diabetes should be assessed individually, taking into account each individual's medical history as well as the potential related risks associated with driving" [69]. With the exception of commercial interstate driving, the rules and regulations on driving and diabetes are governed by individual states and vary considerably. The Federal government in the United States does not impose any specific restrictions regarding driving for people with diabetes who are not treated with insulin. Similar to European regulations, drivers with insulin-treated diabetes may be able to obtain a driving license for commercial vehicles such as large trucks, but may not be able to cross state boundaries. Canada also imposes restrictions on driving licenses that are similar to Europe and the USA [70].

Driving regulations in other countries

Many developing countries, such as most in sub-Saharan Africa, place no restriction on drivers with diabetes, and surprisingly these still do not exist in most advanced countries in the Middle East. The lack of driving regulations in general, and the absence of restrictions for medical disorders that can affect driving, are reflected by the high mortality and accident rate associated with road traffic accidents in these countries.

The Australian National Transport Commission have issued guidelines that promote safe driving for people with diabetes [71]. Drivers who are not insulin-treated are issued with an unconditional driving license, provided certain criteria are met (including co-morbidities). People requiring insulin treatment are issued with a period-restricted (time limited) driving license, which includes professional drivers with the equivalent of Group 2 driving licenses. In contrast with the EU, if a person with diabetes in Australia experiences severe hypoglycemia they must cease driving for a minimum period of six weeks. In addition, any driver who has a persistent loss of hypoglycemia awareness is considered unfit to drive unless their ability to experience early warning symptoms is restored.

Recommendations for safe driving practice have been issued for drivers with diabetes, an example of these is shown in Table 1.

Conclusions

Driving is a complex activity that is both mentally and physically demanding; drivers often underestimate these demands. Diabetes can impair driving performance in several

Table 1 Recommendations for safe driving practice for drivers with insulin-treated diabetes [25, 72]

- Always carry your glucose meter and blood glucose strips with you
- Check your blood glucose no more than 1 h before the start of the first journey and every two hours whilst you are driving
- If driving multiple short journeys, it is not necessary to test before each additional journey as long as you test every 2 h while driving. More frequent testing may be required in circumstances where a greater risk of hypoglycemia is present, e.g., after physical activity or altered meal routine
- Try to ensure that blood glucose is kept above 5.0 mmol/l (90 mg/dl) while driving. If your blood glucose is 5.0 mmol/l or less, have a snack. Do not drive if blood glucose is less than 4.0 mmol/l (72 mg/dl) or you feel hypoglycemic
- If hypoglycemia develops while driving, stop the vehicle in a safe location as soon as possible
- Always keep an emergency supply of fast-acting carbohydrate such as glucose tablets or sweets within easy reach inside the vehicle
- Do not start driving until 45 min after blood glucose has returned to normal (confirmed by measuring blood glucose). It takes time for the brain to recover fully from hypoglycemia
- Carry personal identification to indicate that you have diabetes in case of injury
- Particular care should be taken during changes of insulin regimen, change in lifestyle, following exercise, during travel and during pregnancy
- Take regular meals, snacks and periods of rest on longer journeys. Do not drink alcohol before, or while driving

ways, through short-term metabolic and longer-term complications. Hypoglycemia is a common side effect of insulin or sulfonylurea therapy and may occur during driving. Driving simulator studies have shown a decline in driving performance and impaired judgment during hypoglycemia. Despite the risks associated with hypoglycemia and driving, several surveys have shown that drivers with insulin-treated diabetes continue to embrace unsafe practices.

Many developed countries have instituted restrictions on drivers with diabetes through statutory regulations that limit the duration and scope of driving licenses. Recommendations and guidance for drivers with insulin-treated diabetes and their medical attendants have been developed, but such advice is absent in many parts of the world, where driving regulations are either very limited or non-existent. This remains a serious challenge to road and public safety in these countries and a risk to all road users.

Although the magnitude of the effects of hypoglycemia while driving on accident risk continues to be debated, hypoglycemia undoubtedly does cause road traffic accidents, some of which have a fatal outcome. Patients prone to debilitating hypoglycemia (such as those with impaired awareness of hypoglycemia) should therefore merit special consideration from the licensing authorities. The adoption of a more individualized approach to the assessment of the medical fitness to drive in North America and in Europe has been an enlightened and commendable development in recent years, but still requires further refinement to ensure its safe and effective application.

Competing interests
The authors have no competing interests to declare in relation to this article.

Authors' contributions
AJG performed the literature search and drafted the manuscript. BMF revised the manuscript and provided additional references. Both authors read and approved the final manuscript.

Authors' information
BMF has previously been a member and chair of the Honorary Advisory Panel on Driving and Diabetes to the Secretary of State for the Department for Transport in the UK.

Author details
[1]JJR Macleod Centre for Diabetes & Endocrinology, Aberdeen Royal Infirmary, Foresterhill, Aberdeen AB25 2ZP, UK. [2]The Queen's Medical Research Institute, The University of Edinburgh, Edinburgh EH16 4TJ, UK.

References
1. Sherman FT. Driving: the ultimate IADL. Geriatrics. 2006;61:9–10.
2. Frier BM. Living with hypoglycaemia. In: Frier BM, Heller SR, McCrimmon RJ, editors. Hypoglycaemia in Clinical Diabetes. 3rd ed. Chichester: John Wiley & Sons; 2014. p. 369–8.
3. Ainsworth BE, Haskell WL, Herrmann SD, Meckes N, Bassett Jr DR, Tudor-Locke C, et al. Compendium of Physical Activities: a second update of codes and MET values. Med Sci Sports Exerc. 2011;2011(43):1575–81.
4. Cox DJ, Gonder-Frederick LA, Kovatchev BP, Clarke WL. The metabolic demands of driving for drivers with type 1 diabetes mellitus. Diabetes Metab Res Rev. 2002;18:381–5.
5. Warren RE, Frier BM. Hypoglycaemia and cognitive function. Diabetes Obes Metab. 2005;7:493–503.
6. Graveling AJ, Deary IJ, Frier BM. Acute hypoglycemia impairs executive cognitive function in adults with and without type 1 diabetes. Diabetes Care. 2013;36:3240–6.
7. Frier BM, Matthews DM, Steel JM, Duncan LJ. Driving and insulin-dependent diabetes. Lancet. 1980;315:1232–4.
8. UK Hypoglycaemia Study Group. Risk of hypoglycaemia in types 1 and 2 diabetes: effects of treatment modalities and their duration. Diabetologia. 2007;50:1140–7.
9. Inkster B, Frier BM. The effects of acute hypoglycaemia on cognitive function in type 1 diabetes. Br J Diabetes Vasc Dis. 2012;12:221–6.
10. McCrimmon RJ, Deary IJ, Huntly BJ, MacLeod KJ, Frier BM. Visual information processing during controlled hypoglycaemia in humans. Brain. 1996;119(Pt 4):1277–87.
11. Cox DJ, Gonder-Frederick L, Clarke W. Driving decrements in type I diabetes during moderate hypoglycemia. Diabetes. 1993;42:239–43.
12. Cox D, Gonder-Frederick L, Kovatchev B, Julian D, Clarke W. Progressive hypoglycemia's impact on driving simulation performance. Occurrence, awareness and correction. Diabetes Care. 2000;23:163–70.
13. Cox DJ, Ford D, Ritterband L, Singh H, Gonder-Frederick L. Disruptive effects of hyperglycemia on driving in adults with type 1 and type 2 diabetes. Diabetes Care. 2011;60 Suppl 1:A223.
14. Sommerfield AJ, Deary IJ, Frier BM. Acute hyperglycemia alters mood state and impairs cognitive performance in people with type 2 diabetes. Diabetes Care. 2004;27:2335–40.
15. Cox DJ, Kovatchev BP, Gonder-Frederick LA, Summers KH, McCall A, Grimm KJ, et al. Relationships between hyperglycemia and cognitive performance among adults with type 1 and type 2 diabetes. Diabetes Care. 2005;28:71–7.
16. Tujii T, Kyaw WT, Iwaki H, Nishikawa N, Nagai M, Kubo M, et al. Evaluation of the effect of pregabalin on simulated driving ability using a driving simulator in healthy male volunteers. Int J Gen Med. 2014;7:103–8.
17. Yale SH, Hansotia P, Knapp D, Ehrfurth J. Neurologic conditions: assessing medical fitness to drive. Clin Med Res. 2003;1:177–88.
18. Liew G, Michaelides M, Bunce C. A comparison of the causes of blindness certifications in England and Wales in working age adults (16–64 years), 1999–2000 with 2009–2010. BMJ Open. 2014;4:e004015.
19. Zammitt NN, Warren RE, Deary IJ, Frier BM. Delayed recovery of cognitive function following hypoglycemia in adults with type 1 diabetes: effect of impaired awareness of hypoglycemia. Diabetes. 2008;57:732–6.
20. Carr DB, Ott BR. The older adult driver with cognitive impairment: "It's a very frustrating life". JAMA. 2010;303:1632–41.
21. George CF, Boudreau AC, Smiley A. Simulated driving performance in patients with obstructive sleep apnea. Am J Respir Crit Care Med. 1996;154:175–81.
22. Stradling J. Driving and obstructive sleep apnoea. Thorax. 2008;63:481–3.
23. Orth M, Duchna HW, Leidag M, Widdig W, Rasche K, Bauer TT, et al. Driving simulator and neuropsychological [corrected] testing in OSAS before and under CPAP therapy. Eur Respir J. 2005;26:898–903.
24. Ellen RL, Marshall SC, Palayew M, Molnar FJ, Wilson KG, Man-Son-Hing M. Systematic review of motor vehicle crash risk in persons with sleep apnea. J Clin Sleep Med. 2006;2:193–200.
25. Inkster B, Frier BM. Diabetes and driving. Diabetes Obes Metab. 2013;15:775–83.
26. Stevens AB, Roberts M, McKane R, Atkinson AB, Bell PM, Hayes JR. Motor vehicle driving among diabetics taking insulin and non-diabetics. BMJ. 1989;299:591–5.
27. Songer TJ, LaPorte RE, Dorman JS, Orchard TJ, Cruickshanks KJ, Becker DJ, et al. Motor vehicle accidents and IDDM. Diabetes Care. 1988;11:701–7.
28. Cox DJ, Kovatchev B, Vandecar K, Gonder-Frederick L, Ritterband L, Clarke W. Hypoglycemia preceding fatal car collisions. Diabetes Care. 2006;29:467–8.
29. Songer TJ, Dorsey RR. High risk characteristics for motor vehicle crashes in persons with diabetes by age. Annu Proc Assoc Adv Automot Med. 2006;50:335–51.
30. Cox DJ, Penberthy JK, Zrebiec J, Weinger K, Aikens J, Frier B, et al. Diabetes and driving mishaps: frequency and correlations from a multinational survey. Diabetes Care. 2003;26:2329–34.
31. Lonnen KF, Powell RJ, Taylor D, Shore AC, MacLeod KM. Road traffic accidents and diabetes: insulin use does not determine risk. Diabet Med. 2008;25:578–84.
32. Major HG, Rees SD, Frier BM. Driving and diabetes: DVLA response to Lonnen et al. Diabet Med. 2009;26:191.

8 Diabetes: From Basic Science to Clinical Practice

33. Signorovitch JE, Macaulay D, Diener M, Yan Y, Wu EQ, Gruenberger JB, et al. Hypoglycaemia and accident risk in people with type 2 diabetes mellitus treated with non-insulin antidiabetes drugs. Diabetes Obes Metab. 2013;15:335–41.

34. Redelmeier DA, Yarnell CJ, Thiruchelvam D, Tibshirani RJ. Physicians' warnings for unfit drivers and the risk of trauma from road crashes. N Engl J Med. 2012;367:1228–36.

35. Vingilis E, Wilk P. Medical conditions, medication use, and their relationship with subsequent motor vehicle injuries: examination of the Canadian National Population Health Survey. Traffic Inj Prev. 2012;13:327–36.

36. Skurtveit S, Strom H, Skrivarhaug T, Morland J, Bramness JG, Engeland A. Road traffic accident risk in patients with diabetes mellitus receiving blood glucose-lowering drugs. Prospective follow-up study. Diabet Med. 2009;26:404–8.

37. Bieber-Tregear M, Funmilayo D, Amana A, Connor D, Tregear S. Diabetes and commercial motor vehicle safety. Department of Transportation's Federal Motor Carrier Safety Administration. 2011.

38. Cox DJ, Ford D, Gonder-Frederick L, Clarke W, Mazze R, Weinger K, et al. Driving mishaps among individuals with type 1 diabetes: a prospective study. Diabetes Care. 2009;32:2177–80.

39. Campbell LK, Gonder-Frederick LA, Broshek DK, Kovatchev BP, Anderson S, Clarke WL, et al. Neurocognitive Differences Between Drivers with Type 1 Diabetes with and without a Recent History of Recurrent Driving Mishaps. Int J Diabetes Mellitus. 2010;2:73–7.

40. Cox DJ, Gonder-Frederick LA, Shepard JA, Campbell LK, Vajda KA. Driving safety: concerns and experiences of parents of adolescent drivers with type 1 diabetes. Pediatr Diabetes. 2012;13:506–9.

41. Redelmeier DA, Kenshole AB, Ray JG. Motor vehicle crashes in diabetic patients with tight glycemic control: a population-based case control analysis. PLoS Med. 2009;6:e1000192.

42. Lipska KJ, Warton EM, Huang ES, Moffet HH, Inzucchi SE, Krumholz HM, et al. HbA1c and risk of severe hypoglycemia in type 2 diabetes: the Diabetes and Aging Study. Diabetes Care. 2013;36:3535–42.

43. Cox DJ, Kovatchev BP, Anderson SM, Clarke WL, Gonder-Frederick LA. Type 1 diabetic drivers with and without a history of recurrent hypoglycemia-related driving mishaps: physiological and performance differences during euglycemia and the induction of hypoglycemia. Diabetes Care. 2010;33:2430–5.

44. Cox DJ, Kovatchev BP, Gonder-Frederick LA, Clarke WL. Physiological and performance differences between drivers with type 1 diabetes with and without a recent history of driving mishaps: a exploratory study. Can J Diabetes. 2003;27:23–8.

45. Cox DJ, Singh H, Lorber D. Diabetes and driving safety: science, ethics, legality and practice. Am J Med Sci. 2013;345:263–5.

46. Cox DJ, Gonder-Frederick L, Ritterband L, Clarke WL, Kovatchev BP, Schmidt K. Internet intervention designed to identify and reduce risk of diabetic driving mishaps (260-OR). Diabetes. 2014;63(supplement 1):a6.

47. Bell D, Huddart A, Krebs J. Driving and insulin-treated diabetes: comparing practices in Scotland and New Zealand. Diabet Med. 2010;27:1093–5.

48. Arffa S. The relationship of intelligence to executive function and non-executive function measures in a sample of average, above average, and gifted youth. Arch Clin Neuropsychol. 2007;22:969–78.

49. Eadington DW, Frier BM. Type 1 diabetes and driving experience: an eight-year cohort study. Diabet Med. 1989;6:137–41.

50. Graveling AJ, Warren RE, Frier BM. Hypoglycaemia and driving in people with insulin-treated diabetes: adherence to recommendations for avoidance. Diabet Med. 2004;21:1014–9.

51. Broz J, Donicova V, Brabec M, Janickova Zdarska D, Polak J. Could continuous glucose monitoring facilitate identifying diabetes patients with a higher risk of hypoglycemia during driving? J Diabetes Sci Technol. 2013;7:1644–5.

52. Kerr D, Olateju T. Driving with diabetes in the future: In-vehicle medical monitoring. J Diabetes Sci Technol. 2010;4:464–9.

53. Pramming S, Thorsteinsson B, Bendtson I, Binder C. The relationship between symptomatic and biochemical hypoglycaemia in insulin-dependent diabetic patients. J Intern Med. 1990;228:641–6.

54. Weinger K, Jacobson AM, Draelos MT, Finkelstein DM, Simonson DC. Blood glucose estimation and symptoms during hyperglycemia and hypoglycemia in patients with insulin-dependent diabetes mellitus. Am J Med. 1995;98:22–31.

55. Cox DJ, Clarke WL, Gonder-Frederick L, Pohl S, Hoover C, Snyder A, et al. Accuracy of perceiving blood glucose in IDDM. Diabetes Care. 1985;8:529–36.

56. Stork AD, van Haeften TW, Veneman TF. The decision not to drive during hypoglycemia in patients with type 1 and type 2 diabetes according to hypoglycemia awareness. Diabetes Care. 2007;30:2822–6.

57. Weinger K, Kinsley BT, Levy CJ, Bajaj M, Simonson DC, Cox DJ, et al. The perception of safe driving ability during hypoglycemia in patients with type 1 diabetes mellitus. Am J Med. 1999;107:246–53.

58. Clarke WL, Cox DJ, Gonder-Frederick LA, Kovatchev B. Hypoglycemia and the decision to drive a motor vehicle by persons with diabetes. JAMA. 1999;282:750–4.

59. Watson WA, Currie T, Lemon JS, Gold AE. Driving and insulin-treated diabetes: who knows the rules and recommendations? Practical Diabetes. 2007;24:201–6.

60. Evans ML, Pernet A, Lomas J, Jones J, Amiel SA. Delay in onset of awareness of acute hypoglycemia and of restoration of cognitive performance during recovery. Diabetes Care. 2000;23:893–7.

61. Blackman JD, Towle VL, Lewis GF, Spire JP, Polonsky KS. Hypoglycemic thresholds for cognitive dysfunction in humans. Diabetes. 1990;39:828–35.

62. Gonder-Frederick LA, Cox DJ, Driesen NR, Ryan CM, Clarke WL. Individual differences in neurobehavioral disruption during mild and moderate hypoglycemia in adults with IDDM. Diabetes. 1994;43:1407–12.

63. Pedersen-Bjergaard U, Pramming S, Heller S, Wallace T, Rasmussen A, Jørgensen H, et al. Severe hypoglycaemia in 1076 adult patients with type 1 diabetes: influence of risk markers and selection. Diabetes Metab Res Rev. 2004;20:479–86.

64. The European Parliament and the Council of the European Union. Directive 2006/126/EC of the European Parliament and of the council of 20 December 2006 on driving licences. Off J Eur Union. 2006;L403:18–60.

65. The European Parliament and the Council of the European Union. Commission Directive 2009/113/EC of 25 August 2009 amending Directive 2006/126/EC of the European Parliament and of the Council on driving licences. Off J Eur Union. 2009;L223:31–5.

66. Parkes A, Tong S, Fernandez-Medina K. The forgotten risk of driving with hypoglycaemia in type 2 diabetes. Transport Research Laboratory. 2014.

67. Kilpatrick ES, Rigby AS, Warren RE, Atkin SL. Implications of new European Union driving regulations on patients with Type 1 diabetes who participated in the Diabetes Control and Complications Trial. Diabet Med. 2013;30:616–9.

68. Akram K, Pedersen-Bjergaard U, Borch-Johnsen K, Thorsteinsson B. Frequency and risk factors of severe hypoglycemia in insulin-treated type 2 diabetes: a literature survey. J Diabetes Complications. 2006;20:402–8.

69. American Diabetes A, Lorber D, Anderson J, Arent S, Cox DJ, Frier BM, et al. Diabetes and driving. Diabetes Care. 2014;37 Suppl 1:S97–103.

70. Begg IS, Yale JF, Houlden RL, Rowe RC, McSherry J. Canadian Diabetes Association's Clinical Practice Guidelines for Diabetes and Private and Commercial Driving. Can J Diabetes. 2003;27:128–40.

71. Austroads. Assessing fitness to drive for commercial and private vehicle drivers. 4th ed. Sydney, Australia: Austroads; 2012.

72. DVLA. At a glance guide to the current medical standards of fitness to drive. Swansea: Driver & Vehicle Licensing Agency; 2014.

2

Update on thyroid-associated Ophthalmopathy with a special emphasis on the ocular surface

Priscila Novaes[1†], Ana Beatriz Diniz Grisolia[1†] and Terry J. Smith[1,2,3*]

Abstract

Thyroid-associated ophthalmopathy (TAO) is a condition associated with a wide spectrum of ocular changes, usually in the context of the autoimmune syndrome, Graves' disease. In this topical review, we attempted to provide a roadmap of the recent advances in current understanding the pathogenesis of TAO, important aspects of its clinical presentation, its impact on the ocular surface, describe the tissue abnormalities frequently encountered, and describe how TAO is managed today. We also briefly review how increased understanding of the disease should culminate in improved therapies for patients with this vexing condition.

Keywords: Graves' disease, Ophthalmopathy, Thyroid, Orbit, Ocular surface

Background

Thyroid-associated ophthalmopathy (TAO[a], aka thyroid eye disease or Graves' ophthalmopathy) refers to several ocular manifestations related to the systemic auto-immune process, Graves' disease (GD) [1]. This syndrome has been attributed to the loss of immune tolerance to the thyrotropin receptor (TSHR) and per-haps other auto-antigenic proteins [2, 3]. TAO results from the linked conspiracy of auto-reactivity and tissue remodeling. The factors that over-arch the ocular components of GD with the pathology occurring in the thy-roid have yet to be identified unambiguously. TAO is the most common and serious extra-thyroidal manifestation of GD, with 25–50% in those with the thyroid disease [4–6]. While the majority of individuals with GD be-come hyperthyroid sometime in the course of their dis-ease, TAO can also occur in primary hypothyroidism and in patients who remain euthyroid [7]. Substantial evidence suggests that GD and TAO result from com-plex interplay between genetic susceptibility, epigenetic

* Correspondence: terrysmi@med.umich.edu
†Equal contributors
[1]Department of Ophthalmology and Visual Sciences, Kellogg Eye Center, University of Michigan Medical School, Ann Arbor, MI 48105, USA
[2]Division of Metabolism, Endocrinology, and Diabetes, Department of Internal Medicine, University of Michigan Medical School, Ann Arbor, MI 48105, USA
Full list of author information is available at the end of the article

factors, and several partially characterized environmental triggers [8]. Several recent reviews have addressed TAO; however none has detailed insights of the association and interactions between TAO, the ocular surface (OS) and dry eye syndrome (DES). We have thus included an emphasis on the OS and DES in this review.

Pathogenesis

The central participant in the pathogenesis of TAO is the orbital fibroblast [9, 10]. Orbital fibroblasts from healthy individuals appear to differ from those with TAO [11–13]. They represent a heterogeneous population of cells with divergent capacities for terminal differentiation and gene expression. We now know that a subpopula-tion of orbital fibroblasts in TAO derive from bone mar-row derived fibrocytes [14]. These cells express several thyroid antigens that have been implicated in TAO. Among them is the TSHR. TSHR has been detected in orbital connective tissue and on orbital fibroblasts, albeit at extremely low levels [15, 16] but the basis for its ex-pression has remained uncertain. Fibrocytes were found to infiltrate the TAO orbit and express higher levels of TSHR than those found on orbital fibroblasts [14, 17, 18]. Furthermore, the receptor displayed on fibrocytes is func-tional in that TSH and thyroid-stimulating immunoglobu-lins (TSI) provoke the generation of extremely high levels of inflammatory cytokines. These include IL-6, TNF-α, IL-

8, and IL-1β [19]. How the receptor participates in TAO is less certain. In addition to TSHR, other thyroid autoantigens have also been detected in orbital tissues and expressed by orbital fibroblasts [8]. Persistence of detectable thyroid autoantibodies in patients with therapy-resistant TAO may support a role for these autoantigens in disease pathogenesis [20].

It is unclear how the abnormal behavior of orbital fibroblasts in TAO interplays with the recruited lymphocytes, mast cells and macrophages. Their accumulation in the orbit is characteristic of the disease. Development of their therapeutic targeting is of considerable importance [12, 18]. Subpopulations of orbital fibroblasts may explain, at least in part, the diversity of clinical TAO presentation. The disease can manifest as predominantly fat expansion or with isolated extraocular muscle (EOM) involvement or most commonly a mixture of both [13, 21]. Fibroblasts can be identified on the basis of cell surface markers such as Thy-1 and CD34. Subsets differ in their ability to differentiate into adipocytes or myofibroblasts [13, 22]. Cells from orbital fat differ phenotypically from those of perimysial derivation [23].

TAO is associated with accelerated glycosaminoglycan production, resulting in mechanical embarrassment of the orbital contents [14, 24, 25]. Orbital fibroblast proliferation and differentiation into adipocytes leads to fat tissue expansion. In muscle, increased glycosaminoglycan accumulation can interfere with normal contraction and movement [9, 14, 25]. In advanced stages of the disease, fibrotic changes can affect muscle functions, resulting in restricted eye movement.

Many clinical signs and symptoms of TAO arise from expansion of soft-tissues within the orbit, leading to exophthalmos [9, 25, 26]. Disturbance of the ocular surface is caused by inadequate lid coverage; the increased palpebral fissure width results in accelerated tear evaporation and elevated tear osmolarity [27, 28], perpetuating an inflammatory cycle [29] and contributing to a major source of disease morbidity.

Eyelid structures are also altered in TAO, resulting in retraction of both upper and lower eyelids. Three different mechanisms have been proposed [24]. The cicatricial and restrictive theory is explained by the effects of TAO on EOM and on the elastic components of eyelid retractor muscles. Enlarged inferior rectus muscle dimension and the generalized orbit connective tissue congestion may retract the lower eyelid margin. This is due to increased tension on the lower eyelid complex (inferior oblique muscle, inferior rectus muscle and the capsulopalpebral fascia (CPF). In the upper eyelid, fibrosis of the Müller and *levator palpebrae superioris* muscles (LPS) is variable. Muscle hyperaction results from increased sympathetic stimulation of the inferior tarsal muscle (lower eyelid) or Müller's muscle (upper eyelid). This is thought to be a consequence of direct thyroid hormone actions. The concept of anterior globe displacement as a mechanism for eyelid retraction resulting from proptosis is demonstrated by improvement of eyelid retraction following surgical correction of proptosis [24, 30, 31]. Overall, these theories appear compatible with the variations of clinical disease presentation.

Clinical presentation

The onset of ocular symptoms/signs and hyperthyroidism can occur simultaneously or diverge temporally by months to years [32]. Patients undergo an initial period where inflammation, progressive orbital congestion, and variably worsening proptosis evolve. This stage is termed the active phase. The activity of the disease can be assessed by calculating the clinical activity score (CAS), based on seven signs (Table 1). In addition, clinical severity can be classified using the NOSPECS score (Table 2). According to Rundle's curve, this phase can last from months to several years [33]. Activity gives way to a period of stabilization and ultimately leads to the inactive phase where the disease no longer progresses. This stable phase is seldom associated with a complete normalization of ocular changes [4].

Proptosis or exophthalmos occurs as a consequence of expanding orbital contents being confined within the boney orbit and the naturally occurring decompression resulting from anterior displacement of the globe. TAO is the most common cause of both unilateral and bilateral proptosis in adults. Pseudo-ptosis and true ptosis may be seen in patients with TAO. The former results from contralateral lid retraction but true ptosis occurs when the levator muscle suffers dehiscence or when concurrent myasthenia gravis is manifested. Strabismus is common in TAO, resulting from restrictive extraocular muscle impairment. It can induce head tilt and diplopia. The inferior and medial rectus muscles are most commonly involved in TAO, resulting in horizontal and vertical deviations. The basis for this predilection has not been identified [23]. Diplopia develops from inflammation and swelling of the extraocular muscles and is generally restrictive. It is classified as intermittent (present upon awakening or during fatigue, present at extremes of gaze) or constant when present in primary gaze and/or reading position [4, 9]. One other important sign of EOM involvement is the elevation of IOP in upgaze, due to the restrictive action of the fibrotic inferior rectus muscles and blockade of the episcleral aqueous outflow. Orbital congestion also contributes to this elevation IOP [34, 35]. Attention should be paid to the position of the eye during applanation tonometry, which must be performed in the standard position and in

Table 1 Clinical activity score

GO activity (CAS)	
1	Spontaneous retrobulbar pain
2	Pain on attempted upward or downward gaze
3	Redness of eyelids
4	Redness of conjunctiva
5	Swelling of caruncle or plica
6	Swelling of eyelids
7	Swelling of conjunctiva (chemosis)

down-gaze [36]. Upper-eyelid retraction (Dalrymple sign), often with temporal flare and scleral show, is one the most common ocular signs of TAO and should be differentiated from proptosis. Lid lag on down-gaze (von Graefe sign) is another important feature of the disease, manifesting as a downward saccadic movement with

Table 2 TAO Eye changes classification - NOSPECS

NOSPECS		
Class	Grade	Criteria
1		No physical signs or symptoms
		Only signs (limited to upper lid retraction, stare, and lid lag)
2		Soft tissue involvement (with symptoms and signs)
	0	Absent
	a	Minimal
	b	Moderate
	c	Marked
3		Proptosis ≥3 mm above upper normal limit
	0	Absent
	a	3–4 mm increase over upper normal
	b	5–7 mm increase
	c	≥8 mm increase
4		Extraocular muscle involvement
	0	Absent
	a	Limitation of motion extremes of gaze
	b	Evident restriction of motion
	c	Fixation of a globe or globes
5		Corneal involvement
	0	Absent
	a	Stippling of cornea
	b	Ulceration
	c	Clouding, necrosis, perforation
6		Sight loss (optic nerve involvement)
	0	Absent
	a	Disc pallor or visual field deffect; vision 20/20–20/60
	b	Same as 6a, but vision 20/70–20/200
	c	Blindness, i.e., failure to perceive light, vision < 20/200

reduced amplitude [24]. Anterior segment signs in TAO include superficial punctate keratitis, superior limbic keratoconjunctivitis, conjunctival injection usually over the rectus muscle insertions and chemosis. Severe proptosis can cause corneal ulceration.

Vision disturbances in severe TAO may occur due to compressive optic neuropathy or dysthyroid optic neuropathy (DON). DON is defined as impairment of optic nerve function due to compression [37]. It presents as blurred vision, visual loss, dyschromatopsia, or field loss and can occur in up to 5% of patients with TAO [25, 38]. Visual impairment in TAO, resulting from dysfunction of the optic nerve, is caused by raised intraorbital pressure due to inflammation [39, 40]. Patients with optic nerve compression may not exhibit marked proptosis, but these individuals usually show substantially increased resistance to retropulsion. In addition, most cases of DON occur without visible optic nerve edema, making frequent documentation of visual acuity, color vision, and pupillary light reflex essential [4]. Due to orbital congestion, choroidal folds may also be seen in TAO, among other warning signs. These include corneal opacity, important lagophthalmos, and pale, swollen optic discs, which can signal impending DON [37]. Therefore, these are important to detect when evaluating patients with TAO. DON is the most serious quality of life-threatening condition associated with TAO [41], and requires immediate treatment [37].

The ocular surface in TAO

A frequently underappreciated casualty of TAO is the ocular surface, a functional unit comprising the corneal and conjunctival epithelium, lid margins and tear film. Classically, increased palpebral fissure width and lid alterations caused by TAO have been implicated in the disruption of ocular surface homeostasis. This leads to corneal exposure, tear film instability, accelerated tear evaporation and high tear osmolarity [27, 28]. Eventually, ocular surface inflammation ensues, initiating a vicious cycle which eventually leads to dry eye syndrome (DES) [29].

Exophthalmos, with the resulting increased fissure width, lagophthalmos, and poor Bell's phenomenon can contribute to DES. Inflammation of the OS and dry eye are frequently associated with TAO, sometimes preceding ophthalmic changes [42, 43].

In one report, patients with occult TAO consistently reported symptoms of ocular irritation, including foreign body sensation, redness, and excessive tearing [7]. These individuals were found to have OS inflammation in the absence of exophthalmos, lid retraction, dysmotility, and diplopia. Thus, the earliest forms of TAO may be confined to the OS, well in advance of lid retraction and lid lag.

A significant correlation was found between TAO activity, measured by CAS, and OS damage, detected by lissamine green staining [44]. In that study, the prevalence of dry eye was 65% in patients with TAO, and histopathologic changes in the conjunctiva were consistent with dry eye syndrome.

Gupta et al. [7] detected conjunctival and episcleral inflammation localized over the extraocular muscles in their entire series of patients and considered it to represent a presenting sign of TAO. Subtle widening of the inter-palpebral fissure was found in 48%, meibomian gland dysfunction in 48%, and a decreased tear break-up time (TBUT of less than 10 s) in 31% of these patients. Corneal and conjunctival vital staining, indicators of ocular surface damage, are a frequent sign in patients with TAO [7, 19, 28, 45].

Patients also present with reduced tear break-up time [19, 28], which indicates greater tear film instability. The Schirmer test, which assesses basal and reflex aqueous tear film production, may be normal [28] or reduced [19].

Clinical diagnosis of DES in TAO

Diagnosis of DES can be made using simple, minimally invasive tests that are routinely conducted as part of the ophthalmological examination. These include administration of a questionnaire that assesses symptoms of ocular irritation and environmental triggers, such as the OS disease index (OSDI). TBUT, a procedure involving the instillation of fluorescein on the ocular surface, measures tear stability and exhibits the greatest correlation with other tests for DES diagnosis [44]. The Schirmer test, detects aqueous deficient dry eye with good sensitivity [46]. Fluorescein and lissamine green staining detect de-epithelized and devitalized ocular surface areas, respectively [45].

TAO, lacrimal gland and the ocular surface

Lacrimal gland (LG) involvement in TAO may result from the direct effects of TSI, since acinar cells of the LG express TSHR [47]. Thyroid, salivary and lacrimal glands resemble one another histologically [48]. Further, all are particularly susceptible to immunological damage [49]. Sjögren's syndrome (SS), an autoimmune disease characterized by chronic lymphocytic infiltration of LG and salivary glands [50], frequently affects patients with thyroiditis [49]. Histopathologic lesions in both diseases are infiltrated by T cells [51]. Patients with SS have a 74-fold greater chance of developing GD than the general population [52]. In TAO, TNF-α increases Fas expression on lacrimal cells, resulting in apoptosis and release of a fragment of α-fodrin [53].

Proteomic analysis of tear film can inform pathology occurring within lacrimal glands [54, 55]. Protective factors such as proline-rich proteins (PRPs) and cystatins were markedly down-regulated in patients with TAO

compared to healthy individuals and those with DES [56]. Altered regulation of proinflammatory and protective proteins found in tears may reflect an inflammation-induced dysfunction of the LG in TAO [55]. Tear proteins were markedly different in those with TAO versus other forms of DES. These include proteins involved in inflammatory response, cell-to cell signaling and interaction, cellular motility and cell death. These findings suggest that different mechanisms induce LG and OS alterations in TAO [56].

Levels of IL-1β, IL-2, IL-6, IL-8, IL-10, IL-17, TNF-α and INF-γ were higher in tears from patients with active vs stable TAO. Further, cytokine levels generally correlated with CAS scores and fluorescein staining [19].

Direct autoimmune targeting in active TAO may contribute to the ocular surface disease, as is evidenced by detection of cytokines in tears [19] and active keratocytes, a putative biomarker for OS inflammation [57], respectively.

Diagnostic considerations

The frequency and severity of TAO may be lessening in newly diagnosed GD hyperthyroidism. Further, TAO rarely progresses to more severe disease [58]. On the other hand, some patients, especially those exposed to tobacco, continue to present with severe disease and others manifest reactivation. Even in the absence of clinical ocular manifestations, imaging reveals subtle orbital changes in most patients with GD [4]. In nearly 70% of asymptomatic, hyperthyroid adults with GD, magnetic resonance imaging (MRI) and computed tomographic (CT) scanning reveal extra-ocular-muscle enlargement [9].

The most frequent clinical features of TAO are upper eyelid retraction, periorbital edema/erythema, and proptosis [9]. It is important to differentiate TAO from other common conditions that present similarly. These include orbital and pre-septal cellulitis, carotid cavernous fistula, orbital pseudotumor, and thickened muscles conditions such as sarcoidosis, neoplastic diseases and amyloid.

In most cases, the diagnosis of TAO can be established clinically. However, imaging studies may be required to evaluate orbit structures and aid in formulating an optimal treatment plan. It is possible to evaluate optic nerve compression on MRI and the orbital bony structure on CT. Neuroimaging usually reveals muscle enlargement with tendon sparing and fat expansion. Imaging may also reveal dilated superior ophthalmic veins and apical crowding of the optic nerve [59].

Management of TAO
General principles
Optimal care of patients with TAO requires a multidisciplinary approach. This usually includes both endocrinologists and ophthalmologists who typically provide primary care.

Other specialists should participate as needed [60, 61]. Several academic centers have assembled multidisciplinary teams to facilitate treatment decisions and provide follow-up patient care, education, and family support [60, 61]. This is true here at the University of Michigan.

Restoration and maintenance of the euthyroid state is essential for all patients with TAO since wide swings in thyroid function can negatively impact its course [4, 60, 62]. Anti-thyroid drugs and surgical thyroidectomy are extremely effective for managing hyperthyroidism. Radioiodine treatment confers a small additional risk of exacerbating TAO or provoking its development de novo, particularly in those who smoke tobacco and in patients with severe hyperthyroidism. Immunosuppressive therapies such as B cell depletion with rituximab may prove effective and should be overseen by a collaborating rheumatologist/clinical immunologist [60, 62].

Patients with GD must be given all the necessary resources and guidance to achieve smoking cessation, irrespective of their ocular disease status. It should be considered a primary goal in the therapeutic plan. Exposure to smoke represents the single most modifiable environmental risk factor thus far identified for TAO [4, 60, 61]. Although the mechanisms responsible for its negative impact are not completely clarified, studies suggest that oxidative stress might represent the culprit, by inducing the expression of fibrosis-related genes and the increase of intracellular pro-inflammatory cytokines [63]. Smoking can lead to progression of TAO, smokers generally have more severe disease, and immunosuppressive treatment is typically less effective in smokers [60, 62, 64, 65]. Advanced age of onset, duration and severity of thyrotoxicosis, and smoking are risk factors [66]. Treatment with anti-thyroid medication was negatively correlated with developing TAO but smoking increased statistically the odds for the disease. Older patients with restricted ocular motility, strabismus, and active TAO are at higher risk of DON and may benefit from early medical intervention [66].

Selenium supplementation may provide benefit for mild cases of TAO; some patients experience improved quality of life and reduced eye symptoms [67, 68]. One study reported a positive effect in mild disease after a 6-month exposure to 100 mcg daily dosage [67]. Limitations of that study included a failure to analyze the background dietary intake of selenium and to determine whether the subjects in the study geographic regions were depleted of the element [60, 67, 68]. Another study failed to detect a correlation between decreased serum Selenium levels and increased TAO severity [69].

Treatments for DES and ocular surface disease in TAO should be personalized. Baseline treatment consists of artificial tears, moisturizing ointments, and supportive measures such as moisture chamber glasses, humidifiers, and protection from wind and smoke [60]. Topical anti-inflammatory therapy may prove beneficial in ocular surface disease.

Therapy of active, moderate to severe TAO

Active TAO typically follows a 2 to 3-year course following Rundle's curve that includes inflammatory signs, progression, and becomes "static at a level of incomplete recovery" [33]. Depending on its severity, active TAO can be followed with conservative measures [61]. Ocular surface lubrication must be preserved and artificial tears, gels and topical cyclosporine may be useful [70]. Topical treatment may prove insufficient to ensure corneal protection. In that case, lacrimal punctum occlusion or temporary tarsorrhaphies may become necessary [61, 71].

Glucocorticoid (GC) therapy is well established, although its benefits remain unproven in large prospective studies. The EUGOGO guidelines recommend prophylaxis of 0.3-0.5 ml prednisone/kg body weight in those undergoing radioiodine ablation of the thyroid who are at high risk of progression or de novo development of TAO. Lower risk patients may receive reduced GC doses [60]. GCs continue to be the first-line treatment of moderate-to-severe active TAO with unpredictable results. The recommended cumulative dose of intravenous GCs should not exceed 8.0 g (4.5 g as intermediate-dose and 7.5 g as a high-dose regimen for the worst cases) with carefully controlled diabetes and hypertension [60]. In special situations such as hepatic dysfunction, cardiovascular morbidity or psychiatric disorders, intravenous GCs should be avoided. Patients with severe reduction of visual acuity, visual field deficits, color desaturation or afferent pupillary defects are at risk for DON and must be treated promptly with high-dose systemic corticosteroids. In these cases, EUGOGO recommends intravenous methylprednisolone 500-1000 mg for 3 consecutive days or alternate days during the first week [60]. Should this prove ineffective, emergency orbital decompression surgery may become necessary [61]. GC can be administered orally, intravenously, or locally injected into the orbit [62].

Efficacy of intravenous and oral GCs were compared in moderately severe TAO patients; parenteral steroids were more effective in reducing CAS by at least 3 points, improvement in visual acuity, and decreasing disease activity at 3 months [62, 65]. In another study, GCs induced complete visual recovery in DON, improved visual acuity, color sensitivity, and normalized visual field defects after 2 weeks of treatment [72]. Combined parenteral and oral GCs were effective with a low rate of side-effects [73]. Intravenous administration appears more efficacious and is better tolerated than orally administered GCs [65, 74].

Radiation therapy (RT) has been reassessed recently in combination with GCs and was found to improve

symptoms more than GCs alone [75]. While those results were promising, a controlled study will be
necessary.

The effectiveness of alternative therapies for TAO is
being studied, frequently in pilot, inadequately powered
studies. B and T cell depletion, insulin-like growth
factor-1 (IGF-I) receptor blockers, TSHR antagonists,
and various cytokine antagonists are under scrutiny [76].
Rituximab (RTX), a monoclonal antibody recognizing
targeting CD20+ B cells, has undergone pilot clinical trials with promising results in some studies [77, 78], while
another suggests no benefit [79]. In an uncontrolled
study of GC-resistant patients, RTX appeared to have
benefit [77]. Larger multicenter trials will be necessary
to establish the efficacy of RTX in TAO.

Potential for IGF-I receptor inhibition as therapy for TAO

TSHR involvement in the pathogenesis of GD is well
established, although clarifying its role in TAO remains
to be accomplished. IGF-IR is over-expressed by orbital
fibroblasts, T cell and B cells in GD, and thus may also
participate in the disease [78, 80–83]. Both TSHR and
IGF-IR appear to be activated by immunoglobulins that
have been detected in GD (GD-IgGs). Tsui et al. [81] reported that crosstalk between TSHR and IGF-IR is critical to the downstream signaling initiated by TSHR
activation. Fibrocytes express even higher levels of TSHR
than do orbital fibroblasts [84, 85]. A very recent study
confirmed the cross-talk occurring between IGF-IR and
TSHR [82]. Activating anti-IGF-IR antibodies have been
detected in some studies but not in others, leaving these
concepts controversial [80, 81, 85]. Teprotumumab, an
IGF-IR blocking monoclonal antibody, attenuates the induction by TSH and TSIs of cytokines in fibrocytes [84].
The antibody has been examined for its potential therapeutic benefits in a multicenter, placebo-controlled clinical trial of active, moderate to severe TAO [http://
clinicaltrials.gov/show/NCT01868997]. Results from this
study should be available in the next few months.

Cytokines represent potentially important therapeutic
targets in active TAO [86]. Tocilizumab, a recombinant,
humanized monoclonal antibody that antagonizes the IL-
6 receptor, was administered intravenously to eighteen patients with TAO who had proven refractory to intravenous
GC in an uncontrolled trial [87]. Improvement of CAS
was observed in all subjects, proptosis decreased in 72%,
and ocular motility improved in 83.3%. No severe side effects or relapses of active TAO were observed at the end
of a follow-up period of at least 9 months. One patient
with compressive optic neuropathy improved, avoiding
orbital decompression. Further studies involving well-
controlled, randomized and masked trials of this and other

anti-cytokine candidates will be necessary in determining
whether these approaches might be effective.

Remediation in stable TAO

Most surgical treatments for TAO are reserved for inactive disease. The notable exceptions are active cases
which require urgent orbital decompression surgery for
DON or sight-threatening optical surface damage. Once
the stable phase has been reached, treatments are largely
surgical, aiming at anatomic, functional, and cosmetic
rehabilitation. Surgeries are typically staged and planned
individually, depending on dysfunction and disfigurement
[61]. Decompression surgery, strabismus surgery, lid
lengthening and cosmetic periorbital surgeries, may be required. These should follow this particular sequential
order since the outcome of each procedure may determine
the necessary goals of the next [60].

Different decompression techniques have been developed. Their use should be tailored to the specific therapeutic goals of each case. Bone and fat removal may be
performed separately or combined to maximize decompression. Modern approaches include infero-medial wall,
lateral wall, and combined (balanced) decompressions. In
general, the appropriate decompression procedure is one
that will result in the degree of proptosis reduction that is
sought [4] (Fig. 1). Lateral and medial wall approaches
offer both advantages and drawbacks. For instance, lateral
wall decompression is accompanied by less post-operative
strabismus but a longer convalescence period. Further,
medial wall procedures can frequently accomplish greater
proptosis reduction [88]. Strabismus/diplopia may be
worsened by decompression and thus may require additional intervention. Minimally invasive approaches have
been advocated by some [60, 89]. Endoscopic techniques
may allow decompression with less morbidity, accessing
areas with good visibility and less exposure. Purely endoscopic procedures and intraoperative surgical tailoring
with personalized boney decompression have resulted in
good outcomes [90]. These procedures can reduce intraocular tension and provide pain relief, improve strabismus
and correct postural visual obscuration in patients with
orbital and optic nerve microvasculopathy [90]. The most
common surgical complications include de novo onset or
worsening of preexisting strabismus and globe dystopia
[89, 91]. Despite normalization of visual acuity and resolution of optic nerve head edema, almost half of patients
with substantial nerve damage will manifest persistent visual field defects following adequate decompression [90].
On the other hand, improvement in severe vision loss as
late as 3-month after onset has been reported following
decompression, suggesting that the procedure may be effective in reversing DON in patients with NLP vision [92].

Criteria with which to judge success of strabismus surgery in TAO are poorly defined. These procedures lack

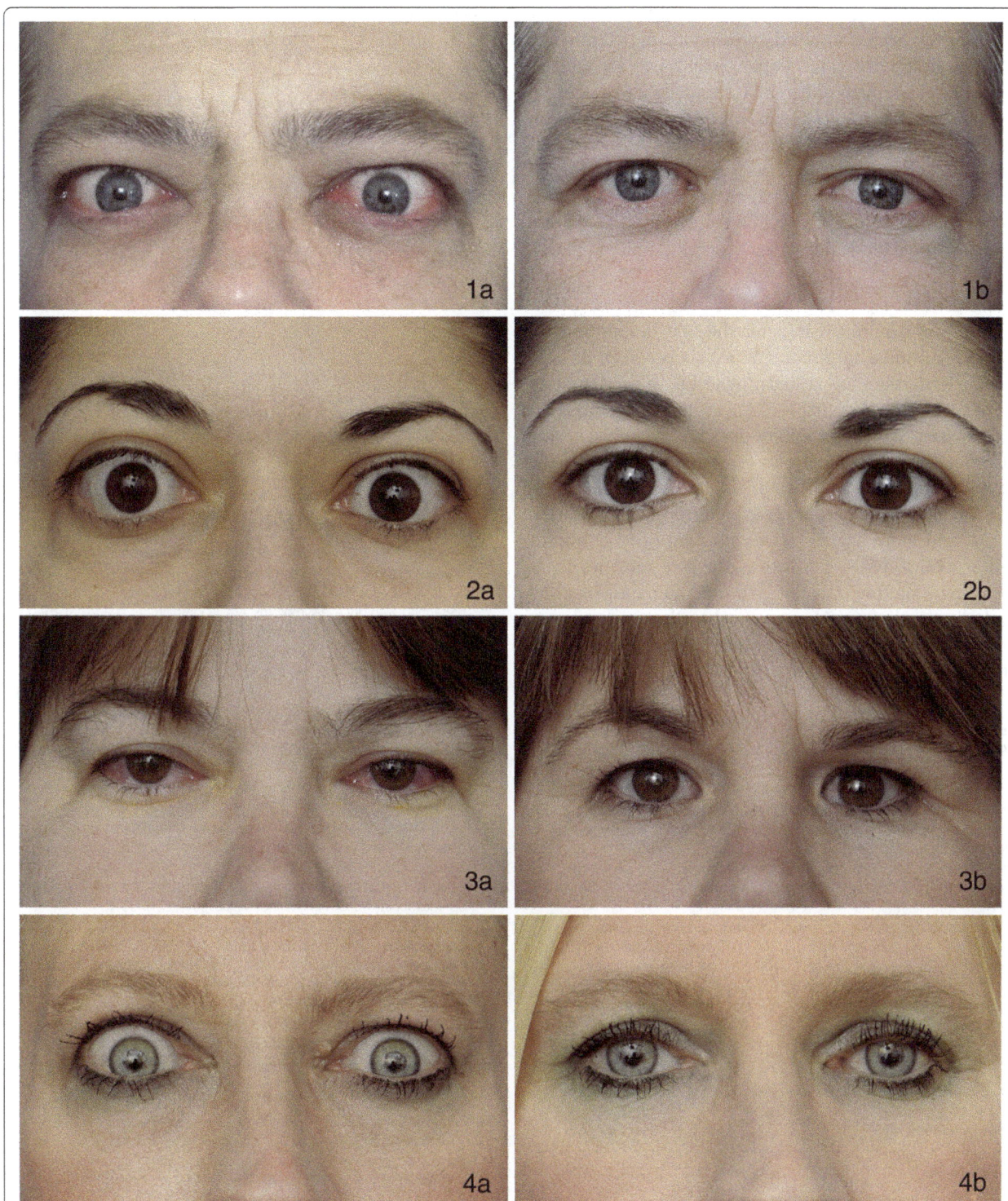

Fig. 1 Patients with thyroid-associated ophthalmopathy before (1**a**, 2**a**, 3**a**, 4**a**) and after (1**b**, 2**b**, 3**b**, 4**b**) surgical treatment. These images exemplify the most common signs of ophthalmopathy, including proptosis, conjunctival hyperemia, periocular edema and upper and lower eyelid retraction. These may improve with treatment. These images were generously provided by Dr. Raymond Douglas, Kellogg Eye Center, University of Michigan, Ann Arbor, USA

standardization, making surgical outcomes difficult to compare. GO-QoL may be useful in assessing surgical outcomes [93]. At least one study demonstrated improved GO-QoL score following strabismus surgery in TAO [94].

Upper eyelid retraction is the most common clinical sign in TAO. It is frequently improved but rarely completely corrected following orbital decompression [62, 71]. Several techniques have been developed for correcting upper eyelid retraction. These aim at weakening retractor muscles, by recession, partial resection, or lengthening [24]. Surgical outcomes in upper eyelid repair are difficult to predict and many different techniques have emerged yielding variable results [24, 62]. Lower eyelid retraction may also be surgically corrected; however, no consensus as to the best approach has been reached. The surgeon's preferences and expertise, anatomical variations, outcome expectations, attitude towards intervention, and disease severity should guide the choice of surgical method [91].

Conclusions

Nearly two hundred years after the first descriptions of GD, we continue to discover more about TAO, its molecular underpinnings, clinical behavior, and attempt to identify improved therapies. Advancing research techniques have led us to clearer insights into this vexing disorder. But substantial barriers remain, including the absence of proven animal models possessing the necessary fidelity to human disease, better access to affected tissue, and more aggressive organization of large, multicenter clinical trials. Ultimately, our goal must focus on restoring immune tolerance to the autoantigens that underlie the disease. That approach will spare many patients the adverse effects of chronic immune suppression and the invasive surgical approaches currently employed.

Abbreviations

CAS: Clinical activity score; CD34: Hematopoietic cell antigen CD34; CPF: Capsulopalpebral fascia; CT: Computed tomography; DES: Dry eye syndrome; DON: Dysthyroid optic neuropathy; EOM: Extraocular muscle; Fas: Apoptosis antigen 1 (CD95); GC: Glucocorticoid; GD: Graves' disease; GO-QoL: Graves' ophthalmopathy quality of life questionnaire; IGF-1R: Insulin-like growth factor-1 receptor; IL-1β: Interleukin 1 Beta; IL-2: Interleukin 2; IL-6: Interleukin 6; IL-8: Interleukin 8; IL-10: Interleukin 10; INF-γ: Interferon gamma; IOP: Intraocular pressure; LG: Lacrimal gland; LPS: *Levator palpebrae superioris* muscle; MRI: Magnetic resonance imaging; NLP: No light perception; OCT: Optical coherence tomography; OS: Ocular surface; OSDI: Ocular surface disease index; POTEI: POTE Ankyrin domain family member I; PRPs: Proline rich proteins; RNFL: Retinal nerve fiber layer; RT: Radiation therapy; RTX: Rituximab; SS: Sjögren's syndrome; TAO: Thyroid-associated ophthalmopathy; TAO-Igs: Thyroid-associated ophthalmopathy immunoglobulins; TBUT: Tear break-up time; Thy-1: Thymocyte antigen 1; TNF-α: Tumor necrosis factor alpha; TSHR: Thyrotropin Receptor; TSI: Thyroid stimulating immunoglobulins

Acknowledgements
The authors are grateful to Ms. Darla Kroft for expert assistance in preparing the manuscript.

Funding
This work was supported in part by National Institutes of Health grants EY008976 and 5UM1AI110557, a Center for Vision grant EY007003 from the National Eye Institute, an unrestricted grant from Research to Prevent Blindness, and by the Bell Charitable Foundation.

Authors contributions
PN and ABDG contributed equally to the manuscript, doing bibliographical research and writing the manuscript. TJS mentored the study, contributed to the writing and reviewed and extensively edited the manuscript. All authors read and approved the final manuscript.

Author details
[1]Department of Ophthalmology and Visual Sciences, Kellogg Eye Center, University of Michigan Medical School, Ann Arbor, MI 48105, USA. [2]Division of Metabolism, Endocrinology, and Diabetes, Department of Internal Medicine, University of Michigan Medical School, Ann Arbor, MI 48105, USA. [3]Department of Ophthalmology and Visual Sciences, Brehm Tower, Room 7112, 1000 Wall Street, Ann Arbor, MI 48105, USA.

References
1. Smith TJ, Hegedus L. Grave's disease. N Engl J Med. 2016;375(16):1552–65.
2. Pujol-Borrell R, et al. Genetics of Graves' disease: special focus on the role of TSHR gene. Horm Metab Res. 2015;47(10):753–66.
3. Wiersinga WM. Thyroid autoimmunity. Endocr Dev. 2014;26:139–57.
4. Bartalena L, Fatourechi V. Extrathyroidal manifestations of Graves' disease: a 2014 update. J Endocrinol Invest. 2014;37(8):691–700.
5. Reddy SV, et al. Prevalence of Graves' ophthalmopathy in patients with Graves' disease presenting to a referral centre in north India. Indian J Med Res. 2014;139(1):99–104.
6. Hiromatsu Y, et al. Graves' ophthalmopathy: epidemiology and natural history. Intern Med. 2014;53(5):353–60.
7. Gupta A, Sadeghi PB, Akpek EK. Occult thyroid eye disease in patients presenting with dry eye symptoms. Am J Ophthalmol. 2009;147(5):919–23.
8. Wang Y, Smith TJ. Current concepts in the molecular pathogenesis of thyroid-associated ophthalmopathy. Invest Ophthalmol Vis Sci. 2014;55(3):1735–48.
9. Bahn RS. Graves' ophthalmopathy. N Engl J Med. 2010;362(8):726–38.
10. Prabhakar BS, Bahn RS, Smith TJ. Current perspective on the pathogenesis of Graves' disease and ophthalmopathy. Endocr Rev. 2003;24(6):802–35.
11. Dik WA, Virakul S, van Steensel L. Current perspectives on the role of orbital fibroblasts in the pathogenesis of Graves' ophthalmopathy. Exp Eye Res. 2016;142:83–91.
12. Shan SJ, Douglas RS. The pathophysiology of thyroid eye disease. J Neuroophthalmol. 2014;34(2):177–85.
13. Smith TJ, et al. Orbital fibroblast heterogeneity may determine the clinical presentation of thyroid-associated ophthalmopathy. J Clin Endocrinol Metab. 2002,07(1).305–92.
14. Douglas RS, et al. Increased generation of fibrocytes in thyroid-associated ophthalmopathy. J Clin Endocrinol Metab. 2010;95(1):430–8.
15. Feliciello A, et al. Expression of thyrotropin-receptor mRNA in healthy and Graves' disease retro-orbital tissue. Lancet. 1993;342(8867):337–8.
16. Heufelder AE, et al. Detection of TSH receptor RNA in cultured fibroblasts from patients with Graves' ophthalmopathy and pretibial dermopathy. Thyroid. 1993;3(4):297–300.
17. Fernando R, et al. Human fibrocytes coexpress thyroglobulin and thyrotropin receptor. Proc Natl Acad Sci U S A. 2012;109(19):7427–32.
18. Smith TJ. TSH-receptor-expressing fibrocytes and thyroid-associated ophthalmopathy. Nat Rev Endocrinol. 2015;11(3):171–81.
19. Huang D, et al. Changes of lacrimal gland and tear inflammatory cytokines in thyroid-associated ophthalmopathy. Invest Ophthalmol Vis Sci. 2014;55(8):4935–43.
20. Eckstein AK, et al. Clinical results of anti-inflammatory therapy in Graves' ophthalmopathy and association with thyroidal autoantibodies. Clin Endocrinol. 2004;61(5):612–8.
21. Garrity JA, Bahn RS. Pathogenesis of graves ophthalmopathy: implications for prediction, prevention, and treatment. Am J Ophthalmol. 2006;142(1):147–53.
22. Smith TJ, et al. Evidence for cellular heterogeneity in primary cultures of human orbital fibroblasts. J Clin Endocrinol Metab. 1995;80(9):2620–5.

23. Mourits MP. Prevention of graves' orbitopathy: early diagnosis of thyroid-associated orbitopathy in Graves' disease. Orbit. 2008;27(6):399–400.

24. Cruz AA, et al. Graves upper eyelid retraction. Surv Ophthalmol. 2013;58(1):63–76.

25. Bartalena L, Wiersinga WM, Pinchera A. Graves' ophthalmopathy: state of the art and perspectives. J Endocrinol Invest. 2004;27(3):295–301.

26. Abramoff MD, et al. Rectus extraocular muscle paths and decompression surgery for Graves orbitopathy: mechanism of motility disturbances. Invest Ophthalmol Vis Sci. 2002;43(2):300–7.

27. Gilbard JP, Farris RL. Ocular surface drying and tear film osmolarity in thyroid eye disease. Acta Ophthalmol. 1983;61(1):108–16.

28. Khurana AK, et al. Tear film profile in Graves' ophthalmopathy. Acta Ophthalmol. 1992;70(3):346–9.

29. DEWS. The definition and classification of dry eye disease: report of the definition and classification subcommittee of the international dry eye workshop (2007). Ocul Surf. 2007;5(2):75–92.

30. Cho RI, et al. The effect of orbital decompression surgery on lid retraction in thyroid eye disease. Ophthal Plast Reconstr Surg. 2011;27(6):436–8.

31. Ribeiro SF, et al. Graves Lower Eyelid Retraction. Ophthal Plast Reconstr Surg. 2016;32(3):161–9.

32. Wiersinga WM, et al. Temporal relationship between onset of Graves' ophthalmopathy and onset of thyroidal Graves' disease. J Endocrinol Invest. 1988;11(8):615–9.

33. Bartley GB. Rundle and his curve. Arch Ophthalmol. 2011;129(3):356–8.

34. Gamblin GT, et al. Prevalence of increased intraocular pressure in Graves' disease–evidence of frequent subclinical ophthalmopathy. N Engl J Med. 1983;308(8):420–4.

35. Fishman DR, Benes SC. Upgaze intraocular pressure changes and strabismus in Graves' ophthalmopathy. J Clin Neuroophthalmol. 1991;11(3):162–5.

36. Kalmann R, Mourits MP. Prevalence and management of elevated intraocular pressure in patients with Graves' orbitopathy. Br J Ophthalmol. 1998;82(7):754–7.

37. Bartalena L, et al. Sight-threatening Grave's orbitopathy. In: De Groot LJ CF, Dungan K, editors. Endotext. South Dartmouth (MA): MDText.com, Inc; 2015.

38. McKeag D, et al. Clinical features of dysthyroid optic neuropathy: a European Group on Graves' Orbitopathy (EUGOGO) survey. Br J Ophthalmol. 2007;91(4):455–8.

39. Mourits MP, et al. Clinical criteria for the assessment of disease activity in Graves' ophthalmopathy: a novel approach. Br J Ophthalmol. 1989;73(8):639–44.

40. Koornneef L. Eyelid and orbital fascial attachments and their clinical significance. Eye (Lond). 1988;2(Pt 2):130–4.

41. Jellema HM, et al. Outcome of inferior and superior rectus recession in Graves' orbitopathy patients. Orbit. 2015;34(2):84–91.

42. Gurdal C, et al. Ocular surface and dry eye in Graves' disease. Curr Eye Res. 2011;36(1):8–13.

43. Bruscolini A, et al. Dry eye syndrome in non-exophthalmic Graves' disease. Semin Ophthalmol. 2015;30(5–6):372–6.

44. Alves M, et al. Comparison of diagnostic tests in distinct well-defined conditions related to dry eye disease. PLoS One. 2014;9(5):e97921.

45. Ismailova DS, Fedorov AA, Grusha YO. Ocular surface changes in thyroid eye disease. Orbit. 2013;32(2):87–90.

46. McGinnigle S, Naroo SA, Eperjesi F. Evaluation of dry eye. Surv Ophthalmol. 2012;57(4):293–316.

47. Eckstein AK, et al. Dry eye syndrome in thyroid-associated ophthalmopathy: lacrimal expression of TSH receptor suggests involvement of TSHR-specific autoantibodies. Acta Ophthalmol Scand. 2004;82(3 Pt 1):291–7.

48. Mason DK, Harden RM, Alexander WD. The salivary and thyroid glands. A comparative study in man. Br Dent J. 1967;122(11):485–9.

49. Jara LJ, et al. Thyroid disease in Sjogren's syndrome. Clin Rheumatol. 2007;26(10):1601–6.

50. Kahaly GJ, et al. Alpha-fodrin as a putative autoantigen in Graves' ophthalmopathy. Clin Exp Immunol. 2005;140(1):166–72.

51. Adamson 3rd TC, et al. Immunohistologic analysis of lymphoid infiltrates in primary Sjogren's syndrome using monoclonal antibodies. J Immunol. 1983;130(1):203–8.

52. Biro E, et al. Association of systemic and thyroid autoimmune diseases. Clin Rheumatol. 2006;25(2):240–5.

53. Martin SJ, et al. Proteolysis of fodrin (non-erythroid spectrin) during apoptosis. J Biol Chem. 1995;270(12):6425–8.

54. Boehm N, et al. Alterations in the tear proteome of dry eye patients–a matter of the clinical phenotype. Invest Ophthalmol Vis Sci. 2013;54(3):2385–92.

55. Matheis N, et al. Proteomics of tear fluid in thyroid-associated orbitopathy. Thyroid. 2012;22(10):1039–45.

56. Matheis N, et al. Proteomics differentiate between thyroid-associated orbitopathy and dry eye syndrome. Invest Ophthalmol Vis Sci. 2015;56(4):2649–56.

57. Villani E, et al. Corneal involvement in Graves' orbitopathy: an in vivo confocal study. Invest Ophthalmol Vis Sci. 2010;51(9):4574–8.

58. Piantanida E, et al. Prevalence and natural history of Graves' orbitopathy in the XXI century. J Endocrinol Invest. 2013;36(6):444–9.

59. Regensburg NI, et al. Densities of orbital fat and extraocular muscles in graves orbitopathy patients and controls. Ophthal Plast Reconstr Surg. 2011;27(4):236–40.

60. Bartalena L, et al. The 2016 European Thyroid Association/European Group on Graves' orbitopathy guidelines for the management of Graves' orbitopathy. Eur Thyroid J. 2016;5(1):9–26.

61. Briceno CA, Gupta S, Douglas RS. Advances in the management of thyroid eye disease. Int Ophthalmol Clin. 2013;53(3):93–101.

62. Rao R, et al. Current trends in the management of thyroid eye disease. Curr Opin Ophthalmol. 2015;26(6):484–90.

63. Kau HC, et al. Cigarette smoke extract-induced oxidative stress and fibrosis-related genes expression in orbital fibroblasts from patients with Graves' ophthalmopathy. Oxid Med Cell Longev. 2016;2016:4676289.

64. Gortz GE, et al. Hypoxia-dependent HIF-1 activation impacts on tissue remodeling in Graves' ophthalmopathy - implications for smoking. J Clin Endocrinol Metab. 2016:jc20161279. Epub ahead of print. doi: http://dx.doi.org/10.1210/jc.2016-1279.

65. Kahaly GJ, et al. Randomized, single blind trial of intravenous versus oral steroid monotherapy in Graves' orbitopathy. J Clin Endocrinol Metab. 2005;90(9):5234–40.

66. Khong JJ, et al. Risk factors for Graves' orbitopathy; the Australian Thyroid-associated Orbitopathy Research (ATOR) Study. J Clin Endocrinol Metab. 2016;101(7):2711–20.

67. Marcocci C, et al. Selenium and the course of mild Graves' orbitopathy. N Engl J Med. 2011;364(20):1920–31.

68. Khong JJ, et al. Serum selenium status in Graves' disease with and without orbitopathy: a case-control study. Clin Endocrinol (Oxf). 2014;80(6):905–10.

69. Dehina N, et al. Lack of association between selenium status and disease severity and activity in patients with Graves' ophthalmopathy. Eur Thyroid J. 2016;5(1):57–64.

70. Foulks GN, et al. Clinical guidelines for management of dry eye associated with Sjogren disease. Ocul Surf. 2015;13(2):118–32.

71. Bartalena L, et al. Consensus statement of the European Group on Graves' orbitopathy (EUGOGO) on management of GO. Eur J Endocrinol. 2008;158(3):273–85.

72. Curro N, et al. Therapeutic outcomes of high-dose intravenous steroids in the treatment of dysthyroid optic neuropathy. Thyroid. 2014;24(5):897–905.

73. Nedeljkovic Beleslin B, et al. Efficacy and safety of combined parenteral and oral steroid therapy in Graves' orbitopathy. Hormones (Athens). 2014;13(2):222–8.

74. Perumal B, Meyer DR. Treatment of severe thyroid eye disease: a survey of the American Society of Ophthalmic Plastic and Reconstructive Surgery (ASOPRS). Ophthal Plast Reconstr Surg. 2015;31(2):127–31.

75. Hahn E, et al. Orbital radiation therapy for Graves' ophthalmopathy: measuring clinical efficacy and impact. Pract Radiat Oncol. 2014;4(4):233–9.

76. Salvi M. Immunotherapy for Graves' ophthalmopathy. Curr Opin Endocrinol Diabetes Obes. 2014;21(5):409–14.

77. Khanna D, et al. Rituximab treatment of patients with severe, corticosteroid-resistant thyroid-associated ophthalmopathy. Ophthalmology. 2010;117(1):133–9. e2.

78. McCoy AN, et al. Rituximab (Rituxan) therapy for severe thyroid-associated ophthalmopathy diminishes IGF-1R(+) T cells. J Clin Endocrinol Metab. 2014;99(7):E1294–9.

79. Stan MN, et al. Randomized controlled trial of rituximab in patients with Graves' orbitopathy. J Clin Endocrinol Metab. 2015;100(2):432–41.

80. Smith TJ, Hegedus L, Douglas RS. Role of insulin-like growth factor-1 (IGF-1) pathway in the pathogenesis of Graves' orbitopathy. Best Pract Res Clin Endocrinol Metab. 2012;26(3):291–302.

81. Tsui S, et al. Evidence for an association between thyroid-stimulating hormone and insulin-like growth factor 1 receptors: a tale of two antigens implicated in Graves' disease. J Immunol. 2008;181(6):4397–405.

82. Krieger CC, et al. TSH/IGF-1 receptor cross talk in Graves' ophthalmopathy pathogenesis. J Clin Endocrinol Metab. 2016;101(6):2340–7.

83. Naik VM, et al. Immunopathogenesis of thyroid eye disease: emerging paradigms. Surv Ophthalmol. 2010;55(3):215–26.

84. Chen H, et al. Teprotumumab, an IGF-1R blocking monoclonal antibody inhibits TSH and IGF-1 action in fibrocytes. J Clin Endocrinol Metab. 2014; 99(9):E1635–40.

85. Douglas RS, et al. Aberrant expression of the insulin-like growth factor-1 receptor by T cells from patients with Graves' disease may carry functional consequences for disease pathogenesis. J Immunol. 2007;178(5):3281–7.

86. Rajaii F, McCoy AN, Smith TJ. Cytokines are both villains and potential therapeutic targets in thyroid-associated ophthalmopathy: From bench to bedside. Expert Rev Ophthalmol. 2014;9(3):227–34.

87. Perez-Moreiras JV, Alvarez-Lopez A, Gomez EC. Treatment of active corticosteroid-resistant graves' orbitopathy. Ophthal Plast Reconstr Surg. 2014;30(2):162–7.

88. Choe CH, Cho RI, Elner VM. Comparison of lateral and medial orbital decompression for the treatment of compressive optic neuropathy in thyroid eye disease. Ophthal Plast Reconstr Surg. 2011;27(1):4–11.

89. Lee KH, et al. Graded decompression of orbital fat and wall in patients with Graves' orbitopathy. Korean J Ophthalmol. 2014;28(1):1–11.

90. Gulati S, et al. Long-term follow-up of patients with thyroid eye disease treated with endoscopic orbital decompression. Acta Ophthalmol. 2015; 93(2):178–83.

91. Eckstein A, Schittkowski M, Esser J. Surgical treatment of Graves' ophthalmopathy. Best Pract Res Clin Endocrinol Metab. 2012;26(3):339–58.

92. Devoto MH, et al. Improvement from no light perception after orbital decompression for graves' optic neuropathy. Ophthalmology. 2014;121(1): 431–2. e1.

93. Jellema HM, et al. Proposal of success criteria for strabismus surgery in patients with Graves' orbitopathy based on a systematic literature review. Acta Ophthalmol. 2015;93(7):601–9.

94. Jellema HM, et al. Quality of life improves after strabismus surgery in patients with Graves' orbitopathy. Eur J Endocrinol. 2014;170(5):785–9.

3

Total costs of basal or premixed insulin treatment in 5077 insulin-naïve type 2 diabetes patients: register-based observational study in clinical practice

Ann-Marie Svensson[1], Vincent Lak[2], MirNabi Pirouzi Fard[1] and Björn Eliasson[2*] (iD)

Abstract

Background: To investigate the costs of treatment with basal insulin (insulin NPH [NPH], insulin glargine [IG], insulin determir [IG]), and premixed insulin (PM) in routine clinical care.

Methods: Cohort study based on data from the Swedish National Diabetes Register, including 5077 insulin-naïve men and women with type 2 diabetes, resident in a distinct geographical region of Sweden. Patients were included between 1 July 2006 and 31 December 2009 and followed for 12 months. All drug- and healthcare-related costs, stratified by diabetes-related or non-diabetes care contacts, were quantified and compared to baseline.

Results: Initiation of insulin treatment generally entails increased diabetes-related health care contacts and treatment costs, and decrease in health care costs. The median changes in costs were generally smaller than the mean changes, reflecting great variations between patients. The treatment costs were higher for IG, ID and PM compared with NPH, although higher age, history cardiovascular disease and diabetes complications as well as higher diabetes-related and other treatment costs were independent predictors. Overall, only PM (but not IG or ID) were associated with higher diabetes-related health care costs, although these were also independently predicted by cardiovascular morbidity and markers of complicated diabetes.

Conclusions: This study demonstrates that the initiation of insulin in patients with type 2 diabetes in clinical practice leads to increased health care contacts, overall and treatment costs, but also generally results in a decrease in health care costs. The diabetes-related treatment cost was lowest using NPH insulin but only premixed insulin was associated with higher diabetes-related health care costs than NPH.

Keywords: Type 2 diabetes, Basal insulin, Cost, Insulin detemir, Insulin glargine, Neutral protamine hagedorn, Premixed insulin

Background

Insulin treatment is commonly used in patients with type 2 diabetes when lifestyle changes and oral hypoglycemic agents (OHA) fail to achieve adequate glycemic control [1, 2]. The medium long-acting NPH (neutral protamine Hagedorn) given at bedtime has been a common first-hand choice, but a long-acting insulin analogue (insulin glargine (IG) or insulin detemir (ID)) is frequently used, particularly in patients experiencing nocturnal hypoglycaemia. Pre-mixed insulin (PM), usually administered twice daily, is another useful treatment option [3].

The clinical effects of these treatment alternatives have been evaluated in randomized clinical trials (RCT) and meta-analyses, and recently also in clinical practice [4, 5]. Overall there are no major differences in the effects on glycemic control, but there can be differences in weight effects, hypoglycemia and insulin doses as well as in

---

* Correspondence: bjorn.eliasson@gu.se
[2]Department of Medicine, Sahlgrenska University Hospital, University of Gothenburg, S-413 45 Göteborg, Sweden
Full list of author information is available at the end of the article

persistence. We recently studied the clinical effects in 5077 insulin-naïve type 2 diabetes patients in a geographically distinct region of Sweden (Region Västra Götaland), who initiated treatment on NPH, IG, ID or PM [6]. The different insulin regimens were found to be equally effective in lowering HbA1c, but PM required 59 % higher and ID 25 % higher insulin doses to achieve a similar HbA1c reduction as NPH. PM was also associated with a significantly greater increase in BMI compared with NPH, and a small but higher number of patients experiencing severe hypoglycemia than the other treatment groups.

The high costs associated with diabetes care have long been recognized, but the number of published studies in this area is low. A recent report based on managed care administrative data in the U.S.A. described in detail the total health care costs for patients with type 2 diabetes [7]. The strongest predictors of high costs for the patients were obesity, comorbidities and hospitalization, but also progression to insulin therapy. There are also very few studies addressing the total costs associated with different insulin regimens, although development programs (RCTs) for new pharmaceutical agents also often include health economic analyses [8]. In clinical practice, the addition of IG, compared with PM, to treatment with oral hypoglycemic agents (OHA) was recently examined, showing better persistence and lower costs [9].

There are no studies available comparing costs of different insulin regimens when added to OHA in unselected cohorts in clinical practice. The aim of this study was therefore to examine health care utilization and costs in our recent study with 5,077 insulin-naïve type 2 diabetes patients, after starting treatment with NPH, IG, ID or PM [6].

Methods

The overall design of this study has recently been described in detail [6]. To summarize, we linked data from four national health registers: the Swedish National Diabetes Register (NDR; clinical data), the Prescribed Drug Register (pharmacological agents, doses), the Cause of Death Register, and the Regional Claims Database (VEGA). The latter contains diagnoses (International Classification of Diseases [ICD]-10 and Diagnosis Related Groups [DRG] codes), procedures performed (Nordic Medico-Statistical Committee [NOMESCO] and local procedure codes) and hospital lengths of stay for inpatient, outpatient, primary, and private care for all inhabitants in the Region Västra Götaland.

Ethics, consent and permissions

All included patients have agreed by informed consent to be registered before inclusion. The Ethics Review Board at the University of Gothenburg approved the study.

Patients, study period, follow-up and censoring

We included insulin-naïve patients with type 2 diabetes, at least 18 years of age. The study period was between 1 July 2005 and 31 December 2010. Patients were not allowed to fill a prescription of insulin from 1 July 2005 to 30 June 2006 to ensure they were previously untreated (data from the Prescribed Drug Register). Patients were required to have their first prescription of insulin filled (index date) between 1 July 2006 and 31 December 2009 to allow for 1 year of follow-up. Patients were thus followed for 12 months or until the occurrence of a censoring event. The mean number days of follow-up were similar in the four treatment groups (352 ± 47 NPH, 358 ± 37 IG, 351 ± 51 ID and 352 ± 47 PM) [6]. Start of follow-up was defined as the date of the first filled insulin prescription (index date) in each patient. In order to ensure continuous insulin use, at least three filled prescriptions of the initiated insulin were required during the follow-up period. Censoring events included a filled prescription of a new type of insulin, death or move out of the Region Västra Götaland.

Costs

Treatment costs (drug-related costs) were retrieved from the Prescribed Drug Register, which has full, nation-wide coverage of all transactions that are made at pharmacies in Sweden, including all drugs (ATC codes A-V) and technical aids (ATC codes W-Y). We used data between 2005-07-01 and 2010-12-31.

Healthcare costs were estimated by using the associated DRG-codes (data from VEGA). To make data comparable, Swedish national DRG-weight lists and costs for 2010 were used (National Board of Health and Welfare, http://www.socialstyrelsen.se/english). VEGA also provided data on outlier costs, which were considered when estimating the final cost per care contact. For outdated DRG-codes, old DRG-weight lists provided by the Swedish National Board of Health and Welfare were used to extract weights, which were used in combination with the 2010 DRG cost. Further, psychiatric DRG-codes were flagged, and the clinic setting where the care contacts occurred, were used to determine whether DRG-weights from the inpatient DRG-list or the psychiatric DRG-list should be applied. For primary care, costs were determined based on the caregiver, where physicians were assumed to have a three times higher rate than other caregivers (e.g. nurses, physiotherapists, etc.). This corresponded to a 1840 SEK cost for a physicians visit, and a 615 SEK cost for all other primary care visits. The approximate value of 100 SEK is currently 12 US dollars (August 2015).

We studied all drug- and health care-related costs, stratified by diabetes-related or non-diabetes care contacts. All costs 12 months before initiation and during follow-up of insulin treatment were recorded. A correlation analysis with costs before and after insulin treatment initiation was performed, to determine whether incremental analysis or pre-index cost adjustment should be undertaken. If the correlation exceeded 0.5, an incremental analysis whereby the prior (baseline) costs are subtracted from the costs observed during follow-up, was recommended. Otherwise, the pre-index costs were included as a covariate in the regression model. Costs are presented in 2010 SEK value after adjusting for consumer price indices provided by Statistics Sweden (www.scb.se/en).

Costs were stratified by whether they were diabetes-related or not, in a mutually exclusive manner, including anti-diabetic treatment costs as well as costs of cardiovascular risk factor treatments (antihypertensive and lipid-lowering treatment, platelet aggregation inhibitors). We also identified all diabetes-related care contacts and their associated costs through the ICD-10 codes E11*, E13*, and E14* (regardless of diagnosis position), as well as cardiovascular disease costs, such as myocardial infarction/ischaemic heart disease (I20-I25), atrial fibrillation (I48), congestive heart failure (I50*), and stroke (I61, I63, I64, I67.9).

Statistical methods

Baseline characteristics are presented as means ± 1 standard deviation (SD) or medians for continuous variables and frequencies for categorical variables with crude significance levels for differences between the groups, when analysed using ANOVA or χ^2 test. For continuous variables with non-normal distribution a Kruskal-Wallis test was performed. All continuous outcome variables were explored for their distribution.

We used generalized linear modeling (GLM) after log transformation to assess potential predictors of diabetes-related health care contacts, health care costs and treatment costs. For each outcome, three models were explored and presented; firstly, unadjusted where outcome was as a function of insulin groups, secondly, including covariates with few missing values (age, gender, level of income, diabetes duration, history of CVD, history of diabetes complications, previous OHA use, and follow-up time), and finally a fully adjusted model including age, gender, level of income, diabetes duration, history of CVD, history of diabetes complications, previous OHA use, follow-up time, pre-index HbA1c, pre-index BMI and weight. Pre-index diabetes-related costs were included as a covariate to account for the patient's type 2 diabetes history and severity. Further, post-index other costs (including cardiovascular costs) were included in the model as a covariate to account for the overall disease burden (comorbidities) of the population, which in turn might affect post-index diabetes-related costs.

Statistical analyses were performed in R (R Foundation for Statistical Computing) or SAS V.9.3 (SAS Institute,

Cary, North Carolina, USA). A two-sided p value <0.05 was considered statistically significant.

Results

As previously reported, 5077 insulin-naïve patients with type 2 diabetes were included in the study [6]. The patients were mostly initiated on NPH (49 %) or PM (34 %), while 13 % and 3 % were initiated on IG and ID. To summarize, there were modest but significant reductions in glycemic control (HbA1c) for patients treated with NPH, IG, ID or PM during one year of follow-up, but the effects of the different regimens did not differ. The weight-adjusted daily insulin doses with ID and PM were 59 % and 25 % higher to achieve similar HbA1c when compared with patients treated with NPH, while the patients treated with PM gained more weight compared with patients treated with other insulin regimens. The recorded number of patients experiencing a hypoglycaemic event was low (only 26 patients in total), but occurred predominantly in patients treated with PM. The mean number of days of follow-up was highest in patients initiating IG.

The numbers of visits in health care before and after starting the insulin treatment are given in Table 1. There was an increase in the number of visits for all four analyzed insulin regimens during the follow-up period. For diabetes-related visits, small differences in the mean number of visits during the pre-index period were observed, such that IG and PM patients had slightly more visits. During the follow-up period, NPH patients had the highest mean number of diabetes-related health care contacts, while ID had the lowest. When diabetes-related care contacts including cardiovascular comorbidities were evaluated, PM had the highest mean number of contacts during the pre-index period, while during the follow-up period, IG, PM, and NPH patients all had close to three contacts. For other care contacts, PM and IG patients had the highest frequency during both the pre-index and the post-index period. For the patients who did have a change in number of contacts (N = 4239), there was no significant difference between the different treatment groups (Additional file 1: Table S1). Adjusting for several covariates emphasized this result, although lower age and use of OHA were independent predictors of less health care contacts. A history of cardiovascular disease, diabetes complications, higher pre-index diabetes-related and other health care costs were independent predictors of more health care contacts.

The costs of health care and treatments before and after starting the insulin treatment are given in Table 2. Diabetes-related costs varied substantially between the treatment groups for all pre-index and post-index treatment and health care costs. The mean pre-index health care costs were considerably higher in the PM patients

Table 1 Number of contacts with the health-care before and after starting insulin treatment

Treatment	Diabetes-related contacts Pre-index Mean ± SD	Post-index Mean ± SD	Diabetes-related contacts including cardiovascular Pre-index Mean ± SD	Post-index Mean ± SD	Other contacts Pre-index Mean ± SD	Post-index Mean ± SD
NPH	2.0 ± 1.8	2.7 ± 2.8	2.2 ± 2.4	3.1 ± 3.7	11.8 ± 15.4	13.9 ± 16.1
IG	2.1 ± 2.4	2.6 ± 3.1	2.3 ± 2.7	2.9 ± 3.3	12.6 ± 14.7	15.0 ± 16.2
ID	1.9 ± 2.1	2.4 ± 2.4	2.1 ± 2.4	2.6 ± 2.6	12.0 ± 13.8	14.2 ± 16.0
PM	2.1 ± 1.9	2.6 ± 2.5	2.4 ± 2.3	3.0 ± 3.3	13.1 ± 15.5	14.8 ± 15.5
p-values	0.003	0.044	0.00004	0.022	0.00002	0.0009

NPH Neutral protamine Hagedorn, IG insulin glargine, ID insulin determir, PM premixed insulin, SD standard deviation

at (SEK 30 990), compared with SEK 22 861 and SEK 19 674 for IG and NPH groups, and SEK 9544 for ID, reflecting differences in clinical characteristics. The mean pre-index treatment costs were around 50 % higher for IG and ID compared with PM and NPH. The health care costs during follow-up were lower for all groups but the ID group, with a similar magnitude of decrease for IG and NPH, while the PM showed the largest decrease. Post-index diabetes-related treatment costs were higher for all groups, compared to pre-index treatment costs, in line with the expectations of a more intense treatment regime after insulin initiation. As expected, the IG and ID still had higher treatment costs, while the proportional cost increase compared to PM and NPH was smaller for IG, at 30 %, compared to 50 % for ID.

For diabetes-related costs where also cardiovascular costs were included (Table 3), similar patterns as for diabetes-related costs were observed. The main differences were that pre-index treatment costs were more similar between groups when CVD treatment was taken into account, and that all treatment groups showed cost

decreases when comparing pre- and post-index health care costs.

The median costs for both health care and treatment in both Tables 2 and 3 were consistently lower than the mean costs, reflecting an asymmetrical cost distribution among the patients with a few patients with very high costs. The discrepancies between the median and the mean costs were more pronounced in the health care costs than the treatment costs. The median increment health care cost was 0 for NPH, IG and ID. For PM there was a small decrement in median health care costs.

For other pre-index health care costs (Table 4), the PM patients consistently showed highest mean costs and ID patients lower costs, and this pattern was repeated also for pre-index treatment costs. For post-index costs, the IG and PM groups showed the highest mean costs, which were also seen for post-index treatment costs ($p < 0.01$). Overall, the differences in incremental other costs between insulin groups were non-significant, while the patterns indicated a moderate increase for treatment costs for all groups.

For patients who did have a change in diabetes-related health care costs (N = 4232), IG and PM increased costs compared with NPH, whereas ID lowered costs in an unadjusted model (Additional file 1: Table S2). In the fully adjusted model only PM was associated with increased health care costs compared with NPH, but higher age, a history of cardiovascular disease, diabetes complications, and pre-index diabetes-related and other health care costs independently predicted higher costs, while previous use of OHA predicted lower diabetes-related health care costs. There were higher treatment costs with IG, ID and PM compared with NPH (Additional file 1: Table S3). ID increased treatment costs more than IG and PM in relation to NPH in both the unadjusted and the adjusted models. In the latter model, higher age, a history of cardiovascular disease, diabetes complications, use of OHA, were independent predictors of lower, while higher municipality income as well as pre-index diabetes-related and other health care costs predicted higher diabetes-related treatment costs.

Table 2 Costs (SEK) of health care and treatments before and after starting the insulin treatment

Treatment	Pre-index Health care Mean/Median	Treatment Mean/Median	Post-index Health care Mean/Median	Treatment Mean/Median	Increment Health care Mean/Median	Treatment Mean/Median	Net cost effect Mean/Median
NPH	19,674/3,228	2,455/1,587	16,570/3,240	8,191/6,840	−3,104/0	5,736/4,528	2,632/4,528
IG	22,861/3,457	2,857/1,959	19,746/3,143	10,818/9,343	−3,115/0	7,962/6,551	4,847/6,551
ID	9,544/2,458	3,041/1,608	11,402/2,647	12,351/10,706	1,858/0	9,310/7,690	11,168/7,690
PM	30,990/4,806	2,155/1,430	22,441/3,681	8,617/7,877	−8,549/−265	6,462/5,972	−2,087/5,707
p-values	<0.0001	<0.0001	0.0001	<0.0001	0.0011	<0.0001	

NPH Neutral protamine Hagedorn, IG insulin glargine, ID insulin determir, PM premixed insulin, SD standard deviation. The approximate value of 100 SEK is currently 12 US dollars (August 2015)

Table 3 Costs (SEK) of health care and treatments (including cardiovascular costs) before and after starting the insulin treatment

Treatment	Pre-index		Post-index		Increment		Net cost effect
	Health care	Treatment	Health care	Treatment	Health care	Treatment	
	Mean/Median	Mean/Median	Mean/Median	Mean/Median	Mean/Median	Mean/Median	Mean/Median
NPH	24,791/3,681	3,449/2,398	19,390/3,681	9,279/7,879	−5,401/0	5,831/4,659	430/4,659
IG	25,197/3,681	3,920/2,679	23,539/3,681	11,967/10,670	−1,658/0	8,047/6,569	6,389/6,569
ID	17,981/2,613	3,815/2,194	13,070/2,955	13,143/11,306	−4,912/0	9,328/7,808	4,416/7,808
PM	36,724/6,366	3,183/2,259	26,388/4,262	9,744/8,800	−10,336/-773	6,560/6,010	−3,776/5,237
p-values	<0.0001	<0.0012	<0.0001	<0.0001	0.0022	<0.0001	

NPH Neutral protamine Hagedorn, IG insulin glargine, ID insulin determir, PM premixed insulin, SD standard deviation. The approximate value of 100 SEK is currently 12 US dollars (August 2015)

Discussion and conclusions

This observational study provides information on costs of the use different types of insulin regimens in patients with type 2 diabetes failing oral glucose-lowering treatment. The results show that although the initiation of insulin treatment generally entails increased diabetes-related health care contacts and treatment costs, it also generally results in a decrease in health care costs, especially when including costs for the treatment and care of cardiovascular diseases. The median changes in costs were generally smaller than the mean changes, reflecting great variations between patients. The treatment costs were higher for IG, ID and PM compared with NPH, although history cardiovascular disease and diabetes complications as well as higher diabetes-related and other treatment costs were independent predictors. Overall, with respect to diabetes-related health care, only PM (but not IG or ID) were associated with higher costs, although these were also independently predicted by cardiovascular morbidity and markers of complicated diabetes.

There are generally differences in clinical characteristics between the patients offered the various treatment options when additional treatment is required on top of OHA in clinical practice. Still, this project including previously presented clinical results [10], provides arguments against the use of PM due to weight gain, higher insulin doses, rates of hypoglycaemia and diabetes–related health care

costs compared with the reference, treatment with NPH. The treatment costs of IG and ID are higher than NPH, but seem to offer other advantages, possibly such as ease of use and low rates of hypoglycaemia, leading to similar overall costs.

Other studies of the costs of initiating basal insulin have reached similar conclusions. A retrospective study on a U.S. population between 2001 and 2006 found that IG compared with NPH had higher drug-related costs, but no significant difference in health-care costs, although both were associated with major cost reductions [11]. Similarly, a UK retrospective primary care register study with data from 1988–2010 found that insulin analogues were associated with higher costs than NPH for the first year but after three years [12]. Contrarily, a Swiss simulation study found IG would be more cost-effective than NPH in the long term [13]. A recent systematic review and meta-analysis concluded that long acting insulin analogues are probably superior to NPH, although the difference is small for HbA1c [14]. The effects of treatment with premixed insulin have also been evaluated [9, 15], leading to careful recommendations of its use [1, 2, 16].

The present study has several strengths. The observational design allows for comparisons of the effectiveness and costs of different types of insulin, and the results are likely to be representative of clinical practice in countries with similar populations, following similar

Table 4 Other costs before and after starting the insulin treatment

Treatment	Pre-index		Post-index		Increment		Net cost effect
	Health care	Treatment	Health care	Treatment	Health care	Treatment	
	Mean/Median	Mean/Median	Mean/Median	Mean/Median	Mean/Median	Mean/Median	Mean/Median
NPH	25,417/9,215	5,209/2,445	24,173/10,439	6,287/2,926	−1,244/755	1,078/125	−166/880
IG	23,533/10,341	5,576/2,784	28,096/12,447	7,063/3,267	4,563/1,225	1,486/224	6,049/1,449
ID	20,297/9,205	4,515/1,455	22,313/10,652	5,300/1,819	2,016/1,717	785/160	2,801/1,877
PM	28,423/10,752	6,380/3,150	26,880/12,191	7,549/3,877	−1,543/883	1,169/283	−374/1,166
p-values	0.0054	<0.00001	0.0010	<0.00001	0.55	0.052	

NPH Neutral protamine Hagedorn, IG insulin glargine, ID insulin determir, PM premixed insulin, SD standard deviation. The approximate value of 100 SEK is currently 12 US dollars (August 2015)

treatment guidelines [17]. All patients fulfilling the inclusion criteria have been included in the calculations, which are based on detailed information from administrative systems with complete coverage. Apart from the general limitations characteristic of observational studies, one weakness in the present study was the limited number of patients on IG and ID, particularly the latter. The lack of reliable data on non-severe hypoglycaemia (i.e., not requiring hospitalization), or patient-reported measures, are important limitations. Furthermore, Analyses did not provide a societal perspective, since neither sick-leave information (productivity gains and losses), nor direct non-medical costs, were considered [18].

This study demonstrates that the initiation of insulin in patients with type 2 diabetes in clinical practice leads to increased health care contacts, overall and treatment costs, but also generally results in a decrease in health care costs. The diabetes-related treatment cost was lowest using NPH insulin but only premixed insulin was associated with higher diabetes-related health care costs than NPH.

Competing interests

B. Eliasson has participated in advisory boards for Sanofi, Eli Lilly and Novo Nordisk and served as a lecturer at educational meetings arranged by these companies. V. Lak, M. Pirouzi Fard and A.M. Svensson declare no conflicts of interest.

Authors' contributions

AMS, MNPF and BE contributed to the conception and design of the study. AMS and MNPF acquired data, and did the statistical analyses. BE and VL drafted the report, and AMS, VL and BE critically revised and finalised it. All authors read and approved the final manuscript.

Author details

[1]Center of Registers in Region Västra Götaland, Göteborg, Sweden.
[2]Department of Medicine, Sahlgrenska University Hospital, University of Gothenburg, S-413 45 Göteborg, Sweden.

References

1. Inzucchi SE, Bergenstal RM, Buse JB, Diamant M, Ferrannini E, Nauck M, et al. Management of hyperglycaemia in type 2 diabetes: a patient-centered approach. Position statement of the American Diabetes Association (ADA) and the European Association for the Study of Diabetes (EASD). Diabetologia. 2012;55:1577–96.
2. Inzucchi SE, Bergenstal RM, Buse JB, Diamant M, Ferrannini E, Nauck M, et al. Management of hyperglycemia in type 2 diabetes, 2015: a patient-centered approach: update to a position statement of the American Diabetes Association and the European Association for the Study of Diabetes. Diabetes Care. 2015;38(1):140–9.
3. DeWitt DE, Hirsch IB. Outpatient insulin therapy in type 1 and type 2 diabetes mellitus: scientific review. JAMA. 2003;289(17):2254–64.
4. Horvath K, Jeitler K, Berghold A, Ebrahim SH, Gratzer TW, Plank J, et al. Long-acting insulin analogues versus NPH insulin (human isophane insulin) for type 2 diabetes mellitus. Cochrane Database Syst Rev. 2007;2, CD005613.
5. Singh SR, Ahmad F, Lal A, Yu C, Bai Z, Bennett H. Efficacy and safety of insulin analogues for the management of diabetes mellitus: a meta-analysis. CMAJ. 2009;180(4):385–97.
6. Eliasson B, Ekström N, Bruce Wirta S, Odén A, Pirouzi Fard M, Svensson A-M. Metabolic effects of basal or premixed insulin treatment in 5077 insulin-naïve type 2 diabetes patients: registry-based observational study in clinical practice. Diabetes Therapy. 2014:in press.
7. Meyers JL, Parasuraman S, Bell KF, Graham JP, Candrilli SD. The high-cost, type 2 diabetes mellitus patient: an analysis of managed care administrative data. Arch Public Health. 2014;72(1):6.
8. Cameron CG, Bennett HA. Cost-effectiveness of insulin analogues for diabetes mellitus. CMAJ. 2009;180(4):400–7.
9. Baser O, Tangirala K, Wei W, Xie L. Real-world outcomes of initiating insulin glargine-based treatment versus premixed analog insulins among US patients with type 2 diabetes failing oral antidiabetic drugs. Clinicoecon Outcomes Res. 2013;5:497–505.
10. Eliasson B, Ekstrom N, Bruce Wirta S, Oden A, Fard MP, Svensson AM. Metabolic effects of Basal or premixed insulin treatment in 5077 insulin-naive type 2 diabetes patients: registry-based observational study in clinical practice. Diabetes Ther. 2014;5(1):243–54.
11. Lee LJ, Yu AP, Johnson SJ, Birnbaum HG, Atanasov P, Buesching DP, et al. Direct costs associated with initiating NPH insulin versus glargine in patients with type 2 diabetes: a retrospective database analysis. Diabetes Res Clin Pract. 2010;87(1):108–16.
12. Idris I, Gordon J, Tilling C, Vora J. A cost comparison of long-acting insulin analogs vs NPH insulin-based treatment in patients with type 2 diabetes using routinely collected primary care data from the UK. J Med Econ. 2015;18(4):273–82.
13. Brandle M, Azoulay M, Greiner RA. Cost-effectiveness of insulin glargine versus NPH insulin for the treatment of Type 2 diabetes mellitus, modeling the interaction between hypoglycemia and glycemic control in Switzerland. Int J Clin Pharmacol Ther. 2011;49(3):217–30.
14. Tricco AC, Ashoor HM, Antony J, Beyene J, Veroniki AA, Isaranuwatchai W, et al. Safety, effectiveness, and cost effectiveness of long acting versus intermediate acting insulin for patients with type 1 diabetes: systematic review and network meta-analysis. BMJ. 2014;349:g5459.
15. Holman RR, Thorne KI, Farmer AJ, Davies MJ, Keenan JF, Paul S, et al. Addition of biphasic, prandial, or basal insulin to oral therapy in type 2 diabetes. N Engl J Med. 2007;357(17):1716–30.
16. Mosenzon O, Raz I. Intensification of insulin therapy for type 2 diabetic patients in primary care: basal-bolus regimen versus premix insulin analogs: when and for whom? Diabetes Care. 2013;36 Suppl 2:S212–8.
17. Force IDFCGT. Global Guideline for Type 2 Diabetes: recommendations for standard, comprehensive, and minimal care. Diabet Med. 2006;23(6):579–93.
18. Gold MR, Siegel JE, Russell LB, Weinstein MC. Cost-Effectiveness in Health and Medicine. New York: Oxford University Press; 1996.

4

Prevalence of Gestational Diabetes Mellitus in urban and rural Tamil Nadu using IADPSG and WHO 1999 criteria (WINGS 6)

Balaji Bhavadharini[1], Manni Mohanraj Mahalakshmi[1], Ranjit Mohan Anjana[1], Kumar Maheswari[1], Ram Uma[2], Mohan Deepa[1], Ranjit Unnikrishnan[1], Harish Ranjani[1], Sonak D Pastakia[3], Arivudainambi Kayal[4], Lyudmil Ninov[4], Belma Malanda[4], Anne Belton[4] and Viswanathan Mohan[1*]

Abstract

Background: To determine the prevalence of Gestational Diabetes Mellitus (GDM) in urban and rural Tamil Nadu in southern India, using the International Association of Diabetes and Pregnancy Study Groups (IADPSG) and the World Health Organization (WHO) 1999 criteria for GDM.

Methods: A total of 2121 pregnant women were screened for GDM from antenatal clinics in government primary health centres of Kancheepuram district ($n = 520$) and private maternity centres in Chennai city in Tamil Nadu ($n = 1601$) between January 2013 to December 2014. Oral glucose tolerance tests (OGTT) were done after an overnight fast of at least 8 h, using a 75 g glucose load and venous samples were drawn at 0, 1 and 2 h. GDM was diagnosed using both the IADPSG criteria as well as the WHO 1999 criteria for GDM.

Results: The overall prevalence of GDM after adjusting for age, BMI, family history of diabetes and previous history of GDM was 18.5 % by IADPSG criteria with no significant urban/rural differences (urban 19.8 % vs rural 16.1 %, $p = 0.46$). Using the WHO 1999 criteria, the overall adjusted prevalence of GDM was 14.6 % again with no significant urban/rural differences (urban 15.9 % vs rural 8.9 %, $p = 0.13$).

Conclusion: The prevalence of GDM by IADPSG was high both using IADPSG as well as WHO 1999 criteria with no significant urban/rural differences. This emphasizes the need for increasing awareness about GDM and for prevention of GDM in developing countries like India.

Keywords: Gestational diabetes mellitus, IADPSG criteria, WHO 1999 criteria, Prevalence, Asian Indians, South Asians

Background

The prevalence of diabetes mellitus (DM) is increasing worldwide and more so in developing countries such as India [1, 2]. Along with the rising tide of the current epidemic of diabetes, the prevalence of gestatimal diabetes mellitus (GDM), defined as any degree of glucose intolerance with onset or first recognition during pregnancy, is also on the rise [3, 4]. GDM increases the risk of complications in both the mother and child and early detection and management improves outcomes for both

* Correspondence: drmohans@diabetes.ind.in
[1]Madras Diabetes Research Foundation, 4, Conran Smith Road, Gopalapuram, Chennai 600 086, India
Full list of author information is available at the end of the article

[5, 6]. In 2013, 6 million women in India had some form of hyperglycemia in pregnancy, of which 90 % were GDM [6]. Racial/ethnic differences in the prevalence of GDM have been documented, with a higher prevalence among Native American, Asian, African-American, and Hispanic populations compared to non-Hispanic Whites [7]. GDM is usually asymptomatic and is most commonly diagnosed by routine screening during pregnancy. Unfortunately, there is little agreement on the best screening and diagnostic tests for GDM. The International Association of Diabetes and Pregnancy Study Group (IADPSG) criteria was introduced in the year 2010 and it has found fairly wide acceptance [8]. However, there have been some reports that it may lead to

inflated prevalence rates of GDM [1, 8–10]. In this paper, we report on the prevalence of GDM in urban and rural Tamil Nadu in southern India using the IADPSG criteria and compare the same with prevalence rates obtained using the World Health Organization (WHO) 1999 criteria for GDM.

Methods

This study is part of the Women in India with GDM Strategy (WINGS) project of the International Diabetes Federation carried out in Chennai city (urban) and rural antenatal clinics in Tamil Nadu in south India. The study was conducted between January 2013 and December 2014. Consecutive pregnant women were screened at their first booking at 15 government primary health centres in Kancheepuram district and 6 private health centres at Chennai city in Tamil Nadu state. Written informed consent was obtained in the local language from all participants and the study was approved by the Institutional Ethics Committee of the Madras Diabetes Research Foundation (MDRF). All procedures followed were in accordance with the ethical standards and in keeping with the Declaration of Helsinki 1975, as revised in 2008. Permission was also obtained from the Directorate of Public Health and the Ministry of Health, Government of Tamil Nadu to conduct the study in the primary health centres. Clinical information including obstetric history, family history of diabetes as well as current and past medications was collected using a structured questionnaire.

Height was measured using a stadiometer (SECA Model 213, Seca Gmbh Co, Hamburg, Germany) to the nearest 0.1 cm and weight was measured with an electronic weighing machine (SECA Model 803, Seca Gmbh Co) to the nearest 0.1 kilogram. The body mass index (BMI) was calculated as weight (kg) divided by height (in metres) squared. Participants were requested to report in the fasting state (at least 8 h of overnight fasting), between 7 and 9 am on the day of blood collection. A fasting venous sample was drawn for plasma glucose estimations. 82.5 g of anhydrous glucose (equivalent to 75 g of monohydrate glucose) was then dissolved in 300 ml of water and was given to the pregnant women who consumed it within 5 min. Further venous samples were drawn at 1 h and 2 h after the ingestion of oral glucose.

Plasma glucose (PG) was estimated by the glucose oxidase–peroxidase method using autoanalyser AU2700 (Beckman, Fullerton, CA). Glycated haemoglobin (HbA1c) was measured using high performance liquid chromatography (HPLC) using Variant machine (BIORAD, Hercules, CA). The intra and inter-assay coefficients of variation (CV) for the glucose and HbA1c ranged from 0.78–1.68 %

and 0.59–1.97 % respectively. All samples were processed in our laboratory which is certified by the College of American Pathologists (CAP) and by the National Accreditation Board for Testing and Calibration Laboratories (NABL), Government of India.

Definitions

GDM was diagnosed by IADPSG criteria, if any one of the fasting, 1 h or 2 h PG values met or exceeded 5.1 mmol/L (≥92 mg/dl), 10.0 mmol/L (≥180 mg/dl) and 8.5 mmol/L (≥153 mg/dl) [11] respectively. As per the IADPSG criteria, in the first trimester, GDM was diagnosed using only the fasting glucose estimations, while in 2nd/3rd trimester, GDM was diagnosed using an oral glucose tolerance test (OGTT).

The World Health Organization (WHO) 1999 criteria [12], which diagnoses GDM using 2 h PG value of 7.7 mmol/l (≥140 mg/dl) was applied to the results, to compare the prevalence rates with those obtained using the IADPSG criteria.

Statistical analysis

All analyses was done using Windows based SPSS statistical package (version 15.0, Chicago, IL). Estimates were expressed as mean ± standard deviation or proportions. To compare continuous variables, t tests were used while chi square tests were used to test differences in proportions. P-value <0.05 was considered significant. A multivariable logistic regression model was developed to identify factors associated with gestational diabetes using GDM diagnosis according to IADSPG criteria as the dependent variable and independent variables were chosen based on p value <0.2 in univariate analysis or were clinically relevant.

Results

A total of 2507 consecutive pregnant women were approached to participate in the WINGS screening programme of whom 2121 consented (84.6 %) which included 520 from rural, and 1601 from urban, centres. As shown in Fig. 1, a total of 488 women underwent screening in the first trimester. GDM was diagnosed in 48 women (9.8 %) using the IADPSG criteria while 6 (1.2 %) had overt diabetes, i.e., fasting PG ≥7 mmol/l (≥126 mg/dl) and/or HbA1c ≥6.5 %. As part of WINGS protocol, in the pilot phase, we did not expect women to return in the 2nd/3rd trimester for repeat OGTT unlike in the Model of Care phase of WINGS where we followed women right through the pregnancy. Nevertheless, of the remaining 434 women, 87 who screened negative in the first trimester, returned for repeat OGTT in the 2nd/3rd trimester. The rest (n = 347) who did not return for a

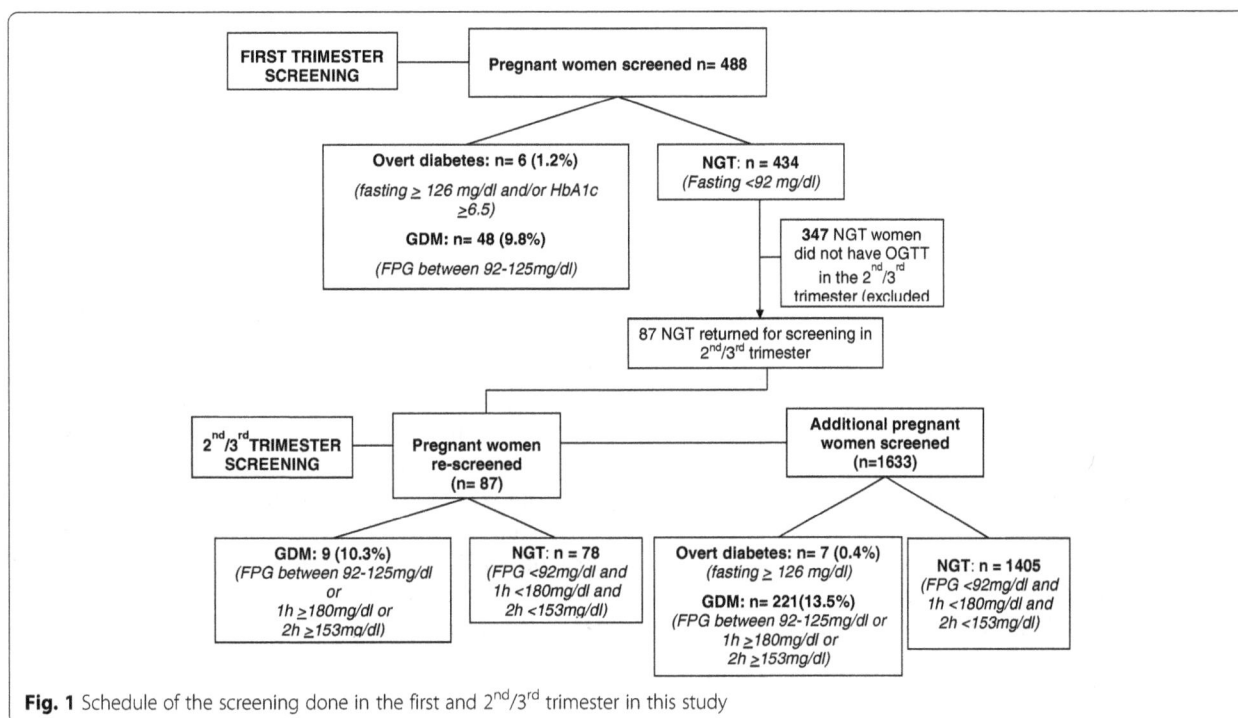

Fig. 1 Schedule of the screening done in the first and 2nd/3rd trimester in this study

repeat OGTT in their 2nd/3rd trimester, were excluded from further analysis.

In the 2nd/3rd trimester, 1633 women who were not screened in the first trimester were screened using the IADPSG criteria. GDM was diagnosed in 221 (13.5 %) women while 7 (0.4 %) women had overt diabetes. Among the 87 women who had normal glucose tolerance (NGT) in the first trimester screening, 9 (10.3 %) developed GDM in the second/third trimester.

In both urban and rural populations, prevalence of GDM was significantly higher by the IADPSG criteria when compared to the WHO 1999 criteria. Table 1 shows that the overall prevalence (unadjusted) of GDM by the IADPSG criteria was 15.7 % ($n = 278$), while in urban areas, it was 16.1 % and in rural areas, 14.4 % ($p = 0.37$). After adjusting for age, BMI, family

history of diabetes and previous history of GDM, the overall prevalence by IADPSG criteria was 18.5 % (urban 19.8 % vs rural 16.1 %, $p = 0.46$).

If the WHO 1999 criteria was used, the unadjusted overall prevalence of GDM was 10.5 % ($n = 186$) [urban 12.4 % ($n = 161$) vs rural 5.3 % ($n = 25$), p < 0.001]. However, after adjusting for age, BMI, family history of diabetes and previous history of GDM, the urban/rural differences disappeared using the WHO 1999 criteria also (urban 15.9 % vs rural 8.9 %, $p = 0.13$).

Of the 278 women identified by IADPSG criteria, 121 (43.5 %) were picked up by the WHO 1999 criteria. Conversely, of the 186 women identified by the WHO 1999 criteria, IADPSG picked up 121 (65.1 %) of GDM (Fig. 2). Thus, 121 pregnant women were diagnosed by both IADPSG and WHO 1999 criteria (agreement, kappa = 0.45).

Table 2 shows the general characteristics of the 1774 study subjects in urban and rural areas. Women with GDM in urban areas were significantly older, had higher BMI and lower levels of fasting and HbA1c ($p < 0.001$) compared to those in rural areas.

Multivariable logistic regression models were used to identify factors associated with gestational diabetes based on the IADPSG criteria (Table 3). The variables that had a p value <0.2 in univariate analysis or were clinically relevant were used in the multiple logistic regression. HbA1c, previous history of GDM, family history of diabetes and age were significantly associated with GDM in this model.

Table 1 Prevalence of gestational diabetes based on IADPSG and WHO 1999 criteria

Criteria	Overall prevalence ($n = 1774$)	Urban ($n = 1301$)	Rural ($n = 473$)
Unadjusted prevalence rates			
IADPSG Criteria	278 (15.7 %)	210 (16.1 %)	68 (14.4 %)
WHO 1999 criteria	186 (10.5 %)	161 (12.4 %)	25 (5.3 %)
Adjusted prevalence rates[a]			
IADPSG Criteria	18.5 %	19.8 %	16.1 %
WHO 1999 criteria	14.6 %	15.9 %	8.9 %

[a]Adjusted for age, BMI, family history of diabetes and previous history of GDM

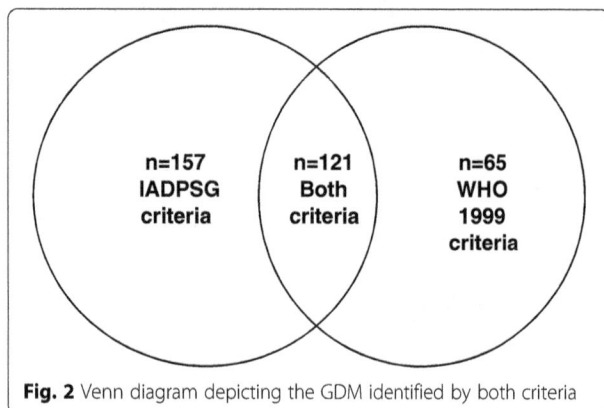

Fig. 2 Venn diagram depicting the GDM identified by both criteria

Discussion

The study reports the following findings:

1. The prevalence of GDM based on the IADPSG criteria, after adjusting for age, BMI, family history of diabetes and previous history of GDM was 18.5 % and based on the WHO 1999 criteria, it was 14.6 %.
2. The prevalence rates of GDM were not significantly different between urban and rural areas both using the IADPSG criteria and WHO 1999 criteria after correcting for the confounders.
3. In the multivariable logistic regression, HbA1c, previous history of GDM, family history of diabetes and age were significantly associated with GDM.

Several criteria for diagnosing GDM have been recommended by various national and international bodies including the American Diabetes Association (ADA), Australasian Diabetes in Pregnancy Study Group (ADIPS), Canadian Diabetes Association (CDA), European Association for the study of Diabetes (EASD), International Association of the Diabetes and Pregnancy Study Groups (IADPSG), International Classification of Diseases (ICD), National Diabetes Data Group (NDDG), the World Health Organization (WHO) and the Diabetes In India Pregnancy Study Group of India (DIPSI). These criteria differ in their requirement for the subject to be in a fasting state, the number of samples needed, the amount of glucose administered and blood glucose thresholds for GDM detection [13]. Not surprisingly, the prevalence rates of GDM also vary according to the criteria used. In this paper, we report on the prevalence of GDM by the IADPSG and the WHO 1999 criteria.

Comparing the prevalence rates with other GDM prevalence studies carried out globally using the IADPSG criteria, a prevalence of 8.9 % has been reported in Sri Lanka [14] and 2.6 % in Thailand [15] and between 2–6 % in Europe [16]. Using the WHO 1999 criteria, a prevalence of 7.2 % was reported in Sri Lanka [15], 9.7 % in Bangladesh [17], 11.4 % in Malaysia [18], 20.6 % in United Arab

Emirates [19] and 16.3 % in Qatar [20]. Table 4 summarizes the prevalence of GDM reported in some of the recent studies conducted worldwide [21–28].

Table 5 and Fig. 3 presents a review of various studies on GDM prevalence carried out in India since 2004. Using the Diabetes in Pregnancy Study Group of India (DIPSI) criteria, which diagnoses GDM based on a non fasting 2 h OGTT, a prevalence of 6.9 % was reported in Jammu [29]. Using the ADA criteria, which recommends a two step procedure, i.e., a 50 g glucose challenge test followed by 100 g confirmatory OGTT, a prevalence of 7.1 % was reported in Haryana [30], 7.7 % in Maharashtra [9] and 8.1 % in Manipur [31] and 3.1 % in Kashmir [32]. Using the IADPSG criteria, a high prevalence (27 %) was reported in Puducherry [10]. Using WHO 1999 criteria, a prevalence of 16.5 % was reported in an earlier study carried out in Chennai [33], and a prevalence of 4.4 % was reported in Kashmir [32]. Recent studies from India by Arora et al. [34] have also reported higher prevalence rates of GDM (34.9 %) using the IADPSG criteria. Though their sample size was large, the authors had used 2 h capillary measurements instead of venous plasma samples albeit with adjustment for the values. This might explain, at least partly, the differences from our study.

The prevalence of GDM in our study was 26.7 % higher by the IADPSG criteria compared to the WHO 1999 criteria. This is similar to the 25 % higher prevalence reported by O'Sullivan et al. [35] [IADPSG–12.4 % vs. WHO–9.4 %]. In another study in Sri Lanka, the prevalence of GDM was 23.6 % higher using IADPSG compared to WHO 1999 criteria [15]. Studies from China showed the prevalence to be higher by IADPSG (19.9 %) when compared to ADA criteria (7.9 %) [36]. A study from Taiwan [37] showed that the IADPSG criteria increased the prevalence of GDM from 4.6 % (by ADA criteria) to 12.4 %. A study from Canada reported an increase in the rates of GDM from 7.9 % using ADA criteria to 9.4 % if IADPSG criteria were used [38]. In Spain, applying the IADPSG criteria was associated with a 3.5-fold increase in GDM prevalence [39]. The higher percentage increase could perhaps to attributed to ethnic differences in fasting hyperglycemia. Earlier studies have shown that Asian Indians have higher fasting hyperglycemia compared to Caucasians [40, 41]. Gopalakrishnan et al. [42] reported 41.9 % prevalence of GDM in their study, of whom 70.5 % had abnormal fasting blood glucose alone. Nayak et al. [43] also showed that 63.8 % of GDM identified by the IADPSG criteria had fasting hyperglycemia. Another study by Moradi et al. [44] showed that 48 % of GDM identified by IADPSG had elevated fasting blood glucose levels alone. Results from our study shows that even among Asian Indians, rural women with GDM have higher fasting hyperglycemia.

Table 2 General characteristics of the GDM and non GDM diagnosed by IADPSG criteria in urban and rural areas

Parameter	URBAN (n = 1301)			p value*	RURAL (n = 473)			p value*	OVERALL (N = 1774)			p value***
	Overall	GDM** (n = 210)	NON GDM (n = 1091)		Overall	GDM** (n = 68)	NON GDM (n = 405)		Overall	GDM (n = 278)	NON GDM (n = 1496)	
Age	26.2 ± 4.1	27.4 ± 4.3	25.9 ± 4.0	<0.001	24 ± 2.9	23.9 ± 2.5	23.9 ± 3.0	<0.001	25.6 ± 3.9	26.5 ± 4.2	25.4 ± 3.8	0.0238
BMI	24.7 ± 4.9	26.2 ± 4.5	24.6 ± 4.9	<0.001	22.1 ± 3.7	22.6 ± 3.9	22.1 ± 3.6	<0.001	24.2 ± 4.7	25.4 ± 4.6	24.0 ± 4.7	<0.001
Family history of T2DM	366 (28.1 %)	82 (39 %)	284 (26 %)	<0.001	51 (10.8 %)	12 (17.6 %)	39 (9.6 %)	<0.001	417 (23.5 %)	94 (33.8 %)	323 (21.6 %)	0.0001
Previous history of GDM	25 (1.9 %)	12 (5.7 %)	13 (1.2 %)	<0.001	1 (0.2 %)	0	1 (0.2 %)	<0.001	26 (1.5 %)	12 (4.3 %)	14 (0.9 %)	0.0062
Fasting (mg/dl)	80 ± 12.8	93 ± 10.4	77 ± 11.6	0.1355	81 ± 12.4	96 ± 11.3	78 ± 10.5	<0.001	80.6 ± 12.6	94.1 ± 10.7	78.0 ± 11.3	<0.001
HbA1c (%)	4.9 ± 0.6	5.1 ± 0.5	4.8 ± 0.5	<0.001	5.1 ± 0.6	5.3 ± 0.6	5.0 ± 0.4	<0.001	4.9 ± 0.53	5.1 ± 0.4	4.9 ± 0.5	<0.001

*p value comparing overall urban vs rural
**p value significant (<0.005), comparing GDM urban vs GDM rural
***p value comparing overall "GDM vs non GDM"

Table 3 Multivariable logistic regression showing factors independently associated with gestational diabetes mellitus diagnosed by IADPSG criteria

Variable	Odds ratio (95 % CI), p value
HbA1c (at booking)	2.91 (1.69–3.12), $p < 0.001$
Previous history of GDM	3.63 (1.48–8.90), $p = 0.005$
Family history of diabetes	1.54 (1.11–2.15), $p = 0.009$
Age (at booking)	1.03 (1.00–1.08), $p = 0.05$
Body mass index (at booking)	1.02 (0.99–1.05), $p = 0.14$
Parity[a]	1.00 (0.74–1.35), $p = 0.99$

[a]Primi mothers as reference

It is interesting to note, that although these women are significantly younger, less heavy, have less family history of diabetes, their fasting plasma glucose levels and HbA1c are higher compared to women with GDM in urban area. This could account for the discrepancy between the prevalence rates by IADPSG and WHO 1999 criteria in the rural population. Given that the two criteria identifies different sets of patients, omitting the fasting criteria (as in the WHO 1999 criteria) would

tend to miss a lot of GDM cases especially in the rural population.

It has also been shown that fasting hyperglycemia by IADPSG criteria is associated with increased perinatal complications [45]. The arguments in favor of using IADPSG criteria are therefore based on pregnancy outcomes, and early screening and diagnosis of GDM helps to initiate treatment earlier (usually medical nutrition therapy) [46, 47]. Thus, whereas on one hand, there is indeed an increase in prevalence of GDM, on the other hand, identifying more women and starting lifestyle changes promises better outcomes [39].

A Sri Lankan study reported 51.1 % agreement between IADPSG and WHO 1999 criteria [15] which is similar to the present study, where 45 % agreement was noted.

We have earlier reported on the necessity for doing fasting OGTTs for diagnosing GDM [48] and also on the need for doing venous plasma samples [49]. In this paper we report on fasting OGTTs using venous plasma samples using both the IADPSG and WHO 1999 criteria.

Table 4 Studies on prevalence of gestational diabetes mellitus–worldwide

Author Name	City/Country	Sample Size	Prevalence	Criteria used for GDM diagnosis
Agarwal et al. (2007)	Al Ain, United Arab Emirates	1172	20.6 %	WHO 1999
Tan et al. (2007)	Malaysia	1600	11.4 %	WHO 1999
Bener et al. (2011)	Doha, Qatar	1608	16.3 %	WHO 1999
Moses et al. (2011)	Australia	1275	9.6 % 13.0 %	ADIPS IADPSG
Dahanayaka et al. (2012)	Sri Lanka	405	8.9 %	IADPSG
Jenum et al. (2012)	Oslo, Norway	823	13 % 31.5 %	WHO 1999 IADPSG
Kalter-Leibovivi et al. (2012)	Israel	3,345	9 %	IADPSG
Reyes-Munoz E et al. (2012)	Mexico	803	10.3 % 30.1 %	ADA 2005 IADPSG
Kanjana et al. (2013)	Thailand	6324	2.6 %	IADPSG
Duran et al. (2014)	Madrid, Spain	1750 1526	10.6 % 35.5 %	Carpenter & Coustan IADPSG
Shang et al. (2014)	China	3083	19.9 % 7.98 %	IADPSG ADA 2005
Liao et al. (2014)	Chengdu, China	5630	11.7 % 24.5 %	ADA 2005 IADPSG
Leng et al. (2015)	Tianjin, China	18589	8.1 % 9.3 %	WHO 1999 IADPSG
Hung et al. (2015)	Taoyuan, China	3056 3641	4.6 % 12.4 %	ADA 2005 IADPSG
Sibartie et al. (2015)	Australia	10103	3.4 % 3.5 %	ADIPS IADPSG
Ethridge et al. (2015)	Ohio, United States of America	8390	4 % 3.3 %	Carpenter & Coustan IADPSG
O'Sullivan et al. (2016)	Galway, Ireland	5500	12.4 % 9.4 %	IADPSG WHO 1999

Table 5 Studies on prevalence of gestational diabetes mellitus in India

Author Name	City/State	Sample Size	Prevalence	Criteria used for GDM diagnosis
Seshiah et al. (2004)	Government Maternity Hospital, Chennai	3674	16.5 %	WHO 1999
Seshiah et al. (2008)	Chennai, South India	4151	Urban-17.8 % Semiurban-13.8 % Rural-9.9 %	WHO 1999
Swami et al. (2008)	Tertiary care hospital in Maharashtra	1225	7.7 %	ADA 2005
Seshiah et al. (2011)	Chennai, South India	1463	13.4 %	DIPSI
Wahi et al. (2011)	Govt Medical College Hospital, Jammu region	2025	6.9 %	DIPSI
Nayak et al. (2013)	Pondicherry Institute of Medical Science	304	27 %	IADPSG
Vanlalhruaii et al. (2013)	Regional Institute of Medical Sciences Manipur	300	8.1 %	ADA 2005
Rajput et al. (2013)	Post Graduate Institute of Medical Sciences Haryana	607	7.1 %	ADA 2005
Zargar et al. (2004)	Sher-i-Kashmir Institute of Medical Sciences	2000	3.1 % 4.4 %	Carpenter & Coustan WHO 1999
Raja et al. (2014)	Government Medical College Srinagar Kashmir valley	306	7.8 %	DIPSI
Rajput et al. (2014)	Rural Haryana	900	13.9 % 9.7 %	WHO 1999 ADA 2005
Kalyani et al. (2014)	Central India	300	8.33 %	WHO 1999
Arora et al. (2015)	Ludhiana, Punjab	5100	34.9 % 9 %	IADPSG WHO 1999
Gopalakrishnan V et al. (2015)	Sanjay Gandhi Postgraduate Institute of Medical Sciences, Lucknow, Uttar Pradesh, India.	332	41.9 %	IADPSG
Present study	Chennai, India	1774	18.5 % 14.6 %	IADPSG WHO 1999

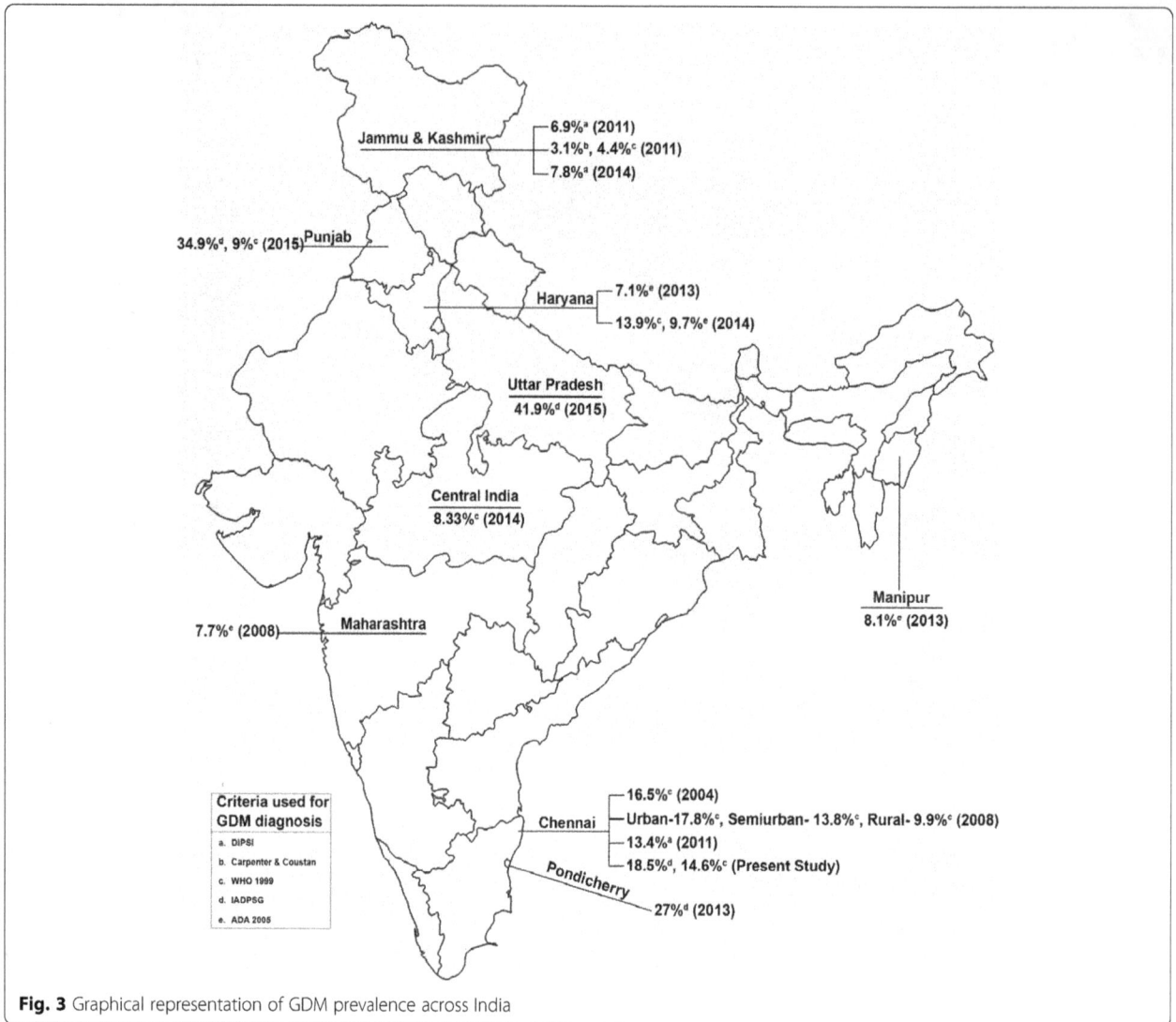

Fig. 3 Graphical representation of GDM prevalence across India

Earlier studies have shown that advanced maternal age, obesity, and family history of diabetes to be associated with GDM [3]. These findings are consistent with the present study findings, which reveals that, HbA1c, previous history of GDM, family history of diabetes and age were found to be associated with GDM diagnosed using the IADPSG criteria.

This study has several strengths: (i) both urban and rural areas were sampled; (ii) large sample size; (iii) this is one of the first studies from India to report on the differences in prevalence of GDM by both IADPSG and WHO 1999 criteria in urban/rural areas (iv) screening was done during the first trimester and in the 2nd/3rd trimester using the IADPSG criteria. Traditionally, screening for GDM is delayed until 2nd or early 3rd trimester since the diabetogenic effects of pregnancy increases with gestational age, and delayed testing would

maximize the detection rate [50, 51]. However, early identification gives time for appropriate intervention which could help reduce complications. Moreover, as shown in our study, screening in the first trimester also provides an opportunity to detect previously undiagnosed overt diabetes as well as GDM. In our study, first trimester screening identified 1.2 % of overt diabetes and 9.8 % GDM. A study from Trichy [52] recently reported GDM prevalence of 13.9 % in first trimester. Data from Oklahoma shows that among American Indians, prevalence of GDM and overt diabetes in first trimester was 24 % and 0.4 % respectively [53]. There is insufficient data from India on the prevalence of overt diabetes in the first trimester and hence the findings from this study are significant. As per the recommendations of IADPSG criteria, women who are labeled as having normal glucose tolerance in the first trimester should undergo a repeat OGTT in the $2^{nd}/3^{rd}$ trimester. However, in our study, only 87 women of the 434 returned for repeat OGTT which is one of the limitations of this study. A recent study by Morikawa et al. [54] from Japan, showed that women who were diagnosed as having normal glucose tolerance (NGT) in the first trimester remained as NGT throughout their pregnancy, despite the significant increase in insulin resistance. In contrast, results from our study shows that among those who returned for a repeat screening ($n = 87$), 10.3 % developed GDM. Similar findings emphasizing the need for repeat screening have been reported earlier in Hungarian women, where the GDM prevalence was noted to increase with advancing gestation [55]. This therefore highlights the importance of repeat screening among women who screened negative in the first trimester in populations like ours which have a higher risk for GDM. Another limitation of the study is that, pregnant women included in the study were from a few selected antenatal clinics in urban and rural areas in Tamil Nadu and hence the results may not be representative of the GDM rates in the country as a whole. Finally, there were some significant differences between the 1774 women who participated and the 386 women who refused to participate, which is yet another limitation (Additional file: 1 Table S1).

Conclusions

The prevalence of GDM in Tamil Nadu was found to be 15.7 % (adjusted 18.5 %) by IADPSG criteria and 10.5 % (adjusted 14.6 %) using the WHO 1999 criteria. There were no urban rural differences using both criteria suggesting that the rural areas in southern India are also fasting catching up with reference to rising GDM prevalence rates. This emphasizes the need for increasing awareness about GDM and taking steps to prevent GDM in India and other developing countries.

Ethical standard

This study was approved by the Institutional Ethics Committee of the Madras Diabetes Research Foundation, Chennai, India [Dated 7th November 2012].

Human and animal rights disclosure

All human rights were observed in keeping with Declaration of Helsinki 2008 (ICH GCP) and the Indian Council of Medical Research (ICMR) guidelines. There are no animal rights issues in this study.

Informed consent disclosure

Written informed consent was obtained from all participants before being included in the study.

Competing interests

Balaji Bhavadharini, Manni Mohanraj Mahalakshmi, Ranjit Mohan Anjana, Kumar Maheswari, Ram Uma, Mohan Deepa, Ranjit Unnikrishnan, Sonak D Pastakia, Arivudainambi Kayal, Lyudmil Ninov, Belma Malanda, Anne Belton, Viswanathan Mohan declare that they have no conflict of interest.

Authors' contributions

VM conceived, initiated, supervised, conducted and commented on all drafts of this paper. BB, MMM, KM and AK coordinated the study and monitored all the data entry. MMM, MD and BB performed the statistical analysis and drafted the paper. RMA, RU, HR, UR, SDP, LN, BM and AB contributed to the interpretative analysis of the data. All authors read and approved the final manuscript.

Acknowledgements

The WINGS programme has been developed through a partnership between the International Diabetes Federation (IDF), the Madras Diabetes Research Foundation (MDRF) in Chennai, India, and the Abbott Fund, the philanthropic foundation of the global healthcare company Abbott. We would also like to place on record our sincere thanks to the Director of Public Health and the Health Secretary, the Government of Tamil Nadu. We also thank the village health nurses and the doctors and study participants for their support. This is the sixth publication from the WINGS project (WINGS-6).

Author details

[1]Madras Diabetes Research Foundation, 4, Conran Smith Road, Gopalapuram, Chennai 600 086, India. [2]Seethapathy Clinic and Hospital, Chennai, India. [3]College of Pharmacy, Purdue University, West Lafayette, IN, USA. [4]International Diabetes Federation, Brussels, Belgium.

References

1. International Diabetes Federation. IDF Diabetes Atlas. 6th ed. Brussels, Belgium: International Diabetes Federation; 2013.
2. Anjana RM, Pradeepa R, Deepa M, Datta M, Sudha V, Unnikrishnan R, et al. Prevalence of diabetes and prediabetes (impaired fasting glucose or/and impaired glucose tolerance) in rural and urban India: Phase 1 results of the Indian Council of Medical Research-INdia DIABetes (INDIAB) study. Diabetologia. 2011;54:3022–7.
3. Seshiah V, Balaji V, Balaji MS, Paneerselvam A, Arthi T, Thamizharasi M, et al. Prevalence of gestational diabetes mellitus in South India (Tamil Nadu)-a community based study. J Assoc Physicians India. 2008;56:329–33.
4. Nallaperumal S, Bhavadharini B, Mahalakshmi MM, Maheswari K, Jalaja R, Moses A, et al. Comparison of the World Health Organization and the International Association of Diabetes and Pregnancy Study Groups criteria in diagnosing gestational diabetes mellitus in South Indians. Indian J Endocrinol Metab. 2013;17:906–9.
5. Crowther CA, Hiller JE, Moss JR, McPhee AJ, Jeffries WS, Robinson JS, Australian Carbohydrate Intolerance Study in Pregnant Women (ACHOIS) Trial Group. Effect of treatment of gestational diabetes mellitus on pregnancy outcomes. N Engl J Med. 2005;352:2477–86.
6. American Diabetes Association. Gestational diabetes mellitus. Diabetes Care. 2004;27(1):S88–90.
7. Centers for Disease Control and Prevention. (2006). Diabetes and women's health across the life stages: A public health perspective. Available: http://www.cdc.gov/diabetes/pubs/pdf/women.pdf.
8. Benhalima K, Hanssens M, Devlieger R, Verhaeghe J, Mathieu C. Analysis of Pregnancy Outcomes Using the New IADPSG recommendation compared with the Carpenter and Coustan criteria in an area with a low prevalence of gestational diabetes. Int J Endocrinol. 2013;2013:248121.
9. Swami SR, Mehetre R, Shivane V, Bandgar TR, Menon PS, Shah NS, et al. Prevalence of carbohydrate intolerance of varying degrees in pregnant

females in western India (Maharashtra)-a hospital-based study. J Indian Med Assoc. 2008;106:712–4.

10. Nayak PK, Mitra S, Sahoo JP, Daniel M, Mathew A, Padma A. Feto-maternal outcomes in women with and without gestational diabetes mellitus according to the International Association of Diabetes and Pregnancy Study Groups (IADPSG) diagnostic criteria. Diabetes Metab Syndr. 2013;7:206–9.

11. International Association of Diabetes and Pregnancy Study Group Consensus Panel. International Association of Diabetes and Pregnancy Study Groups recommendations on the diagnosis and classification of hyperglycemia in pregnancy. Diab Care. 2010;33:676–82.

12. World Health Organization. Definition, diagnosis and classification of diabetes mellitus and its complications. Report of a WHO consultation. Geneva: WHO Department of Non communicable Disease Surveillance; 1999.

13. Linnenkamp U, Guariguata L, Beagley J, Whiting DR, The CNH, IDF. Diabetes Atlas methodology for estimating global prevalence of hyperglycaemia in pregnancy. Diabetes Res Clin Pract. 2014;103:186–96.

14. Dahanayaka NJ, Agampodi SB, Ranasinghe OR, Jayaweera PM, Wickramasinghe WA, Adhikari AN, et al. Inadequacy of the risk factor based approach to detect gestational diabetes mellitus. Ceylon Med J. 2012;57:5–9.

15. Kanjana K, Wiyada L, Petch W, Sinart P, Buppa S. Prevalence of Gestational Diabetes Mellitus and Pregnancy Outcomes in Women with Risk Factors Diagnosed by IADPSG Criteria at Bhumibol Adulyadej Hospital. Thai J Obstet Gynaecol. 2013;21:4.

16. Buckley BS, Harreiter J, Damm P, Corcoy R, Chico A, Simmons D, et al. Gestational diabetes mellitus in Europe: prevalence, current screening practice and barriers to screening. A review. Diabet Med. 2012;29:844–54.

17. Jesmin S, Akter S, Akashi H, Al-Mamun A, Rahman MA, Islam MM, et al. Screening for gestational diabetes mellitus and its prevalence in Bangladesh. Diabetes Res Clin Pract. 2014;103:57–62.

18. Tan PC, Ling LP, Omar SZ. Screening for gestational diabetes at antenatal booking in a Malaysian university hospital: the role of risk factors and threshold value for the 50-g glucose challenge test. Aust N Z J Obstet Gynaecol. 2007;47:191–7.

19. Bener A, Saleh NM, Al-Hamaq A. Prevalence of gestational diabetes and associated maternal and neonatal complications in a fast-developing community: global comparisons. Int J Womens Health. 2011;3:367–73.

20. Agarwal MM, Dhatt GS, Zayed R, Bali N. Gestational diabetes: relevance of diagnostic criteria and preventive strategies for Type 2 diabetes mellitus. Arch Gynecol Obstet. 2007;276:237–41.

21. Reyes-Muñoz E, Parra A, Castillo-Mora A, Ortega-González C. Effect of the diagnostic criteria of the International Association of Diabetes and Pregnancy Study Groups on the prevalence of gestational diabetes mellitus in urban Mexican women: a cross-sectional study. Endocr Pract. 2012;18(2):146–51.

22. Jenum AK, Mørkrid K, Sletner L, Vangen S, Torper JL, Nakstad B, Voldner N, Rognerud-Jensen OH, Berntsen S, Mosdøl A, Skrivarhaug T, Vårdal MH, Holme I, Yajnik CS, Birkeland KI. Impact of ethnicity on gestational diabetes identified with the WHO and the modified International Association of Diabetes and Pregnancy Study Groups criteria: a population-based cohort study. Eur J Endocrinol. 2012;166(2):317–24.

23. Moses RG, Morris GJ, Petocz P, San Gil F, Garg D. The impact of potential new diagnostic criteria on the prevalence of gestational diabetes mellitus in Australia. Med J Aust. 2011;194(7):338–40.

24. Liao S, Mei J, Song W, Liu Y, Tan YD, Chi S, Li P, Chen X, Deng S. The impact of the International Association of Diabetes and Pregnancy Study Groups (IADPSG) fasting glucose diagnostic criterion on the prevalence and outcomes of gestational diabetes mellitus in Han Chinese women. Diabet Med. 2014;31(3):341–51.

25. Leng J, Shao P, Zhang C, Tian H, Zhang F, Zhang S, Dong L, Li L, Yu Z, Chan JC, Hu G, Yang X. Prevalence of gestational diabetes mellitus and its risk factors in Chinese pregnant women: a prospective population-based study in Tianjin, China. PLoS One. 2015;10(3):e0121029.

26. Ethridge Jr JK, Catalano PM, Waters TP. Perinatal outcomes associated with the diagnosis of gestational diabetes made by the international association of the diabetes and pregnancy study groups criteria. Obstet Gynecol. 2014; 124(3):571–8.

27. Sibartie P, Quinlivan J. Implementation of the International Association of Diabetes and Pregnancy Study Groups Criteria: Not Always a Cause for Concern. J Pregnancy. 2015;2015:754085.

28. Kalter-Leibovici O, Freedman LS, Olmer L, Liebermann N, Heymann A, Tal O, Lerner-Geva L, Melamed N, Hod M. Screening and diagnosis of gestational diabetes mellitus: critical appraisal of the new International Association of Diabetes in Pregnancy Study Group recommendations on a national level. Diabetes Care. 2012;35(9):1894–6.

29. Wahi P, Dogra V, Jandial K, Bhagat R, Gupta R, Gupta S, et al. Prevalence of gestational diabetes mellitus (GDM) and its outcomes in Jammu region. J Assoc Physicians India. 2011;59:227–30.

30. Rajput R, Yadav Y, Nanda S, Rajput M. Prevalence of gestational diabetes mellitus & associated risk factors at a tertiary care hospital in Haryana. Indian J Med Res. 2013;137:728–33.

31. Vanlalhruaii, Ranabir S, Prasad L, Singh NN, Singh TP. Prevalence of gestational diabetes and its correlation with blood pressure in Manipuri women. Indian J Endocrinol Metab. 2013;17:957–61.

32. Zargar AH, Sheikh MI, Bashir MI, Masoodi SR, Laway BA, Wani AI, et al. Prevalence of gestational diabetes mellitus in Kashmiri women from the Indian subcontinent. Diabetes Res Clin Pract. 2004;66:139–45.

33. Seshiah V, Balaji V, Balaji MS, Sanjeevi CB, Anders G. Gestational Diabetes Mellitus in India. J Assoc Physicians India. 2004;52:707.

34. Arora GP, Thaman RG, Prasad RB, Almgren P, Brøns C, Groop LC, Vaag AA. Prevalence and risk factors of gestational diabetes in Punjab, North India: results from a population screening program. Eur J Endocrinol. 2015; 173(2):257–67.

35. O'Sullivan EP, Avalos G, O'Reilly M, Dennedy MC, Gaffney G, Dunne F. Atlantic DIP collaborators. Atlantic Diabetes in Pregnancy (DIP): the prevalence and outcomes of gestational diabetes mellitus using new diagnostic criteria. Diabetologia. 2011;54:1670–5.

36. Shang M, Lin L. IADPSG criteria for diagnosing gestational diabetes mellitus and predicting adverse pregnancy outcomes. J Perinatol. 2014; 34(2):100–4.

37. Hung T-H, Hsieh TT. The Effects of Implementing the International Association of Diabetes and Pregnancy Study Groups Criteria for Diagnosing Gestational Diabetes on Maternal and Neonatal Outcomes. PLoS One. 2015;10:3.

38. Kong JM, Lim K, Thompson DM. Evaluation of the International Association of theDiabetes In Pregnancy Study Group new criteria: gestational diabetes project. Can J Diabetes. 2015;39(2):128–32.

39. Duran A, Sáenz S, Torrejón MJ, Bordiú E, Del Valle L, Galindo M, Perez N, Herraiz MA, Izquierdo N, Rubio MA, Runkle I, Pérez-Ferre N, Cusihuallpa I, Jiménez S, García de la Torre N, Fernández MD, Montañez C, Familiar C, Calle-Pascual AL. Introduction of IADPSG criteria for the screening and diagnosis of gestational diabetes mellitus results in improved pregnancy outcomes at a lower cost in a large cohort of pregnant women: the St. Carlos Gestational Diabetes Study. Diabetes Care. 2014;37(9):2442–50.

40. Raji A, Seely EW, Arky RA, Simonson DC. Body fat distribution and insulin resistance in healthy Asian Indians and Caucasians. J Clin Endocrinol Metab. 2001;86(11):5366–71.

41. Khoo CM, Sairazi S, Taslim S, Gardner D, Wu Y, Lee J, van Dam RM, Shyong Tai E. Ethnicity modifies the relationships of insulin resistance, inflammation, and adiponectin with obesity in a multiethnic Asian population. Diabetes Care. 2011;34(5):1120–6.

42. Gopalakrishnan V, Singh R, Pradeep Y, Kapoor D, Rani AK, Pradhan S, Bhatia E, Yadav SB. Evaluation of the prevalence of gestational diabetes mellitus in North Indians using the International Association of Diabetes and Pregnancy Study Groups (IADPSG) criteria. J Postgrad Med. 2015; 61(3):155–8.

43. Nayak PK, Mitra S, Sahoo JP, Daniel M, Mathew A, Padma A. Feto-maternal outcomes in women with and without gestational diabetes mellitus according to the International Association of Diabetes and Pregnancy Study Groups (IADPSG) diagnostic criteria. Diabetes and Metabolic Syndrome. J Clin Res Rev. 2013;7:206–9.

44. Moradi S, Shafieepour MR, Mortazavi M, Pishgar F. Prevalence of gestational diabetes mellitus in Rafsanjan: a comparison of different criteria. Med J Islam Repub Iran. 2015;29:209.

45. Zawiejska A, Wender-Ozegowska E, Radzicka S, Brazert J. Maternal hyperglycemia according to IADPSG criteria as a predictor of perinatal complications in women with gestational diabetes: a retrospective observational study. J Matern Fetal Neonatal Med. 2014;27(15):1526–30.

46. Hadar E, Yogev Y. Translating the HAPO study into new diagnostic criteria for GDM? From HAPO to IADPSG and back to O'Sullivan. Clin Obstet Gynecol. 2013;56:758–73.

47. Visser GH, De Valk HW. Is the evidence strong enough to change the diagnostic criteria for gestational diabetes now? Am J Obstet Gynecol. 2013; 208:260–4.

48. Mohan V, Mahalakshmi MM, Bhavadharini B, Maheswari K, Kalaiyarasi G, Anjana RM, Uma R, Usha S, Deepa M, Unnikrishnan R, Pastakia SD, Malanda B, Belton A, Kayal A. Comparison of screening for gestational diabetes mellitus by oral glucose tolerance tests done in the non-fasting (random) and fasting states. Acta Diabetol. 2014;51(6):1007–13.
49. Bhavadharini B, Mahalakshmi MM, Maheswari K, Kalaiyarasi G, Anjana RM, Deepa M, Ranjani H, Priya M, Uma R, Usha S, Pastakia SD, Malanda B, Belton A, Unnikrishnan R, Kayal A, Mohan V. Use of capillary blood glucose for screening for gestational diabetes mellitus in resource-constrained settings. Acta Diabetol. 2015. Apr 28. [Epub ahead of print].
50. Lind T. Metabolic changes in pregnancy relevant to diabetes mellitus. Postgrad Med J. 1979;55:353–7.
51. Nahum GG, Wilson SB, Stanislaw H. Early-pregnancy glucose screening for gestational diabetes mellitus. J Reprod Med. 2002;47:656–62.
52. Neelakandan R, Sethu PS. Early universal screening for gestational diabetes mellitus. J Clin Diagn Res. 2014;8(4):12–4.
53. Azar M, Stoner JA, Dao HD, Stephens L, Goodman JR, Maynard J, Lyons TJ. Epidemiology of Dysglycemia in Pregnant Oklahoma American Indian Women. J Clin Endocrinol Metab. 2015;100(8):2996–3003.
54. Morikawa M, Yamada T, Yamada T, Kojima T, Nishida R, Cho K, Minakami H. Clinical significance of second-trimester 50-g glucose challenge test among Japanese women diagnosed as normoglycemic after first-trimester 75-g glucose tolerance test. Taiwan J Obstet Gynecol. 2016;55(1):16–9.
55. Bitó T, Nyári T, Kovács L, Pál A. Oral glucose tolerance testing at gestational weeks < or=16 could predict or exclude subsequent gestational diabetes mellitus during the current pregnancy in high risk group. Eur J Obstet Gynecol Reprod Biol. 2005;121(1):51–5.

5

Hypophysitis: Evaluation and Management

Alexander Faje

Abstract

Hypophysitis is the acute or chronic inflammation of the pituitary gland. The spectrum of hypophysitis has expanded in recent years with the addition of two histologic subtypes and recognition as a complication of treatment with immune checkpoint inhibitors. Despite the increased number of published cases, the pathogenesis of hypophysitis is poorly understood, and treatment strategies are diverse and controversial. The diagnosis of hypophysitis generally requires histopathologic confirmation. The presentation and clinical course of hypophysitis varies. Hypophysitis can resolve spontaneously, relapse may occur, and some cases can be refractory to treatment.

Keywords: Hypophysitis, Hypopituitarism, Diabetes insipidus

Abbreviations: ADCC, Antibody-dependent cell-mediated cytotoxicity; CTLA-4, Cytotoxic T-lymphocyte antigen-4; ECD, Erdheim-Chester disease; IIF, Indirect immunofluorescence; LCH, Langerhans cell histiocytosis; MRI, Magnetic resonance imaging; PD-1, Programmed cell death 1

Background

Hypophysitis has gained greater clinical recognition over time. Several histologic variants and causative agents have been identified. Although hypophysitis remains a rare diagnosis, the number of published cases has increased substantially and expanded to involve a more gender and age diverse population. The quantity and quality of available information is limited, however, and consensus, especially regarding treatment, has been elusive. Prospective studies are necessary to better define optimal diagnostic and management strategies.

Hypophysitis can be classified according to etiology, morphology, and/or histopathology. Etiology refers to primary or secondary cases of hypophysitis. Primary hypophysitis refers to isolated inflammation of the pituitary not associated with medications, systemic inflammatory disorders, infections, or other diseases. Secondary hypophysitis includes cases associated with immunotherapy (interleukin 2, interferon, and medications targeting cytotoxic T-lymphocyte antigen-4 [CTLA-4] or programmed cell death 1 [PD-1]) [1–6], rupture of sellar cysts (Rathke's cleft cysts and craniopharyngiomas), and rarely, pituitary adenomas [7–15]. Some authors utilize the term secondary hypophysitis more broadly and also include systemic inflammatory processes which may

involve the pituitary gland (such as sarcoidosis, Wegener's granulomatosis, Crohn's disease, Takayasu's arteritis, Cogan's syndrome), inflammatory cell proliferative disorders (Langerhans cell histiocytosis [LCH] and Erdheim-Chester disease [ECD]), infections (tuberculosis, syphilis, Whipple's disease, mycoses), and tumor-associated inflammatory infiltrate (germinoma).

Morphologic categorization is made according to whether inflammation involves the anterior pituitary gland (adenohypophysitis), posterior gland and stalk (infundibuloneurohypophystis), or entire gland (panhypophysitis).

Histologic subtypes of hypophysitis include the following: lymphocytic, granulomatous, xanthomatous, and plasmacytic (Table 1). Occasionally, mixed histology is encountered [16]. Necrotizing hypophysitis has also been proposed as an additional variant, but it has only been reported in 3 cases [17, 18]. Lymphocytic hypophysitis is characterized by diffuse lymphocyte infiltration (primarily T cells) of the pituitary gland. Lymphoid follicles can be observed and occasional plasma cells, eosinophils, and fibroblasts may also be present [19]. Granulomatous hypophysitis shows large numbers of multinucleated giant cells and histiocytes with granuloma formation [20, 21]. Xanthomatous hypophysitis demonstrates lipid-laden "foamy" histiocytes without the presence of granulomas [22, 23]. Plasmacytic hypophysitis, also termed IgG4-related hypophysitis, has extensive gland infiltration by plasma cells with a high degree of IgG4

Correspondence: afaje@partners.org
Neuroendocrine Unit, Massachusetts General Hospital and Harvard Medical School, 55 Fruit Street, Boston, MA 02114, USA

Table 1 Histologic subtypes of hypophysitis and patient characteristics

	Gender predominance	Association with pregnancy	Mean age of presentation
Lymphocytic	Female, ~3:1	Yes	4th decade
Granulomatous	Female, ~3:1	No	5th decade
Xanthomatous	Female, ~3:1	No	4th decade
Plasmacytic (IgG4-related)	Male, ~2:1	No	7th decade

Mixed histology is observed occasionally, and necrotizing hypophysitis has been proposed as an additional category. Data abstracted from references [20, 23, 25, 27, 66]

positivity [24–26]. Pituitary gland fibrosis and atrophy may occur in later stages of these hypophysitis variants.

Precise usage of the term hypophysitis is important. Loose or inconsistent application (such as grouping germinoma-associated inflammation and primary lymphocytic hypophysitis) can cause reader confusion and suggest inappropriate treatments rather than provide diagnostic clarification. Unfortunately, such cases have been mixed with primary hypophysitis in some review paper data sets [27]. Unless otherwise stated, further discussion in this manuscript will focus on patients with primary hypophysitis. A caveat exists for IgG4-related hypophysitis, which is often a manifestation of systemic disease with involvement of multiple organs. Most authors have not grouped IgG4-related hypophysitis in the general category of secondary hypophysitis, though it may be reasonable to do so. This manuscript does include an examination of IgG4-related hypophysitis. Given the expanding applications of immune checkpoint inhibitors and increasing frequency of this form of secondary hypophysitis, brief discussion will also be devoted to immunotherapy-associated hypophysitis.

Epidemiology

The annual incidence of hypophysitis is estimated to be 1 in 7–9 million. Hypophysitis accounts for approximately 0.4 % of pituitary surgery cases (based on a group of large surgical series totaling nearly 10,000 procedures at 5 centers) [28–32].

Lymphocytic hypophysitis was first reported in 1962 [33], and granulomatous hypophysitis was described in the early twentieth century [34, 35]. The first cases of xanthomatous hypophysitis and IgG4-related hypophysitis were published more recently in 1998 and 2004, respectively [22, 36].

Lymphocytic hypophysitis is the most common histologic variant, with over 390 cases reported. Granulomatous hypophysitis is the next most frequent subtype, followed by xanthomatous and IgG4-related hypophysitis [25]. Lymphocytic hypophysitis was initially thought to occur only in adult women, but cases were

subsequently described in men [37] and children [38–40]. Lymphocytic hypophysitis does occur more frequently in women compared to men (approximately 3:1 ratio of cases [27]), in large part because of its association with pregnancy [41]. Though recent series have not shown as strong a relationship [42, 43], the majority of cases among reproductive-aged women appear to occur during the end of pregnancy or the first few months after delivery [16, 27]. The incidence of lymphocytic hypophysitis peaks during the fourth decade of life and is uncommon in children and the elderly.

Granulomatous and xanthomatous hypophysitis also occur more frequently in women (approximately 3:1 ratio of cases), but neither form is linked with pregnancy. Xanthomatous hypophysitis and lymphocytic hypophysitis have a similar mean age of presentation, but granulomatous hypophysitis is diagnosed more often at a slightly later timepoint in the fifth decade [20, 23]. IgG4-related hypophysitis occurs more frequently in men and tends to develop at a more advanced age in the seventh decade of life. IgG4-related hypophysitis also does not have an association with pregnancy [25, 26].

Immunotherapy-associated hypophysitis occurs in up to 10–15 % of patients receiving agents targeting CTLA-4, on average 2–3 months after starting therapy. Older age and male gender may be risk factors for the development of hypophysitis with anti-CTLA-4 medications. Hypophysitis is comparatively rare following treatment with anti-PD-1 agents. Hypophysitis has also been reported very rarely after treatment with interleukin 2 and interferon [6].

Clinical presentation

Patients with hypophysitis present with symptoms related to mass effect from pituitary gland enlargement and pituitary/hypothalamic dysfunction. Headache is the most common presenting symptom, occurring in about half of patients. Visual symptoms due to compression of the optic nerves and/or cranial nerves III, IV, and VI in the cavernous sinuses can occur in a substantial minority of patients [16, 27, 42]. Cavernous carotid artery occlusion is a rare complication of hypophysitis [31, 44–46]. The onset of symptoms, including headache, can be insidious, subacute, or acute even mimicking apoplexy [42, 47, 48].

The majority of patients with hypophysitis have multiple anterior pituitary hormone deficiencies, and anterior panhypopituitarism is not uncommon. The severity of hormone deficiencies may appear to be out of proportion to radiographic findings. Serum prolactin levels may be low, normal, or elevated [16, 19, 27, 42]. Unlike what is observed in clinically nonfunctioning pituitary adenomas [49], there is not a clear hierarchy of anterior pituitary hormone deficiencies in hypophysitis patients. Hypothalamic pituitary adrenal axis dysfunction is frequently present. Diabetes insipidus is also common and may occur in up to half of patients [16, 19, 27, 42].

Immunotherapy-associated hypophysitis often presents with headache and anterior hypopituitarism. The degree of pituitary enlargement is typically mild, and compression of the optic apparatus is very rare. Unlike other forms of hypophysitis, diabetes insipidus is extremely unusual in patients with immunotherapy-associated hypophysitis [6].

Diagnosis

The differential diagnosis for primary hypophysitis is broad, and ultimately histopathology (which is not always possible to obtain) is required for confirmation. Alternative diagnostic considerations include anatomic variants (a small/narrow sella turcica with specious pituitary enlargement) and congenital malformations, pituitary hyperplasia, solid and cystic sellar/suprasellar lesions (such as pituitary adenomas with or without apoplexy, Rathke's cleft cyst, craniopharyngioma, pituitcyte-derived tumors, hamartoma, dermoid or epidermoid cyst, gangliocytoma, lipoma), malignancies (central nervous system germinoma, lymphoma, glioma, metastatic lesions, LCH, ECD), systemic inflammatory disorders (sarcoidosis, Wegener's granulomatosis, Crohn's disease, Takayasu's arteritis, Cogan's syndrome), and infections (tuberculosis, syphilis, Whipple's disease, mycoses). A thorough evaluation is necessary to accurately diagnose hypophysitis, especially in the absence of tissue confirmation. In the largest series of pituitary stalk lesions published to date, only 4 % of pathology-proven diagnoses represented primary hypophysitis (and only one-third of cases were inflammatory disorders of any type). Significantly, more than half of the confirmed stalk lesions represented neoplastic processes, and half of these cases were metastatic lesions [50]. A positive response to glucocorticoids, often interpreted as supporting evidence for hypophysitis, is not specific for inflammatory processes. Glucocorticoids are part of standard treatment regimens for LCH and ECD [51, 52], and temporary treatment responses can be observed in lymphoma and intracranial germinomas [53–55]. Treatment responses in the latter are likely due to effects on tumor infiltrating lymphocytes. This lymphoid infiltrate can be significant enough that misdiagnosis can even occur after tissue biopsy due to sampling error [56–58].

Certain radiology findings may support a diagnosis of hypophysitis. These imaging characteristics include homogenous enhancement of the pituitary, diffuse symmetric gland enlargement, midline stalk thickening, absence of a posterior pituitary bright spot, normal sellar size, dural thickening, parasellar T2-weighted hypointensity, and parasellar mucosal thickening. One group described a radiologic scoring model with an apparent high ability to distinguish hypophysitis from pituitary adenomas [59]. This model was not assessed for its discriminatory value against other potential diagnoses. Ultimately, radiologic findings are not specific for hypophysitis, especially compared to nonadenomatous sellar lesions.

Diagnostic criteria have been proposed for IgG4-related hypophysitis. These include the following: 1) pituitary histopathology demonstrating mononuclear infiltration with greater than 10 IgG4-positive cells per high-powered field, 2) magnetic resonance imaging (MRI) showing a sellar mass and/or stalk thickening plus biopsy-proven IgG4-related disease at another tissue site, or 3) sellar mass and/or stalk thickening plus a serum IgG4 level > 140 mg/dl and a radiologic and clinical response to treatment with glucocorticoids [24]. These proposed criteria may be inadequate in some circumstances. Recent studies have shown that neither serum IgG4 levels [60, 61] nor IgG4-positive tissue staining [62–65] are necessarily sensitive nor specific for IgG4-related disease. According to more recent international consensus criteria, diagnoses of IgG4-related disease are primarily based upon pathology demonstrating 2 of 3 major histopathological features (dense lymphoplasmacytic infiltrate, storiform fibrosis [a cartwheel or whirled pattern of fibrosis, at least focally], and obliterative phlebitis) with appropriate clinicopathologic correlation. IgG4 serum levels and tissue staining have important secondary roles [66]. Published cases of IgG4-related hypophysitis typically do not comment on the presence or absence of such histologic features [26]. When it is described, storiform fibrosis has been reported in some [67] but not all cases of IgG4-related hypophysitis [68] following tissue analysis. Obliterative phlebitis has not been reported in any case of IgG4-related hypophysitis. As Ngaosuwan et al. noted, the diagnosis of IgG4-related hypophysitis is difficult without the presence of other organ involvement [69]. Although only a minority of reported IgG4-related hypophysitis cases have included histopathology, almost all patients had other organ involvement [70].

No case of immunotherapy-associated hypophysitis has been confirmed by pituitary gland biopsy. Diagnoses are established clinically based upon the close temporal relationship of immunotherapy treatment and the development of hypopituitarism with reversible pituitary enlargement [6, 71]. The relationship of lymphocytic hypophysitis with pregnancy [27, 41] may also allow a clinical diagnosis to be made with a reasonable degree of confidence in some pregnant or early postpartum women without tissue confirmation when appropriate imaging and biochemical findings are present with an otherwise negative thorough diagnostic evaluation.

Patient demographics and coexistent medical conditions may also help focus diagnostic considerations. For example, intracranial germinomas have a peak incidence in the second decade of life and are extremely rare after the age of 30 [72]. LCH can be diagnosed at any age, but the incidence of this disease progressively declines throughout life [73, 74].

Given the broad differential diagnosis for hypophysitis, caution and close follow up is strongly advised for the treatment of presumed cases lacking histopathologic confirmation.

Treatment

No prospective controlled studies have examined the treatment of hypophysitis, and a limited number of cases detail the natural history of untreated disease. Available retrospective data sets are confounded by reporting and treatment selection biases and likely encompass a heterogeneous group of diseases due to the lack of histologic confirmation in many cases and variable clinical evaluation. Medical therapies differ significantly by the type of agent, dosage, and duration of treatment.

Symptoms from mass effect, such as optic nerve compression and other cranial nerve palsies, and severe headache are general indications for the treatment of hypophysitis (Fig. 1). Practice patterns vary for less clinically severe cases. It is unclear whether treatment with immune suppressing medications improves pituitary function outcomes compared to supportive therapy.

Spontaneous resolution of pituitary enlargement has been observed in a number of published cases of hypophysitis [19]. One group recently reported regression of radiologic findings in 15/15 patients receiving supportive therapy [43]. A large recent retrospective review of hypophysitis cases in Germany noted radiologic improvement or stability in 16/22 cases without active treatment [75]. Pituitary surgery (gross total resection or partial resection) and glucocorticoid therapy appeared to be somewhat more effective at mass reduction in that study. Surgery (generally patients undergoing gross total resection) was associated with less improvement and greater loss of pituitary function. Patients receiving glucocorticoid therapy had a significant risk of relapsing pituitary enlargement and experienced frequent side effects from treatment. Approximately one-quarter of patients receiving supportive therapy demonstrated improvement in pituitary function, and 82 % of that group had stable or improved function. Similar results were reported in the patients treated with pharmacologic doses of glucocorticoids. Headache resolution was similar in all three groups [75]. Comparable rates of pituitary function recovery were reported following supportive therapy by Khare et al. [43]. A review by Lupi et al. suggested that pituitary function improvement may occur in approximately one-half of patients treated with glucocorticoids. Importantly, histopathology was available in only 22 % of these patients [76]. Similarly, a minority of patients had tissue confirmation in the study from Germany. Moreover, evaluation for secondary causes of hypophysitis was limited in the majority of those patients [42, 75]. Limited clinical evaluations were also frequent in the largest review of granulomatous hypophysitis cases [20].

Other immunosuppressive agents such as methotrexate, azathioprine, rituximab, infliximab, cyclosporine, and mycophenolate mofetil have been utilized in a small number of patients with hypophysitis [75–82]. Treatment with stereotactic radiosurgery and fractionated radiotherapy has been reported in a few patients, typically with refractory disease. Radiation dosages ranged from low levels to higher amounts used to treat pituitary adenomas [31, 83, 84].

Patients with immunotherapy-associated hypophysitis have been treated with physiologic to high-dose glucocorticoids. Although it is unclear whether pharmacologic

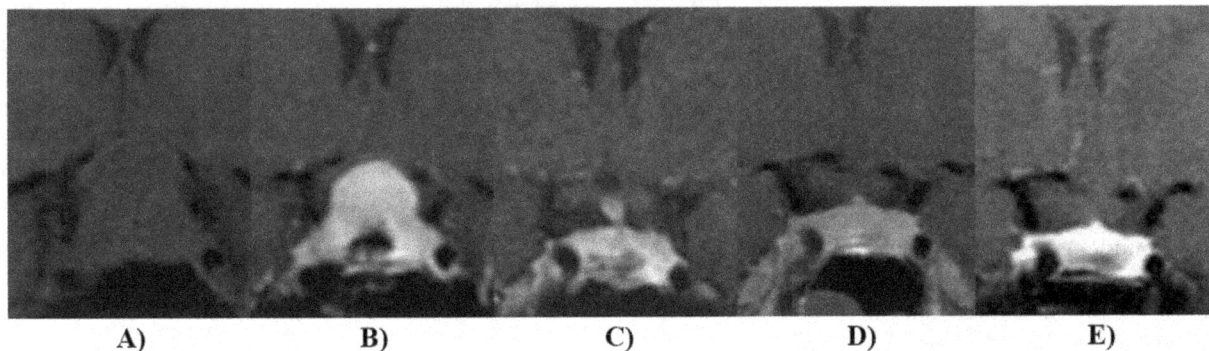

Fig. 1 Hypophysitis was diagnosed in a 30 year old during the late third trimester of pregnancy. The patient presented with 3 weeks of progression vision loss. Panel **a** depicts a coronal pre-contrast T1-weighted image of the pituitary. Transsphenoidal biopsy (Panel **b**) demonstrated lymphocytic hypophysitis and glucocorticoid therapy was begun with prednisone 60 mg daily. Following delivery, the pituitary gland decreased in size (Panel **c**) and remained stable 2 months (Panel **d**) and 5 months (Panel **e**) after glucocorticoid taper and discontinuation

dosages of glucocorticoids improve patient outcomes, higher doses do not appear to negatively impact the anti-tumor efficacy of immunotherapy or patient survival [6]. Improvement of pituitary function occurs in some patients following the resolution of hypophysitis; thyroidal and gonadal axis normalization occurs more frequently than adrenal recovery. The development of hypophysitis may be associated with improved patient survival in melanoma patients treated with Ipilimumab [71, 85].

Pathogenesis

The mechanisms underlying the development of hypophysitis are unknown. Other autoimmune diseases coexist in a portion of patients with hypophysitis. Unlike many of these other conditions, pituitary autoantigens in hypophysitis have not yet been clearly identified. Several candidates have been proposed, including growth hormone, pituitary gland specific factors 1a and 2 [86, 87], alpha-enolase and gamma-enolase [88, 89], secretogrannin II [90], chorionic somatomammotropin, CGI-99 [91], and corticotroph-specific transcription factor [92]. Measurements of antibodies to these proteins, however, do not have sufficient sensitivity and specificity to be diagnostically useful [16, 93]. Given the lack of clinically validated autoantigens, many studies have utilized indirect immunofluorescence (IIF) to detect the presence of pituitary autoantibodies. Ricciuti et al. systematically described methodologic limitations of IIF in the assessment of anti-pituitary antibodies, their potential effects on data interpretation, and methods to optimize results [94].

The pathogenic role of IgG4 in IgG4-related disease, including hypophysitis, is unclear, and it has been suggested that elevation of these antibodies may represent a bystander phenomenon [95]. IgG4 predominance often correlates with immune downregulation, in part due to its ability to participate in fragment antigen binding arm exchange [96].

Immunotherapy agents presumably can activate an autoimmune process directed against unidentified pituitary antigens. Pituitary autoantibodies were detected in patients who developed hypophysitis following treatment with Ipilimumab (a monoclonal antibody targeting CTLA-4), but these antibodies were not present in patients without hypophysitis. CTLA-4 is also expressed by the pituitary gland, and treatment with Ipilimumab may directly target pituitary cells via activation of the classical complement pathway and antibody-dependent cell-mediated cytotoxicity (ADCC) [97–99]. Pituitary CTLA-4 expression levels appear to vary widely [100] and may affect the risk of developing hypophysitis following treatment with Ipilimumab. In support of this hypothesis, hypophysitis has not been reported in patients with germline CTLA-4 mutations, although many of these patients had other severe autoimmune diseases which can occur following treatment with Ipilimumab [101, 102]. It is unknown whether PD-1 is expressed by the pituitary gland. Notably, anti-PD-1 agents are IgG4-based antibodies, which can not activate the classical complement pathway and are not effective mediators for ADCC [96, 103–105].

Conclusions

Currently, the diagnosis of primary hypophysitis typically requires a thorough evaluation for other potential neoplastic lesions, infiltrative diseases, infection, and systemic inflammatory processes plus histopathologic confirmation. In some cases, tissue biopsy may not be feasible. Cases of immunotherapy-associated hypophysitis and lymphocytic hypophysitis associated with pregnancy may potentially be diagnosed with some degree of confidence without surgery. Cranial nerve deficits due to mass effect from pituitary gland enlargement and severe headache are general indications for treatment with medical therapy and/or surgery. It is unclear whether active treatment improves clinical outcomes compared to supportive therapy for more mild cases of hypophysitis, and the therapies may be associated with side effects. Pituitary gland debulking rather than gross total resection is more commonly performed. Glucocorticoids (at variable dosages and duration) are the most frequent choice for medical therapy, though many other immunosuppressive agents have been utilized in the treatment of hypophysitis. Even when treatment is initially successful, disease recurrence is not uncommon. Radiation therapy appears promising, especially for refractory cases of hypophysitis, but the available published data consists of only a handful of patients.

Hypophysitis is an increasingly recognized but rare and poorly understood heterogeneous disease. The pathogenesis of primary hypophysitis is not yet known, and clinically validated disease markers have not been identified. In the absence of more detailed knowledge, various etiologic, morphologic, and histologic categories have been proposed, but the clinical utility of such schemas is limited. Inconsistent usage of terminology and variable diagnostic evaluations have also clouded data interpretation. Available studies are largely limited to retrospective series that likely include patients with diverse pathologies. Clinical investigation is constrained by the rarity of the disease. The acquisition of sufficient controlled prospective data will require multicenter collaboration. Until such investigations take place, optimal management strategies will remain largely undefined and controversial.

Acknowledgements
None.

Funding
None.

References

1. Chan WB, Cockram CS. Panhypopituitarism in association with interferon-alpha treatment. Singapore Med J. 2004;45:93–4.
2. Concha LB, Carlson HE, Heimann A, Lake-Bakaar GV, Paal AF. Interferon-induced hypopituitarism. Am J Med. 2003;114:161–3.
3. Ridruejo E, Christensen AF, Mando OG. Central hypothyroidism and hypophysitis during treatment of chronic hepatitis C with pegylated interferon alpha and ribavirin. Eur J Gastroenterol Hepatol. 2006;18:693–4.
4. Sakane N, Yoshida T, Yoshioka K, Umekawa T, Kondo M, Shimatsu A. Reversible hypopituitarism after interferonalfa therapy. Lancet. 1995;345:1305.
5. Tebben PJ, Atkinson JL, Scheithauer BW, Erickson D. Granulomatous adenohypophysitis after interferon and ribavirin therapy. Endocr Pract. 2007;13:169–75.
6. Faje A. Immunotherapy and hypophysitis: clinical presentation, treatment, and biologic insights. Pituitary. 2016;19:82–92.
7. Albini CH, MacGillivray MH, Fisher JE, Voorhess ML, Klein DM. Triad of hypopituitarism, granulomatous hypophysitis, and ruptured Rathke's cleft cyst. Neurosurgery. 1988;22:133–6.
8. Daikokuya H, Inoue Y, Nemoto Y, Tashiro T, Shakudo M, Ohata K. Rathke's cleft cyst associated with hypophysitis: MRI. Neuroradiology. 2000;42:532–4.
9. Wearne MJ, Barber PC, Johnson AP. Symptomatic Rathke's cleft cyst with hypophysitis. Br J Neurosurg. 1995;9:799–803.
10. Hama S, Arita K, Tominaga A, Yoshikawa M, Eguchi K, Sumida M, Inai K, Nishisaka T, Kurisu K. Symptomatic Rathke's cleft cyst coexisting with central diabetes insipidus and hypophysitis: case report. Endocr J. 1999;46:187–92.
11. Puchner MJ, Ludecke DK, Saeger W. The anterior pituitary lobe in patients with cystic craniopharyngiomas: three cases of associated lymphocytic hypophysitis. Acta Neurochir (Wien). 1994;126:38–43.
12. McConnon JK, Smyth HS, Horvath E. A case of sparsely granulated growth hormone cell adenoma associated with lymphocytic hypophysitis. J Endocrinol Invest. 1991;14:691–6.
13. Jenkins PJ, Chew SL, Lowe DG, Afshart F, Charlesworth M, Besser GM, Wass JA. Lymphocytic hypophysitis: unusual features of a rare disorder. Clin Endocrinol (Oxf). 1995;42:529–34.
14. Moskowitz SI, Hamrahian A, Prayson RA, Pineyro M, Lorenz RR, Weil RJ. Concurrent lymphocytic hypophysitis and pituitary adenoma. Case report and review of the literature. J Neurosurg. 2006;105:309–14.
15. Holck S, Laursen H. Prolactinoma coexistent with granulomatous hypophysitis. Acta Neuropathol. 1983;61:253–7.
16. Caturegli P, Lupi I, Landek-Salgado M, Kimura H, Rose NR. Pituitary autoimmunity: 30 years later. Autoimmun Rev. 2008;7:631–7.
17. Ahmed SR, Aiello DP, Page R, Hopper K, Towfighi J, Santen RJ. Necrotizing infundibulo-hypophysitis: a unique syndrome of diabetes insipidus and hypopituitarism. J Clin Endocrinol Metab. 1993;76:1499–504.
18. Gutenberg A, Caturegli P, Metz I, Martinez R, Mohr A, Bruck W, Rohde V. Necrotizing infundibulo-hypophysitis: an entity too rare to be true? Pituitary. 2012;15:202–8.
19. Beressi N, Beressi JP, Cohen R, Modigliani E. Lymphocytic hypophysitis. A review of 145 cases. Ann Med Interne (Paris). 1999;150:327–41.
20. Hunn BH, Martin WG, Simpson Jr S, McLean CA. Idiopathic granulomatous hypophysitis: a systematic review of 82 cases in the literature. Pituitary. 2014;17:357–65.
21. Doniach I, Wright EA. Two cases of giant-cell granuloma of the pituitary gland. J Pathol Bacteriol. 1951;63:69–79.
22. Folkerth RD, Price Jr DL, Schwartz M, Black PM, De Girolami U. Xanthomatous hypophysitis. Am J Surg Pathol. 1998;22:736–41.
23. Hanna B, Li YM, Beutler T, Goyal P, Hall WA. Xanthomatous hypophysitis. J Clin Neurosci. 2015;22:1091–7.
24. Leporati P, Landek-Salgado MA, Lupi I, Chiovato L, Caturegli P. IgG4-related hypophysitis: a new addition to the hypophysitis spectrum. J Clin Endocrinol Metab. 2011;96:1971–80.
25. Caturegli P, Iwama S. From Japan with love: another tessera in the hypophysitis mosaic. J Clin Endocrinol Metab. 2013;98:1865–8.
26. Shimatsu A, Oki Y, Fujisawa I, Sano T. Pituitary and stalk lesions (infundibulo-hypophysitis) associated with immunoglobulin G4-related systemic disease: an emerging clinical entity. Endocr J. 2009;56:1033–41.
27. Caturegli P, Newschaffer C, Olivi A, Pomper MG, Burger PC, Rose NR. Autoimmune hypophysitis. Endocr Rev. 2005;26:599–614.
28. Imber BS, Lee HS, Kunwar S, Blevins LS, Aghi MK. Hypophysitis: a single-center case series. Pituitary. 2015;18:630–41.
29. Buxton N, Robertson I. Lymphocytic and granulocytic hypophysitis: a single centre experience. Br J Neurosurg. 2001;15:242–5. discussion 245–246.
30. Sautner D, Saeger W, Ludecke DK, Jansen V, Puchner MJ. Hypophysitis in surgical and autoptical specimens. Acta Neuropathol. 1995;90:637–44.
31. Leung GK, Lopes MB, Thorner MO, Vance ML, Laws Jr ER. Primary hypophysitis: a single-center experience in 16 cases. J Neurosurg. 2004;101:262–71.
32. Honegger J, Fahlbusch R, Bornemann A, Hensen J, Buchfelder M, Muller M, Nomikos P. Lymphocytic and granulomatous hypophysitis: experience with nine cases. Neurosurgery. 1997;40:713–22. discussion 722–713.
33. Goudie RB, Pinkerton PH. Anterior hypophysitis and Hashimoto's disease in a young woman. J Pathol Bacteriol. 1962;83:584–5.
34. Brissaud HH, Gougerot H, Gy A. Nevrite localised avec troubles trophiques a la suite de coupure de pouce. Rev Neurol. 1908;13:645.
35. Simmonds M. U¨ber das Vorkommen von Riesenzellen in der Hypophyse. Virchows Arch. 1917;223(3):281–90.
36. van der Vliet HJ, Perenboom RM. Multiple pseudotumors in IgG4-associated multifocal systemic fibrosis. Ann Intern Med. 2004;141:896–7.
37. Guay AT, Agnello V, Tronic BC, Gresham DG, Freidberg SR. Lymphocytic hypophysitis in a man. J Clin Endocrinol Metab. 1987;64:631–4.
38. Levine SN, Benzel EC, Fowler MR, Shroyer 3rd JV, Mirfakhraee M. Lymphocytic adenohypophysitis: clinical, radiological, and magnetic resonance imaging characterization. Neurosurgery. 1988;22:937–41.
39. Hoshimaru M, Hashimoto N, Kikuchi H. Central diabetes insipidus resulting from a nonneoplastic tiny mass lesion localized in the neurohypophyseal system. Surg Neurol. 1992;38:1–6.
40. Gellner V, Kurschel S, Scarpatetti M, Mokry M. Lymphocytic hypophysitis in the pediatric population. Childs Nerv Syst. 2008;24:785–92.
41. Landek-Salgado MA, Gutenberg A, Lupi I, Kimura H, Mariotti S, Rose NR, Caturegli P. Pregnancy, postpartum autoimmune thyroiditis, and autoimmune hypophysitis: intimate relationships. Autoimmun Rev. 2010;9:153–7.
42. Honegger J, Schlaffer S, Menzel C, Droste M, Werner S, Elbelt U, Strasburger C, Stormann S, Kuppers A, Streetz-van der Werf C, et al. Diagnosis of primary hypophysitis in Germany. J Clin Endocrinol Metab. 2015;100:3841–9.
43. Khare S, Jagtap VS, Budyal SR, Kasaliwal R, Kakade HR, Bukan A, Sankhe S, Lila AR, Bandgar T, Menon PS, Shah NS. Primary (autoimmune) hypophysitis: a single centre experience. Pituitary. 2015;18:16–22.
44. Peruzzotti-Jametti L, Strambo D, Sangalli F, De Bellis A, Comi G, Sessa M. Bilateral intracavernous carotid artery occlusion caused by invasive lymphocytic hypophysitis. J Stroke Cerebrovasc Dis. 2012;21:918. e919-911.
45. Ikeda J, Kuratsu J, Miura M, Kai Y, Ushio Y. Lymphocytic adenohypophysitis accompanying occlusion of bilateral internal carotid arteries–case report. Neurol Med Chir (Tokyo). 1990;30:346–9.
46. Melgar MA, Mariwalla N, Gloss DS, Walsh JW. Recurrent lymphocytic hypophysitis and bilateral intracavernous carotid artery occlusion. an observation and review of the literature. Neurol Res. 2006;28:177–83.
47. Minakshi B, Alok S, Hillol KP. Lymphocytic hypophysitis presenting as pituitary apoplexy in a male. Neurol India. 2005;53:363–4.
48. Husain Q, Zouzias A, Kanumuri VV, Eloy JA, Liu JK. Idiopathic granulomatous hypophysitis presenting as pituitary apoplexy. J Clin Neurosci. 2014;21:510–2.
49. Kravarusic J, Molitch ME. Lymphocytic hypophysitis and other inflammatory conditions of the pituitary. In: Oxford Textbook of Endocrinology and Diabetes. New York: Oxford University Press; 2011. p. 259–66.

50. Turcu AF, Erickson BJ, Lin E, Guadalix S, Schwartz K, Scheithauer BW, Atkinson JL, Young Jr WF. Pituitary stalk lesions: the Mayo Clinic experience. J Clin Endocrinol Metab. 2013;98:1812–8.

51. Cives M, Simone V, Rizzo FM, Dicuonzo F, Cristallo Lacalamita M, Ingravallo G, Silvestris F, Dammacco F. Erdheim-Chester disease: a systematic review. Crit Rev Oncol Hematol. 2015;95:1–11.

52. Monsereenusorn C, Rodriguez-Galindo C. Clinical characteristics and treatment of langerhans cell histiocytosis. Hematol Oncol Clin North Am. 2015;29:853–73.

53. Strowd RE, Burger P, Holdhoff M, Kleinberg L, Okun MS, Olivi A, Pardo-Villamizar C, Schiess N. Steroid-responsive intracranial germinoma presenting as Holmes' tremor: importance of a tissue diagnosis. J Clin Neurosci. 2015;22:911–3.

54. Si SJ, Khatua S, Dhall G, Nelson MD, Gonzalez-Gomez I, Finlay JL. Regression of primary central nervous system germinoma after dexamethasone administration: a case report. Pediatr Hematol Oncol. 2010;27:237–43.

55. Mascalchi M, Roncaroli F, Salvi F, Frank G. Transient regression of an intracranial germ cell tumour after intravenous steroid administration: a case report. J Neurol Neurosurg Psychiatry. 1998;64:670–2.

56. Gutenberg A, Bell JJ, Lupi I, Tzou SC, Landek-Salgado MA, Kimura H, Su J, Karaviti LP, Salvatori R, Caturegli P. Pituitary and systemic autoimmunity in a case of intrasellar germinoma. Pituitary. 2011;14:388–94.

57. Konno S, Oka H, Utsuki S, Kondou K, Tanaka S, Fujii K, Yagishita S. Germinoma with a granulomatous reaction. Problems of differential diagnosis. Clin Neuropathol. 2002;21:248–51.

58. Endo Y, Kumabe T, Ikeda H, Shirane R, Yoshimoto T. Neurohypophyseal germinoma histologically misidentified as granulomatous hypophysitis. Acta Neurochir (Wien). 2002;144:1233–7.

59. Gutenberg A, Larsen J, Lupi I, Rohde V, Caturegli P. A radiologic score to distinguish autoimmune hypophysitis from nonsecreting pituitary adenoma preoperatively. AJNR Am J Neuroradiol. 2009;30:1766–72.

60. Khosroshahi A, Cheryk LA, Carruthers MN, Edwards JA, Bloch DB, Stone JH. Brief Report: spuriously low serum IgG4 concentrations caused by the prozone phenomenon in patients with IgG4-related disease. Arthritis Rheumatol. 2014;66:213–7.

61. Wallace ZS, Deshpande V, Mattoo H, Mahajan VS, Kulikova M, Pillai S, Stone JH. IgG4-Related Disease: Clinical and Laboratory Features in One Hundred Twenty-Five Patients. Arthritis Rheumatol. 2015;67:2466–75.

62. Chang SY, Keogh KA, Lewis JE, Ryu JH, Cornell LD, Garrity JA, Yi ES. IgG4-positive plasma cells in granulomatosis with polyangiitis (Wegener's): a clinicopathologic and immunohistochemical study on 43 granulomatosis with polyangiitis and 20 control cases. Hum Pathol. 2013;44:2432–7.

63. Nishioka H, Shibuya M, Haraoka J. Immunohistochemical study for IgG4-positive plasmacytes in pituitary inflammatory lesions. Endocr Pathol. 2010;21:236–41.

64. Bando H, Iguchi G, Fukuoka H, Taniguchi M, Kawano S, Saitoh M, Yoshida K, Matsumoto R, Suda K, Nishizawa H, et al. A diagnostic pitfall in IgG4-related hypophysitis: infiltration of IgG4-positive cells in the pituitary of granulomatosis with polyangiitis. Pituitary. 2015;18:722–30.

65. Ohkubo Y, Sekido T, Takeshige K, Ishi H, Takei M, Nishio S, Yamazaki M, Komatsu M, Kawa S, Suzuki S. Occurrence of IgG4-related hypophysitis lacking IgG4-bearing plasma cell infiltration during steroid therapy. Intern Med. 2014;53:753–7.

66. Deshpande V, Zen Y, Chan JK, Yi EE, Sato Y, Yoshino T, Kloppel G, Heathcote JG, Khosroshahi A, Ferry JA, et al. Consensus statement on the pathology of IgG4-related disease. Mod Pathol. 2012;25:1181–92.

67. Bando H, Iguchi G, Fukuoka H, Taniguchi M, Yamamoto M, Matsumoto R, Suda K, Nishizawa H, Takahashi M, Kohmura E, Takahashi Y. The prevalence of IgG4-related hypophysitis in 170 consecutive patients with hypopituitarism and/or central diabetes insipidus and review of the literature. Eur J Endocrinol. 2014;170:161–72.

68. Tauziede-Espariat A, Polivka M, Bouazza S, Decq P, Robert G, Laloi-Michelin M, Adle-Biassette H. The prevalence of IgG4-positive plasma cells in hypophysitis: a possible relationship to IgG4-related disease. Clin Neuropathol. 2015;34:181–92.

69. Ngaosuwan K, Trongwongsa T, Shuangshoti S. Clinical course of IgG4-related hypophysitis presenting with focal seizure and relapsing lymphocytic hypophysitis. BMC Endocr Disord. 2015;15:64.

70. Sosa GA, Bell S, Christiansen SB, Pietrani M, Glerean M, Loto M, Lovazzano S, Carrizo A, Ajler P, Fainstein Day P. Histologically confirmed isolated IgG4-related hypophysitis: two case reports in young women. Endocrinol Diabetes Metab Case Rep. 2014;2014:140062.

71. Faje AT, Sullivan R, Lawrence D, Tritos NA, Fadden R, Klibanski A, Nachtigall L. Ipilimumab-induced hypophysitis: a detailed longitudinal analysis in a large cohort of patients with metastatic melanoma. J Clin Endocrinol Metab. 2014;99:4078–85.

72. Jennings MT, Gelman R, Hochberg F. Intracranial germ-cell tumors: natural history and pathogenesis. J Neurosurg. 1985;63:155–67.

73. Howarth DM, Gilchrist GS, Mullan BP, Wiseman GA, Edmonson JH, Schomberg PJ. Langerhans cell histiocytosis: diagnosis, natural history, management, and outcome. Cancer. 1999;85:2278–90.

74. Stalemark H, Laurencikas E, Karis J, Gavhed D, Fadeel B, Henter JI. Incidence of Langerhans cell histiocytosis in children: a population-based study. Pediatr Blood Cancer. 2008;51:76–81.

75. Honegger J, Buchfelder M, Schlaffer S, Droste M, Werner S, Strasburger C, Stormann S, Schopohl J, Kacheva S, Deutschbein T, et al. Treatment of primary hypophysitis in Germany. J Clin Endocrinol Metab. 2015;100:3460–9.

76. Lupi I, Manetti L, Raffaelli V, Lombardi M, Cosottini M, Iannelli A, Basolo F, Proietti A, Bogazzi F, Caturegli P, Martino E. Diagnosis and treatment of autoimmune hypophysitis: a short review. J Endocrinol Invest. 2011;34:e245–252.

77. Schreckinger M, Francis T, Rajah G, Jagannathan J, Guthikonda M, Mittal S. Novel strategy to treat a case of recurrent lymphocytic hypophysitis using rituximab. J Neurosurg. 2012;116:1318–23.

78. Xu C, Ricciuti A, Caturegli P, Keene CD, Kargi AY. Autoimmune lymphocytic hypophysitis in association with autoimmune eye disease and sequential treatment with infliximab and rituximab. Pituitary. 2015;18:441–7.

79. Lecube A, Francisco G, Rodriguez D, Ortega A, Codina A, Hernandez C, Simo R. Lymphocytic hypophysitis successfully treated with azathioprine: first case report. J Neurol Neurosurg Psychiatry. 2003;74:1581–3.

80. Li HT, Wang ST, Qiu MC. Gynecomastia, obesity and underdeveloped testis and penis: suspected hypophysitis successfully cured with low dose of cyclosporine A. Chin Med J (Engl). 2009;122:2791–3.

81. Ward L, Paquette J, Seidman E, Huot C, Alvarez F, Crock P, Delvin E, Kampe O, Deal C. Severe autoimmune polyendocrinopathy-candidiasis-ectodermal dystrophy in an adolescent girl with a novel AIRE mutation: response to immunosuppressive therapy. J Clin Endocrinol Metab. 1999;84:844–52.

82. Louvet C, Maqdasy S, Tekath M, Grobost V, Rieu V, Ruivard M, Le Guenno G. Infundibuloneurohypophysitis associated with sjogren syndrome successfully treated with mycophenolate mofetil: a case report. Medicine (Baltimore). 2016;95:e3132.

83. Ray DK, Yen CP, Vance ML, Laws ER, Lopes B, Sheehan JP. Gamma knife surgery for lymphocytic hypophysitis. J Neurosurg. 2010;112:118–21.

84. Selch MT, DeSalles AA, Kelly DF, Frighetto L, Vinters HV, Cabatan-Awang C, Wallace RE, Solberg TD. Stereotactic radiotherapy for the treatment of lymphocytic hypophysitis. Report of two cases. J Neurosurg. 2003;99:591–6.

85. Eatrides J, Weber J, Egan K, Acierno M, Schell M, Lillienfeld H, Creelan B: Autoimmune hypophysitis is a marker of favorable outcome during treatment of melanoma with ipilimumab. AACR: Advances in Melanoma: From Biology to Therapy 2014, abstract.

86. Takao T, Nanamiya W, Matsumoto R, Asaba K, Okabayashi T, Hashimoto K. Antipituitary antibodies in patients with lymphocytic hypophysitis. Horm Res. 2001;55:288–92.

87. Tanaka S, Tatsumi KI, Kimura M, Takano T, Murakami Y, Takao T, Hashimoto K, Kato Y, Amino N. Detection of autoantibodies against the pituitary-specific proteins in patients with lymphocytic hypophysitis. Eur J Endocrinol. 2002;147:767–75.

88. Tanaka S, Tatsumi KI, Takano T, Murakami Y, Takao T, Yamakita N, Tahara S, Teramoto A, Hashimoto K, Kato Y, Amino N. Anti-alpha-enolase antibodies in pituitary disease. Endocr J. 2003;50:697–702.

89. O'Dwyer DT, Clifton V, Hall A, Smith R, Robinson PJ, Crock PA. Pituitary autoantibodies in lymphocytic hypophysitis target both gamma- and alpha-Enolase - a link with pregnancy? Arch Physiol Biochem. 2002;110:94–8.

90. Bensing S, Hulting AL, Hoog A, Ericson K, Kampe O. Lymphocytic hypophysitis: report of two biopsy-proven cases and one suspected case with pituitary autoantibodies. J Endocrinol Invest. 2007;30:153–62.

91. Lupi I, Broman KW, Tzou SC, Gutenberg A, Martino E, Caturegli P. Novel autoantigens in autoimmune hypophysitis. Clin Endocrinol (Oxf). 2008;69:269–78.

92. Smith CJ, Bensing S, Burns C, Robinson PJ, Kasperlik-Zaluska AA, Scott RJ, Kampe O, Crock PA. Identification of TPIT and other novel autoantigens in lymphocytic hypophysitis: immunoscreening of a pituitary cDNA library and development of immunoprecipitation assays. Eur J Endocrinol. 2012;166:391–8.

93. Falorni A, Minarelli V, Bartoloni E, Alunno A, Gerli R. Diagnosis and classification of autoimmune hypophysitis. Autoimmun Rev. 2014;13:412–6.

94. Ricciuti A, De Remigis A, Landek-Salgado MA, De Vincentiis L, Guaraldi F, Lupi I, Iwama S, Wand GS, Salvatori R, Caturegli P. Detection of pituitary antibodies by immunofluorescence: approach and results in patients with pituitary diseases. J Clin Endocrinol Metab. 2014;99:1758–66.

95. Wallace ZS, Stone JH. An update on IgG4-related disease. Curr Opin Rheumatol. 2015;27:83–90.

96. Vidarsson G, Dekkers G, Rispens T. IgG subclasses and allotypes: from structure to effector functions. Front Immunol. 2014;5:520.

97. Iwama S, De Remigis A, Callahan MK, Slovin SF, Wolchok JD, Caturegli P. Pituitary expression of CTLA-4 mediates hypophysitis secondary to administration of CTLA-4 blocking antibody. Sci Transl Med. 2014;6:230ra245.

98. Romano E, Kusio-Kobialka M, Foukas PG, Baumgaertner P, Meyer C, Ballabeni P, Michielin O, Weide B, Romero P, Speiser DE. Ipilimumab-dependent cell-mediated cytotoxicity of regulatory T cells ex vivo by nonclassical monocytes in melanoma patients. Proc Natl Acad Sci U S A. 2015;112:6140–5.

99. Laurent S, Queirolo P, Boero S, Salvi S, Piccioli P, Boccardo S, Minghelli S, Morabito A, Fontana V, Pietra G, et al. The engagement of CTLA-4 on primary melanoma cell lines induces antibody-dependent cellular cytotoxicity and TNF-alpha production. J Transl Med. 2013;11:108.

100. Faje A, Ma J, Wang X, Swearingen B, Tritos NA, Nachtigall L, Zhang X, Klibanski A: Cytotoxic T-lymphocyte antigen-4 gene expression in human pituitary adenomas. ENDO 2015, abstract.

101. Kuehn HS, Ouyang W, Lo B, Deenick EK, Niemela JE, Avery DT, Schickel JN, Tran DQ, Stoddard J, Zhang Y, et al. Immune dysregulation in human subjects with heterozygous germline mutations in CTLA4. Science. 2014;345:1623–7.

102. Schubert D, Bode C, Kenefeck R, Hou TZ, Wing JB, Kennedy A, Bulashevska A, Petersen BS, Schaffer AA, Gruning BA, et al. Autosomal dominant immune dysregulation syndrome in humans with CTLA4 mutations. Nat Med. 2014;20:1410–6.

103. Garred P, Michaelsen TE, Aase A. The IgG subclass pattern of complement activation depends on epitope density and antibody and complement concentration. Scand J Immunol. 1989;30:379–82.

104. Michaelsen TE, Garred P, Aase A. Human IgG subclass pattern of inducing complement-mediated cytolysis depends on antigen concentration and to a lesser extent on epitope patchiness, antibody affinity and complement concentration. Eur J Immunol. 1991;21:11–6.

105. Bruhns P, Iannascoli B, England P, Mancardi DA, Fernandez N, Jorieux S, Daeron M. Specificity and affinity of human Fcgamma receptors and their polymorphic variants for human IgG subclasses. Blood. 2009;113:3716–25.

Detemir plus aspart and glulisine induced lipoatrophy

Sima Saberi[1], Nazanene H. Esfandiari[2]*, Mark P. MacEachern[3] and Meng H. Tan[2]

Abstract

Background: In the first and only literature review, conducted in 2009, of human insulin analog- induced lipoatrophy, there were 12 published cases, including 1 with aspart, 1 with detemir, 1 with NovoMix 30 and none with detemir plus aspart. It is perceived that insulin analog induced-lipoatrophy is increasing. We conducted a 2015 literature review of published reports of lipoatrophy induced by aspart, detemir, detemir plus aspart, and NovoMix30. We also report a new case of detemir plus aspart and glulisine induced lipoatrophy.

Methods: Our focused literature searches (limited to 1995–2014) in PubMed, Embase, and Web of Science, using a combination of insulin analog and lipoatrophy terminology, was conducted in early January 2015.

Results: From the 520 unique citations there were 33 (from 13 papers and 9 abstracts) lipoatrophy cases induced by detemir (n = 5), aspart (n = 21), detemir plus aspart (n = 4) and NovoMix 30 (n = 3), representing 30 new cases since 2009. Many of these reported cases were females (76 %), had type 1 diabetes mellitus (T1DM) (94 %) and were in young persons (61 %). A 41-year-old T1DM woman developed lipoatrophy on her upper thighs, arms and abdomen 14 months after injecting detemir plus aspart at the same sites. Later on, after a year on continuous subcutaneous insulin infusion (CSII) using aspart and then glulisine, she developed lipoatrophy at the infusion sites. When CSII insulin was switched to lispro she did not develop lipoatrophy after 10 months. Meanwhile, the original lipoatrophy sites significantly improved.

Conclusions: Our literature review uncovered 30 new published cases of aspart, detemir, aspart plus detemir and NovoMix 30-induced lipoatrophy since 2009. The largest increase in cases was in aspart- induced lipoatrophy. Recent surveys showed most rapid acting insulin analog-induced lipoatrophy were associated with CSII. In our review of the reported cases, 85.7 % cases of aspart-induced lipoatrophy were associated with CSII. As in previous reports, we showed lipoatrophy was more common in females, T1DM and young persons. Our patient may be the 5th published case of detemir plus aspart-induced lipoatrophy and possibly the first case report of glulisine induced lipoatrophy. She believed both detemir plus aspart and glulisine induced the lipoatrophy.

Keywords: Lipoatrophy, Aspart, Detemir, Aspart plus detemir, NovoMix 30, Glulisine, Continuous subcutaneous insulin infusion

* Correspondence: nazanene@med.umich.edu
[2]Division of Metabolism, Endocrinology and Diabetes, University of Michigan, Lobby C, 24 Frank Lloyd Wright Drive, Ann Arbor, MI 48106, USA
Full list of author information is available at the end of the article

Background

Insulin-induced lipoatrophy was a very common cutaneous complication of insulin therapy, found in 25- 55 % of patients injecting bovine and porcine insulin [1]. It became less common (<10 %) with purer animal and human insulin [1]; and uncommon (about 1 %) after human insulin analogs became available [2]. Lipoatrophy has been reported in patients using basal (glargine [3] and detemir [4]), rapid-acting (lispro [5], aspart [6] and glulisine [7]) and mixture [8] insulin analogs injections. In the first and only literature review of human insulin analog-induced lipoatrophy, done in November 2009 [9], there were 12 cases, including 1 with aspart, 1 with detemir, 1 with NovoMix 30 (Biphasic aspart – 30 % aspart 70 %, NPH insulin) and none with detemir plus aspart. Insulin analog induced lipoatrophy is perceived to be increasing in prevalence [2]. In this paper we report a literature review conducted in early January 2015 of published reports of lipoatrophy induced by aspart, detemir, detemir plus aspart, and NovoMix30 injections and report a new case of lipoatrophy induced by detemir plus aspart as well as glulisine injection. We will not cover lipoatrophy induced by lispro, lispro mixtures, and glargine in detail.

Methods

We conducted focused literature searches in early January 2015 in PubMed, Embase, and Web of Science using a combination of insulin analog and lipoatrophy terminology. We used MeSH and EMTREE controlled terms when appropriate for broad concepts, such as "insulin analog" [mesh] and lipodystrophy [mesh:noexp]. We supplemented each controlled term with a comparable set of title/abstract keywords, going so far as to include all individual insulin analogs ('lispro', 'humalog', 'aspart', 'novolog', 'detemir', 'levemir', 'glulisine', 'apidra', and 'glargine', 'lantus'). We also conducted a similar search in Web of Science to primarily identify conference abstracts that were not found in PubMed or Embase. We limited all searches to articles and abstracts published between 1995 (when the first insulin analog was launched) and 2014, and deliberately designed the searches to miss, when possible, citations pertaining to HIV-related lipoatrophy. We exported citations into Endnote X6 (Thomson Reuters) and used its functionality to eliminate duplicates.

We report a new case of a female type 1 diabetes mellitus (T1DM) patient who developed lipoatrophy when injecting detemir plus aspart in the same site. Later on, when using continuous subcutaneous insulin infusion (CSII) to deliver aspart and then glulisine, she also developed lipoatrophy at the infusion sites. We obtained written informed consent from the patient for publication of this case report and the images.

We requested information on lipoatrophy associated with aspart and/or detemir injections from the manufacturer of these insulin analogs.

Results

Literature search

The literature search of PubMed, EMBASE and Web of Science yielded 273, 252 and 119 citations respectively, giving a combined total of 644 citations (Fig. 1). After the duplicates were eliminated, we had 520 unique citations. Two authors (MT and NE) reviewed each of the 520 citations and concurred on those identified as lipoatrophy induced by insulin analog aspart, detemir, detemir plus aspart and NovoMix 30 injections. We found 33 reported cases from 18 citations (13 papers/letters/observations/vignette and 9 abstracts). From the references of 13 papers, pearling was done to determine whether they included other published abstracts/papers on lipoatrophy induced by aspart, detemir, detemir plus aspart, NovoMix 30 and glulisine injections. We found none.

The 33 lipoatrophy cases are induced by detemir (n = 5) [4, 10, 11], aspart (n = 21) [6, 10, 12–22], detemir plus aspart (n = 4) [11, 23, 24], and NovoMix 30 (n = 3) [8, 10] injections (Table 1). One of the detemir cases [4], one of the aspart cases [6] and one of the NovoMix30 cases [8] were previously described in the 2009 literature review [9], giving 30 new cases since then: 4 detemir cases [10, 11], 20 aspart cases [10, 12–22], 2 NovoMix 30 [10], and 4 detemir plus aspart cases [11, 23, 24]. The characteristics of the 33 cases are:

Gender

Of the 5 patients with detemir-induced lipoatrophy, the gender of 4 was stated. All were females. Of the 21 patients with aspart-induced lipoatrophy, the gender of 20 was stated. Of these, 13 were females and 7 were males. All 4 patients with detemir plus aspart-induced lipoatrophy were females. Of the 3 patients with NovoMix 30-induced lipoatrophy, 1 was female and the gender of the other 2 was not stated.

Type of diabetes

All 5 patients with detemir-induced lipoatrophy had T1DM. Twenty of the 21 patients with aspart-induced lipoatrophy had T1DM and one had type 2 diabetes mellitus (T2DM). Among the 4 adult female patients with detemir plus aspart-induced lipoatrophy, 2 had T1DM and 2 had T2DM. All 3 patients with NovoMix 30-induced lipoatrophy had T1DM.

Age

Four of the 5 patients with detemir-induced lipoatrophy were adults and 1 was an adolescent. Fourteen of the 21

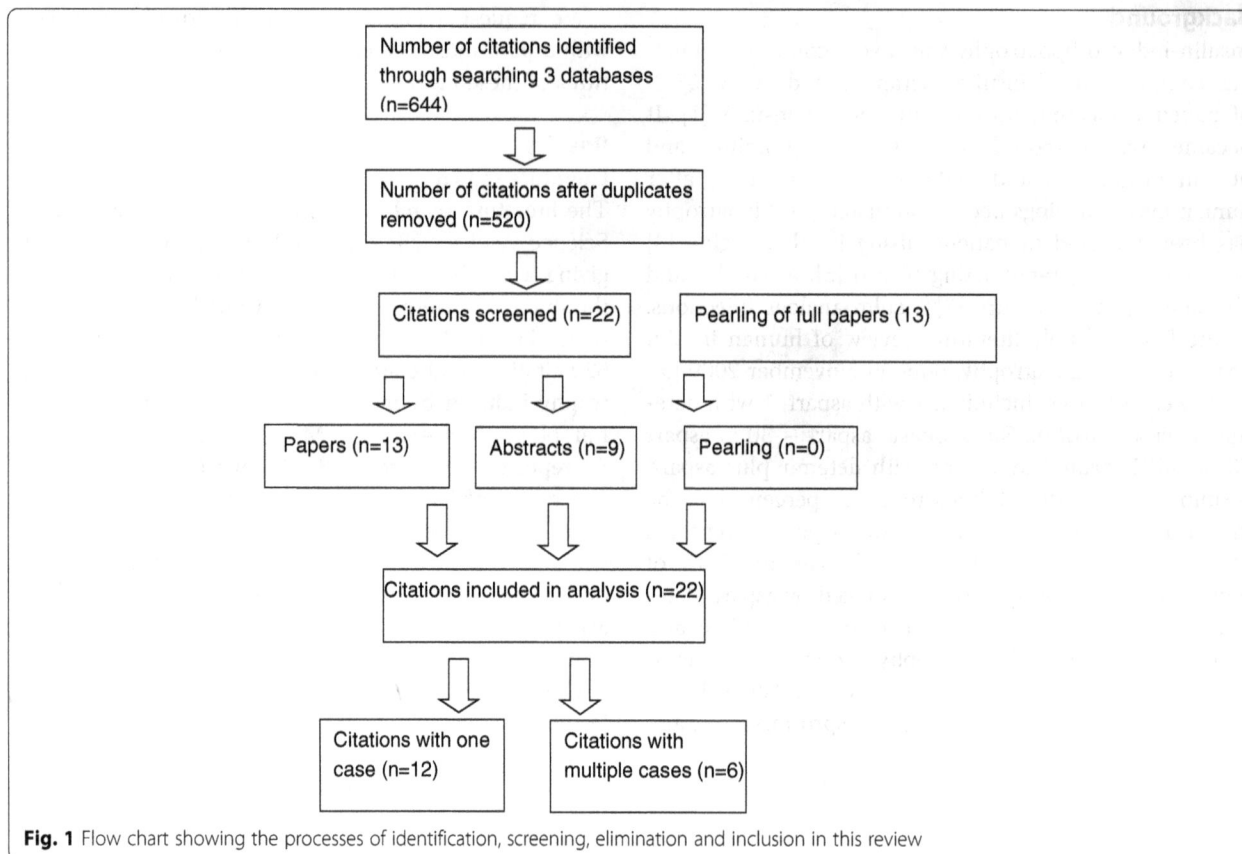

Fig. 1 Flow chart showing the processes of identification, screening, elimination and inclusion in this review

patients with aspart-induced lipoatrophy were children, 3 were adults, 3 adolescents and 1 had no age mentioned. All 4 patients with detemir plus aspart- induced lipoatrophy were adults. Two patients with Novo-Mix 30-induced lipoatrophy were children and 1 an adult.

Case

We report a 41-year-old Caucasian woman with T1DM diagnosed in April 2010 who developed lipoatrophy on her upper thighs, arms and abdomen injection sites in June 2011 after being on multiple daily insulin regimen of detemir plus aspart for 14 months (Fig. 2). Her Hemoglobin A1c improved from 10.9 % at diagnosis to 6.4-7.4 % after starting these insulin analogs. She injected both insulin analogs in the same sites and could not specify which insulin analog was the cause of these indentations. In September 2011 she started CSII using Omnipod with aspart. New lipoatrophy developed at the infusion sites within a year. In November 2012 glulisine was used instead of aspart. When the infusion was above or below the lipoatrophy thigh sites, the lipoatrophy worsened. Therefore, she switched to abdominal sites and developed new lipoatrophy there. She was then evaluated by allergists at 2 different tertiary centers. One recommended steroid therapy and the other recommended observation. She chose clinical observation without steroid treatment.

In February 2014 lispro was used instead of glulisine because the original lipoatrophy sites were not improving. In December 2014, 10 months after switching to lispro and using abdominal sites only, no new lipoatrophy had appeared at infusion sites. Her latest A1C in December 2014 was 7.2 %. Meanwhile the original lipoatrophy sites in the upper thighs, upper arms and abdomen improved significantly (Fig. 3).

Information from the manufacturer

In their response to our request for information on lipoatrophy induced by detemir, aspart, detemir plus aspart the manufacturer stated they did not have incidence data on lipoatrophy associated with these insulin analogs [25].

Lipoatrophy induced by other insulin analogs

In the same literature search 17 cases of lispro, 2 cases of lispro mixture, and 7 cases of glargine induced lipoatrophy were reported. No reported case of glulisine-induced lipoatrophy was found. These cases are not described in detail in this paper; but their details can be obtained from the authors. Our new case of detemir plus aspart induced lipoatrophy also developed lipoatrophy when using glulisine, making it the first published reported case of glulisine induced lipoatrophy.

Table 1 Thirty-three lipoatrophy cases induced by detemir, aspart, detemir plus aspart, and NovoMix30

Year published and country	Detemir	Aspart	Detemir plus aspart	NovoMix30 (30 % aspart plus 70 % NPH)	Glulisine
Literature Search 2009 (9)					
Hussein et al. UK 2007 [8]				65 yo Caucasian female with late-onset T1DM started on NovoMix 30. LA in both thighs (onset not mentioned). When switched to abdomen, new LA developed. Did not resolve.	
Szypowska et al. Poland 2008 [6]		32 mo Caucasian boy with T1DM using Asp in CSII. LA at infusion sites in buttocks 10 months later. Switched to Lispro and LA reported at new infusion sites.			
Del Olmo et al. Spain 2008 [4]	30 yo female T1DM. Detemir 10 u hs. LA appear on thighs "several" months after initiation. No LA with NPH, Mixtard 30 or Actrapid used earlier.				
Literature Search 2015					
Kesavadev J et al. India 2008 [12]		55 yo Indian male with T2DM (?) on CSII using Asp developed LA at infusion sites 2 months after initiating therapy.			
Bocca et al. Netherlands 2009 [13]		7 yo girl with T1DM since age 1 yr. Started on CSII using Asp at age 5 yrs. At age 7 yrs LA developed at infusion sites on buttocks and thighs.			
Chang YT et al. USA 2010 [14]		11 yo girl with T1DM on CSII using Asp. Developed LA at infusion sites after 1 yr. Previously on MDI using Asp + glargine with lipohypertrophy at injection sites. Switched to lispro and applied sodium cromoglicate cream with little effect.			
Ninnikoski et al. Finland 2010 [15]		7 yo boy with T1DM on CSII using Asp. Developed LA in infusion site on buttocks within a year of starting Asp. Switched to lispro and used a different site. Applied pimecrolimus cream with little effect on LA.			

Table 1 Thirty-three lipoatrophy cases induced by detemir, aspart, detemir plus aspart, and NovoMix30 (Continued)

Reference	Description	
Ninnikoski et al. Finland 2010 [15]	15 yo boy with T1DM on CSII using Asp. Developed LA in infusion site on thighs within a year of starting Asp. Switched to glulisine and changed site. LA did not disappear.	
Ninnikoski et al. Finland 2010 [15]	10 yo girl with T1DM since age 5 years on CSII using Asp. Developed LA in infusion sites on thighs 4 yrs later. Switched to lispro and changed site. Applied Na cromoglycate with some improvement in LA.	
Babiker et al. UK 2011 [10]		4 yo Caucasian T1DM NovoMix 30. LA 2-3 yrs after insulin. LA in new injection sites when site changed
Babiker et al. UK 2011 [10]		5 yo Caucasian T1DM NovoMix 30. LA 3 yrs after insulin. LA in new injection sites with Lispro 25/75
Babiker et al. UK 2011 [10]	12 yo Caucasian T1DM Novorapid+ glargine. LA 3 yrs after insulin. Novorapid site only. Resolved when site changed	
Babiker et al. UK 2011 [10]	14 yo Caucasian T1DM Novorapid+detemir. LA 3 yrs after insulin. Detemir site only. LA when detemir changed to glargine.	
George PS et al. UK 2011 [16]	? yo woman with T1DM on CSII using Asp. Developed LA at infusion sites 2 years after initiation. Previously on MDI using glargine and Asp without LA.	
Yazdanyar S et al. Denmark 2011 [17]	17 yo girl with T1DM developed lipoatrophy at aspart infusion sites 1.5 years after starting CSII. Previously used Biphasic Asp. Switched to glulisine without lipoatrophy.	
Yazdanyar S et al. Denmark 2011 [17]	8 yo boy with T1DM developed LA as aspart infusion sites soon after starting CSII Previously used aspart, Biphasic aspart and glulisine without LA.	

Table 1 Thirty-three lipoatrophy cases induced by detemir, aspart, detemir plus aspart, and NovoMix30 (Continued)

Reference	Description
Yazdanyar S et al. Denmark 2011 [17]	7 yo girl with T1DM developed LA at Aspart infusion sites 10 months after starting CSII. Previously used Asp and Biphasic Asp without LA.
Tavare AN et al. UK 2011 [23]	53 yo Indian woman with T2DM developed LA at Asp + Det injection sites. Previously on NovoMix 30 with itching and erythema. Also developed LA (onset not stated) and local reaction to Lispro, Lispro 25/75, glargine and Human Mixtard 30.
Peteiro-Gonzalez D et al. Spain 2011 [18]	39 yo woman with T1DM on MDI-glargine and Asp. LA at Asp sites (thighs) 2 years after Asp therapy. Also had primary hypothyroidism and psoriasis. Biopsy and TNFα elevated.
Salma et al. France 2011 [19]	42 yo man with T1DM since age 7 yrs. After CSII for 14 months, he developed LA. Applied Na Cromoglycate and switshed to glulisine.
Swelheim et al. Netherlands 2012 [20]	7 yo female with T1DM CSII aspart. LA (few months later) in buttocks and thighs. Substituted with lispro with no benefit.
Suththanantha J et al. UK 2012 [21]	7 yo girl with T1DM developed LA at Asp infusion site when on CSII. Onset not mentioned.
Suththanantha et al. UK 2012 [21]	17 yo boy with T1DM developed LA at Asp injection sites (on MDI). Onset not mentioned. Had hypothyroidism and Addison's disease.
Agha et al. UK 2013 [11]	54 yo female with T1DM. Detemir in her thighs and Aspart in her abdomen. Lipoatrophy in her thighs. Hypoglycemia improved when injection site changed to abdomen.
Agha et al. UK 2013 [11]	29 yo female with T1DM. Detemir in her thighs and Aspart in her abdomen. Lipoatrophy in her thighs after 2.5 years.

Table 1 Thirty-three lipoatrophy cases induced by detemir, aspart, detemir plus aspart, and NovoMix30 (*Continued*)

Agha et al. UK 2013 [11]	26 yo T1DM woman on detemir and aspart developed LA at injection sites on her thighs. LA onset not mentioned
Agha et al. UK 2013 [11]	32 yo T1DM woman on detemir plus aspart developed LA at injection sites on her thighs. LA onset not mentioned.
Agha et al. UK 2013 [11]	64 yo female with T1DM. Detemir in her thighs for 8 years. LA in thighs 2-3 years after starting it.
Breznik et al. Slovenia 2013 [24]	62 yo T2DM woman on detemir plus aspart developed LA 5.5 yrs after starting insulin. Did not resolve spontaneously. Biopsy findings
Simeonovic M et al. UK and Australia 2014 [22]	3 yo girl with T1DM developed LA at Asp infusion site (buttock) when on CSII (after 1-3 yrs).
Simeonovic M et al. UK and Australia 2014 [22]	7 yo girl with T1DM developed LA at Asp infusion site (abdomen) when on CSII (1-3 yrs later).
Simeonovic M et al. UK and Australia 2014 [22]	8 yo girl with T1DM developed LA at Asp infusion site (thigh) when on CSII (after 1-3 yrs).
Simeonovic M et al. UK and Australia 2014 [22]	10 yo girl with T1DM developed LA at Asp infusion site (abdomen) when on CSII (after 1-3 yrs).
Saberi et al. USA 2014 (our report)	41 yo T1DM woman developed LA at injection sites on thighs, upper arms and abdomen 14 months after starting aspart and detemir MDI. When switched to CSII (Omnipod) using aspart LA developed within a year. When switched to CSII using glulisine LA developed after a year. When switched to CSII using lispro no new LA after 10 months. The original LA began to fill in when left alone.

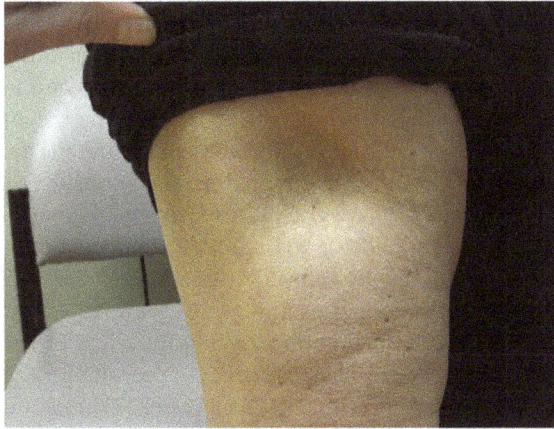

Fig. 2 Lipoatrophy on thigh in November 2012

Discussion

Based on our 2015 literature search of published reports, our adult female patient with T1DM may be the 5th published case of detemir plus aspart-induced lipoatrophy. Aspart was launched in 2000 and detemir in 2006. The first published report on detemir plus aspart-induced lipoatrophy in 2011 was followed by 3 more cases in 2013. Among the previously reported 4 adult female patients with detemir plus aspart-induced lipoatrophy, 2 had T1DM [11] and 2 had T2DM [23, 24]. When both detemir and aspart are injected in the same site, it is difficult to identify whether one or both of these insulin analogs induced the lipoatrophy as either can cause it. According to our patient, she injected aspart and detemir in the same sites and could not determine which insulin analog induced the lipoatrophy. When she was on CSII using aspart and then glulisine she also developed lipoatrophy at the infusion sites.

In the past, CSII was reported to treat lipoatrophy induced by human insulin [26]. Today, lipoatrophy induced

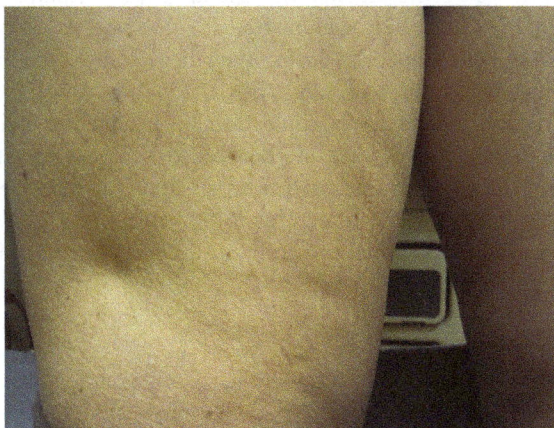

Fig. 3 Improved lipoatrophy on thigh in December 2014

by rapid-acting insulin analog is often associated with CSII. Two recent surveys reported 83.3 % [27] and 87 % [2] of patients with lipoatrophy induced by rapid-acting insulin analogs use CSII. In our report 18 of the 21 (85.7 %) cases of aspart-induced lipoatrophy were associated with CSII and only 3 cases injected aspart. The infusion may cause the lipoatrophy [22]. Together continuous exposure to insulin and continuous mechanical irritation by the infusion catheter may trigger events that lead to lipoatrophy. Some patients did not develop lipoatrophy when injecting aspart but did so when infusing aspart via CSII [17, 22]. Others develop lipoatrophy with both injection and infusion implying the delivery method does not matter. Our patient had aspart-induced lipoatrophy within a year at the infusion sites when on CSII. She also developed lipoatrophy at the infusion sites when infusing glulisine via CSII after a year. Ten months after infusing lispro via CSII, she has not developed lipoatrophy at the infusion sites. This may be because she has not infused lispro long enough (one year or longer) as lipoatrophy can develop from 4 weeks [9] to 5.5 years [24] after starting insulin. It may also be because lispro does not induce lipoatrophy in her. Although all 5 insulin analogs can induce lipoatrophy, some patients have lipoatrophy induced by one but not another [17].

Clinical presentation

Lipoatrophy is the loss of subcutaneous fat at insulin injection/infusion sites as demonstrated by biopsy [18, 28] and MRI [29]. In the past, 10 - 55 % of diabetic patients injecting impure bovine or porcine insulin developed lipoatrophy [1, 30]. With the availability of purer animal and human insulin, the prevalence of lipoatrophy decreased to 0.2-1.4 % [30, 31]. With insulin analog injections/infusions, the prevalence of lipoatrophy had been reported to be 2.5 % in a single center study [27] and 1.1 % in a multicenter survey [2].

There are no reported objective data for exact onset of insulin-induced lipoatrophy. The reported first observed onsets of insulin-induced lipoatrophy range from 4 weeks to 2 years [9], 2–3 to 23 months [26] to 6–24 months [1] after initiation of insulin therapy. In our literature search the first observed onsets of lipoatrophy range from 2 months to 5.5 years.

Lipoatrophy is more common in females in reported cases of lipoatrophy. In our review, the gender of 29 patients was identified. Of these 22 (75.8 %) were females and 7 males. Our patient is female. Why lipoatrophy is more prevalent in women remains unclear. There may be a reporting bias in this female gender predominance as this data is based on case reports and not clinical trials or MedWatch reports.

Lipoatrophy can overlap with other autoimmune diseases [21, 32]. Female T1DM patients with lipoatrophy have a higher risk of developing Hashimoto's thyroiditis and celiac disease [32]. Autoimmune diseases affect 8 % of the population and of these 78 % are females [33]. Whether lipoatrophy and autoimmune diseases in females share a common etiology remains to be established. In females with T1DM and insulin-induced lipoatrophy, the physician should screen for other autoimmune disease(s). Our patient has Hashimoto's thyroiditis with hypothyroidism; she does not have celiac disease or primary adrenal insufficiency.

Many of the reported cases of lipoatrophy induced by insulin analogs are in the pediatric population. Why this is remains unanswered. In our review, 20 (60.6 %) of the 33 cases were in the pediatric age group: 1 with detemir, 17 with aspart, and 2 with NovoMix 30. Like the previous 4 reported cases of lipoatrophy induced by detemir plus aspart injections, our case is an adult. Similarly, 4 of the 5 cases of lipoatrophy induced by detemir were adults. This probably reflects the age of patients using detemir plus aspart and detemir alone. Lipoatrophy more commonly occurs in T1DM partly because many cases are in the pediatric age group and possibly due to a potential immune-mediated inflammation causing lipoatrophy in patients with autoimmune type 1 diabetes. In our report, 31 of the 33 patients had T1DM and 2 had T2DM. Our patient has T1DM.

Lipohypertrophy sites from insulin injection can lead to impaired insulin absorption [34, 35]. To the best of our knowledge there are no published insulin absorption studies done in insulin analog-induced lipoatrophy sites. But, it is reasonable to expect variable insulin absorption in lipoatrophy sites with loss of adipose tissue, making glycemic control challenging. Some patients improved their glycemic control when insulin injection site is changed from the lipohypertrophy to an unaffected site [36]. One patient with lipoatrophy had improved glycemic control when the injection site was changed [11]. Another patient improved his glycemic control when given intraperitoneal insulin suggesting that the lipoatrophy may have been causing poor insulin absorption [37]. Changing the injection or cannula site in our patient did not significantly affect her glycemic control. Clinically, insulin-induced lipoatrophy can be cosmetically distressing and disfiguring to the patient. For these reasons, the clinician should inspect the insulin injection/infusion sites regularly to identify lipodystrophy (lipohypertrophy and/or lipoatrophy), especially in patients with erratic glycemic control, so measures to manage the problem and prevent the development of further areas of lipoatrophy can be implemented.

As all these are reported cases, the number of cases of lipoatrophy induced by each insulin analog cannot be compared. However, all insulin analogs can induce lipoatrophy.

Etiology

Many possible etiologies have been considered for insulin-induced lipoatrophy. These include cresol preservative in insulin, alcohol used for sterilization of syringes and needles, injury to the fat cells, glycolytic ferments in the insulin, possible nerve injury [38], mechanical trauma from repeat injections, and cryotrauma from cold insulin [10]. Immune etiologies have also been suggested - immune reaction to insulin [39, 40] and immune complex mediated inflammation [26]. Lipoatrophic lesions occurred in individuals using animal insulins who have high levels of circulating anti-insulin antibodies and the edges of lipoatrophy lesions were characterized by deposition of immunologic proteins within dermal vessel [39]. Although this had been questioned, a strong relationship between lipoatrophy and insulin antibodies was recently reported in adults with T2DM on recombinant human insulin or insulin analogs [41]. The immune-complex mediated inflammatory response involves local macrophage release of tumor necrosis factor α causing adipocyte dedifferentiation [26, 42] in patients using both animal and recombinant human insulin. Increased numbers of degranulating mast cells that stain positively for tryptase and chymase antibodies have also been seen in skin biopsies of patients with lipoatrophic sites of insulin analogs [43]. Histology has shown small adipocyte lobules with hyperplastic capillaries, loss of adipose tissue, areas of membranous lipodystrophy usually lined by an acellular homogeneous eosinophilic material and a focal lymphoid cell infiltration abutting hypodermis blood vessels [26, 44] in patients using both animal and human insulins. Although several studies have demonstrated a possible immune basis to the etiology of lipoatrophy, there are others which do not. Jermendy et al. reported absence of inflammatory cells and no local immune mechanisms in the biopsy specimen [44]. Milan et al. suggested that adipose tissue metabolic changes play a role in lipoatrophy as they did not identify any inflammatory cells in the skin biopsy specimens of their three T1DM patients with lipoatrophy by insulin analogs [28]. This study demonstrated a decrease in fat cell volume with adipocytes losing their lipid content leading to the hypothesis that adipocytes chronically exposed to high local insulin levels could develop insulin resistance resulting in an increase in the lipolytic process causing lipoatrophy. A significant down-regulation of leptin expression along with an increase in free fatty acid was also seen which was thought to result in the recruitment of fat cell precursors [28].

Treatment

A change in insulin formulation, avoiding injections in the lipoatrophy sites (our patient noted this when the Omnipod was used near the sites), and changing the insulin needle daily have helped resolve lipoatrophy in some patients [3]. There are also case reports of adding glucocorticoid therapy such as dexamethasone or beta-methasone to the insulin analog [20, 45]; but this can cause blood glucose fluctuations if the betamethasone/insulin analog solution becomes inhomogenous resulting in erratic insulin administration [20]. Administering low-dose oral glucocorticoid such as prednisone 5–10 mg daily [46, 47] has also been used to improve lipoatrophy. Corticosteroids are able to induce differentiation of adi-pocytes and have immune-modulating properties [45]. However, addition of glucocorticoid therapy can result in worsening glycemic control and increased insulin re-quirements [20]. Our patient declined the recommen-dation of using steroids. Yet, with time and not using the lipoatrophy sites, the original lipoatrophy began to improve (Fig. 3).

Changing the mode of insulin delivery, such as using CSII, can potentially improve lipoatrophy in patients using human insulin injections [48]. However, in our literature review, 18 of the 21 cases of lipoatrophy in-duced by aspart were associated with CSII which has been hypothesized to contribute to the development of lipoatrophy [22]. Why the largest increase in aspart-induced lipoatrophy occurred in those on CSII remains unclear. There may be a reporting bias in this group as this data is based on case reports and not clinical trials and Medwatch reports. Our patient developed lipoatro-phy when on CSII using aspart and glulisine.

In 2 small studies topical 4 % sodium cromolyn in pet-rolatum solvent was partially effective therapy for early lipoatrophy areas and prevention of the development of new such areas [43, 49]. Our literature review described 2 other cases of lipoatrophy induced by aspart which im-proved with sodium cromolyn therapy [15, 19]. Cromolyn stabilizes mast cells that are tryptase-positive/chymase-positive and prevents the release of histamine in the pres-ence of antigen-IgE antibody reactions [43].

Finally, 2 case reports described treatment of insulin-induced lipoatrophy. The first one is treating lipoatrophy successfully with an insulin jet –injector [50]. In an extremely refractory case Noud et al. used intraperito-neal insulin delivered by Diaport [37]. Inhaled insulin can potentially be used in patients with lipoatrophy in-duced by injected insulin. Lipoatrophy was not described as an adverse event in the Afreeza® product monograph [51]. We are aware that in Afreeza® trials high anti-insulin antibodies titers were documented. To the best of our knowledge no case of insulin lipoatrophy has been described in the Afreeza® clinical trials. Possible explanations for this include [a] without repeated injec-tions of insulin no atrophy occurs despite the high insu-lin antibodies tiers; [b] an uncommon complication like insulin induced lipoatrophy may not appear in the lim-ited number of patients who have used Afreeza thus far;

and [c] the association of high insulin antibodies titers and injected insulin lipoatrophy does not imply a cause-effect association.

Conclusion

Our case may be the 5th case of detemir plus aspart in-duced lipoatrophy and possibly the first published case report of glulisine induced lipoatrophy. In prescribing in-formation for Apidra [7] lipoatrophy was mentioned. There are 30 new published cases of aspart, detemir, dete-mir plus aspart and NovoMix induced lipoatrophy since 2009. These represent only a percentage of the cases of lipoatrophy induced by these insulin analogs. The ISPAD survey [2], the single center study [27] and the recent Rosenbloom recidivus [38] mentioned many cases (some due to these insulin analogs) which have not been pub-lished. To better understand insulin analog-induced lipoa-trophy, more research on the prevalence of this cutaneous complication of insulin therapy, its etiology, pathogenesis and management need to be conducted. It is unrealistic to expect every case of insulin analog induced lipoatrophy to be published. But, sharing of data on reported, but not published, cases can be helpful.

Competing interests
The authors declare that they have no competing interests.

Authors' contributions
SS, NHE, MHT all wrote the manuscript. MM did the literature search. MHT and NHE reviewed each of the 520 citations and concurred on those identified as lipoatrophy induced by insulin analog aspart, detemir, detemir plus aspart and NovoMix 30 injections. All authors read and approved the final manuscript.

Author details
[1]Ann Arbor Endocrinology and Diabetes, PC, Ypsilanti, Michigan, USA. [2]Division of Metabolism, Endocrinology and Diabetes, University of Michigan, Lobby C, 24 Frank Lloyd Wright Drive, Ann Arbor, MI 48106, USA. [3]Taubman Health Sciences Library, University of Michigan, Ann Arbor, Michigan, USA.

References
1. Richardson T, Kerr D. Skin-Related Complications of Insulin Therapy. Epidemiology and Emerging Management Strategies. Am J Clin Dermatol. 2003;4:661–7.
2. Forsander GA, Malmodin OC, Kordonouri O, Ludvigsson J, Klingensmith G, Beaufort CD. An ISPAD survey of insulin-induced lipoatrophy [Abstract]. Pediatr Diabetes. 2013;14 Suppl 18:20.
3. Ampudia-Blasco FJ, Girbes J, Carmena R. A case of lipoatrophy with insulin glargine: Long-acting insulin analogs are not exempt from this complication. Diabetes Care. 2005;28:2983.
4. del Olmo MI, Campos V, Abellan P, Merino-Torres JF, Pinon F. A case of lipoatrophy with insulin detemir. Diabetes Res and Clin Pract. 2008;80:e20–1.
5. Griffin ME, Feder A, Tambolane WV. Lipoatrophy Associated With Lispro Insulin In Insulin Pump Therapy. An old complication, a new cause? Diabetes Care. 2001;24:174.
6. Szypowska A, Skórka A, Pańkowska E. Lipoatrophy associated with rapid-acting insulin analogues in young patients with Type 1 diabetes mellitus. Endokrynol Diabetol Chor Przemiany Materii Wieku Rozw. 2008;14:117–8.
7. Apidra Prescribing Information http://products.sanofi.us/apidra/apidra.html Accessed January 17, 2015.

8. Hussein SF, Siddique H, Coates P, Green. Lipoatrophy is a thing of the past, or is it? Diabet Med. 2007;24:1470–2.

9. Holstein A, Stege H, Kovacs P. Lipoatrophy associated with the use of insulin analogues: a new case associated with the use of insulin glargine and review of the literature. Expert Opin Drug Saf. 2010;9:225–31.

10. Babiker A, Datta V. Lipoatrophy with insulin analogues in type 1 diabetes. Arch Dis Child. 2011;96:101–2.

11. Agha A, Duffield E, Elrishi M. Detemir insulin related lipoatrophy: a case series. Pract Diabetes. 2013;30:296.

12. Kesavadev J, Kumar A, Ahammed S, Dinkar G, Jothydev S. Insulin Aspart Induced Lipoatrophy in a Patient on Insulin Pump [Abstract]. Diabetes. 2008;57 Suppl 1:578.

13. Bocca G, Westerlaken C. Good result for betamethasone added to an insulin analog, as treatment for insulin analog induced lipoatrophy. Report of a case [Abstract]. Horm Res. 2009;72:501–2.

14. Chang YT, Evans B, D'Arcangelo MR, Milstein MT, Gabbay RA. Lipoastrophy in a girl after switching insulin analog injection to a pump [Abstract]. Diabetes. 2010;59:A695.

15. Niinikoski H, Nanto-Salonen K, Ruusu P, Kinnala A, Putto-Launla A, Keskinen JTJP. Insuliinhoiden lapsille ainheuttama lipoatrofia. Duodecim. 2010;126:1328–32.

16. George PS, Robertson M, Grant L, Mackie ADR. Lipoatrophy associated with insulin aspart in continuous subcutaneous insulin infusion. Pract Diab Int. 2011;28:108.

17. Yazdanyar S, Dolmer BS, Strauss G. Three children with lipoatrophy associated with human rapid-acting insulin analogues. Eur J Pediat Dermatol. 2011;21:11–5.

18. Peteiro-Gonzalez D, Fernandez-Rodriguez B, Cabezas-Agricola JM, Araujo-Vilar D. Severe localized lipoatrophy related to therapy with insulin analogs in type 1a diabetes mellitus. Diab Res Clin Prac. 2011;91:e61–3.

19. Salma B, Plat F, Bourrel F, Sanchez M, Bernamo E. Succes d'un traitement par chromoglycate de sodium dans un cas de lipoatrophie insulinique sous pompe externe a insulin [Abstract]. Diabetes Metab. 2011;37:A97.

20. Swelheim HT, Westerlaken C, van Pinxteren-Nagler E, Bocca G. Lipoatrophy in a girl with type 1 diabetes mellitus: Beneficial effect of treatment with a glucocorticoid added to an insulin analog. Diabetes Care. 2012;35, e2.

21. Suththarantha J, Puthi VR, Walton S. Severe lipoatrophy complicating insulin analogue treatment: first reported case of lipoatrophy complicating the administration of insulin aspart via continuous subcutaneous insulin infusion (CSII) [Abstract]. Horm Res. 2012;78 Suppl 1:163–4.

22. Simeonovic M, Anuar A, Edge J, Makaya T. Lipoatrophy: re-emerging with analogue insulins, Is there a link with CSII? Pract Diabetes. 2014;31:164–6.

23. Tavare AN, Doolittle HJ, Baburaj R. Pan-insulin allergy and severe lipoatrophy complicating type 2 diabetes. Diabet Med. 2011;28:500–3.

24. Breznik V, Kokol R, Luzar B, Miljkovic J. Insulin-induced localized lipoatrophy. Acta Dermatovenerol APA. 2013;22:83–5.

25. Patel C, Koenig S. Medical Information Novo Nordisk Inc. Novemeber 12, 2014 (personal communication).

26. Radermecker RP, Pierard GE, Scheen AJ. Lipodystrophy Reactions to Insulin: Effects of Continuous Insulin Infusion and New Insulin Analogs. Am J Clin Dermatol. 2007;8:21–8.

27. Schnell K, Biester T, Tsioli C, Datz N, Danne T, Kordonouri O. Lipoatrophy in a large pediatric diabetes outpatient service [Abstract]. Pediatr Diabetes. 2013;14(Suppl18):20.

28. Milan G, Murano I, Costa S, Pianta A, Tiengo C, Zulato E, et al. Lipoatrophy Induced by Subcutaneous Insulin Infusion: Ultrastructural Analysis and Gene Expression Profiling. J Clin Endocrinol and Metab. 2010;95:3126–32.

29. Sackey AH. Injection-Site Lipoatrophy. N Engl J Med. 2009;361:19 e41.

30. Schernthaner G. Immunogenicity and Allergenic Potential of Animal and Human Insulins. Diabetes Care. 1993;16 Suppl 3:155–65.

31. Hajheydari Z, Kashi Z, Akha O, Akbarzadeh S. Frequency of lipodysdrophy induced by recombinant human insulin. Eur Rev Med Pharmacol. 2011;15:1196–201.

32. Salgin B, Meissner T, Beyer P, Haberland H, Borkenstein M, Fussenegger J, et al. Lipoatrophy is Associated with an Increased Risk of Hashimoto's thyroiditis and Coeliac Disease in Female Patients with Type 1 Diabetes. Horm Res Paediatr. 2013;79:368–72.

33. Fairweather DL, Frisancho-Kiss S, Rose NR. Sex differences in Autoimmune Disease from a Pathological Perspective. Am J Pathol. 2008;173:600–9.

34. Johansson UB, Amsberg S, Hannerz L, Wredling R, Admason U, Arnqvist HJ, et al. Impaired Absorption of Insulin Aspart From Lipohypertrophic injection sites. Diabetes Care. 2005;28:2025–7.

35. Heinemann L. Insulin Absorption from Lipodystrophic Areas: A (Neglected) Source of Trouble for Insulin Therapy. J Diab Sci Technology. 2010;4:750–3.

36. Chowdhury TA, Escudier V. Poor glycemic control caused by insulin-induced lipohypertrophy. Br Med J. 2003;327:383–4.

37. Noud MN, Renard E, McBride C, Cotterill AM, Harris M. Benefits of intra-peritoneal insulin administration in a child with severe insulin-induced lipoatrophy [Abstract]. Pediat Diabetes. 2009;10 Suppl 11:100.

38. Rosenbloom AL. Insulin Injection Lipoatrophy Recidivus. Pediat Diabetes. 2014;15:73–4.

39. Reeves WG, Allen BR, Tatterstall RB. Insulin induced lipoatrophy: evidence for an immune pathogenesis. Br Med J. 1980;280:1500–3.

40. Raile K, Noelle V, Landgraf R, Schwarz HP. Insulin antibodies are associated with lipoatrophy but also with lipohypertrophy in children and adolescents with type 1diabetes. Exp Clin Endocrinol Diab. 2001;109:393–6.

41. Takahashi K, Hakozaki A, Narazaki M, Takebe N, Ishigaki Y. Insulin antibodies are associated with lipoatrophy in adults with type 2 diabetes mellitus [Abstract]. Diabetologia. 2014;57 Suppl 1:S396.

42. Atlan-Gepner C, Bongrand P, Farnarier C, Xerri L, Choux R, Gauthier JF, et al. Insulin-induced Lipoatrophy in Type 1 Diabetes: A possible tumor necrosis factor- α- mediated dedifferentiation of adiposities. Diabetes Care. 1996;19:1283–5.

43. Lopez X, Castells M, Ricker A, Velazquez EF, Mun E, Goldfine A. Human Insulin Analog-Induced Lipoatrophy. Diabetes Care. 2008;31(3):442–4.

44. Jermendy G, Nadas J, Sapi Z. "Lipoblastoma-like" lipoatrophy induced by human insulin: morphological evidence for dedifferentiation of adipocytes? Diabetologia. 2000;43:955–6.

45. Ramos AJS, Farias MA. Human Insulin-Induced Lipoatrophy: A successful treatment with glucocorticoid. Diabetes Care. 2006;29:926–7.

46. Chantelau EA, Praetor R, Praetor J, Poll LW. Relapsing insulin-induced lipoatrophy, cured by prolonged low-dose oral prednisone: a case report. Diabetol Metab Syndr. 2011;3:33–7.

47. Chantelau EA, Prator R, Prator J. Insulin-induced localized lipoatrophy preceded by shingles (herpes zoster): a case report. J of Med Case Rep. 2014;8:223–8.

48. Chantelau E, Reuter M, Schotes S, Stark AA. Severe lipoatrophy with human insulin successfully treated by CSII. Diabet Med. 1993;10:580–1.

49. Phua EJ, Lopez X, Ramus J, Goldfine AB. Cromoyln Sodium for Insulin-Indueced Lipoatrophy: Old Drug, New Use. Diabetes Care. 2013;36:e204–5.

50. Logwin S, Conget L, Jansa M, Vidal M, Nicolau C, Gomis R. Human Insulin Induced Lipoatrophy, Successful treatment with a jet-injection device. Diabetes Care. 1996;19:255–6.

51. Afreeza Prescribing Information. http://products.sanofi.us/afrezza/afrezza.html. Accessed June 21 2015.

7

Can a single interactive seminar durably improve knowledge and confidence of hospital diabetes management?

Timothy W. Bodnar[2], Jennifer J. Iyengar[3], Preethi V. Patil[3] and Roma Y. Gianchandani[1,3*]

Abstract

Background: Safe and effective diabetes management in the hospital is challenging. Inadequate knowledge has been identified by trainees as a key barrier. In this study we assess both the short-term and long-term impact of an interactive seminar on medical student knowledge and comfort with hospital diabetes management.

Methods: An interactive seminar covering hospital diabetes management and utilizing an audience response system was added to the third-year medical student curriculum. Students were given a multiple choice assessment immediately before and after the seminar to assess their comprehension of the material. Students were also asked to rate their confidence on this topic. Approximately 6 months later, students were given the same assessment to determine if the improvements in hospital diabetes knowledge and confidence were durable over time. Students from the preceding medical school class, who did not have a hospital diabetes seminar as a part of their curriculum, were used as a control.

Results: Fifty–three students participated in the short-term assessment immediately before and after the seminar. The mean score (maximum 15) was 7.7 +/- 2.7 (51%) on the pre-test and 11.4 +/- 1.8 (76%) on the post-test ($p < 0.01$). 75 students who attended the seminar completed the same set of questions 6 months later with mean score of 9.2 ± 2.3 (61%). The control group of 100 students who did not attend seminar had a mean score of 8.8 ± 2.5 (58%). The difference in scores between the students 6-months after the seminar and the control group was not significantly different ($p = 0.30$).

Conclusions: Despite initial short-term gains, a single seminar on hospital diabetes management did not durably improve trainee knowledge or confidence. Addition of repeated and focused interactions during clinical rotations or other sustained methods of exposure need to be evaluated.

Keywords: Diabetes, Glycemic Management, Medical Education, Medical Students

Background

Patients with diabetes account for a disproportionally high percentage of inpatient stays, estimated at 22% of hospital inpatient days in the United States [1]. Both hyperglycemia and hypoglycemia remain common problems among admitted patients with diabetes and have been associated with poor clinical outcomes [2, 3]. Therefore, effective glycemic management in the hospital is an important safety and quality care measure for patient outcomes. The management of diabetes in the inpatient setting poses several unique challenges including fluctuating nutritional status, confounding medications, and presence of other acute and chronic illnesses. Insulin is one of the most common drugs implicated in preventable adverse drug events in the hospital [4]. As the prevalence of diabetes continues to grow, it is imperative that trainees, regardless of fields of practice, are well versed in diabetes management.

Although resident physicians acknowledge the importance of glycemic management in the hospital, there are several identifiable barriers to the attainment of target glucose levels [5–7]. One of the cited barriers to

* Correspondence: romag@umich.edu
[1]24 Frank Lloyd Wright Drive, P.O. Box 482, Ann Arbor, MI 48106, USA
[3]University of Michigan Health System, Ann Arbor, MI, USA
Full list of author information is available at the end of the article

improved inpatient glycemic management among residents is lack of knowledge of appropriate insulin regimens [6, 7]. A survey of medicine residents found that less than half reported that hospital diabetes management was explicitly addressed in their residency and 97% of responded that they would like this training to be included in the curriculum [8]. This finding is not unique to a single instituition or even the United States, with several studies nationally and internationally noting concerns about the comfort and preparedness of physicians and trainees to manage inpatient diabetes [9–11].

Several previously published interventions have targeted trainees at resident physician level in an effort to improve trainee knowledge of inpatient glycemic management. Such interventions have incorporated a variety of educational formats including the use of computer-based modules [12, 13], case-based training [14], mobile device-based educational tool [15], and a comprehensive longitudinal curriculum [16]. While many of these studies had positive outcomes as measured by improvement in diabetes knowledge and comfort among trainees or improvements in measured glycemic control on the wards, there is a limited data on the long-term durability of any improvements. Similarly, short-term medical education interventions have been studied for non-diabetes topics, but have also failed to examine long-term retention [17–19]. Many of the previous diabetes studies focused only on internal medicine resident physicians, despite evidence that trainees in other specialities demonstrate less knowledge of hospital diabetes management [10]. Given the rise of diabetes and hyperglycemia in the hospital, it is increasingly important that trainees of many specialties become knowledgeable and comfortable with hospital diabetes management.

We hypothesized that targeting students earlier in their medical training would help reduce the gap in hospital diabetes knowledge across specialties. However, in order for such an intervention to be effective beyond medical school, students would need gains in knowledge and confidence to be durable. Similar to studies of trainees at the resident physician level, there is evidence that medical students also lack knowledge in hospital diabetes. A study by Landsang et al of fourth year medical students found notable knowledge gaps including failure to recognize stress hyperglycemia and frequent recommendation the use of sliding scale insulin without scheduled basal bolus insulin [20]. This study also found students were less likely to provide appropriate management of diabetes than they were to other commonly encountered clinical problems such as chest pain or hypertension. A well-designed study by MacEwen et al found that a "Diabetes Day" with lectures and learning tutorials improved diabetes knowledge

and comfort in medical students in the UK [21]. However, they did not look at long-term maintenance of knowledge. We developed an interactive seminar on hospital diabetes management for the third-year medical student curriculum and evaluated if this would durably improve knowledge and confidence related to this topic.

Methods
Setting and population
The University of Michigan Medical School (UMMS), in Ann Arbor, MI, USA, enrolls approximately 170–175 students per class per year, for a combined enrollment between 650 and 710 students during a particular academic year. In-state students vary between approximately 45–55% for a given class, and the percentage of female students has ranged from 45 to 55% over fiscal years 2011–2015 [22]. UMMS students match into a wide variety of postgraduate training programs, with the top 5 (in descending order) from 2008-2012 being: Internal Medicine, Pediatrics, Emergency Medicine, Anesthesiology, and Family Practice [23].

Through at least the 2013–2014 academic year, the curriculum at UMMS consists of 2 years of preclinical training (in classroom and laboratory settings) and 2 years of clinical training (in patient care settings) including required clerkships such as Surgery, Obstetrics & Gynecology, Psychiatry, and Internal Medicine. During the entirety of the M3 year, M3 students have protected time on Friday afternoons for a mandatory lecture series entitled, "The M3 Seminar Series." All M3 students, regardless of current clerkship or rotation, meet for a series of seminars on important medical and humanistic topics. The curriculum for the M3 Seminar Series has evolved over time in response to changing educational needs, student evaluations of individual seminars, and student and faculty requests for individual topics. The first seminar given on hospital diabetes management was given during the 2012–2013 academic year, meaning that the M3 students graduating in 2014 attended this seminar, while the M4 students graduating in 2013 (who were M3 students during the 2011–2012 academic year) did not experience this seminar or anything similar.

The M3 seminar covering hospital diabetes management is the only formal didactic experience on this topic that all UMMS students receiving during their clinical training (M3 and M4 years). All other training on this topic is less formal and more experiential ("on the job" training during clinical clerkships, subinternships, and electives), and thus, may be more variable from student to student.

Intervention

The authors created an approximately 90-min interactive session, utilizing didactic slides covering important concepts necessary for safe and effective hospital diabetes management (including an evidence-based approach) of non-critically ill patients, as well as a series of interactive cases to illustrate some key concepts. The interactive cases incorporated an electronic audience remote response system to encourage audience participation. This presentation underwent a series of edits amongst the authorship group, with input from colleagues in the Division of Metabolism, Endocrinology, and Diabetes within the Department of Internal Medicine at UMMS. This seminar had a didactic component taught by an endocrinology faculty member (RYG) and the cases by endocrinology trainees (TWB and JJI). This presentation has been published online [24]. The educational objectives of the seminar are listed in Fig. 1 using Bloom's Taxonomy.

Assessment

The assessment tool was also developed by the authors. Although several excellent assessment tools have been published in the past by other groups [13, 16, 21, 25, 26], the authors felt it was important to tailor the content of the assessment to the material in the presentation, which covered non-acute inpatient diabetes management and did not include acute topics like DKA or HHS or more advanced resident-level topics like peripartum glycemic management. The 15 multiple-choice questions (each with one correct answer choice and 3 incorrect answer choices) were formulated to cover critical pieces of knowledge as deemed important by the authors and colleagues, with combined decades of experience managing diabetes in the hospital setting. The 3 questions asking participants to rate their confidence managing diabetes, blood pressure, and electrolyte disturbances in the hospital were chosen to assess whether the addition of the seminar improved confidence managing diabetes (experimental group compared to control group) and whether any improvement was seen relative to other problems often managed in the hospital setting (but which, like type 2 diabetes, are much less often the primary reason for admission).

Questions were vetted through the assistance of the Medical Education Scholars Program, a faculty development seminar for expertise in medical education at UMMS. Writing quiz/survey questions is a key part of the curriculum for this group. Questions deemed confusing or vague by the group (consisting of UMMS

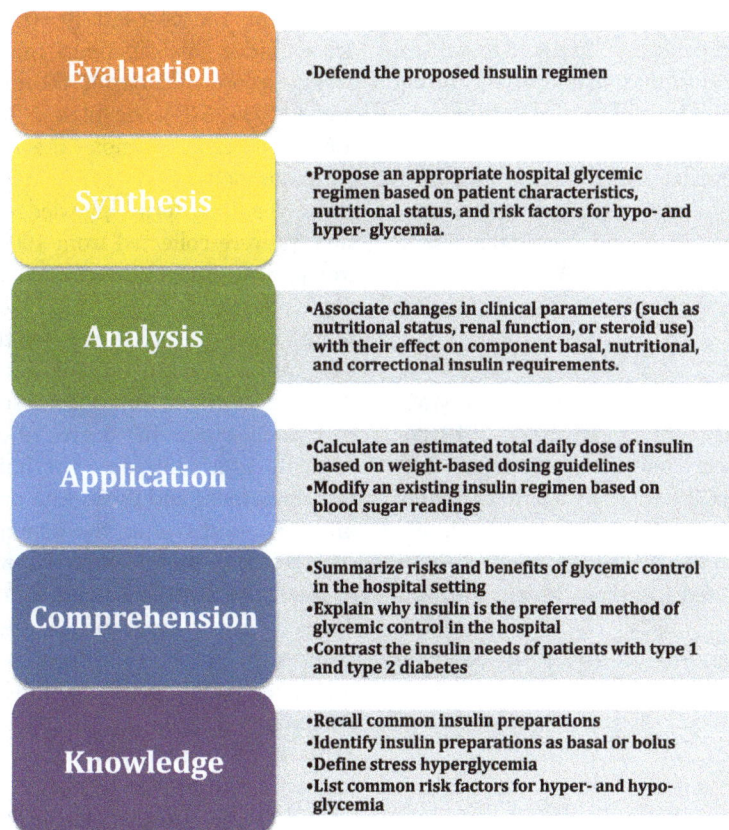

Evaluation
•Defend the proposed insulin regimen

Synthesis
•Propose an appropriate hospital glycemic regimen based on patient characteristics, nutritional status, and risk factors for hypo- and hyper- glycemia.

Analysis
•Associate changes in clinical parameters (such as nutritional status, renal function, or steroid use) with their effect on component basal, nutritional, and correctional insulin requirements.

Application
•Calculate an estimated total daily dose of insulin based on weight-based dosing guidelines
•Modify an existing insulin regimen based on blood sugar readings

Comprehension
•Summarize risks and benefits of glycemic control in the hospital setting
•Explain why insulin is the preferred method of glycemic control in the hospital
•Contrast the insulin needs of patients with type 1 and type 2 diabetes

Knowledge
•Recall common insulin preparations
•Identify insulin preparations as basal or bolus
•Define stress hyperglycemia
•List common risk factors for hyper- and hypo- glycemia

Fig. 1 Educational objectives for the seminar organized by Bloom's Taxonomy

faculty members in a variety of medical specialties) were re-written or discarded. Finally, colleagues in the Division of Metabolism, Endocrinology, and Diabetes within the Department of Internal Medicine at UMMS also reviewed the questions. See Additional file 1 for multiple choice questions, answer choices, and correct answers.

Experimental group

The experimental group consisted of students at UMMS during the 2013–2014 academic year (2013–2014 cohort) who attended the M3 seminar covering hospital diabetes management. Short-term changes in knowledge among the experimental group were assessed by administering the assessment tool immediately before and after the seminar, with responses collected using an audience reponse system. Although students were required to attend the seminar as part of their M3 curriculum, participation in the pre- and post- assessment was voluntary. In order to assess the long-term impact of the seminar, students who attended the M3 seminar were recruited via group email approximately 6-months after seminar completion for reassessment. Any student who attended the seminar was allow to complete the long-term assessment, not just those who have previously participated in pre- and post-test assessment. These students, now in their M4 year, were given the same 18-question assessment used in the pre- and post- test. In order to control for improvement in diabetes that might occur during sub-interships training or other clinical rotations, the long-term assessment was timed such that it was administered after the majority of students would have completed their subinternship training (similar to the control group). Students completing the long-term assessment were entered into a raffle for $25 Amazon.com gift cards to encourage participation.

Control group

The control group consisted of M4 students at UMMS during the 2012–2013 academic year (2012–2013 cohort). These students, recruited via group email during the 2nd half of their 4th year of medical school (2012–2013 school year), did not have hospital diabetes management as a formal component of their curriculum. They completed the same 18-question assessment tool as the experimental group and were also incentivized for participation with a $25 Amazon.com gift card raffle.

Statistical analysis

For the knowledge-based questions, the score was calculated by summing the number of correct responses out of a maximum possible score of 15. For the confidence questions, responses were scored using a range from 1–4, 1: extremely unconfident and 4: extremely confident. The short-term (pre- and post-test) responses for the experimental group were compared using a two-tailed paired t-test. To compare the experiemental group to the control group, a student's T-test and Wilcoxon Mann Whitney test were used. Comparison of responses on individual questionnaire items were made using a Fischer's exact test.

Finally, to determine the relationship between the knowledge score and confidence score a proportional odds model was fitted to the data. The model included the main effects group and aggregate knowledge score and the interaction terms. All statistical analysis was performed using the statistical software SPSS version 19 or the Real Statistics Resource Pack for Excel.

Results

With regards to the short-term knowledge assessment, 69 students participated in the pre- and post-test assessment using the audience reponse system. Of these, the 53 students who completed at least half of both the pre- and post-test questions were included the in the analysis; on average students included in the study attemped 13.2 +/- 1.8 pre-test questions and 14.2 +/- 1.4 post-test questions. The mean score out of 15 questions was 7.7 +/- 2.7 (51.2%) on the pre-test and 11.4 +/- 1.8 (75.7%) on the post-test ($p < 0.01$). If missing responses are excluded this difference remains significant with an average score of 58% for the pre-test and 80% for the post-test ($p < 0.01$). See Table 1 for the percentage correct for individual item among the 15 multiple-choice knowledge questions.

For the long-term knowledge durability assessment, surveys were collected from 100 students from the control group (2012–2013 cohort) and 75 students in the experimental group (2013–2014 cohort). This represented a 60% response rate for the control group and a 44% response rate from the experimental group. Given that the audience response system is annonymous we cannot determine the degree of overlap between the the students who completed the immediate pre- and post-test assessment and those who participated in the assessment 6-months after the seminar. However, both are representative samples out of the estimated 175 students in total who attended the seminar. The mean number of correct answers (out of 15 questions) in the control group was 8.8 ± 2.5 (58%) compared to 9.2 ± 2.3 (61%) in the experimental group at 6-months after the seminar. Percentage correct for individual items are listed in Table 1. The experimental group in the immediate post-test scored significantly higher than the control group with $p < 0.01$. However, there was no significant difference between the experimental group at 6-months and the control group. ($p = 0.30$).

Table 1 Percentage of correct responses to individual questions according to group

	Experimental Group			Control Group	P-value
	Pre-Test	Post-Test	6 months-Post	M4 Controls	6 months-Post vs Control
Which answer choice contains *only* basal insulin?	60	92	85	84	0.84
Which answer choice contains *only* bolus insulin?	66	85	84	83	1
What is the difference between prandial insulin and correction insulin?	68	89	92	94	0.76
What is the difference between basal insulin and bolus insulin?	83	87	87	88	0.82
When a patient is made NPO, which type of insulin order should *always* be held?	58	91	80	80	1
For a patient with Type 1 Diabetes, which type of insulin order should *never* be completely held?	66	98	88	81	0.29
Upon admitting a patient with Type 2 Diabetes to a general care unit, what is the appropriate initial strategy for oral anti-diabetes medications?	49	94	72	51	*0.01*
What is the approximate duration of action of regular insulin?	25	30	24	36	0.1
What is the approximate duration of action of insulin aspart/Novo log and lispro/Humalog?	13	23	28	24	0.6
What is the approximate duration of action of insulin glargine/Lantus?	55	89	65	65	1
What is the approximate duration of action of NPH insulin?	51	42	40	32	0.34
As a starting point, which range of calculations can you use to estimate insulin total daily dose (TDD) for a patient with diabetes?	47	92	52	39	0.09
As a starting point, how should total daily dose (TDD) of insulin be divided?	60	83	59	59	1
What is 70/30 insulin?	51	60	47	56	0.23
Systemic steroids impact all blood sugars the *greatest* impact is on which?	15	81	12	4	0.08
Overall	51	76	61	58	0.3

There was also no significant difference in student-reported confidence in managing type 2 diabetes between the experimental group at 6-months after the seminar and the control group. Confidence scores for managing type 2 diabetes trailed scores for managing blood pressure and electrolyte imbalances in the hospital (Table 2). Confidence level in treating type 2 diabetes in the hospital increased with increasing knowledge score for the 15 diabetes knowledge questions (OR = 1.84, P = 0.02) across cohorts. There was no similar increase in the confidence level in treating electrolyte imbalance and blood pressure.

Table 2 Mean student-reported confidence scores

	Control group (n = 100)	Experimental group (n = 75)	P-value
Confidence level			
Managing Type 2 Diabetes	2.01 ± 0.77	2.17 ± 0.76	0.16
Managing electrolyte imbalances	2.48 ± 0.70	2.56 ± 0.70	0.57
Managing blood pressure	2.73 ± 0.55	2.80 ± 0.68	0.45

Items assessed on a scale of 1–4, where 1 = extremely UNconfident/always need supervisor assistance, 2 = somewhat UNconfident/often need supervisor assistance, 3 = somewhat confident/occasionally need supervisor assistance, 4 = extremely confident/almost never need supervisor assistance
P–value was obtained by Wilcoxon Mann Whitney test

Discussion

The addition of an interactive seminar as a madantory part of the 3rd year medical school curriculum resulted in short-term improvement in knowledge of hospital diabetes management, as evidenced by a significant improvement in scores on multiple choice questions from the pre-test to the post-test assessment. Students on the post-test also scored significantly higher than the control group of students from the preceding medical school class who did not participate in the seminar. However, when students were given the same set of questions 6 months later, scores declined, and were no better than the control group. Several previous studies assessing short-term educational interventions and exclusively evaluating short-term outcomes have reported similar findings [15, 21, 27, 28]. This may represent effective presentations and/or the advantages of short-term memory.

Very few studies have evaluated the long-term impact of an intervention on trainee knowledge of hospital diabetes management. Our study suggests that evaluating only short-term post-intervention data can overestimate the impact of a single-session of educational intervention. We were asked to bolster the medical student curriculum by specifically focusing on hospital diabetes management. The authors (TWB, JJI, RYG) had noticed a lack of knowledge and comfort managing diabetes in the hospital amongst trainees in our institution, so we chose to assess not only the short-term gains in knowledge and confidence, but also the long-term gains. Despite an immediate improvement, students scored no better when reassesed 6 months later in comparison to the control cohort (which did not have the inpatient diabetes seminar in their curriculum).

Our study fills an important gap in the existing literature by demonstrating a lack of durability of improvement following an interactive seminar. This may explain the disconnect between the positive findings in many of the educational intervention studies and the fact that many trainees still report feeling ill-equipped to manage the diabetes scenarios they encounter in the hospital. Since the hospital teams are not comfortable managing diabetes there is not much opportunity to address this gap during medical student clerkships on the inpatient floors.

Our study results also that medical educational interventions in hospital diabetes should should consider a more longitudinal addition to the curriculum, perhaps with an even greater component of active learning, an idea reflected in the findings of a qualitative study of medical student learning by Luscombe and Montgomery [29]. We point out that diabetes and hyperglycemia is ubiquitous in the hospital environment, and despite ongoing exposure to the topic, knowledge gains after our interactive seminar were not durable. One could hypothesize that topics encountered less frequently may suffer more from loss of knowledge gains. It may not be reassuring, but rather alarming, to learn that putting substantial effort into bolstering a curriculum with a single seminar may not "move the needle" much in the long run.

To our knowledge there has only been one previously published study which examined the durability of a short-term educational intervention to improve inpatient diabetes knowledge. Tamler and colleagues used computer-based modules to educate internal medicine residents on hospital diabetes management. While they did find their intervention durably improved scores on a multiple choice question assessment, they were unique in that they administered a refresher course to residents several months after completing the initial course. They noted that topics that were not included in the refresher and not frequently encountered on the wards had declining scores over time. Their study supports our data and suggests that the addition of a refresher course could be one way to improve the durability of our initial knowledge gains [30].

The longest follow up after an intervention associated with hospital diabetes management education was a study using a two-pronged approach. One was an endocrinologist rounding with general medicine residents two times a day for 2 weeks on the diabetes patients admitted to the hospital. The second was to provide medicine residents with pocket cards outlining hospital diabetes management guidelines. Their dual effort improved diabetes knowledge and also reduced hyperglycemia in hospitalized diabetes patients over a 12 month period. This approach delivered continuous inpatient diabetes education over a sustained period of time and therefore had the ability to cover and reinforce various glucose management scenrios [31].

Our study indeed has limitations. It is a single-center study evaluating a single educational intervention and targets third year medical students. Results may not be broadly generalizable to other institutions, types of short-term interventions, or levels of trainees. For example, it may be that our efforts to target the diabetes knowledge and confidence gap across disciplines was targeted too early in their training to fully engage our learners, who did not yet have broad clinical experience with hospital diabetes management. An additional limitation is that response rates were low but still are acceptable rates for survey literature. We also did not have the authority to mandate 100% audience participation during the seminar with using the audience response system, nor the authority to mandate completion of the survey 6 months later.

Future studies are needed to address more broadly (at multiple institutions, various methods of instruction and learning, different groups of trainees) educational interventions that reinforce knowledge and lead to *durable* gains. Additionally, we suggest that this problem is not limited to the topic of hospital diabetes management, but is more pervasive in medical education. It may also be useful to randomize groups of learners to variable interventions differing in scope, target audience and longitudinal nature.

Conclusions

Adding a single seminar on hospital diabetes management in the M3 year boosted immediate post-seminar performance compared to pre-seminar knowledge. This intervention did not durably improve medical student knowledge or change confidence levels at a 6-month evaluation. Repetative interactions with greater focus on the topic during clinical rotation and other sustained methods of exposure need to be evaluated. Furthermore, knowledge and confidence managing diabetes in the hospital go hand in hand, suggesting the possibility that interventions that increase one may help the other.

Abbreviations
M3 year: 3rd year of medical school; M4 year: 4th year of medical school; UMMS: University of Michigan Medical School

Acknowledgements
The authors would like to thank the UMMS medical students who participated in the study. The authors would like to thank Arno K. Kumagai, MD, for his review of the manuscript.

Funding
TWB was supported by the University of Michigan Fellowship in Metabolism, Endocrinology, and Diabetes.

Authors' contributions
RYG was responsible for starting the seminar and the didactic and cases were based on hospital diabetes management service guidelines at the University of Michigan. TWB, JJI and RYG designed the study. TWB, JJI and RYG prepared and delivered the seminar teaching on hospital diabetes management. PVP conducted statistical analysis and JJI assisted. TWB was the primary author. JJM, RYG and PVP also contributed to the text. RYG supervised the study and reviewed and finalized the manuscript. All authors read and approved the final manuscript

Authors information
Timothy W. Bodnar is now a practicing endocrinologist with Ann Arbor Endocrinology & Diabetes Associates in Ypsilanti, MI and is a Key Faculty member of the Internal Medicine Residency Program at St. Joseph Mercy Hospital in Ypsilanti, MI. This research was conducted during his fellowship in Metabolism, Endocrinology, and Diabetes at the University of Michigan. Jennifer J. Iyengar is now a fellow in Metabolism, Endocrinology, and Diabetes at the University of Michigan. This research was conducted during her residency in Internal Medicine at the University of Michigan. Preethi V. Patil is a research analyst at the University of Michigan. Roma Y. Gianchandani is an Associate Professor of Internal Medicine in the Division of Metabolism, Endocrinology, and Diabetes at the University of Michigan. She is also the Director of the Hospital Intensive Insulin Program at the University of Michigan.

Author details
[1]24 Frank Lloyd Wright Drive, P.O. Box 482, Ann Arbor, MI 48106, USA. [2]Ann Arbor Endocrinology & Diabetes Associates P.C., Ypsilanti, MI, USA. [3]University of Michigan Health System, Ann Arbor, MI, USA.

References
1. American Diabetes Association. Economic costs of diabetes in the U.S. In 2007. Diabetes Care. 2008;31:596–615.
2. Wexler DJ, Meigs JB, Cagliero E, Nathan DM, Grant RW. Prevalence of Hyper- and Hypoglycemia Among Inpatients With Diabetes. Diabetes Care. 2007;30:367–9.
3. Moghissi ES, Korytkowski MT, DiNardo M, Einhorn D, Hellman R, Hirsch IB, et al. American Association of Clinical Endocrinologists and American Diabetes Association Consensus Statement on Inpatient Glycemic Control. Diabetes Care. 2009;32:1119–31.
4. Winterstein AG, Hatton RC, Gonzalez-Rothi R, Johns TE, Segal R. Identifying clinically significant preventable adverse drug events through a hospital's database of adverse drug reaction reports. Am. J. Health-Syst. Pharm. AJHP Off. J. Am. Soc. Health-Syst. Pharm. 2002;59:1742–9.
5. Latta S, Alhosaini MN, Al-Solaiman Y, Zena M, Khasawneh F, Eranki V, et al. Management of inpatient hyperglycemia: assessing knowledge and barriers to better care among residents. Am J Ther. 2011;18:355–65.
6. Cook CB, McNaughton DA, Braddy CM, Jameson KA, Roust LR, Smith SA, et al. Management of inpatient hyperglycemia: assessing perceptions and barriers to care among resident physicians. Endocr Pract Off J Am Coll Endocrinol Am Assoc Clin Endocrinol. 2007;13:117–24.
7. Cheekati V, Osburne RC, Jameson KA, Cook CB. Perceptions of resident physicians about management of inpatient hyperglycemia in an urban hospital. J Hosp Med. 2009;4:E1–8.
8. Peterson AA, Charney P, Rennert NJ. Eliminating Inpatient Sliding-Scale Insulin: A Reeducation Project With Medical House Staff. Diabetes Care. 2005;28:2987.
9. George JT, Warriner D, McGrane DJ, Rozario KS, Price HC, Wilmot EG, et al. Lack of confidence among trainee doctors in the management of diabetes: the Trainees Own Perception of Delivery of Care (TOPDOC) Diabetes Study. QJM Mon J Assoc Physicians. 2011;104:761–6.
10. Trepp R, Wille T, Wieland T, Reinhart WH. Diabetes-related knowledge among medical and nursing house staff. Swiss Med Wkly. 2010;140:370–5.
11. Zyl D van, Rheeder P. Survey on knowledge and attitudes regarding diabetic in-patient management by medical and nursing staff at Kalafong hospital. J. Endocrinol. Metab. Diabetes South Afr. [Internet]. 2008 [cited 2016 Oct 23];13. Available from: http://www.ajol.info/index.php/jemdsa/article/view/34716. Accessed 19 Nov 2016.
12. Cook CB, Wilson RD, Hovan MJ, Hull BP, Gray RJ, Apsey HA. Development of Computer-Based Training to Enhance Resident Physician Management of Inpatient Diabetes. J Diabetes Sci Technol. 2009;3:1377–87.
13. Vaidya A, Hurwitz S, Yialamas M, Min L, Garg R. Improving the management of diabetes in hospitalized patients: the results of a computer-based house staff training program. Diabetes Technol Ther. 2012;14:610–8.
14. Tamler R, Green DE, Skamagas M, Breen TL, Looker HC, Babyatsky M, et al. Effect of case-based training for medical residents on inpatient glycemia. Diabetes Care. 2011;34:1738–40.
15. Desimone ME, Blank GE, Virji M, Donihi A, DiNardo M, Simak DM, et al. Effect of an educational Inpatient Diabetes Management Program on medical resident knowledge and measures of glycemic control: a randomized controlled trial. Endocr Pract Off J Am Coll Endocrinol Am Assoc Clin Endocrinol. 2012;18:238–49.
16. Rubin DJ, McDonnell ME. Effect of a diabetes curriculum on internal medicine resident knowledge. Endocr Pract Off J Am Coll Endocrinol Am Assoc Clin Endocrinol. 2010;16:408–18.
17. Nayak L, Erinjeri JP. Audience response systems in medical student education benefit learners and presenters. Acad Radiol. 2008;15:383–9.
18. Dhaliwal HK, Allen M, Kang J, Bates C, Hodge T. The effect of using an audience response system on learning, motivation and information retention in the orthodontic teaching of undergraduate dental students: a cross-over trial. J Orthod. 2015;42:123–35.
19. Karbownik MS, Wiktorowska-Owczarek A, Kowalczyk E, Kwarta P, Mokros Ł, Pietras T. Board game versus lecture-based seminar in the teaching of pharmacology of antimicrobial drugs–a randomized controlled trial. FEMS Microbiol Lett. 2016;363:1–9.
20. Lansang MC, Harrell H. Knowledge on Inpatient Diabetes Among Fourth-Year Medical Students. Diabetes Care. 2007;30:1088–91.
21. MacEwen AW, Carty DM, McConnachie A, McKay GA, Boyle JG. A "Diabetes Acute Care Day" for medical students increases their knowledge and confidence of diabetes care: a pilot study. BMC Med. Educ. [Internet]. 2016 [cited 2016 Oct 16];16. Available from: http://www.ncbi.nlm.nih.gov/pmc/articles/PMC4784451/. Accessed 19 Nov 2016.
22. Medical School Facts & Figures — through FY16 | University of Michigan Medical School [Internet]. [cited 2016 Oct 16]. Available from: https://medicine.umich.edu/medschool/about/facts-figures-rankings. Accessed 19 Nov 2016.
23. UM Grads Go Blue and Beyond [Internet]. [cited 2016 Oct 16]. Available from: http://www.med.umich.edu/medschool/admissions/info_grads/. Accessed 19 Nov 2016.
24. Gianchandani R, Bodnar T. Management of Inpatient Hyperglycemia - An Interactive Seminar. MedEdPORTAL Publ. [Internet]. 2014 [cited 2016 Oct 16]; Available from: https://www.mededportal.org/publication/9816. Accessed 19 Nov 2016.
25. Gosmanova A, Gosmanov N. Assessing diabetes-related knowledge among internal medicine residents using multiple-choice questionnaire. Am J Med Sci. 2009;338:348–52.
26. Derr RL, Sivanandy MS, Bronich-Hall L, Rodriguez A. Insulin-Related Knowledge Among Health Care Professionals in Internal Medicine. Diabetes Spectr. 2007;20:177–85.
27. Herring R, Pengilley C, Hopkins H, Tuthill B, Patel N, Nelson C, et al. Can an interprofessional education tool improve healthcare professional confidence, knowledge and quality of inpatient diabetes care: a pilot study? Diabet Med J Br Diabet Assoc. 2013;30:864–70.

28. Engel SS, Crandall J, Basch CE, Zybert P, Wylie-Rosett J. Computer-assisted diabetes nutrition education increases knowledge and self-efficacy of medical students. Diabetes Educ. 1997;23:545–9.

29. Luscombe C, Montgomery J. Exploring medical student learning in the large group teaching environment: examining current practice to inform curricular development. BMC Med Educ. 2016;16:184.

30. Tamler R, Green DE, Skamagas M, Breen TL, Lu K, Looker HC, et al. Durability of the effect of online diabetes training for medical residents on knowledge, confidence, and inpatient glycemia. J Diabetes. 2012;4:281–90.

31. Baldwin D, Villanueva G, McNutt R, Bhatnagar S. Eliminating Inpatient Sliding-Scale Insulin. Diabetes Care. 2005;28:1008–11.

8

Diabetes and other endocrine-metabolic abnormalities in the long-term follow-up of pancreas transplantation

Marcio W Lauria and Antonio Ribeiro-Oliveira Jr*

Abstract

Pancreas transplantation (PTX) has been demonstrated to restore long-term glucose homeostasis beyond what can be achieved by intensive insulin therapy or islet transplants. Moreover, PTX has been shown to decrease the progression of the chronic complications of diabetes. However, PTX patients require chronic use of immunosuppressive drugs with potential side effects. The long-term follow-up of PTX patients demands special care regarding metabolic deviations, infectious complications, and chronic rejection. Diabetes and other endocrine metabolic abnormalities following transplantation are common and can increase morbidity and mortality. Previous recipient-related and donor-related factors, as well as other aspects inherent to the transplant, act together in the pathogenesis of those abnormalities. Early recognition of these disturbances is the key to timely treatment; however, adequate tools to achieve this goal are often lacking. In a way, the type of PTX procedure, whether simultaneous pancreas kidney or not, seems to differentially influence the evolution of endocrine and metabolic abnormalities. Further studies are needed to define the best approach for PTX patients. This review will focus on the most common endocrine metabolic disorders seen in the long-term management of PTX: diabetes mellitus, hyperlipidemia, and bone loss. The authors here cover each one of these endocrine topics by showing the evaluation as well as proper management in the follow-up after PTX.

Keywords: Pancreas transplantation, Diabetes, Hyperlipidemia, Bone loss

Background

During the past decades, pancreas transplantation (PTX) has evolved into a procedure mainly reserved for type 1 diabetes patients undergoing simultaneously kidney transplantation, although it has also been performed as an isolate procedure [1]. Importantly, it has significantly improved diabetes related quality of life as well as life expectancy when compared to kidney only recipients [2]. However, there is a paucity of publications as related to the endocrine follow-up evaluation and management to this population of diabetic patients after pancreas transplantation.

A Pubmed search was conducted searching for terms "pancreas transplantation AND metabolism", "pancreas transplantation AND diabetes", "pancreas transplantation AND hyperlipidemia", "pancreas transplantation AND bone disease". We have included only English written articles, and we have tried to prioritize prospective studies. However, due to the lack of available data concerning pancreas transplantation and metabolic abnormalities, we have also included retrospective, transversal and case reports studies.

Main text

PTX is the implantation of a healthy pancreas (usually from a deceased donor) into a patient who typically has type 1 diabetes. More than 35,000 PTXs have been reported worldwide [3]. Eighty-four percent of PTX procedures are performed along with kidney transplantation (both organs coming from the same donor) in diabetic patients with renal failure. This is referred to as simultaneous pancreas-kidney (SPK) transplantation. Nine percent of PTXs are performed after a previous successful kidney transplantation, which is termed pancreas-after-kidney transplantation (PAK). The remaining 7 % of cases are performed as pancreas transplantation alone

---

* Correspondence: antoniorojr@gmail.com
Department of Internal Medicine (Endocrinology section and Transplantation unit), Federal University of Minas Gerais, Rua Alfredo Balena, 190, 30130-100 Belo Horizonte, MG, Brazil

(PTA) in nonuremic patients with very labile difficult to manage diabetes.

The number of US PTX has declined by over 20 %, while the overall number of pancreas transplants performed outside the US has increased since 2010. The decline in US numbers is predominantly due to the decline in PTA and PAK. With the decline in the number of transplants, a change towards better pancreas donor selection has been observed [3]. Furthermore, the number of PTX in patients with type 2 diabetes and end-stage renal disease has increased, and accounted for 9 % of all SPK recipients in 2010–14 [3].

Pancreas transplantation is superior to intensive insulin therapy with respect to glycated hemoglobin (A1C) normalization and shows the additional physiological property of proinsulin and C-peptide release [4]. With new advances in immunosuppression and changes in surgical techniques, patient survival and pancreas graft function have been improving, with PTX being widely employed as a treatment modality for patients with diabetes,especially those with established nephropathy [1, 3]. Nevertheless, PTX remains a complex procedure, which is still associated with high general surgical morbidity. In addition, graft failure, side effects of immunosuppressive agents, opportunistic infections, and cardio- and cerebrovascular problems can increase morbidity and mortality following transplantation [1, 5, 6].

Diabetes and other metabolic abnormalities have frequently been observed after PTX, which can influence its long-term outcomes. These disorders have been related to various factors such as immunosuppressive drug side effects, chronic rejection, and recipient lifestyle after transplantation. Early recognition of these abnormalities can provide for more opportune treatment [1, 4, 5].

This review will focus on the most common endocrine and metabolic disorders related to PTX, such as diabetes, hyperlipidemia, and bone loss. It is noteworthy to mention that due to the absence of clinical guidelines developed through the GRADE approach to this population, our suggested evaluation and follow-up may eventually show variations from other centers, although we have tried to summarize them through the best available sources.

Diabetes after pancreas transplantation
Glucose metabolism disorders
No other insulin delivery regimen can achieve the level of physiologic glycemic regulation than that obtained with PTX. It has proved more effective in lowering A1C than intensive insulin treatment or islet transplants [1, 5–7]. Restoration of β-cell secretory capacity, improvement in glucose counter-regulation, and return to hypoglycemia awareness can all be achieved with a successful PTX [8]. Normalization of A1C occurs within weeks to months and can last for more than

15 years [9]. Transient hyperglycemia may occur within the first six months due to acute or chronic rejection, pancreatitis, or a marked increase in insulin resistance due to weight gain. Immunosuppressant medication effects [5, 6], such as steroids, calcineurin inhibitors (tacrolimus, in particular), sirolimus, and mycophenolate have also been linked to posttransplantation hyperglycemia [10].

Hypoglycemia may also occur following PTX [11, 12]; however, severe episodes (with or without symptom awareness) are rare. By 3 months after PTX, glucagon secretion and hepatic glucose production in response to hypoglycemia also return to normal [13]. Although epinephrine and growth hormone responses to hypoglycemia improve after pancreas transplant, these do not return to normal [14].

Hyperinsulinism is frequently observed after PTX, as are elevated C-peptide and proinsulin concentrations. One likely explanation for these abnormalities—among other reasons, such as the side effects of immunosuppression—is the systemic release of insulin via the iliac vein, as there is no first-pass effect of insulin through the liver [15]. It has been reported that drainage of the venous effluent of the pancreas transplant via the superior mesenteric or portal vein (portal venous drainage) allows comparable blood glucose control but lower insulin levels, as well as possible advantages in metabolic control over systemic venous drainage. However, this mechanism has not been accepted by all authors [16, 17]. Interestingly, a recent report [18] in SPK patients at 1 and 5 years posttransplantation showed that peripheral insulin resistance with homeostatic model assessment (HOMA-IR) >4 was related to decreased pancreatic graft survival. However, data from HOMA-IR in transplanted patients is lacking and needs to be interpreted cautiously.

The prevalence of diabetes after pancreas transplantation is variable, depending on the frequency of assessment, duration of follow-up, and, most importantly, the case definition for diabetes or glucose intolerance. The estimates of this prevalence is rather imprecise as some have taken insulin use as the definition for diabetes while others excluded technical failures or acute rejection to this assessment.

Hyperglycemia after PTX may have more than one of the following explanations: graft failure (due to rejection, thrombosis, or pancreatitis), new-onset diabetes (type 2 or secondary to corticosteroids or immunosuppressive drugs), immunosuppressant-induced islet cell toxicity (particularly tacrolimus in high doses), or recurrent autoimmune type 1 diabetes [19].

Interestingly, the recurrence of type 1 diabetes has been related to the presence of the autoantibodies to the zinc transporter 8 and cannot be explained by genetically encoded amino acid sequence donor-recipient mismatches for this autoantigen [20].

Most cases of late hyperglycemia are attributed to chronic rejection, which, along with technical failure, is the most common cause of hyperglycemia following PTX. Chronic rejection accounts for approximately 50 % (or more) of the grafts that survive over five years [21]. Pancreas failure in the long term can be related to the donor, to the surgical manipulation of the graft, or to the recipient (Table 1).

Neidlinger et al. [22] analyzed 674 PTX recipients over a 10-year period, with mean follow-up of more than 6 years. The incidence of posttransplant diabetes mellitus (PTDM) was 14 % and 25 % at 3 and 10 years after PTX, respectively. Higher recipient body mass index and posttransplant weight gain, donor age, and donor-positive with recipient-negative CMV status were associated with PTDM after controlling for possible confounding factors [22]. Dean et al. also found a relationship between PTDM, high pretransplant insulin requirements and episodes of acute rejection [6]. Hilling et al. demonstrated that recipient factors are more important in explaining differences in pancreas graft survival than donor factors [23]. Interestingly, the incidence of post-transplant diabetes after successful PTX is lower than that for other solid organ transplants despite the use of the same immunosuppressive drugs [24].

Both PAK and PTA entail higher incidence of graft loss from chronic rejection compared with SPK [3]. For the PAK and PTA categories, such risk remains high even after 1 year posttransplantation, thus requiring greater doses of immunosuppressive drugs and increasing toxicity risks [25]. In one study developed by our group comparing long-term follow-up between PTA and SPK patients, we showed that PTA patients exhibited higher tacrolimus levels and worse renal function [26].

Evaluation

Fasting glucose and A1C should be ordered at all consultations. If A1C is elevated or fasting glucose exceeds 100 mg/dl, unassociated with a recent rejection episode, an oral glucose tolerance test (OGTT) should be performed [27].

Table 1 Related risk factors for diabetes mellitus following pancreas transplantation

- Donor: older age and high body mass index
- Surgical procedure: extensive manipulation of the graft and long ischemic period
- Recipient: higher body mass index and posttransplant weight gain; donor age, hepatitis C virus and donor-positive with recipient-negative CMV status
- Type of pancreas transplantation: pancreas transplantation alone and pancreas after kidney transplantation
- Immunosuppressive regimen: prolonged use of glucocorticoids and use of tacrolimus
- Follow-up: number of acute rejection episodes, loss of the kidney graft in pancreas-kidney transplantation, and long duration of the transplant

There are no specific criteria to diagnose diabetes after pancreas transplantation and so it is recommended to adopt the Second International Consensus of Post -Transplant Diabetes Mellitus [28]. The threshold to define diabetes is based on data from non-transplant patients: fasting glucose ≥ 126 mg/dl on more than one occasion, random glucose ≥200 mg/dl with symptoms or a 2-h glucose level after a 75-g oral glucose tolerance test ≥200 mg/dl [27]. Although A1C ≥ 6.5 % can be used to diagnose diabetes in the general population, it should not be used alone in post-transplant diabetes mellitus, particularly in the first year after transplantation [28].

Pancreas transplantation recipients presenting with recurrent hyperglycemia should have their C-peptide levels measured and undergo pancreas biopsy to distinguish between rejection, recurrence of type 1 diabetes, and onset of type 2 diabetes [4]. Duplex sonographic scanning of the allograft could be helpful in excluding thrombosis and rejection. However, sonography is less accurate than biopsy to diagnose rejection [29, 30]. Ultrasound-guided pancreas biopsy is otherwise considered the gold standard for the diagnosis of an allograft dysfunction.

Unfortunately, hyperglycemia is a late marker of chronic graft rejection. Although plasma glucose has high specificity (90 % to 95 %), it is the least sensitive marker of rejection [31]. Hence, identification of the subjects at risk of returning to the diabetic state due to graft loss or any other cause is difficult and often delayed. Consequently, appropriate treatment becomes unfeasible.

Several tests have been proposed to identify patients at high risk for all-cause pancreatic graft failure. Slight alterations in glucose metabolism seem to appear earlier and might be predictive of pancreatic graft failure. Pfeffer et al. performed OGTT 1.7 years after SPK transplantation on average and showed that impaired glucose tolerance predicted risk of graft failure in 10 years [32]. Battezzati et al., taking blood samples at 2 h intervals for plasma glucose, serum insulin, and C-peptide levels, reported that mean 24-h glucose greater than 127 mg/dL at 1 year posttransplantation was the best predictive index of return to a diabetic state [33]. The intravenous glucose tolerance test and the arginine-induced insulin secretion test have also been used as rejection markers [34, 35]. In islet transplantation patients, glucose variability and a higher frequency of glucose levels above 140 mg/dL determined by the continuous glucose monitoring system (CGMS) have proved useful early indicators of graft dysfunction [36]. We have also demonstrated that 72 h mean glucose measured by CGMS in PTX patients with normal oral glucose tolerance was associated with chronic rejection in a 5 year follow-up [37]. Recently, Hiratsuka et al. have described the utility of peripheral plasma fasting serum C-peptide response to 1 mg of glucagon intravenously to predict insulin-free treatment [38]. However, further studies are warranted, since biochemical parameters and imaging tools still lack diagnostic accuracy to detect early graft failure, especially for PTA and PAK.

In SPK recipients, serum creatinine levels have been used to diagnose rejection, since kidney graft rejection usually precedes or is concurrent with rejection of the pancreas graft [19].

Urinary amylase levels can be monitored in pancreas recipients with bladder-drained exocrine secretions [39, 40]. An analysis result of a 12-h or 24-h urine collection in which amylase levels have declined 50 % or more from baseline suggests rejection or pancreatitis. Serum amylase and lipase levels provide additional means for following pancreas function, especially in the case of enterically drained grafts. However, they lack the sensitivity and specificity of urinary amylase measures [4]. Long-term graft survival is greater for SPK vs PAK or PTA transplants, which partly explains the decrease in the number of these two last transplant modalities in the past decade [41]. Indeed, in SPK the pancreas and kidney are usually obtained from the same deceased donor and, therefore, changes in kidney function can be used to monitor whether rejection is occurring at either organ.

Table 2 summarizes the recommended tests for identifying patients at risk for pancreatic graft dysfunction.

Management
Strict glycemic control is the cornerstone of therapy, which can preserve residual β-cell function and eventually recover it when glucotoxicity is corrected. Blood glucose levels should be less than 110 mg/dL before meals and less than 180 mg/dL postprandial [42].

Insulin therapy is generally preferred because of its superior results in controlling diabetes, in addition to being more predictable and rapidly titrated. Insulin therapy is mandatory in the setting of ketoacidosis or metabolic decompensation with unintended weight loss. Furthermore, insulin should be used when hyperglycemia derives from rejection or other causes of graft failure. Further, insulin therapy is mandatory when hyperglycemia derives from rejection or other causes of graft

Table 2 Tests for identifying pancreas graft dysfunction

- Urinary amylase levels (only for bladder- drained transplants)
- Serum amylase and lipase levels
- Fasting glucose levels (consider OGTT if >100 mg/dl)
- A1C
- Creatinine (in SPK patients)
- Duplex sonographic scanning of the allograft (when thrombosis and/or rejection are suspected)
- Ultrasound- guided biopsy (gold standard for rejection)

failure. Despite extensive clinical experience with a variety of insulin types, no prospective studies have addressed the relative efficacy of specific insulin regimens for treating posttransplant diabetes [42].

When the cause of hyperglycemia is new-onset type 2 diabetes, oral agents can be used, although this has not been clearly defined for PTX. They should be attempted in patients with mild hyperglycemia with preserved/robust c-peptide. Metformin improves insulin sensitivity, most notably in the liver. Given the risk of metformin-induced lactic acidosis, this agent is contraindicated for patients with severe renal or hepatic dysfunction. Sulfonylureas stimulate insulin secretion and can be an option. However, these drugs are associated with an increased risk of hypoglycemia and can also contribute to β-cell exhaustion. Thiazolidinediones, which primarily target insulin resistance at the level of skeletal muscles and adipocytes, have been evaluated as a potential therapeutic option and seem to be a safe and effective treatment. Special attention must be given to the side effects of thiazolidinediones, such as weight gain, hepatotoxicity, edema, cardiac failure, and increased fracture risk. Agonists of GLP-1 and oral dipeptidyl peptidase inhibitors have not been consistently investigated and thus cannot be recommended, although they might have a positive effect by stimulating insulin secretion in transplant recipients [43].

Although current clinical evidence is largely anecdotal, tailoring of immunosuppression should be considered in patients with poorly controlled diabetes despite therapeutic lifestyle changes and pharmacologic interventions. In this context, therapeutic options include reduction in corticosteroid and/or calcineurin inhibitors dose, and conversion from tacrolimus to cyclosporine or sirolimus [44, 45].

Steroid avoidance or withdrawal for PTX patients has been a matter of debate. A recent review by Montero et al. [46] concluded that the available data, including randomized controlled trials, are still insufficient to firmly infer on the harms and benefits of steroid withdrawal in pancreas transplantation. A study by Amodu et al. [47] showed that steroid maintenance is not associated with the risk of death or graft failure although increasing the risk of infectious complications.

Hyperlipidemia after pancreas transplantation
Lipid metabolism disorders
Hyperlipidemia after solid organ transplantation occurs in 60 % to 80 % of recipients of immunosuppressive therapy [48]. High triglycerides and low density lipoprotein cholesterol (LDL-c) levels are two of the most important lipid disorders found in those patients. Combined hyperlipidemia is also common. Many risk factors can contribute to the development of dyslipidemia after PTX, such as older

age, obesity, posttransplantation weight gain, pretransplantation hyperlipidemia, male gender, graft dysfunction, proteinuria, new-onset diabetes, prednisone dosage, and the type of immunosuppression regimen (Table 3).

Sirolimus has been found to be associated with greater increases in triglycerides and cholesterol, although tacrolimus and cyclosporine also have deleterious effects on lipid metabolism [5, 10].

The majority of PTX patients have preexisting dyslipidemia, since they are generally poorly controlled diabetes patients, most of them with advanced nephropathy. Compared to preoperative levels, patients who underwent SPK experience improvements in their lipid profile, while those submitted to PTA remain with stable lipid levels [49]. Patients who underwent PTA exhibit similar lipid levels to SPK patients posttransplantation, which suggests that the contrasting clinical course seen between these two groups is attributable to preoperative lipid profile differences [26]. Relative to PTA patients, SPK patients have significantly lower levels of LDL-c and use significantly fewer lipid-lowering medications [50]. Portal venous instead of systemic venous drainage of the pancreas allograft does not seem to impact lipid metabolism in the long-term follow-up [17]. Steroid withdrawal regimens have been related to lower prevalence of hyperlipidemia after PTX [51].

Qualitatively, a persisting profile of potentially atherogenic alterations in lipoprotein lipase, cholesteryl ester transfer, and lipoprotein composition has been reported after PTX [52]. However, the findings and interpretation of those data have been questioned by others [53].

Evaluation
In the first 3 months following PTX, lipid levels are quite unstable because of high doses of immunosuppressive drugs [54]. After that, levels usually stabilize during the first year posttransplantation. It is important to avoid misleading situations when interpreting the results, such as acute stress conditions and secondary causes of dyslipidemia.

Table 3 Risk factors contributing to the development of dyslipidemia following pancreas transplantation

- Older age
- Obesity/Overweight
- Weight gain after transplantation
- Pretransplantation hyperlipidemia
- Male gender
- Graft dysfunction
- Proteinuria
- New-onset diabetes
- Prednisone dosage
- Immunosuppressive agents: sirolimus (particularly), tacrolimus, cyclosporine

Monitoring lipid profile at least every 6 months following transplantation is advisable.

Management
Due to the high incidence of atherosclerotic disease events and the absence of specific studies, PTX patients should be considered high risk and treated to maintain LDL-c <100 mg/dl, according to published guidelines for kidney transplant patients [55].

A diet-oriented approach should be the first line treatment in hyperlipidemia [56]; changes in the immunosuppression regimen should also be considered. Tacrolimus appears to have fewer adverse effects on lipids than cyclosporine, which is not explained by concomitant steroid administration. Cross-over studies with renal transplant patients have shown improvement in lipid profile after conversion from cyclosporine to tacrolimus [57, 58].

Statins are considered the cornerstone of drug therapy in posttransplantation hypercholesterolemia. The outcomes and benefits of statins based on heart and kidney clinical studies provide a solid rationale to support their use in organ transplantation. Furthermore, statins can potentially exert cholesterol-independent immunosuppressive effects [59]. Use of statins in PTA patients may lead to improved outcomes. Whether this is due to cardiovascular protection or other factors unrelated to lipid lowering remains unclear [60].

Similarly to kidney transplant, statin treatment has uncertain effects on overall mortality, stroke, kidney function, and toxicity outcomes in PTX recipients. Further studies would improve our knowledge of the benefits and harms of statin treatment regarding cardiovascular events in this clinical setting [61].

Since statins can cause hepatotoxicity, it is important to monitor liver function after statin introduction. Moreover, we should be cautious about the myotoxic effects of statins and the risk of rhabdomyolysis due to interaction with drugs that inhibit the cytochrome P450 isoenzyme and thus increase statin levels [62]. Regarding associations between statins and tacrolimus, animal studies have shown a pronounced interaction, similar to that described for cyclosporine. Not all statins are metabolized by the same enzyme; therefore, they exhibit a different drug interaction and safety profile [63]. Statin-induced dysglycemia is another concern that has recently been described in kidney transplants [64]. The choice of a statin should be based on individual patient requirements and adapted according to treatment response. Pravastatin and fluvastatin have been considered the safest statins to be used in transplanted patients [65]. However, given their low potency, a high-potency statin may be necessary in patients with significant dyslipidemia [66, 67].

Concerning hypertriglyceridemia, fibrates should be used cautiously, since they may induce renal dysfunction. Gemfibrozil seems to be devoid of this side-effect [68]. Interestingly, in the Fenofibrate Intervention and Event Lowering in Diabetes (FIELD), fenofibrate reduced albuminuria and slowed estimated renal function loss over 5 years, despite initially and reversibly increasing plasma creatinine. Confirmatory studies are merited [69].

Bone diseases following pancreas transplantation
Calcium and bone metabolism disorders
Bone complications are another major source of late morbidity for PTX patients. Fractures after SPK transplant are common: 45 to 49 % within the first 2 years, which is one of the highest fracture rates reported for any organ transplant [70]. Cortical osteoporosis is prevalent in SPK recipients at the time of transplantation and shows early progression after transplantation [71]. Over the long term, bone densitometry values and fracture risk seem to stabilize or improve, especially in steroid sparing protocols and/or aggressive osteoporosis treatment [71, 72].

The disturbances in bone and mineral metabolism observed after transplantation are largely determined by preexisting factors at the time of transplantation (advanced age, female gender, long duration of pretransplant kidney failure, history of pretransplant fracture) and by factors inherent to the transplant status, such as kidney function and use of immunosuppressive agents [73, 74] (Table 4).

Compared to PTA recipients, kidney transplant recipients have the disadvantage of presenting for transplantation with preexisting osteodystrophy, which is difficult to predict from routine laboratory or radiologic investigations and it may persist, improve, or worsen after transplantation [75]. Interestingly, SPK has been associated with a significant 31 % reduction in fracture risk compared to kidney alone transplantation in men with type 1 diabetes after adjustment for fracture covariates [76]. It is not known whether the apparent benefit of SPK is due to improved bone strength or fewer falls observed with the restoration of euglycemia. Furthermore, a recent study by Rocha et al. [77] showed that, in SPK patients followed for at about 3 years, a gain in BMI was significantly predictive

Table 4 Factors related to bone and mineral metabolism disturbances following pancreas transplantation

- Preexisting: older age, female gender, long duration of pretransplant kidney failure, history of pretransplant fracture, severity of hyperparathyroidism secondary to kidney disease
- Inherent to transplant status: kidney function, use of immunosuppressive agents (especially glucocorticoids and calcineurin inhibitors)
- Other factors commonly observed after transplantation: hypogonadism, vitamin D deficiency, persistent parathyroid disease, thyroid abnormalities

of bone mass improvement whereas an increasing in serum levels of alkaline phosphatase was significantly associated with a decrease in the same parameter.

After kidney transplantation, many laboratory features of chronic kidney disease improve; however, abnormally high or low bone turnover rates have been reported in bone biopsy studies [78, 79].

Corticosteroids exacerbate bone loss by suppressing osteoblastic activity and activating osteoclastic resorption. Calcineurin inhibitors also have direct negative effects on bone [80–82]. Factors such as hypogonadism, vitamin D deficiency, adynamic bone disease, previous or ongoing parathyroid disease, previous uncontrolled diabetes, and thyroid function abnormalities can also contribute to bone loss [19]. Persistently increased PTH concentrations can be found in as many as 75 % of patients at 1 year posttransplantation; this is largely due to failure of the enlarged glands to involute. Elevated FGF23 levels and decreased Klotho expression in the parathyroid gland may play a role in the pathogenesis of hyperparathyroidism after kidney transplantation [83]. A major determinant of persistent posttransplant hyperparathyroidism is its severity at the time of transplantation, corresponding to pretransplantation PTH levels [84, 85]. Persistent hyperparathyroidism is a major risk factor for fractures after kidney transplantation [86]. The foot and ankle are the most common fracture sites after PTX, accounting for over 50 % of the cases. This suggests that preexisting diabetes-related deformities could be an etiologic factor. Charcot neuroarthropathy has been diagnosed in 4.6 % of SPK recipients during the first year posttransplantation [87, 88]. In addition, a variety of other anatomic sites are affected [89].

Evaluation
No clinical trial data to inform clinical recommendations for bone disease in PTX patients are available. Most data is limited to before-after data or registry studies. In view of this, guidance for renal transplantation patients is taken as a reference, although it needs to be applied cautiously [55].

Close monitoring of serum calcium, phosphate, 25-hydroxy-vitamin D (25 OH-D), and PTH concentrations are recommended for SPK and PAK recipients [19]. Bone mineral density should be measured in the first 3 months after transplantation, when patients have a calculated clearance of creatinine above 30 mL/min, and then repeated on a regular basis [55]. The work-up should also include periodical determination of thyroid and sex hormone status in eligible populations [4]. Biomarkers of bone turnover could be useful in individualizing therapy to prevent or treat bone loss after transplantation [90]. For PTA recipients, evaluation should be done considering the presence of other fracture risk factors such as peripheral neuropathy, poor muscle strength, balance impairment, visual acuity reduction, and propensity to falls.

Management

Vitamin D deficiency and insufficiency should be corrected by using treatment strategies recommended for the general population to achieve a serum 25 OH-D concentration of at least 20 ng/mL to prevent and treat osteometabolic diseases [55]. Low 25 OH-D has been independently associated with an increased risk of all-cause mortality in kidney transplantation [91]. Pleotropic effects of vitamin D, such as immune response regulation, and protective effects from cardiovascular disease, cancer, and infections seem to be very attractive to the transplanted population. However, more solid data are needed to confirm this and to set the optimal level of serum Vitamin D supplementation in order to attain the best clinical outcome [92]. Calcium supplementation (500 mg elemental calcium daily) appears to lower bone resorption after transplantation and should be routinely prescribed—especially in regimens with high doses of immunosuppressive drugs [93]. Calcium dietary intake of at least 1 g daily should also be advised.

In patients with established osteoporosis (presence of densitometric osteoporosis or fractures associated with osteopenia), anti-resorption therapy, usually with bisphosphonates orally or intravenously, is warranted [90, 94]. Bisphosphonates may also be beneficial to prevent bone loss after transplant, although this needs to be more clearly established.

In patients with persistent hyperparathyroidism after transplantation, calcitriol may provide additional benefits in reducing bone loss [94]. A calcium sensor blocker (Cinacalcet) has not yet been approved for use in transplanted patients and evidence of its safety in this clinical setting is still incomplete. In refractory and persistent cases of hyperparathyroidism, parathyroidectomy should be considered [95].

Other endocrine and metabolic diseases

Thyroid diseases are common in the general population and, therefore, can be often observed in the pancreas transplanted population. Furthermore, patients with type 1 diabetes show increased incidence of autoimmune thyroid diseases. However, no relationship between pancreas transplantation and thyroid disesases has been described. Thus, screening and management of thyroid diseases in pancreas transplanted patients is not different from the general population.

Hypogonadism in men and women have been reported before and after pancreas transplantation, mainly in those patients with SPK and probably due to the effects of the end stage renal disease in the hypothalamic-gonadotroph axis function. Immunosupressive drugs may play a role in these disorders. However, in the majority of the cases, gonadal function actually recovers after transplantation [96]. Glucocorticoid metabolism alterations may occur in transplanted patients and are related to its chronic use to prevent organ rejection. These patients should be advised to increase or reassume glucocorticoid therapy during stress to avoid adrenal insufficiency.

Conclusions

Disturbances in the metabolism of carbohydrates, lipids, and bone mineral are prevalent problems observed in the follow-up of PTX patients. In addition to causing morbidity, such disturbances can indirectly increase the risk of death associated with cardiovascular diseases and fractures. Previous recipient-related and donor-related factors and others inherent to the transplant act together in the pathogenesis of these abnormalities. Early recognition of such disturbances is the key to timely treatment; however, adequate tools to achieve this goal are frequently lacking. Further studies are needed to define the best approach for PTX patients.

PTX is a technically demanding procedure which is associated with the above-mentioned abnormalities in the endocrine system beyond infectious and rejection complications. Furthermore, patient follow-up is complex due to multiple interfering factors, where immunosuppressive drugs play an important role. Therefore, despite the good outcomes recently achieved in centers with a specialized transplantation unit as well as recent advances to the field, PTX should still be considered the last resort treatment in patients whose diabetic complications have become life-threatening or enough burdensome to be maintained with the current available diabetes treatment.

Abbreviations
PTX, pancreas transplantation; SPK, simultaneous pancreas kidney transplantation; PAK, pancreas after kidney transplantation; PTA, pancreas transplantation alone; A1C, glycated hemoglobin; HOMA-IR, homeostatic model assessment; PTDM, posttransplant diabetes mellitus; OGTT, oral glucose tolerance test; CGMS, continuous glucose monitoring system; LDL-c, low density lipoprotein cholesterol; 25 OH-D, 25hydroxy vitamin D

Funding
This work is funded by FAPEMIG (Fundação Estadual para o Desenvolvimento da Pesquisa do Estado de Minas Gerais) and CNPq (Conselho Nacional de Desenvolvimento Científico e Tecnológico).

Authors' contributions
Both authors contributed to the conceptual development of the review, references, drafting, editing, and the final approval of the manuscript.

References

1. Niclauss N, Morel P, Volonte F, Bosco D, Berney T. Pancreas and islets of Langerhans transplantation: current status in 2009 and perspectives. Rev Med Suisse. 2009;5:1266.
2. Sureshkumar KK, Mubin T, Mikhael N, Kashif MA, Nghiem DD, Marcus RJ. Assessment of quality of life after simultaneous pancreas-kidney transplantation. Am J Kidney Dis. 2002;39:1300.
3. Gruessner A, Gruessner R. Pancreas Transplantation of US and Non-US Cases from 2005 to 2014 as Reported to the United Network for Organ Sharing (UNOS) and the International Pancreas Transplant Registry (IPTR). Rev Diabet Stud. 2016;14:e2016002 [Epub ahead of print].
4. Mai M, Ahsan N, Gonwas T. The long-term management of pancreas transplantation. Transplantation. 2006;82:991.
5. Rangel EB. The metabolic and toxicological considerations for immunosuppressive drugs used during pancreas transplantation. Expert Opin Drug Metab Toxicol. 2012;8:1531.
6. Dean PG, Kudva YC, Larson TS, Kremers WK, Stegall MD. Posttransplant diabetes mellitus after pancreas transplantation. Am Journ of Transplant. 2008;8:175.
7. The Diabetes Control and Complications Trial Research Group. The effect of intensive treatment of diabetes on the development and progression of long-term complications in insulin-dependent diabetes mellitus. N Engl J Med. 1993;329:977.
8. Rickels M. Recovery of endocrine function after islet and pancreas transplantation. Curr Diab Rep. 2012;12:587.
9. Robertson RP, Sutherland DE, Lanz KJ. Normoglycemia and preserved insulin secretory reserve in diabetic patients 10–18 years after pancreas transplantation. Diabetes. 1999;48:1737.
10. Subramanian S, Trence D. Immunosuppressive Agents: effects on glucose and lipid metabolism. Endocrinol Metabol Clin N Am. 2007;36:891.
11. Battezzati A, Bonfatti D, Benedini S, et al. Spontaneous hypoglycaemia after pancreas transplantation in Type 1 diabetes mellitus. Diabet Med. 1998;15:991.
12. Redmon J, Teuscher A, Robertson R. Hypoglycemia after pancreas transplantation. Diabetes Care. 1998;21:1944.
13. Barrou Z, Seaquist E, Robertson R. Pancreas transplantation in diabetic humans normalizes hepatic glucose production during hypoglycemia. Diabetes. 1994;43:661.
14. Bolinder J, Wahrenberg H, Persson A, et al. Effect of pancreas transplantation on glucose counterregulation in insulin-dependent diabetic patients prone to severe hypoglycaemia. J Intern Med. 1991;230:527.
15. Diem P, Abid M, Redmon J, Sutherland D, Robertson R. Systemic venous drainage of pancreas allografts as independent cause of hyperinsulinemia in type I diabetic recipients. Diabetes. 1990;39:534.
16. Petruzzo P, Laville M, Badet L, Lefrançois N, Bin-Dorel S, Chapuis F, et al. Effect of venous drainage site on insulin action after simultaneous pancreas-kidney transplantation. Transplantation. 2004;77:1875.
17. Bazerbachi F, Selzner M, Marquez M, Norgate A, Aslani N, McGilvray ID, et al. Portal venous versus systemic venous drainage of pancreas grafts: impact on long-term results. Am J Transplant. 2012;12:226.
18. de Mier Pendón-Ruiz V, Navarro Cabello MD, Martínez Vaquera S, Lopez-Andreu M, Aguera Morales ML, Rodriguez-Benot A, et al. Index high insulin resistance in pancreas-kidney transplantation contributes to poor long-term survival of the pancreas graft. Transplant Proc. 2015;47:117.
19. Larsen J. Pancreas transplantation: Indications and consequences. Endocr Rev. 2004;25:919.
20. Vendrame F, Hopfner YY, Diamantopoulos S, Virdi SK, Allende G, Snowhite IV et al. Risk Factors for Type 1 Diabetes Recurrence in Immunosuppressed Recipients of Simultaneous Pancreas-Kidney Transplants. Am J Transplant. 2015. doi: 10.1111/ajt.13426.
21. Wakil K, Sugawara Y, Kokudo N, Kadowaki T. Causes of graft failure in simultaneous pancreas-kidney transplantation by various time periods. Clin Transpl. 2012;27:23.
22. Neidlinger N, Singh N, Klein C, Odorico J, del Rio Munoz A, Becker Y, et al. Incidence of and risk factors for posttransplant diabetes mellitus after pancreas transplantation. Am J Transplant. 2010;9:1.
23. Hilling D, Baranski A, Haasnoot A, van der Boog P, Terpstra O, van de Marang-Mheen P. Contribution of donor and recipient characteristics to short- and long-term pancreas graft survival. Ann Transplant. 2012;17:28.
24. First M, Dhadda S, Croy R, Holman J, Fitzsimmons W. New-onset diabetes after transplantation (NODAT): an evaluation of definitions in clinical trials. Transplantation. 2013;96:58.
25. Gruessner AC, Sutherland DE, Gruessner RW. International Pancreas Transplant Registry. In: Gruessner RW, Sutherland DE, editors. Transplantation of the pancreas. New York: Springer; 2004. p. 539.
26. Lauria M, Figueiro J, Machado L, Sanches M, Nascimento G, Lana A, et al. Metabolic Long-Term Follow-Up of Functioning Simultaneous Pancreas-Kidney Transplantation Versus Pancreas Transplantation Alone: Insights and Limitations. Transplantation. 2010;89:83.
27. American Diabetes Association. Classification and diagnosis of diabetes. In: 2016 Standards of Medical Care in Diabetes. Diabetes Care. 2016;39:S13.
28. Sharif A, Hecking M, de Vries AP, Porrini E, Hornum M, Rasoul-Rockenschaub S, et al. Proceedings from an international consensus meeting on posttransplantation diabetes mellitus: recommendations and future directions. Am J Transplant. 2014;14:1992.
29. Wong J, Krebs T, Klassen D, Daly B, Simon E, Bartlett S, et al. Sonographic evaluation of acute pancreatic transplant rejection: morphology-Doppler analysis versus guided percutaneous biopsy. Am J Roentgenol. 1996;166:803.
30. Tolat PP, Foley WD, Johnson C, Hohenwalter MD, Quiroz FA. Pancreas transplant imaging: how I do it. Radiology. 2015;275:14.
31. Abendroth D, Capalbo M, Illner WD, Landgraf R, Land W. Critical analysis of rejection markers sIL-2R, urinary amylase, and lipase in whole-organ pancreas transplantation with exocrine bladder drainage. Transplant Proc. 1992;24:786.
32. Pfeffer F, Nauck M, Drognitz O, Benz S, von Dobschuetz E, Hopt U. Postoperative oral glucose tolerance and stimulated insulin secretion: a predictor of endocrine graft function more than 10 years after pancreas-kidney transplantation. Transplantation. 2003;76:1427.
33. Battezzati A, Benedini S, Caldara R, Calori G, Secchi A, Pozza G, et al. Prediction of the long-term metabolic success of the pancreatic graft function. Transplantation. 2001;71:1560.
34. Elmer D, Hathaway D, Bashar Abdulkarim A, Hughes T, Shokouh-Amiri H, Gaber L, et al. Use of glucose disappearance rates (kG) to monitor endocrine function of pancreas allografts. Clin Transplant. 1998;12:56.
35. Teuscher A, Seaquist E, Robertson R. Diminished insulin secretory reserve in diabetic pancreas transplant and non diabetic kidney transplant recipients. Diabetes. 1994;43:593.
36. Faradji R, Monroy K, Riefkohl A, Lozano L, Gorn L, Froud T, et al. Continuous glucose monitoring system for early detection of graft dysfunction in allogenic islet transplant recipients. Transplant Proc. 2006;38:3274.
37. Lauria M, Figueiró J, Sanches M, Gontijo R, Mariano B, Lana A, et al. Glucose control in pancreas transplantation assessed by 72-h continuous glucose monitoring. Transplantation. 2012;94:e2.
38. Hiratsuka I, Suzuki A, Kondo-Ando M, Hirai H, Maeda Y, Sekiguchi-Ueda S, et al. Utility of glucagon stimulation test in type 1 diabetes after pancreas transplantation. Transplant Proc. 2014;46:967.
39. Jönsson P, Källén R, Borgström A, Ohlsson K. Exocrine pancreatic proteins in serum during pancreatic allograft rejection. Pancreas. 1994;9:244.
40. Newell K, Bruce D, Cronin D, Woodle E, Millis J, Piper J, et al. Comparison of pancreas transplantation with portal venous and enteric exocrine drainage to the standard technique utilizing bladder drainage of exocrine secretions. Transplantation. 1996;62:1353–4.
41. Israni A, Skeans M, Gustafson S, Schnitzler M, Wainright J, Carrico R, et al. OPTN/SRTR 2012 Annual Data Report: pancreas. Am J Transplant. 2014;14(S1):45.
42. Goldberg P. Comprehensive management of post-transplant diabetes mellitus: from intensive care to home care. Endocrinol Metabol Clin N Am. 2007;36:905.
43. Ghofaili K, Fung M, Ao Z, Meloche M, Shapiro R, Warnock G, et al. Effect of Exenatide on [beta] Cell Function After Islet Transplantation in Type 1 Diabetes. Transplantation. 2007;83:24.
44. Emre S, Genyk Y, Schluger L, Fishbein T, Guy S, Sheiner P, et al. Treatment of tacrolimus-related adverse events by conversion to cyclosporine in liver transplant patients. Transplant Int. 2000;13:73.
45. Troppmann C. Nonimmunologic endocrine graft dysfunction. In: Gruessner RW, Sutherland DER, editors. Transplantation of the pancreas. New York: Springer; 2004. p. 249.
46. Montero N, Webster AC, Royuela A, Zamora J, Crespo Barrio M, Pascual J. Steroid avoidance or withdrawal for pancreas and pancreas with kidney transplant recipients. Cochrane Database Syst Rev. 2014;15(9):CD007669.
47. Amodu LI, Tiwari M, Levy A, Akerman M, Rehman S, Kressel A, et al. Steroid maintenance is associated with an increased risk of infections but has no effect on patient and graft survival in pancreas transplantation: A retrospective review of the UNOS database. Pancreatology. 2015;15:554.

48. Miller LW. Cardiovascular toxicities of immunosuppressive agents. Am J Transplant. 2002;2:807.

49. Lauria M, Figueiró J, Machado L, Sanches M, Lana A, Ribeiro-Oliveira A. The impact of functioning pancreas-kidney transplantation and pancreas alone transplantation on the lipid metabolism of statin-naïve diabetic patients. Clin Transplant. 2009;23:199.

50. Luan F, Miles C, Cibrik D, Ojo A. Impact of simultaneous pancreas and kidney transplantation on cardiovascular risk factors in patients with type I diabetes mellitus. Transplantation. 2007;84:541.

51. Malheiro J, Martins L, Fonseca I, Gomes A, Santos J, Dias L, et al. Steroid withdrawal in simultaneous pancreas-kidney transplantation: a 7-year report. Transplant Proc. 2009;41:909.

52. Bagdade J, Teuscher A, Ritter M, Eckel R, Robertson R. Alterations in cholesteryl ester transfer, lipoprotein lipase, and lipoprotein composition after combined pancreas-kidney transplantation. Diabetes. 1998;47:113.

53. Föger B, Königsrainer A, Ritsch A, Lechleitner M, Steurer W, Margreiter R, et al. Pancreas transplantation modulates reverse cholesterol transport. Transplant Int. 1999;12:360.

54. Larsen J, Stratta R, Ozaki C, Taylor R, Miller S, Duckworth W. Lipid status after pancreas kidney transplantation. Diabetes Care. 1992;15:35.

55. Kasiske B, Zeier M, Craig J, Ekberg H, Garvey C, Green M, et al. KDIGO clinical practice guideline for the care of kidney transplant recipients. Am J Transplant. 2009;9 Suppl 3:S1.

56. Markowski D, Larsen J, McElligott M, Walter G, Miller S, Frisbie K, et al. Diet after pancreas transplantation. Diabetes Care. 1996;19:735.

57. Steinmüller T, Gräf K, Schleicher J, Leder K, Bechstein W, Mueller A, et al. The effect of FK 506 versus cyclosporine on glucose and lipid metabolism- a randomized trial. Transplantation. 1994;58:669.

58. Baid-Agrawal S, Delmonico FL, Tolkoff-Rubin N, Farrell M, Williams WW, Shih V, et al. Cardiovascular risk profile after conversion from cyclosporine A to tacrolimus in stable renal recipients. Transplantation. 2004;77:1199.

59. Kobashigawa J. Statins in solid organ transplantation – is there an immunosuppressive effect? Am J Transplant. 2004;4:1013.

60. Scalea J, Cooper M. A possible role for statin therapy in solitary pancreas transplantation? Transplant Proc. 2013;45:3348.

61. Palmer S, Navaneethan S, Craig J, Perkovic V, Johnson D, Nigwekar S, et al. HMG CoA reductase inhibitors (statins) for kidney transplant recipients. Cochrane Database Syst Rev. 2014;1:CD005019.

62. Mück W, Neal D, Boix O, Voith B, Hasan R, Alexander G. Tacrolimus/cerivastatin interaction study in liver transplant recipients. J Clin Pharmacol. 2001;52:213.

63. Stirling C, Isles C. Rhabdomyolysis due to simvastatin in a transplant patient: are some statins safer than others? Nephrol Dial Transplant. 2001;16:873.

64. Choe E, Wang H, Kwon O, Cho Y, Huh K, Kim M. HMG CoA reductase inhibitor treatment induces dysglycemia in renal allograft recipients. Transplantation. 2014;97:419.

65. Mucha K, Foroncewicz B, Oldakowska-J U, Soldacki D, Kryst P, Paczek L. How to Choose a Statin After Kidney Transplantation: Case Analyses. Transplant Proc. 2006;38:161.

66. Riella L, Gabardi S, Chandraker A. Dyslipidemia and its therapeutic challenges in renal transplantation. Am J Transplant. 2012;12:1975.

67. Robertsen I, Asberg A, Granseth T, Vethe N, Akhlaghi F, Ghareeb M, et al. More potent lipid-lowering effect by rosuvastatin compared with fluvastatin in everolimus-treated renal transplant recipients. Transplantation. 2014;97:1266.

68. Broeders N, Knoop C, Antoine M, Tielemans C, Abramowicz D. Fibrate-induced increase in blood urea and creatinine: is gemfibrozil the only innocuous agent? Nephrol Dial Transplant. 2000;15:1993.

69. Davis TM, Ting R, Best JD, Donoghoe MW, Drury PL, Sullivan DR, et al. Effects of fenofibrate on renal function in patients with type 2 diabetes mellitus: the Fenofibrate Intervention and Event Lowering in Diabetes (FIELD) Study. Diabetologia. 2011;54:280.

70. Chiu M, Sprague S, Bruce D, Woodle E, Thistlethwaite J, Josephson M. Analysis of fracture prevalence in kidney pancreas allograft recipients. J Am Soc Nephrol. 1998;9:677.

71. Smets Y, de Fijter J, Ringers J, Lemkes H, Hamdy N. Long-term follow-up study on bone mineral density and fractures after simultaneous pancreas-kidney transplantation. Kidney Int. 2004;66:2070.

72. Pereira S, Pedroso S, Martins L, Santos P, Almeida M, Freitas C, et al. Bone mineral density after simultaneous kidney-pancreas transplantation: four years follow-up of 57 recipients. Transplant Proc. 2010;42:555.

73. Nisbeth U, Lindh E, Ljunghall S, Backman U, Fellström B. Increased fracture rate in diabetes mellitus and females after renal transplantation. Transplantation. 1999;67:1218.

74. Vautour L, Melton L, Clarke B, Achenbach S, Oberg A, McCarthy J. Long-term fracture risk following renal transplantation: a population-based study. Osteoporos Int. 2004;15:160.

75. Hamdy N. Calcium and bone metabolism pre- a post-kiney transplantation. Endocrinol Metabol Clin N Am. 2007;36:923.

76. Nikkel L, Iyer S, Mohan S, Zhang A, McMahon D, Tanriover B, et al. Pancreas-kidney transplantation is associated with reduced fracture risk compared to kidney alone transplantation in men with type 1 diabetes. Kidney Int. 2013;83:471.

77. Rocha A, Martins S, Malheiro J, Dores J, Santos C, Henriques C. Changes in bone mineral density following long-term simultaneous pancreas-kidney transplantation. J Bone Miner Metab. 2015; in print.

78. Monier-Faugere M, Mawad H, Qi Q, Friedler R, Malluche H. High prevalence of low bone turnover and occurrence of osteomalacia after kidney transplantation. J Am Soc Nephrol. 2000;11:1093.

79. Rojas E, Carlini R, Clesca P, Arminio A, Suniaga O, De Elguezabal K, et al. The pathogenesis of osteodystrophy after renal transplantation as detected by early alterations in bone remodeling. Kidney Int. 2003;63:1915.

80. Julian B, Laskow D, Dubovsky J, Dubovsky E, Curtis J, Quarles L. Rapid loss of vertebral mineral density after renal transplantation. N Engl J Med. 1991;325:544.

81. Fornoni A, Cornacchia F, Howard G, Roos B, Striker G, Striker L. Cyclosporin A affects extracellular matrix synthesis and degradation by mouse MC3T3–E1 osteoblasts in vitro. Nephrol Dial Transplant. 2001;16:500.

82. Stempfle H, Werner C, Siebert U, Assum T, Wehr U, Rambeck W, et al. The role of tacrolimus (FK506)-based immunosuppression on bone mineral density and bone turnover after cardiac transplantation: a prospective, longitudinal, randomized, double-blind trial with calcitriol. Transplantation. 2002;73:547.

83. Hong Y, Choi D, Lim S, Yang C, Chang Y. Decreased parathyroid Klotho expression is associated with persistent hyperparathyroidism after kidney transplantation. Transplant Proc. 2013;45:2957.

84. Alsina J, Gonzalez M, Bonnin R, Ricart Y, Castelao A, Gonzalez C, et al. Long-term evolution of renal osteodystrophy after renal transplantation. Transplant Proc. 1989;21:2151.

85. Messa P, Sindici C, Cannella G, Miotti V, Risaliti A, Gropuzzo M, et al. Persistent secondary hyperparathyroidism after renal transplantation. Kidney Int. 1998;54:1704.

86. Perrin P, Caillard S, Javier R, Braun L, Heibel F, Borni-Duval C, et al. Persistent hyperparathyroidism is a major risk factor for fractures in the five years after kidney transplantation. Am J Transplant. 2013;13:2653.

87. Rangel E, Sá J, Gomes S, Carvalho A, Melaragno C, Gonzalez A, et al. Charcot neuroarthropathy after simultaneous pancreas-kidney transplant. Transplantation. 2012;94:642.

88. Holmes C, Schmidt B, Munson M, Wrobel JS. Charcot stage 0: A review and considerations for making the correct diagnosis early. Clinical Diabetes and Endocrinology. 2015;1:18.

89. Bouillon R. Diabetic bone disease. Calcif Tissue Int. 1991;49:155.

90. Mainra R, Elder GJ. Individualized therapy to prevent bone mineral density loss after kidney and kidney-pancreas transplantation. Clin J Am Soc Nephrol. 2010;5:117.

91. Keyzer C, Riphagen IJ, Joosten MM, Navis G, Muller Kobold AC, Kema IP, et al. Associations of 25(OH) and 1,25(OH)2 vitamin D with long-term outcomes in stable renal transplant recipients. J Clin Endocrinol Metab. 2015;100:81.

92. Hesketh C, Knoll G, Molnar A, Tsampalieros A, Zimmerman D. Vitamin D and kidney transplant outcomes: a protocol for a systematic review and meta-analysis. Syst Rev. 2014;3:64.

93. Yu R, Faull R, Coates PT, Coates PS. Calcium supplements lower bone resorption after renal transplant. Clin Transplant. 2012;26:292.

94. Ebeling P. Approach to the patient with transplantation-related bone loss. J Clin Endocrinol Metab. 2009;94:1483.

95. Messa P, Regalia A, Alfieri C, Cresseri D, Forzenigo L, Gandolfo M, et al. Current indications to parathyroidectomy in CKD patients before and after renal transplantation. Nephrol. 2013;26:1025.

96. Mack-Shipman LR, Ratanasuwan T, Leone JP, Miller SA, Lyden ER, Erickson JM, et al. Reproductive hormones after pancreas transplantation. Transplantation. 2000;70:1180.

9

Temporal changes in frequency of severe hypoglycemia treated by emergency medical services in types 1 and 2 diabetes: a population-based data-linkage cohort study

Huan Wang[1*], Peter T. Donnan[1], Callum J. Leese[2], Edward Duncan[3], David Fitzpatrick[3,4], Brian M. Frier[5] and Graham P. Leese[6]

Abstract

Background: Almost 20 years ago, the frequencies of severe hypoglycemia requiring emergency medical treatment were reported in people with types 1 and 2 diabetes in the Tayside region of Scotland. With subsequent improvements in the treatment of diabetes, concurrent with changes in the provision of emergency medical care, a decline in the frequency of severe hypoglycemia could be anticipated. The present population-based data-linkage cohort study aimed to ascertain whether a temporal change has occurred in the incidence rates of hypoglycemia requiring emergency medical services in people with types 1 and 2 diabetes.

Methods: The study population comprised all people with diabetes in Tayside, Scotland over the period 1 January 2011 to 31 December 2012. Patients' data from different healthcare sources were linked anonymously to measure the incidence rates of hypoglycemia requiring emergency medical services that include treatment by ambulance staff and in hospital emergency departments, and necessitated hospital admission. These were compared with data recorded in 1997–1998 in the same region.

Results: In January 2011 to December 2012, 2029 people in Tayside had type 1 diabetes and 21,734 had type 2 diabetes, compared to 977 and 7678, respectively, in June 1997 to May 1998. In people with type 2 diabetes, the proportion treated with sulfonylureas had declined from 36.8 to 22.4% ($p < 0.001$), while insulin-treatment had increased from 11.7 to 18.7% ($p < 0.001$). The incidence rate of hypoglycemia requiring emergency medical treatment had significantly fallen from 0.115 (95% CI: 0.094–0.136) to 0.082 (0.073–0.092) events per person per year in type 1 diabetes ($p < 0.001$), and from 0.118 (0.095–0.141) to 0.037 (0.003–0.041) in insulin-treated type 2 diabetes ($p = 0.008$). However, the absolute annual number of hypoglycemia events requiring emergency treatment was 1.4-fold higher.

Conclusions: Although from 1998 to 2012 the incidences of hypoglycemia requiring emergency medical services appeared to have declined by a third in type 1 diabetes and by two thirds in insulin-treated type 2 diabetes, because the prevalence of diabetes was higher (2.7 fold), the number of severe hypoglycemia events requiring emergency medical treatment was greater.

Keywords: Diabetes, Hypoglycemia, Emergency medical care, Insulin, Sulfonylurea

* Correspondence: hwang@dundee.ac.uk
[1]Dundee Epidemiology and Biostatistics Unit, Population Health Sciences, University of Dundee, The Mackenzie Building, Kirsty Semple Way, Dundee DD2 4BF, UK
Full list of author information is available at the end of the article

Background

Hypoglycemia remains a common side-effect of the treatment of diabetes with insulin despite the introduction of novel insulins, formulations and methods of delivery, coupled with advances in glycemic monitoring. The epidemiology of severe hypoglycemia (defined as any event requiring help for recovery) has been well documented in western countries [1], but is much more common in many parts of the world than had been recognised previously [2], as is non-severe (self-treated) hypoglycemia, particularly during sleep [1]. In unselected populations with type 1 diabetes in northern Europe the incidence of severe hypoglycemia has been reported to vary from 1.1 to 3.2 events per person per year [1, 3–8]. Population-based studies of emergency medical services utilisation [9] have reported the incidence of hypoglycemia requiring emergency treatment in people with type 1 diabetes to be between 0.08 and 0.49 events per person per year. Severe hypoglycemia events in people with diabetes account for 0.5% to 1.02% of all emergency ambulance call outs in the UK per annum [10–13] where the frequency of severe hypoglycemia and its treatment by emergency medical services has been surveyed by opportunistic examination of ambulance records [10, 11]. However, the accuracy and validity of many such surveys were limited by inadequate study design and retrospective review of incomplete data.

Almost 20 years ago, the frequencies of severe hypoglycemia events that required the assistance of emergency medical services from primary care, ambulance, hospital emergency and inpatient medical services were recorded prospectively in detail over a 12-month period (June 1997 to May 1998 inclusive) in people with types 1 and 2 diabetes in the region of Tayside in Scotland [12]. The incidences of severe hypoglycemia events requiring emergency medical treatment were 0.115 events per person per year in type 1 diabetes, 0.118 in insulin-treated type 2 diabetes and 0.009 in people with type 2 diabetes taking sulfonylureas, with respective prevalence of 7.1%, 7.3%, and 0.8%. Many more self-reported hypoglycemia events are treated by family members, friends or colleagues who do not request help from the emergency medical services [3, 12] and an incidence of 1.15 events per person per year in type 1 diabetes and 0.35 events per person per year in insulin-treated type 2 diabetes [12], were reported in the same region. Around 63% to 73% people who experienced severe hypoglycemia events remain at home following treatment by ambulance paramedics [10, 11, 13], which influences the frequency of treatment in hospital emergency departments (EDs) and hospital admission. With subsequent improvements in the treatment of diabetes, combined with changes in methods of providing emergency medical care, it could be anticipated that the frequency of severe hypoglycemia events requiring emergency treatment would have declined despite more intensive management of diabetes being applied to attain stricter glycemic control.

The present study aimed to re-measure the incidence rates of severe hypoglycemia in types 1 and 2 diabetes that had required emergency medical services in the same region of Tayside over the period 1 January 2011 to 31 December 2012, and by comparison with the incidence rates documented in 1997–1998, to ascertain whether these had changed significantly over time.

Methods

Data sources and linkage

Data were derived from several sources. The Scottish Care Information-Diabetes (SCI-Diabetes) provides an integrated shared electronic patient record to support the management of people with diabetes within the National Health Service (NHS) in Scotland. It includes information on type of diabetes, date of diagnosis and treatment modality. The Scottish Ambulance Service electronic patient records comprise the date of the event, the symptoms, diagnosis of hypoglycemia and treatment administered by ambulance clinicians to individual patients, which can identify emergency call-outs related to hypoglycemia. Data on admissions to EDs with hypoglycemia were obtained from Information Services Division Scotland. The Scottish Morbidity Register (SMR01) dataset collects episode level data on hospital inpatient and day case admissions from hospitals in Scotland. It provides information on dates of admission and discharge, and medical conditions, which can be used to identify hospital admission associated with hypoglycemia. Prescribing data were linked with diabetes drugs with British National Formulary (BNF) codes, to provide detailed information on the drugs dispensed. Data on social deprivation were available for the 2011–12 cohort using the Scottish index of multiple deprivation (SIMD) which is derived from the postcode via the community health index register [14]. The SIMD categories patients into five divisions of deprivation.

Data were collected and collated by the Health Informatics Centre in University of Dundee that conforms to ISO27001. Data was linked using the Community Health Index number that is used universally in the NHS with over 99% of accuracy for people with diabetes in Scotland.

Study design and statistical analyses

The period of study was from 1 January 2011 to 31 December 2012, inclusive, and similar methodology was used to that employed in the previous study [12], enabling direct comparisons of incidence rates of severe hypoglycemia to be made with 1997–1998. The study population comprised all people with diabetes in

Tayside, Scotland. All events of hypoglycemia that required emergency medical services (ambulance, ED attendance, and hospital admission) during the study period were identified. The incidence of hypoglycemia was analysed separately by type of diabetes. Type 1 diabetes was defined by requiring insulin within 6 months of diagnosis and not taking any oral glucose-lowering medication other than metformin. All other participants were considered to have type 2 diabetes and were further classified by the type of medications being prescribed in order of their propensity to induce hypoglycemia:

a) Agents that do not usually cause hypoglycemia, (i.e. metformin, pioglitazone, dipeptidyl peptidase-4 (DPP-4) inhibitors, sodium-glucose co-transporter-2 (SGLT-2) inhibitors, glucagon-like peptide-1 (GLP-1) agonists).
b) Oral medications that may cause hypoglycemia, i.e. sulfonylureas or glinides. This could be in combination with medication in category a).
c) Treatment with insulin. This could be in combination with a medication in either category a) or b).

The incidence rates were expressed as events per person per year. The 95% confidence intervals were calculated based on the maximum likelihood method for Poisson-distributed observations. The incidence rate ratios (IRRs) along with their 95% confidence intervals and p values were calculated to assess the significance of differences between the two populations in the same region but at a different time period. All the analyses were conducted in R version 3.2.5.

Results
Study cohort
A substantial increase in the prevalence of diabetes had occurred in Tayside, Scotland during the 14 years

separating the two surveys. In June 1997 to May 1998, of the 367,051 residents of Tayside, 8655 people had diabetes (crude overall prevalence = 2.4%), with 977 of 8655 (11.3%) having type 1 diabetes and 7678 (88.7%) having type 2 diabetes (Table 1). The present study examined data from 23,763 people with diabetes (mid-year population estimate in Tayside in 2012 = 411,749, crude overall prevalence of diabetes during the 2 years from 1 January 2011 to 31 December 2012 = 5.8%), which included 2029 with type 1 diabetes (8.5%) and 21,734 with type 2 diabetes (91.5%).

Between June 1997 and May 1998, 69 of 977 people with type 1 diabetes had experienced 112 hypoglycemia events requiring emergency medical services, while 91 of 7678 people with type 2 diabetes had been treated for 132 events. From 1 January 2011 to 31 December 2012, a total of 702 events of hypoglycemia requiring emergency medical services were recorded in 467 people with diabetes (Table 1). Some individuals had experienced recurrent episodes of hypoglycemia; 187 people with type 1 diabetes had experienced 319 events and 280 people with type 2 diabetes had experienced 383 events.

From June 1997 to May 1998, among the 7678 people with type 2 diabetes, 901 (11.7%) were being treated with insulin (Table 2), 2823 (36.8%) were being treated with sulfonylureas (group b), and 3954 (51.5%) were being treated with non-insulin secretagogues alone (group a). From 1 January 2011 to 31 December 2012, a significantly higher proportion of people with type 2 diabetes were receiving treatment with non-secretagogues (58.9%) or insulin (18.7%), but fewer were being treated with secretagogues (22.4%).

Incidence of severe hypoglycemia
The overall annual incidence rates of severe hypoglycemia events requiring treatment by the emergency medical services during the 2 years of the survey are shown for the

Table 1 People with diabetes and number of hypoglycemia events requiring emergency medical services in Tayside, Scotland

	Type 1 diabetes	Type 2 diabetes	Total
June 1997 – May 1998			
People with diabetes	977 (11.3%)	7678 (88.7%)	8655 (100%)
Mean age at study	33	66	–
Mean duration of diabetes (years)	17	8	–
People with severe hypoglycemia	69	91	160
Severe hypoglycemia events	112	132	244
1 January 2011–31 December 2012			
People with diabetes	2029 (8.5%)	21,734 (91.5%)	23,763 (100%)
Mean age at study	40	68	–
Mean duration of diabetes (years)	18	7	–
People with severe hypoglycemia	187	280	467
Severe hypoglycemia events	319	383	702

Table 2 Number of people (%) with type 2 diabetes and different types of treatment, including a) non-secretagogues e.g. metformin, pioglitazone, DPP-4 inhibitor, SGLT-2 inhibitor, GLP-1 agonist; b) secretagogues e.g. sulfonylureas and glinides; and insulin treated type 2 diabetes

Group of people with type 2 diabetes	Number of people (%)		Proportion difference (95% CI)	P value
	June 1997 – May 1998 (n = 7678)	1 Jan 2011–31 Dec 2012 (n = 21,734)		
a)	3954 (51.5%)	12,812 (58.9%)	0.075 (0.062–0.087)	< 0.001
b)	2823 (36.8%)	4859 (22.4%)	−0.144 (−0.156 – −0.132)	< 0.001
Insulin	901 (11.7%)	4063 (18.7%)	0.070 (0.061–0.078)	< 0.001

different treatment groups in Table 3. This was highest in people with type 1 diabetes (0.082 events per person per year, 95% CI: 0.073–0.092) and lowest in those with type 2 diabetes who were taking oral glucose-lowering medications that were not insulin secretagogues (group a). Among people with type 2 diabetes, the insulin-treated patients had a much higher incidence than those receiving other types of treatment. By comparison with the period of June 1997 to May 1998, significantly lower incidence were observed in people with type 1 diabetes (IRR = 0.720, 95% CI: 0.580–0.892, p < 0.001) and people with type 2 diabetes receiving insulin (IRR = 0.314, 95% CI: 0.249–0.395, p = 0.008). The IRRs for the groups receiving secretagogues (group a) and non-secretagogues (group b) were not calculated because the number of hypoglycemia events in these two groups were not currently available for the data from June 1997 to May 1998.

No information was available on ethnicity but the prevalence of ethnic minorities is low at ≤3% in Tayside, Scotland, and has not changed in the time between these two surveys in what is a very stable population. Data on social deprivation were not available from 1997 to 1998, but data from 2011 to 2012 showed an increasing trend in the incidence rate of severe hypoglycemia in association with social deprivation in type 1 diabetes (Table 4), but a similar trend was not observed for different social deprivation categories in insulin-treated type 2 diabetes.

Emergency medical services utilized
The number of hypoglycemia events requiring different emergency medical services from 1 January 2011 to 31 December 2012 are shown in Fig. 1. Of the 702 events, 512 required emergency attendance by the ambulance service, 150 were treated in the hospital emergency department, and 175 events resulted in direct or indirect hospital admission. Any combination of these three emergency medical services was utilized in 116 hypoglycemia events. The proportion requiring inpatient hospital treatment had slightly increased from 21% (52 of 244 events) in 1997–1998 to 25% (175 of 702 events) in the period from 1 January 2011 to 31 December 2012, whereas usage of the ambulance service and of treatment in an emergency department was less frequent, decreasing from 91% (223 of 244) and 63% (153 of 244), respectively, to 73% (512 of 702) and 21% (150 of 702). Overall, 124 of 383 (32%) events in type 2 diabetes and 51 of 319 (16%) events in type 1 diabetes resulted in hospital admission. In general, a 1.4-fold increase in the total number of severe hypoglycemia events (244 events in 1997–1998 to an average of 351 events per year in 2011 and 2012) was recorded, compared to a 2.7-fold increase in the total

Table 3 Incidence rates of hypoglycemia requiring emergency medical services. (Rates for patients with type 1 diabetes, type 2 diabetes treated with a) non-secretagogues, b) secretagogues, or insulin)

Group	June 1997–May 1998	1 January 2011–31 December 2012			
	Incidence rate[a] (95% CI)	Events (person-years)	Incidence rate[a] (95% CI)	IRR[b] (95% CI)	P value
Type 1	0.115 (0.094–0.136)	319 (3867.35)	0.082 (0.073–0.092)	0.720 (0.580–0.892)	< 0.001
Type 2 a)	0.001 (0.000–0.002)	50 (22,100.36)	0.002 (0.002–0.003)	–	–
b)	0.009 (0.006–0.013)	51 (9318.80)	0.005 (0.004–0.007)	–	–
Insulin	0.118 (0.095–0.141)	282 (7601.69)	0.037 (0.033–0.041)	0.314 (0.249–0.395)	0.008
All type 2	0.017 (0.014–0.020)	383 (39,020.86)	0.010 (0.009–0.011)	0.571 (0.468–0.696)	< 0.001

[a]Incidence rate is expressed as events per person per year. [b]IRR incidence rate ratio

Table 4 Incidence rates of hypoglycemia requiring emergency medical services in people with type 1 and insulin-treated type 2 diabetes across different categories of Scottish index of multiple deprivation

Social deprivation	Incidence rates of severe hypoglycemia (95% CI)	
	Type 1 diabetes	Insulin-treated type 2 diabetes
1 (most deprived)	0.120 (0.093–0.147)	0.044 (0.033–0.054)
2	0.103 (0.078–0.128)	0.048 (0.036–0.059)
3	0.089 (0.069–0.108)	0.024 (0.016–0.031)
4	0.066 (0.051–0.081)	0.037 (0.029–0.045)
5 (least deprived)	0.041 (0.025–0.058)	0.032 (0.021–0.044)

diabetes population during the same period from 8655 to 23,763.

Discussion

While severe hypoglycemia remains a major clinical problem, particularly for people treated with insulin, this may be declining in some patient groups. The present population-based, data-linkage study within a single region of Scotland has demonstrated that a lower incidence rate of severe hypoglycemia had required treatment by emergency medical services compared to the frequency observed 14 years earlier. While the incidence rate of severe hypoglycemia in people with type 1 diabetes had declined by about 30% (IRR = 0.720, 95% CI: 0.580–0.892, $p < 0.001$), a more prominent fall was observed in people with insulin-treated type 2 diabetes, which was almost 70% lower (IRR = 0.314, 95% CI: 0.249–0.395, $p = 0.008$). However, although the incidence of severe hypoglycemia had declined, the absolute number of events had increased by 1.4 fold, in association with a 2.7-fold rise in the size of the diabetes population in Tayside. A similar finding of a lower incidence of severe hypoglycemia but a higher absolute number requiring treatment in hospital was observed over a 10-year period in a study in England [15], while a

higher absolute number of severe hypoglycemia events was also reported in a German study [16]. This indicates that the overall demand on the emergency medical services to treat severe hypoglycemia is rising, despite a decline in the incidence rate of severe hypoglycemia requiring emergency medical treatment.

The prevalence of diabetes in Tayside, Scotland in 1997–1998 was identified from an accurately recorded population-based data-linkage study [17]. While the greater number of people with diabetes in 2011 and 2012 compared to 1997–1998 probably reflects a genuine increase in prevalence of the disorder, it may partly result from better case ascertainment, with fewer people having undiagnosed diabetes and the observed prevalence is consistent with national prevalence statistics. The mean duration of type 2 diabetes has also declined from 1998 to 2011 and 2012, from 8 to 7 years, consistent with earlier diagnosis.

The lower incidence rate of severe hypoglycemia in type 1 diabetes that has now been observed may be a consequence of more intensive diabetes education in Tayside since 1998 [18] along with the greater use of glucose monitoring and insulin pumps, and the introduction of newer insulin analogues, which are associated with a lower rate of hypoglycemia [19], particularly at night. Although an overall reduction in the incidence rate of severe hypoglycemia may have been offset by greater efforts to improve glycemic control, the mean HbA1c in people with hypoglycemia in 2011–2012 were higher than in 1997–1998 for both type 1 and type 2 diabetes (Table 5). Poorer average glycemic control could be one explanation as to why the incidence rate of severe hypoglycemia events had declined, although in recent years no deterioration in glycemic control has been evidence in all patients with type 1 diabetes in Scotland [20]. The more likely explanation is that it may be easier to achieve good glycemic control without suffering

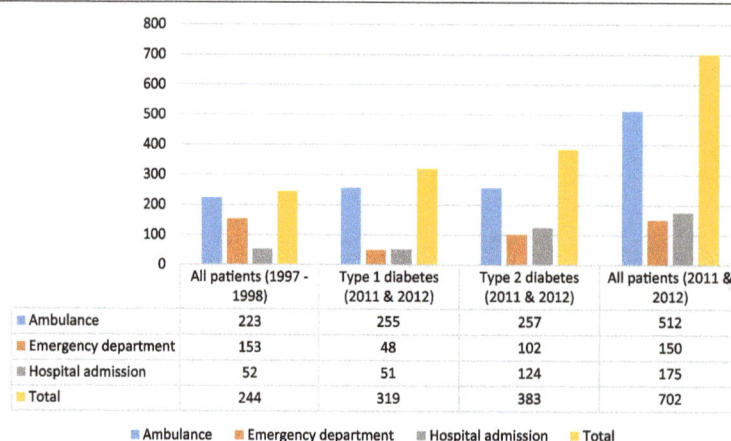

	All patients (1997 - 1998)	Type 1 diabetes (2011 & 2012)	Type 2 diabetes (2011 & 2012)	All patients (2011 & 2012)
■ Ambulance	223	255	257	512
■ Emergency department	153	48	102	150
■ Hospital admission	52	51	124	175
■ Total	244	319	383	702

Fig. 1 Number of hypoglycemia events requiring emergency medical services

Table 5 Mean HbA1c levels with 95% confidence intervals in groups of people with types 1 or 2 diabetes who have had (or have not had) hypoglycemia events requiring emergency medical services. b) Secretagogues e.g. sulfonylureas and glinides

	Severe hypoglycemia	June 1997–May 1998		January 2011–December 2012	
		Number of people	Mean HbA1c (95% CI)	Number of people	Mean HbA1c (95% CI)
Type 1	No	908	7.93 (7.76–8.10)	1671	9.19 (5.45–12.93)
	Yes	69	7.77 (7.29–8.25)	182	9.00 (5.76–12.23)
Type 2 b)	No	2800	7.16 (7.08–7.23)	4772	7.93 (4.81–11.05)
	Yes	23	8.00 (7.10–8.91)	47	7.60 (4.72–10.48)
Insulin	No	835	8.23 (8.09–8.37)	3390	8.86 (5.16–12.56)
	Yes	66	7.87 (7.47–8.28)	183	8.49 (4.97–12.02)
All diabetes	No	8495	7.19 (7.14–7.24)	20,953	7.67 (4.21–11.13)
	Yes	160	7.85 (7.57–8.14)	454	8.47 (4.98–11.95)

hypoglycemia, and thus hypoglycemia is relatively more common in patients with erratic control and higher mean HbA1c. The assumption that an inverse linear relationship exists between the frequency of severe hypoglycemia and HbA1c concentration is not supported by cross-sectional studies of both type 1 [21] or type 2 diabetes [22], in which many people who experience recurrent severe hypoglycemia have elevated HbA1c concentrations. This is consistent with severe hypoglycemia being relatively common in people whose glycemic control is poor.

In addition, the mean HbA1c values for 1997–98 and 2011–12 are not directly comparable as the ascertainment of HbA1c measurements were approximately 80% and 91% respectively, and patients not engaging with medical services are more likely to have poor glycemic control and are less likely to have HbA1c measured regularly. The explanation for the increasing age of patients with type 1 diabetes having hypoglycemia may be similar, with a greater proportion of younger patients receiving more modern insulins and or using continuous subcutaneous insulin infusion with an insulin pump.

In the 14 years between the two studies the proportion of people with type 2 diabetes treated with insulin had risen significantly from 11.7 to 18.7% (Table 2), and the absolute number of severe hypoglycemia events had increased from 132 to an average of 191 events per year. Despite the increase in the absolute number of events, the incidence rate of severe hypoglycemia in people with insulin-treated type 2 diabetes requiring emergency medical treatment was significantly lower and may have been promoted by changes in clinical management. These include more comprehensive patient education, the earlier use of insulin while significant β-cell function is still preserved, which is associated with a lower risk of hypoglycemia [23], and the earlier use of basal insulin in combination with oral agents, including DPP-4 inhibitors and GLP-1 agonists, which have a low risk of inducing hypoglycemia. The duration of insulin therapy is

closely related to hypoglycemia risk in type 2 diabetes, which rises progressively as pancreatic β-cell function fails [3, 4, 24].

The incidence rate of severe hypoglycemia also declined in people with type 2 diabetes treated with sulfonylureas. This was associated with a decline in the use of sulfonylureas from 36.8 to 22.4%, and may reflect avoidance of their use in people at high risk of hypoglycemia. People with type 2 diabetes who experienced severe hypoglycemia were twice as likely to require hospital admission than those with type 1 diabetes (32% vs 16%), which has been reported by another British study [25]. People with type 2 diabetes are more likely to be older and more frail, both being risk factors that are associated with severe hypoglycemia [26, 27].

During the period of the present study, the ambulance service treated more episodes of severe hypoglycemia without the need to transfer patients to hospital. The increase in non-conveyance may have resulted from the introduction in non-conveyance clinical guidelines for post-hypoglycemia patients in 2005 [28].

The present study has some limitations. If an ambulance had been called after a self-treated episode of hypoglycemia had resolved, such an incident may not have been recorded as a severe hypoglycemia event. Hypoglycemia treated by General Practitioners (GP) would not have been recorded. Some cases may have been missed if the patients who had experienced severe hypoglycemia had presented with another principal complaint such as chest pain or the consequences of trauma, and blood glucose had not been measured.

The present study indicates that around 9% (187 of 2029) of people with type 1 diabetes experienced severe hypoglycemia that required emergency medical services, which compares to 13% in a recent large prospective study [29] that relied on self-reported data. When using self-reported data the incidence rate of severe hypoglycemia in type 2 diabetes has varied between 0.1 and 0.7 events per person per year [1, 3, 6, 10, 24, 30]. This compares to incidence rates of emergency medical treatment in the present study of 0.01 events per person per year for all people with type 2 diabetes and 0.037 events per person per year for those with insulin-treated type 2 diabetes (Table 3). In other studies, the reported rates were much lower at 0.017 events [31] and 0.003 events [32] per person per year, respectively.

Conclusions

The present large population-based study over a 2-year period has used data from different sources, and describes routine experience of the involvement of emergency medical services in the treatment of severe hypoglycemia. It suggests that the incidence rates of severe hypoglycemia requiring emergency medical services are declining both in types 1 and 2 diabetes, although the absolute number of events requiring emergency treatment is rising. While the burden on the emergency medical services is greater, with less duplication of service utilization and a significant reduction of the number of people attending hospital for treatment, provision may be more efficient than in previous years.

Abbreviations

DPP-4: Dipeptidyl peptidase-4; GLP-1: Glucagon-like peptide-1; NHS: National Health Service; SCI-Diabetes: Scottish Care Information-Diabetes; SGLT-2: Sodium-glucose co-transporter-2; SMR: Scottish Morbidity Register

Acknowledgments

We acknowledge Richard Combe, a senior data analyst in Scottish Ambulance Service, who extracted the date of ambulance service for this study. We also thank the editor and reviewers for their constructive comments for this manuscript.

Funding

Funding was received from Novo Nordisk for the support of a research fellow (HW) and data-linkage costs, and support of the Health Informatics Centre (HIC) in University of Dundee for managing and supplying the anonymised data.

Authors' contributions

HW researched the data and wrote the manuscript. CJL contributed to the discussion. ED and DF provided advice on ambulance clinical data. PTD, ED, and DF reviewed and revised the manuscript. GPL and BMF participated in conceptual design, contributed to the discussion, and revised the manuscript. All authors read and approved the final manuscript.

Competing interests

The authors declare that they have no competing interests.

Author details

[1]Dundee Epidemiology and Biostatistics Unit, Population Health Sciences, University of Dundee, The Mackenzie Building, Kirsty Semple Way, Dundee DD2 4BF, UK. [2]University of Edinburgh, Faculty of Medicine, Edinburgh, UK. [3]NMAHP Research Unit, University of Stirling, Stirling, UK. [4]Scottish Ambulance Service, National Headquarters, Edinburgh, UK. [5]BHF Centre for Cardiovascular Science, The Queen's Medical Research Institute, University of Edinburgh, Edinburgh, UK. [6]School of Medicine, Ninewells Hospital and Medical School, Dundee, UK.

References

1. Frier BM. Hypoglycaemia in diabetes mellitus: epidemiology and clinical implications. Nat Rev Endocrinol. 2014;10(12):711–22.
2. Khunti K, Alsifri S, Aronson R, Cigrovski Berkovic M, Enters-Weijnen C, Forsen T, et al. Rates and predictors of hypoglycaemia in 27 585 people from 24 countries with insulin-treated type 1 and type 2 diabetes: the global HAT study. Diabetes Obes Metab. 2016;18(9):907–15.
3. Donnelly LA, Morris AD, Frier BM, Ellis JD, Donnan PT, Durrant R, et al. Frequency and predictors of hypoglycaemia in Type 1 and insulin-treated Type 2 diabetes: a population-based study. Diabet Med. 2005;22(6):749–55.
4. Group UH. Risk of hypoglycaemia in types 1 and 2 diabetes: effects of treatment modalities and their duration. Diabetologia. 2007;50(6):1140–7.
5. Pramming S, Thorsteinsson B, Bendtson I, Binder C. Symptomatic hypoglycaemia in 411 type 1 diabetic patients. Diabet Med. 1991;8(3):217–22.
6. MacLeod KM, Hepburn DA, Frier BM. Frequency and morbidity of severe hypoglycaemia in insulin-treated diabetic patients. Diabet Med. 1993;10(3):238–45.
7. Pedersen-Bjergaard U, Pramming S, Heller SR, Wallace TM, Rasmussen AK, Jorgensen HV, et al. Severe hypoglycaemia in 1076 adult patients with type 1 diabetes: influence of risk markers and selection. Diabetes Metab Res Rev. 2004;20(6):479–86.
8. Kristensen PL, Hansen LS, Jespersen MJ, Pedersen-Bjergaard U, Beck-Nielsen H, Christiansen JS, et al. Insulin analogues and severe hypoglycaemia in type 1 diabetes. Diabetes Res Clin Pract. 2012;96(1):17–23.
9. Giorda CB, Ozzello A, Gentile S, Aglialoro A, Chiambretti A, Baccetti F, et al. Incidence and risk factors for severe and symptomatic hypoglycemia in type 1 diabetes. Results of the HYPOS-1 study. Acta Diabetol. 2015;
10. Farmer AJ, Brockbank KJ, Keech ML, England EJ, Deakin CD. Incidence and costs of severe hypoglycaemia requiring attendance by the emergency medical services in South Central England. Diabet Med. 2012;29(11):1447–50.
11. Khunti K, Fisher H, Paul S, Iqbal M, Davies MJ, Siriwardena AN. Severe hypoglycaemia requiring emergency medical assistance by ambulance services in the East Midlands: a retrospective study. Prim Care Diabetes. 2013;7(2):159–65.
12. Leese GP, Wang J, Broomhall J, Kelly P, Marsden A, Morrison W, et al. Frequency of severe hypoglycemia requiring emergency treatment in type 1 and type 2 diabetes: a population-based study of health service resource use. Diabetes Care. 2003;26(4):1176–80.
13. Brackenridge A, Wallbank H, Lawrenson RA, Russell-Jones D. Emergency management of diabetes and hypoglycaemia. Emerg Med J. 2006;23(3):183–5.
14. Scottish Index of Multiple Deprivation 2004: Summary Technical Report. Scottish Executive; 2004.
15. Zaccardi F, Davies MJ, Dhalwani NN, Webb DR, Housley G, Shaw D, et al. Trends in hospital admissions for hypoglycaemia in England: a retrospective, observational study. Lancet Diabetes Endocrinol. 2016;4(8):677–85.
16. Holstein A, Patzer OM, Machalke K, Holstein JD, Stumvoll M, Kovacs P. Substantial increase in incidence of severe hypoglycemia between 1997-2000 and 2007-2010: a German longitudinal population-based study. Diabetes Care. 2012;35(5):972–5.
17. Morris AD, Boyle DI, MacAlpine R, Emslie-Smith A, Jung RT, Newton RW, et al. The diabetes audit and research in Tayside Scotland (DARTS) study: electronic record linkage to create a diabetes register. DARTS/MEMO Collaboration. Br Med J. 1997;315(7107):524–8.

Temporal changes in frequency of severe hypoglycemia treated by emergency medical services in types 1 and 2...

79

18. Jordan LV, Robertson M, Grant L, Peters RE, Cameron JT, Chisholm S, et al. The Tayside insulin management course: an effective education programme in type 1 diabetes. Int J Clin Pract. 2013;67(5):462–8.

19. Pedersen-Bjergaard U, Kristensen PL, Beck-Nielsen H, Norgaard K, Perrild H, Christiansen JS, et al. Effect of insulin analogues on risk of severe hypoglycaemia in patients with type 1 diabetes prone to recurrent severe hypoglycaemia (HypoAna trial): a prospective, randomised, open-label, blinded-endpoint crossover trial. Lancet Diabetes Endocrinol. 2014;2(7):553–61.

20. Scottish Diabetes Survey Monitoring Group. Scottish diabetes survey 2015. NHS Scotland, 2015.

21. Weinstock RS, Xing D, Maahs DM, Michels A, Rickels MR, Peters AL, et al. Severe hypoglycemia and diabetic ketoacidosis in adults with type 1 diabetes: results from the T1D Exchange clinic registry. J Clin Endocrinol Metab. 2013;98(8):3411–9.

22. Lipska KJ, Warton EM, Huang ES, Moffet HH, Inzucchi SE, Krumholz HM, et al. HbA1c and risk of severe hypoglycemia in type 2 diabetes: the Diabetes and Aging Study. Diabetes Care. 2013;36(11):3535–42.

23. Chow LS, Chen H, Miller ME, Marcovina SM, Seaquist ER. Biomarkers related to severe hypoglycaemia and lack of good glycaemic control in ACCORD. Diabetologia. 2015;58(6):1160–6.

24. Henderson JN, Allen KV, Deary IJ, Frier BM. Hypoglycaemia in insulin-treated Type 2 diabetes: frequency, symptoms and impaired awareness. Diabet Med. 2003;20(12):1016–21.

25. Heller SR, Frier BM, Herslov ML, Gundgaard J, Gough SC. Severe hypoglycaemia in adults with insulin-treated diabetes: impact on healthcare resources. Diabet Med. 2016;33(4):471–7.

26. Shorr RI, Ray WA, Daugherty JR, Griffin MR. Incidence and risk factors for serious hypoglycemia in older persons using insulin or sulfonylureas. Arch Intern Med. 1997;157(15):1681–6.

27. Fu H, Curtis BH, Xie W, Festa A, Schuster DP, Kendall DM. Frequency and causes of hospitalization in older compared to younger adults with type 2 diabetes in the United States: a retrospective, claims-based analysis. J Diabetes Complicat. 2014;28(4):477–81.

28. Scottish Ambulance Service. Scottish Ambulance Service annual report. 2005.

29. Cariou B, Fontaine P, Eschwege E, Lievre M, Gouet D, Huet D, et al. Frequency and predictors of confirmed hypoglycaemia in type 1 and insulin-treated type 2 diabetes mellitus patients in a real-life setting: results from the DIALOG study. Diabetes Metab. 2015;41(2):116–25.

30. Akram K, Pedersen-Bjergaard U, Carstensen B, Borch-Johnsen K, Thorsteinsson B. Frequency and risk factors of severe hypoglycaemia in insulin-treated Type 2 diabetes: a cross-sectional survey. Diabet Med. 2006;23(7):750–6.

31. Davis TM, Brown SG, Jacobs IG, Bulsara M, Bruce DG, Davis WA. Determinants of severe hypoglycemia complicating type 2 diabetes: the Fremantle diabetes study. J Clin Endocrinol Metab. 2010;95(5):2240–7.

32. Khalid JM, Raluy-Callado M, Curtis BH, Boye KS, Maguire A, Reaney M. Rates and risk of hospitalisation among patients with type 2 diabetes: retrospective cohort study using the UK General Practice Research Database linked to English Hospital Episode Statistics. Int J Clin Pract. 2014;68(1):40–8.

10

Thyroid dysfunction in metabolic syndrome patients and its relationship with components of metabolic syndrome

Saroj Khatiwada[1]*, Santosh Kumar Sah[2], Rajendra KC[3], Nirmal Baral[4] and Madhab Lamsal[4]

Abstract

Background: A growing body of evidence suggests that metabolic syndrome is associated with endocrine disorders including thyroid dysfunction. Thyroid dysfunction in metabolic syndrome patients may further add to cardiovascular disease risk thereby increasing mortality. This study was done to assess thyroid function in metabolic syndrome patients and evaluate its relationship with the components of metabolic syndrome.

Methods: A cross sectional study was carried out among 169 metabolic syndrome patients at B P Koirala Institute of Health Sciences, Dharan, Nepal. Anthropometric measurements (height, weight, waist circumference) and blood pressure were taken. Fasting blood samples were analysed to measure glucose, triglyceride, high density lipoprotein (HDL) cholesterol and thyroid hormones (triiodothyronine, thyroxine and thyroid stimulating hormone).

Results: Thyroid dysfunction was seen in 31.9 % ($n = 54$) metabolic syndrome patients. Subclinical hypothyroidism (26.6 %) was the major thyroid dysfunction followed by overt hypothyroidism (3.5 %) and subclinical hyperthyroidism (1.7 %). Thyroid dysfunction was much common in females (39.7 %, $n = 29$) than males (26 %, $n = 25$) but not statistically significant ($p = 0.068$). The relative risk of having thyroid dysfunction in females was 1.525 (CI: 0.983–2.368) as compared to males. Significant differences ($p = 0.001$) were observed in waist circumference between patients with and without thyroid dysfunction and HDL cholesterol which had significant negative correlation with thyroid stimulating hormone.

Conclusions: Thyroid dysfunction, particularly subclinical hypothyroidism is common among metabolic syndrome patients, and is associated with some components of metabolic syndrome (waist circumference and HDL cholesterol).

Keywords: Metabolic syndrome, Nepal, Subclinical hypothyroidism, Thyroid dysfunction

Background

Metabolic syndrome constitutes a cluster of risk factors characterized by hypertension, atherogenic dyslipidemia, hyperglycemia, prothrombotic and proinflammatory conditions [1]. This cluster of metabolic abnormalities is associated with increased risk for atherosclerotic cardiovascular disease and type 2 diabetes mellitus [2]. The prevalence of metabolic syndrome is increasing all over the world with distinct evidence of high prevalence in India and other South Asian countries [3].

Thyroid dysfunction, prominently subclinical hypothyroidism has been observed more frequently in metabolic syndrome patients than general population [3]. Both metabolic syndrome and hypothyroidism are independent risk factors for cardiovascular diseases (CVD). Presence of both conditions may be compounded to increase the risk for CVD and a considerable overlap occurs in the pathogenic mechanisms of atherosclerotic cardiovascular disease by metabolic syndrome and hypothyroidism [4]. There are reports about higher thyroid stimulating hormone (TSH) level in metabolic syndrome patients than in healthy ones, and high prevalence of metabolic syndrome in subjects with TSH level higher than normal as compared to those with normal TSH level [5, 6]. However the association between

* Correspondence: khatiwadasaroj22@gmail.com
This study was done at the Department of Biochemistry of B P Koirala Institute of Health Sciences (BPKIHS) Dharan, Nepal.
[1]Department of Pharmacy, Central Institute of Science and Technology (CIST) College, Pokhara University, Kathmandu, Nepal
Full list of author information is available at the end of the article

thyroid dysfunction and components of metabolic syndrome is still debatable [7].

There is evidence that thyroid function may need to be assessed in patients with metabolic syndrome who are also at higher risk for CVD. Thyroid dysfunction is common in Nepal, and the prevalence of diabetes mellitus and metabolic syndrome has been rising steadily. Reports suggest that 20.7 % of the Nepalese population have metabolic syndrome based on National Cholesterol Education Program (NCEP) criteria [8, 9]. However, thyroid function in such patients is not well studied. A study by Gyawali et al. in the central region of Nepal reported thyroid dysfunction in 31.8 % of metabolic syndrome patients [3]. We conducted the present study among metabolic syndrome patients in the eastern region of Nepal to assess the rate of thyroid dysfunction and explore the potential relationship between components of metabolic syndrome and thyroid function, and provide evidence for the better clinical management of metabolic syndrome patients. The present study aims to evaluate the pattern of thyroid dysfunction in Nepalese metabolic syndrome patients.

In this study, we assessed thyroid function and examined the association between components of metabolic syndrome and thyroid function in Nepalese population with metabolic syndrome.

Methods

A cross-sectional study was conducted among metabolic syndrome patients at the department of biochemistry of B P Koirala Institute of Health Sciences (BPKIHS), Dharan, Nepal from September 2013 to September 2014. One hundred sixty nine metabolic syndrome patients aged ≥20 years were selected from the hospital during the study period. The sample size was calculated by taking prevalence of thyroid dysfunction as 15 % (approximate) in this region. Metabolic syndrome was diagnosed based on modified Asian NCEP-ATP III panel criteria [10]. The exclusion criteria was patients receiving medication that may alter thyroid functions or lipid levels, pregnant women, and patients with a cardiovascular disease, corticosteroid use, active liver disease, and renal dysfunction. After taking informed consent from each patient, height, weight, waist circumference and blood pressure was taken from each subject. The study protocol was approved by the institute review board of B P Koirala Institute of Health Sciences. Fasting venous blood samples (5 ml) were collected and analyzed for blood glucose, triglycerides, high density lipoprotein (HDL) cholesterol, free triiodothyronine (T3), free thyroxine (T4) and thyroid stimulating hormone (TSH). Blood glucose and triglycerides were measured by enzymatic method (kits from AGAPPE diagnostics by Biolyzer 100) and HDL cholesterol by homogeneous, direct method (kits from Gesan by

Biolyzer 100). Serum free T3, free T4 and TSH were measured by using fluorescent immunoassay (VIDAS, biomeriux SA, France).

Metabolic syndrome patients were considered to have thyroid dysfunction if patients thyroid hormones level fell outside the reference range (free T3 (4.0–8.3 pmol/L), free T4 (9.0–20.0 pmol/L) and TSH level (0.25–5 mIU/L)). Patients were said to be euthyroid if all thyroid hormone levels fell within reference range. Overt hypothyroidism was defined as TSH > 5 mIU/L and free T3 < 4.0 pmol/L and free T4 < 9.0 pmol/L. Subclinical hypothyroidism was considered if TSH > 5 mIU/L and free T3 and free T4 within reference range. Subclinical hyperthyroidism was defined as TSH < 0.25 mIU/L and free T3 and free T4 within reference range. The data generated from study was analyzed using SPSS version 11.0. Continuous variables were expressed as mean ± SD values. Independent sample t test and one way ANOVA was applied for continuous variables and chi square test for categorical variables at 95 % confidence interval. Pearson correlation coefficients were calculated to find relationship between the components of metabolic syndrome and thyroid profile parameters at 95 % confidence interval. Relative risk with 95 % confidence interval (CI) was used to assess the risk factors for thyroid dysfunction in metabolic syndrome.

Results

The study population consisted of 56.8 % ($n = 96$) males and 43.2 % ($n = 73$) females, with mean age of 47 ± 12.5 years. Height, weight, body mass index (BMI), waist circumference, systolic BP and diastolic BP were 157.4 ± 8 cm, 70.7 ± 7.9 Kg, 28.6 ± 3.3 Kg/m^2, 102.5 ± 6.7 cm, 129.3 ± 13.6 mmHg and 84.9 ± 11.5 mmHg respectively. Similarly, levels of biochemical parameters; fasting blood glucose, triglyceride, HDL cholesterol, free T3, free T4 and TSH were 126.2 ± 50.4 mg/dL, 198.2 ± 90.8 mg/dL, 49.9 ± 15.3 mg/dL, 5.1 ± 1.0 pmol/L, 12.0 ± 2.9 pmol/L and 4.2 ± 3.4 mIU/L respectively. Thyroid dysfunction was found in 31.9 % ($n = 54$) patients. Subclinical hypothyroidism (26.6 %) was the major thyroid dysfunction followed by overt hypothyroidism (3.5 %) and subclinical hyperthyroidism (1.7 %). Components of metabolic syndrome according to thyroid dysfunction type are shown in Table 1. Waist circumference and blood glucose was significantly different across the thyroid dysfunction groups. Thyroid dysfunction was more common among females 39.7 % ($n = 29$) than males 26 % ($n = 25$) but not statistically significant ($p = 0.068$). Among males, 23 had subclinical hypothyroidism, 1 had overt hypothyroidism and 1 had subclinical hyperthyroidism. Similarly among females, 22 had subclinical hypothyroidism, 5 had overt hypothyroidism and 2 had subclinical hyperthyroidism. The relative risk of having

Table 1 Components of metabolic syndrome among different thyroid dysfunction group

Parameters	Euthyroid N = 115	Overt hypothyroid N = 6	Subclinical hypothyroid N = 45	Subclinical hyperthyroid N = 3
Systolic BP (mmHg)	129.7 ± 12.7	130 ± 10.9	128.2 ± 16.6	131.6 ± 2.8
Diastolic BP (mmHg)	85.5 ± 10.9	85.8 ± 15.3	83.7 ± 12.5	76.7 ± 15.2
Waist circumference (Cm)	103.7 ± 6.4	99.3 ± 8.5	100.6 ± 6.4	92.3 ± 4.6
Blood glucose (mg/dL)	123 ± 51	106.1 ± 32.2	131.5 ± 44.4	209.6 ± 75.1
Triglyceride (mg/dL)	190.5 ± 75.7	201.6 ± 69	220.1 ± 123	158 ± 75.7
HDL cholesterol (mg/dL)	51 ± 17	50 ± 12.4	47 ± 10.9	49.3 ± 1.1

thyroid dysfunction in females was 1.525 (0.983–2.368; $p = 0.068$) as compared to males. When metabolic syndrome parameters were compared between the patients subgroups (with TSH < 5 mIU/L and TSH ≥ 5 mIU/L), then systolic BP, diastolic BP, waist circumference, blood glucose, triglyceride and HDL cholesterol were 129.7 ± 12.6 mmHg versus 128.4 ± 16 mmHg; $p = 0.602$, 85.3 ± 11 mmHg versus 84 ± 12.8 mmHg; $p = 0.513$, 103.4 ± 6.6 cm versus 100.5 ± 6.6 cm; $p = 0.008$, 125.2 ± 53.2 mg/dL versus 128.6 ± 43.7 mg/dL; $p = 0.692$, 189.7 ± 75.5 mg/dL versus 217.9 ± 117.6 mg/dL; $p = 0.119$ and 51 ± 16.8 mg/dL versus 47.4 ± 11 mg/dL; $p = 0.103$ respectively. Correlation between the components of metabolic syndrome and TSH and free T4 is shown in Table 2. HDL cholesterol showed significant negative correlation with TSH level. BMI had negative correlation with free T3 ($r = -0.161$, $p = 0.037$) and free T4 ($r = -0.15$, $p = 0.052$) and weak positive correlation with TSH ($r = 0.105$, $p = 0.174$).

Discussion

Metabolic syndrome can be associated with endocrine and non-endocrine disorders and has widespread consequences. Alterations in thyroid functions, though well known, are not recognized clinically and there is inconsistency in thyroid functions in metabolic syndrome [11]. The present study identifies thyroid dysfunction as a common endocrine disorder in metabolic syndrome patients; subclinical hypothyroidism (26.6 %) was the commonest followed by overt hypothyroidism (3.5 %) and subclinical hyperthyroidism (1.7 %). Our findings

are consistent with previous studies investigating thyroid function in metabolic syndrome patients. A study by Gyawali et al. in Kavre district of central Nepal reported thyroid dysfunction in 31.84 % of metabolic syndrome patients, the most common dysfunction was subclinical hypothyroidism (29.32 %) followed by overt hypothyroidism (1.67 %) and subclinical hyperthyroidism (0.83 %) [3]. Previous studies in eastern Nepal have also reported higher rate of thyroid dysfunction. Though, thyroid function status of adult population from cross-sectional studies in community settings are unavailable, hospital based studies by Baral et al. and Khatiwada et al. have reported higher rate of thyroid disorders [8, 12]. Study by Baral et al. in eastern Nepal reported hyperthyroid and hypothyroid in 13.68 % and 17.19 % of the general population respectively. Similarly, Khatiwada et al. observed thyroid dysfunction in 36 % of diabetes mellitus patients in a tertiary hospital of eastern Nepal. Prevalence of higher rates of thyroid dysfunction in this region may be due to higher rate of thyroid autoimmunity, iodine deficiency or iodine excess [12]. Recent findings about iodine nutrition among children of this region indicate excess iodine intake in these areas as revealed by excess urinary iodine excretion [13]. A study in India by Shantha et al. found subclinical hypothyroidism in 21.9 % and overt hypothyroidism in 7.4 % metabolic syndrome patients [1]. Similarly, a study by Meher et al. showed a high prevalence of subclinical hypothyroidism (22 %) and overt hypothyroidism (4 %) in the metabolic syndrome patients [14]. We observed thyroid dysfunction to be more common in females (39.7 %) than males (26 %) patients, and this has been observed in a number of studies including the general population [1].

The TSH level of metabolic syndrome patients in our study was in upper normal range, which suggests some degree of thyroid dysfunction in such patients. In a case control study assessing CVD risk factors in an eastern Nepalese population, the mean TSH level of a healthy control population was 2.35 ± 1.07 mIU/L, which is lower than the mean TSH of this present study [15]. The TSH level was above the reference range for normal population in the study of Gyawali et al., and they also observed significantly higher TSH level in metabolic syndrome patients as compared to controls [3]. A positive association has also been reported, between a higher TSH level

Table 2 Correlation of components of metabolic syndrome with TSH and free T4

Components	TSH		Free T4	
	R	P value	R	P value
Systolic BP (mmHg)	-0.001	0.985	0.062	0.421
Diastolic BP (mmHg)	0.077	0.321	-0.141	0.068
Waist circumference (Cm)	-0.121	0.117	-0.056	0.469
Blood glucose (mg/dL)	0.059	0.444	-0.051	0.513
Triglyceride (mg/dL)	0.064	0.408	-0.035	0.65
HDL cholesterol (mg/dL)	-0.174	0.024	0.1	0.195

within the euthyroid reference range and the prevalence of the metabolic syndrome [5]. A study in Korea indicated that higher levels of TSH may predict the metabolic syndrome in the study subjects, suggesting that the influence of thyroid function on metabolic abnormality extends into subjects without metabolic syndrome [16]. In the present study, subclinical hyperthyroid patients had highest systolic BP and fasting blood glucose, overt hypothyroid patients had highest diastolic BP and euthyroid patients had highest waist circumference. Highest triglyceride and lowest HDL cholesterol was seen in patients with subclinical hypothyroidism. It has been observed that subclinically hypothyroid patients have higher systolic BP, diastolic BP, fasting blood glucose and triglycerides compared to euthyroid patients [17]. In our previous case control study, we observed that subclinical hypothyroidism patients have significantly higher diastolic BP, total cholesterol, LDL cholesterol and hs-CRP than euthyroid controls [15]. Our current findings may be due to small number of thyroid dysfunction patients (overt hypothyroidism and subclinical hyperthyroidism). Hypothyroidism is associated with factors of metabolic syndrome such as dyslipidemia, hypertension, obesity, and often insulin resistance. It has been reported that 95 % of newly diagnosed hypothyroid patients have increased levels of cholesterol and 5 % of have hypertriglyceridemia. Hypothyroidism also leads to increased level of LDL cholesterol. All these factors directly contribute to accelerated atherosclerosis [18].

The correlation between subclinical hypothyroidism and metabolic syndrome and its components varies in different studies and seems to be influenced by age, gender and race of study participants [19]. In the present study, waist circumference was significantly different ($p = 0.001$) between patients with and without thyroid dysfunction, and HDL cholesterol had significant negative association with TSH level, however, other components of metabolic syndrome had no significant relationships with thyroid dysfunction. Thyroid hormones affect lipid metabolism and thus the components of metabolic syndrome, and there is positive relation between TSH and LDL cholesterol, whereas negative relation between TSH and HDL cholesterol [15]. Our findings are similar to previous study, where no significant relationship between components of metabolic syndrome and thyroid dysfunction were found except for waist circumference [3]. There are contrasting reports about the association between various metabolic syndrome parameters and thyroid function. In a study in Nigeria, metabolic syndrome was significantly associated with higher free T4 levels [2]. In a study in India, subclinical hypothyroidism was significantly associated with metabolic syndrome and a linear association was observed between TSH levels and total cholesterol, triglycerides, LDL, and HDL cholesterol levels across the metabolic syndrome group [14]. However, in a study in Turkey, TSH was not related with any metabolic syndrome parameters [20].

In the present study, we observed negative association of BMI with free T3 and free T4 and weak positive correlation with TSH. In a study in Germany, euthyroid subjects with TSH in the upper normal range (2.5–4.5 mU/L) were more obese (BMI > 30 Kg/m^2), had higher triglyceride levels, and an increased likelihood of having metabolic syndrome [21].

High prevalence of overt and subclinical hypothyroidism in metabolic syndrome as seen in our study may have harmful effect on cardiovascular health. Hypothyroidism will lead to increased lipid levels and hypertension leading to increased risk for CVD. The effects due to metabolic syndrome and hypothyroidism may be compounded to increase risk for CVD [1]. Thus, assessing thyroid function in metabolic syndrome patients may help identify patients at high risk for CVD. However, it is still unclear whether patients with subclinical hypothyroidism should be treated, and the distinct benefit of prescribing levothyroxine for cardiovascular benefits in these patients is still debatable [15]. The present study has however several limitations. First the sample size was small, which may have affected the correlation between components of metabolic syndrome and thyroid function. Second, the iodine nutrition status in the patients was not assessed. It has been found that both iodine deficiency and excess can lead to thyroid disorder particularly subclinical hypothyroidism. Also, the presence of thyroid autoimmunity in the study population may lead to higher rate of thyroid dysfunction [12].

Conclusions

In conclusion, the study finds thyroid dysfunction specifically subclinical hypothyroidism is a common endocrine disorder in Nepalese patients with metabolic syndrome, and thyroid function is associated with certain components of metabolic syndrome (waist circumference and HDL cholesterol).

Abbreviations
BMI: Body mass index; BP: Blood pressure; CVD: Cardiovascular disease; Free T3: Free triiodothyronine; Free T4: Free thyroxine; hs-CRP: High sensitivity C reactive protein; HDL: High density lipoprotein; LDL: Low density lipoprotein; NCEP: National Cholesterol Education Program; NCEP-ATP III: National Cholesterol Education Program, Adult Treatment Panel III; TSH: Thyroid stimulating hormone.

Author's contribution
SK, SKS, RKC, NB and ML designed the study. SKS and RKC performed laboratory analysis. SK performed statistical analysis and wrote manuscript. SKS, RKC, NB and ML reviewed manuscript draft. All authors read and approved the final version of the manuscript.

Acknowledgements
We kindly acknowledge Department of Biochemistry of B P Koirala Institute of Health Sciences for providing resources for the study.

Author details

[1]Department of Pharmacy, Central Institute of Science and Technology (CIST) College, Pokhara University, Kathmandu, Nepal. [2]Department of Biochemistry, Universal College of Medical Sciences, Bhairahawa, Nepal. [3]Department of Medical Laboratory Technology, Modern Technical College, Satdobato, Lalitpur, Nepal. [4]Department of Biochemistry, B P Koirala Institute of Health Sciences, Dharan, Nepal.

References

1. Shantha GP, Kumar AA, Jeyachandran V, Rajamanickam D, Rajkumar K, Salim S, et al. Association between primary hypothyroidism and metabolic syndrome and the role of C reactive protein: a cross-sectional study from South India. Thyroid Res. 2009;2(1):2. doi:10.1186/1756-6614-2-2.

2. Udenze I, Nnaji I, Oshodi T. Thyroid function in adult Nigerians with metabolic syndrome. Pan Afr Med J. 2014;18:352. doi:10.11604/pamj.2014.18.352.4551.

3. Gyawali P, Takanche JS, Shrestha RK, Bhattarai P, Khanal K, Risal P, et al. Pattern of thyroid dysfunction in patients with metabolic syndrome and its relationship with components of metabolic syndrome. Diabetes Metab J. 2015;39(1):66–73.

4. Kota SK, Meher LK, Krishna S, Modi K. Hypothyroidism in metabolic syndrome. Indian J Endocrinol Metab. 2012;16 Suppl 2:S332–3.

5. Waring AC, Rodondi N, Harrison S, Kanaya AM, Simonsick EM, Miljkovic I, et al. Thyroid Function and Prevalent and Incident Metabolic Syndrome in Older Adults: The Health, Aging, and Body Composition Study. Clin Endocrinol (Oxf). 2012;76(6):911–8.

6. Heima NE, Eekhoff EM, Oosterwerff MM, Lips PT, van Schoor NM, Simsek S. Thyroid function and the metabolic syndrome in older persons: a population-based study. Eur J Endocrinol. 2012;168(1):59–65.

7. Mehran L, Amouzegar A, Tohidi M, Moayedi M, Azizi F. Serum free thyroxine concentration is associated with metabolic syndrome in euthyroid subjects. Thyroid. 2014;24(11):1566–74.

8. Baral N, Lamsal M, Koner BC, Koirala S. Thyroid dysfunction in eastern Nepal. Southeast Asian J Trop Med Public Health. 2002;33:638–41.

9. Sharma SK, Ghimire A, Radhakrishnan J, Thapa L, Shrestha NR, Paudel N, et al. Prevalence of hypertension, obesity, diabetes, and metabolic syndrome in Nepal. Int J Hypertens. 2011;2011:821971.

10. Misra A, Khurana L. The metabolic syndrome in South Asians: epidemiology, determinants, and prevention. Metab Syndr Relat Disord. 2009;7:497–514.

11. Chugh K, Goyal S, Shankar V, Chugh SN. Thyroid function tests in metabolic syndrome. Indian J Endocrinol Metab. 2012;16(6):958–61.

12. Khatiwada S, Kc R, Sah SK, Khan SA, Chaudhari RK, Baral N, et al. Thyroid Dysfunction and Associated Risk Factors among Nepalese Diabetes Mellitus Patients. Int J Endocrinol. 2015;2015:570198. doi:10.1155/2015/570198.

13. Khatiwada S, Gelal B, Shakya PR, Lamsal M, Baral N. Urinary Iodine Excretion among Nepalese School Children in Terai Region. Indian J Pediatr. 2015. doi:10.1007/s12098-015-1755-x.

14. Meher LK, Raveendranathan SK, Kota SK, Sarangi J, Jali SN. Prevalence of hypothyroidism in patients with metabolic syndrome. Thyroid Res Pract. 2013;10:60–4.

15. Kc R, Khatiwada S, Deo Mehta K, Pandey P, Lamsal M, Majhi S. Cardiovascular Risk Factors in Subclinical Hypothyroidism: A Case Control Study in Nepalese Population. J Thyroid Res. 2015;2015:305241. doi:10.1155/2015/305241.

16. Park SB, Choi HC, Joo NS. The Relation of Thyroid Function to Components of the Metabolic Syndrome in Korean Men and Women. J Korean Med Sci. 2011;26(4):540–5.

17. Garduño-Garcia Jde J, Alvirde-Garcia U, López-Carrasco G, Padilla Mendoza ME, Mehta R, Arellano-Campos O, et al. TSH and free thyroxine concentrations are associated with differing metabolic markers in euthyroid subjects. Eur J Endocrinol. 2010;163(2):273–8.

18. Gluvic Z, Sudar E, Tica J, Jovanovic A, Zafirovic S, Tomasevic R, et al. Effects of levothyroxine replacement therapy on parameters of metabolic syndrome and atherosclerosis in hypothyroid patients: a prospective pilot study. Int J Endocrinol. 2015;2015:147070.

19. Tehrani FR, Tohidi M, Dovom MR, Azizi F. A Population Based Study on the Association of Thyroid Status with Components of the Metabolic Syndrome. J Diabetes Metab. 2011;2:156. doi:10.4172/2155-6156.1000156.

20. Tarcin O, Abanonu GB, Yazici D, Tarcin O. Association of metabolic syndrome parameters with TT3 and FT3/FT4 ratio in obese Turkish population. Metab Syndr Relat Disord. 2012;10(2):137–42.

21. Ruhla S, Weickert MO, Arafat AM, Osterhoff M, Isken F, Spranger J, et al. A high normal TSH is associated with the metabolic syndrome. Clin Endocrinol (Oxf). 2010;72(5):696–701.

The cost-effectiveness of diabetes prevention: results from the Diabetes Prevention Program and the Diabetes Prevention Program Outcomes Study

William H. Herman

Abstract

Background: The Diabetes Prevention Program (DPP) was a randomized, controlled clinical trial. It demonstrated that among high-risk individuals with impaired glucose tolerance, diabetes incidence was reduced by 58 % with lifestyle intervention and 31 % with metformin compared to placebo. During the Diabetes Prevention Program Outcomes Study (DPPOS), all DPP participants were unmasked to their treatment assignments, the original lifestyle intervention group was offered additional lifestyle support, the metformin group continued metformin, and all three groups were offered a group-implemented lifestyle intervention. Over the 10 years of combined DPP/DPPOS follow-up, diabetes incidence was reduced by 34 % in the lifestyle group and 18 % in the metformin group compared to placebo. The purpose of this article is to review and synthesize analyses published by the DPP/DPPOS Research Group that have described the cost-effectiveness of diabetes prevention.

Methods: We describe the resource utilization and costs of the DPP and DPPOS interventions, the costs of non-intervention-related medical care, the impact of the interventions on diabetes progression and quality-of-life, and the cost-effectiveness of the interventions from health system and societal perspectives. Cost-effectiveness analyses were performed with a 3-year time horizon using DPP data, a lifetime time horizon that simulated 3-year DPP data, and a 10-year time horizon using combined DPP/DPPOS data.

Results: Although more expensive than the placebo intervention, the greater costs of the lifestyle and metformin interventions were offset by reductions in the costs of nonintervention-related medical care. Every year after randomization, quality-of-life was better for participants in the lifestyle intervention compared to those in the metformin or placebo intervention. In both the simulated lifetime analysis and the 10-year within trial economic analysis, lifestyle and metformin were extremely cost-effective (that is, improved outcomes at a low incremental cost) or even cost-saving (that is, improved outcomes and reduced total costs) compared to the placebo intervention.

Conclusions: The implementation of diabetes prevention programs in high-risk individuals will result in important health benefits and represents a good value for money.

Keywords: Cost, Quality-of-life, Cost-utility

Correspondence: dppmail@bsc.gwu.edu
Diabetes Prevention Program Coordinating Center, The Biostatistics Center, George Washington University, 16110 Executive Blvd., Suite 750, Rockville, MD 20852, USA

Introduction

The Diabetes Prevention Program (DPP) was a multi-center clinical trial designed to determine whether modest weight loss through dietary changes and increased physical activity or treatment with the oral antihyperglycemic medication metformin could delay or prevent the development of type 2 diabetes in high-risk individuals [1]. The DPP enrolled 3234 participants with glucose intolerance who were at least 25 years of age and had a body mass index of 24 kg/m^2 or higher (22 kg/m^2 in Asian-Americans). Mean age of participants was 51 years and mean BMI was 34.0 kg/m^2. Sixty-eight percent of participants were women and 45 % were members of minority groups.

The goals for participants randomized to the intensive lifestyle intervention were to achieve and maintain a weight reduction of at least 7% of initial body weight through a low-calorie, low-fat diet and physical activity of moderate intensity, such as brisk walking for at least 150 min per week [2]. A 16-lesson core curriculum addressing diet, physical activity, and behavior modification was implemented to help participants achieve these goals. The curriculum, taught by case managers on a one-to-one basis during the first 24 weeks after enrollment, was flexible, culturally sensitive, and individualized. Subsequent individual sessions (usually monthly) and group sessions were designed to reinforce the behavioral changes.

The medication interventions (metformin and placebo) were initiated at a dose of 850 mg taken orally once a day [3]. At one month, the dose of metformin or placebo was increased to 850 mg twice daily unless gastrointestinal symptoms warranted a longer titration period. Participants were seen by case managers and adherence to the treatment regimen was reinforced quarterly. The standard lifestyle recommendations for the medication groups were provided in an annual 20 to 30 min individual session. The DPP demonstrated that compared to the placebo intervention, the intensive lifestyle intervention reduced the incidence of type 2 diabetes by 58 %, and the metformin intervention reduced the incidence of type 2 diabetes by 31 % over 3 years [1].

At the conclusion of DPP, participants were enrolled in the Diabetes Prevention Program Outcomes Study (DPPOS). DPPOS was designed to assess the long-term effects of the interventions on health [4]. During DPPOS, participants originally randomized to the lifestyle and metformin interventions were encouraged to continue those interventions and all participants were offered a group lifestyle intervention. The incidence of diabetes during the 10-year average follow-up after DPP randomization was reduced by 34 % in those initially randomized to lifestyle and 18 % in those initially randomized to metformin compared to placebo [4].

To date, we have reported the resources used and the costs of care, and the cost-effectiveness of the lifestyle and metformin interventions relative to the placebo intervention over the 3 year timeframe of the randomized controlled clinical trial [5, 6]. We also used data collected during the 3 years of the DPP and a computer model to simulate the cost-effectiveness of the interventions over a lifetime [7]. Although we [7] and others [8, 9] suggested that the DPP interventions would be cost-effective or even cost-saving over the long term, one analysis suggested that they might be too expensive to be routinely implemented [10]. To better address the longer-term cost-effectiveness of the DPP interventions, we subsequently performed a within-trial analysis spanning the combined 10-years of DPP/DPPOS [11]. In this report, we synthesize and discuss the results of these published reports.

Review
Methods

We described the direct medical costs, direct non-medical costs, and indirect costs incurred by participants in the lifestyle, metformin, and placebo intervention groups during DPP [5] and DPPOS [11]. In general, we calculated the direct medical costs of the interventions by assessing resources used and applying standard unit costs [5]. We excluded from the analysis the resources used and costs of developing the interventions and collecting outcomes to evaluate the interventions [5]. The direct costs of medical care received outside the study and indirect costs were determined annually from patient self-report. Direct non-medical costs were assessed once during DPP and once during DPPOS, and costs were annualized. All costs were adjusted to 2000 or 2010 U.S. dollars using the Consumer Price Index and the Medical Consumer Price Index.

In our analyses, we adopted two separate perspectives: the perspective of a large health system and the perspective of society. In the analyses that adopted the perspective of a health system, we considered the direct medical costs of the DPP/DPPOS interventions and the direct medical costs of care received outside the study. In the analyses adopting the perspective of society, we considered direct medical costs, direct non-medical costs, and indirect costs.

Direct medical costs represent expenditures for medical services and products that are usually paid by health systems. These costs include the costs of hospital days, emergency room visits, urgent care (immediate care for injuries and illnesses in a medical facility outside of a traditional emergency room) visits, outpatient visits, calls to providers, supplies, laboratory tests, and prescription medications. In estimating direct medical costs, we considered the costs of the interventions and the costs of non-intervention-related medical care received outside the DPP/DPPOS. Direct non-medical costs represent expenditures arising as a result of medical treatment or illness but not involving the purchase of medical services or products. Since these costs do not represent health care expenditures, they are not usually paid by health systems. They do, however, represent "out-of-pocket" costs to patients and costs to society. In DPP/DPPOS, direct non-medical costs included the value of the time that participants spent traveling to and attending appointments, exercising, shopping, and cooking; the costs of exercise classes, exercise equipment, special foods, and food preparation items; and the costs of transportation to and from appointments. Indirect costs are another cost to society that arise from illness-related morbidity and mortality. Indirect costs from morbidity arise from being absent from work due to medical treatment, illness, or long-term disability. Indirect mortality costs arise from lost productivity due to premature death.

We performed cost-utility analyses by comparing costs to outcomes across intervention groups. When an intervention costs less and improves outcomes relative to an alternative treatment, it is called cost-saving. When an intervention costs more but improves outcomes relative to an alternative treatment at a cost per unit outcome considered to represent a good value for the money spent, it is termed cost-effective. Outcomes were expressed in terms of quality-adjusted life-years (QALYs) [6]. QALYs measure length of life adjusted for quality of life. Mathematically, QALYs are calculated as the sum of the product of the number of years of life and the quality-of-life in each of those years. The numerical value assigned to quality of life is called a health utility score. By convention, health utility scores are placed on a continuum where perfect health is assigned a value of 1.0 and health judged equivalent to death is assigned a value of 0.0. We assessed health utility scores from the perspective of the general public using the Self-Administered Quality of Well-Being Index (QWB-SA) which was administered to DPP participants annually.

At the end of DPP, we performed a 3-year within trial economic analysis of the DPP and used a simulation model to estimate the lifetime cost-effectiveness of the interventions. The simulation model was originally developed by the Centers for Disease Control and Prevention and Research Triangle Institute International to assess the progression from impaired glucose tolerance to the onset of diabetes to clinically diagnosed diabetes to diabetes with complications and comorbidities to death [12]. The model has a Markov structure and includes annual transition probabilities between disease states. In addition to disease progression, the model tracks costs and QALYs. For our analyses, we modified the model to include data from the DPP on progression, costs, and quality of life associated with impaired

glucose tolerance; data from the United Kingdom Prospective Diabetes Study (UKPDS) on diabetes progression, complications, and comorbidities; and new data on the cost and quality of life associated with diabetes. To estimate the costs of type 2 diabetes, we applied a multiplicative prediction model that estimates annual direct medical costs according to demographic characteristics, diabetes treatments, cardiovascular risk factors, and microvascular and macrovascular complications and comorbidities [13]. To estimate health utility scores associated with type 2 diabetes, we applied an additive prediction model that estimates health utility scores according to demographic characteristics, treatments, and disease state variables [14]. We then modeled the interventions as they were implemented in the DPP and projected year 3 DPP intervention costs, health utility scores, and intervention effectiveness into the future. We assessed simulated lifetime costs and QALYs and calculated cost-effectiveness ratios by dividing incremental costs adjusted to year 2000 U.S. dollars by incremental QALYs. We discounted both costs and QALYs at 3 % per year.

In sensitivity analyses, we assessed how robust the results of the lifetime simulation were to plausible changes in the inputs. First, we modeled the interventions by age group. Then, we modeled the interventions as they might be implemented in routine clinical practice and assessed the effect of reducing the costs of the interventions. Specifically, we recalculated the cost of the lifestyle intervention, assuming that the core curriculum, supervised activity sessions, and lifestyle group sessions were administered as a closed group of 10 participants and that costs were reduced accordingly. Similarly, we recalculated the cost of the metformin intervention by using the cost of generic metformin priced at 25 % the cost of Glucophage (Bristol-Myers Squibb, Princeton, New Jersey). Then, we evaluated the impact of reduced participant adherence by reducing the effectiveness of the lifestyle and metformin interventions by 20 % and 50 % after year 3. Finally, we evaluated the impact of both reduced costs and reduced effectiveness on lifetime cost-effectiveness.

In the 10-year within trial economic analysis, we calculated the total direct medical costs and QALYs for participants over 10 years according to their original DPP randomization groups and assessed cost-effectiveness without simulation modeling but using the empiric data [11]. As a sensitivity analysis, we again estimated what the cost of the lifestyle intervention might have been if it had been administered during DPP in a group format rather than individually (DPP group lifestyle intervention). Although metformin was implemented with brand name metformin (Glucophage), we again assumed that it was implemented with generically-priced DPPOS/DPPOS.

Results

Direct medical costs of the DPP/DPPOS interventions

During both DPP and DPPOS, the lifestyle and metformin interventions were substantially more expensive than the placebo intervention. Table 1 shows the undiscounted per capita direct medical costs of the DPP/DPPOS interventions by intervention group and study year [5]. The costs of the lifestyle intervention were less during DPPOS than during DPP because of the change from an individual- to a group- implemented intervention and because fewer visits took place [11]. The costs of the placebo intervention were higher during DPPOS than during DPP because placebo participants engaged in the group lifestyle intervention [11]. The cumulative undiscounted per participant cost of the lifestyle intervention ($4572) was substantially greater than the metformin intervention ($2881) or the placebo intervention ($752). The estimated cost of the DPP group lifestyle intervention ($2995) was approximately one-third less than that of the lifestyle intervention.

Direct medical costs of care received outside the DPP/DPPOS interventions

To estimate the costs of medical care outside the DPP/DPPOS, we assessed the mean per capita cost of hospital days, emergency room visits, urgent care visits, outpatient visits, calls to providers, supplies, laboratory tests, and prescription medications within the intervention groups [5]. Table 2 shows the undiscounted per capita direct medical costs of care outside the DPP/DPPOS. Cumulative per capita direct medical costs of care outside the DPP/DPPOS were least for the lifestyle group ($24,563), intermediate for the metformin group ($25,615), and highest for the placebo group ($27,468) indicating that metformin and lifestyle participants used fewer medical resources outside the DPP/DPPOS

Table 1 Undiscounted per capita direct medical costs of the DPP/DPPOS interventions by intervention group and study year ($)

Year	Lifestyle	Metformin	Placebo	DPP Group Lifestyle[a]
1-DPP	1,826	584	87	898
2-DPP	887	294	50	563
3-DPP	915	299	47	590
4 (Bridge)	173	301	220	173
5-DPPOS	126	138	62	126
6-DPPOS	112	136	61	112
7-DPPOS	139	137	59	139
8-DPPOS	138	132	55	138
9-DPPOS	126	131	55	126
10-DPPOS	130	130	55	130
Total	4,572	2,281	752	2,995

[a]Sensitivity analysis. Assumes that the core curriculum and follow-up visits were conducted as group sessions with ten participants during the 3 years of DPP

Table 2 Undiscounted per capita direct medical costs of care outside the DPP/DPPOS by intervention group and study year, and distribution of undiscounted per capita 10-year direct medical costs of care outside the DPP/DPPOS by intervention group and type ($)

Costs by year	Lifestyle	Metformin	Placebo
1-DPP	1,423	1,517	1,617
2-DPP	1,780	1,837	2,045
3-DPP	1,979	1,854	2,018
4 (Bridge)	2,059	2,087	2,330
5-DPPOS	2,015	2,174	2,543
6-DPPOS	2,519	2,493	2,636
7-DPPOS	2,645	3,061	2,875
8-DPPOS	3,444	3,607	3,319
9-DPPOS	3,291	3,298	3,265
10-DPPOS	3,406	3,686	4,822
TOTAL	24,563	25,615	27,468
Costs by category	Lifestyle	Metformin	Placebo
Outpatient visits	6,845	7,145	7,325
Inpatient care	5,631	5,817	6,856
ER visits	1,941	1,690	1,825
Urgent care visits	1,697	1,945	1,811
Calls to physicians	712	742	712
Prescription medications	6,490	6,619	6,959
Self-monitoring supplies and laboratory tests for diabetes	1,248	1,628	1,978
TOTAL	24,563	25,615	27,468

interventions than participants randomized to the placebo intervention [5]. The cumulative per-participant direct medical costs of non-intervention-related medical care increased substantially over time. The direct medical costs of non-intervention related medical care were substantially greater than the costs of the interventions and by 3 years, the cumulative costs of non-intervention-related medical care exceeded the 10-year cumulative direct medical costs of the interventions [11]. The greater cost of non-intervention-related medical care for the placebo group was largely driven by greater use of outpatient and inpatient services, prescription medications, and by the greater rate of conversion to diabetes with the attendant costs of self-monitoring and laboratory tests (Table 2). Across treatment groups, the direct medical costs of non-intervention-related medical care were 34 to 44 % higher among diabetic participants compared to nondiabetic participants.

Total direct medical costs

By year 10, the cumulative undiscounted, per capita, total direct medical costs of the interventions and non-intervention-related medical care were higher for lifestyle

($29,135) than for placebo ($28,040) but were lower for metformin ($27,896) than for placebo ($28,040). They were also lower for the DPP group lifestyle ($27,558).

Direct Non-medical costs

Participants randomized to the three intervention groups reported that they spent different amounts of time attending appointments and traveling to and from appointments, exercising, shopping, and cooking and that they received different levels of enjoyment from leisure-time physical activity [5, 11]. They also reported different out-of-pocket costs related to purchases of services and products related to physical activity and diet, different expenditures for food, and different transportation costs [5, 11].

Diet-related costs were substantial but did not differ among intervention groups. As might be expected, physical activity-related costs were greatest for lifestyle. Transportation-related costs were also substantially higher for lifestyle and metformin, due to the greater number of study visits. Total diet-related, physical activity-related, and transportation-related costs were greatest for lifestyle but similar for metformin and placebo.

Participant time contributed substantially to direct nonmedical costs. Participant time related to the interventions (time spent traveling to study visits, at study visits, and for intervention-related calls) was greater for lifestyle and metformin than for the placebo. Participant time related to medical care outside of the interventions was generally greater for placebo than for metformin or lifestyle. Time spent shopping and cooking was the largest component of participant time but differed little across intervention groups. Although lifestyle subjects spent more time exercising, the adjusted value of the time they spent exercising was less than for either metformin or placebo because of their greater enjoyment of leisure time physical activity and the lower opportunity cost.

The total per capita 10-year direct nonmedical costs including the costs of participant time were lowest for metformin ($144,143) and similar for placebo and lifestyle ($147,043 and $147,493 respectively) [11].

Indirect costs

Participants in the three intervention groups reported small differences in time lost from school, work, or usual activities as a result of study visits, illness, or injury. In general, participants in the placebo and metformin groups reported more time lost than participants in the lifestyle group [11].

Health utility scores

Every year after randomization, quality-of-life was better for participants in the lifestyle intervention than for those in the metformin or placebo interventions [11].

Across treatment groups, quality-of-life was worse among participants who developed diabetes [11]. Since more placebo participants developed diabetes, the cumulative, undiscounted, per-participant QALYs-gained over 10 years was greatest for lifestyle (6.81), intermediate for metformin (6.69), and least for placebo (6.67) [11].

Within DPP 3-year cost-effectiveness analysis

From the perspective of a health system and compared to the placebo intervention, the lifestyle intervention cost $31,500 per QALY-gained and the metformin intervention cost $99,600 per QALY-gained [6]. From the perspective of society and compared to the placebo intervention, the lifestyle intervention cost $51,600 per QALY-gained and the metformin intervention cost $99,200 per QALY-gained [6]. The lifestyle intervention was more cost-effective than the metformin intervention from the perspective of both a health system and society.

Simulated lifetime cost-effectiveness of the DPP interventions

The Fig. 1 illustrates the simulated lifetime cumulative incidence of type 2 diabetes by intervention group based on analysis of 3 years of data from the DPP [7]. With the placebo intervention, approximately 50 % of participants would develop diabetes within 7 years. In contrast, it would take approximately 18 years for 50 % of lifestyle participants to develop diabetes and 10 years for 50 % of metformin participants to develop diabetes. Thus, compared with the placebo intervention, the lifestyle intervention delayed the onset of diabetes by 11 years and metformin delayed the onset of diabetes by 3 years. Over a lifetime, 83 % of participants treated with the placebo intervention would develop diabetes, as compared to 63 % of those treated with the lifestyle intervention and 75 % of those treated with the metformin intervention. Thus, compared with the placebo intervention, the lifestyle intervention reduced the absolute risk of developing diabetes by 20 % and the metformin intervention reduced the risk of developing diabetes by 8 %. The number needed to treat (NNT), that is, the number of individuals that would need to be treated to prevent one additional case of diabetes over a lifetime, was 5 for the lifestyle intervention and 13 for the metformin intervention. The relative risk reductions were 24 % and 10 %, respectively.

Table 3 summarizes the simulated economic outcomes from the lifetime simulation. Compared with the placebo intervention, the lifestyle intervention cost $635 more over a lifetime and produced a gain of 0.57 QALY [7]. The cost per QALY (Δ cost/Δ QALY) was approximately $1100 [7]. Compared to the placebo intervention, the metformin intervention cost $3922 more over a lifetime and resulted 0.13 QALY-gained [7]. Thus, compared to

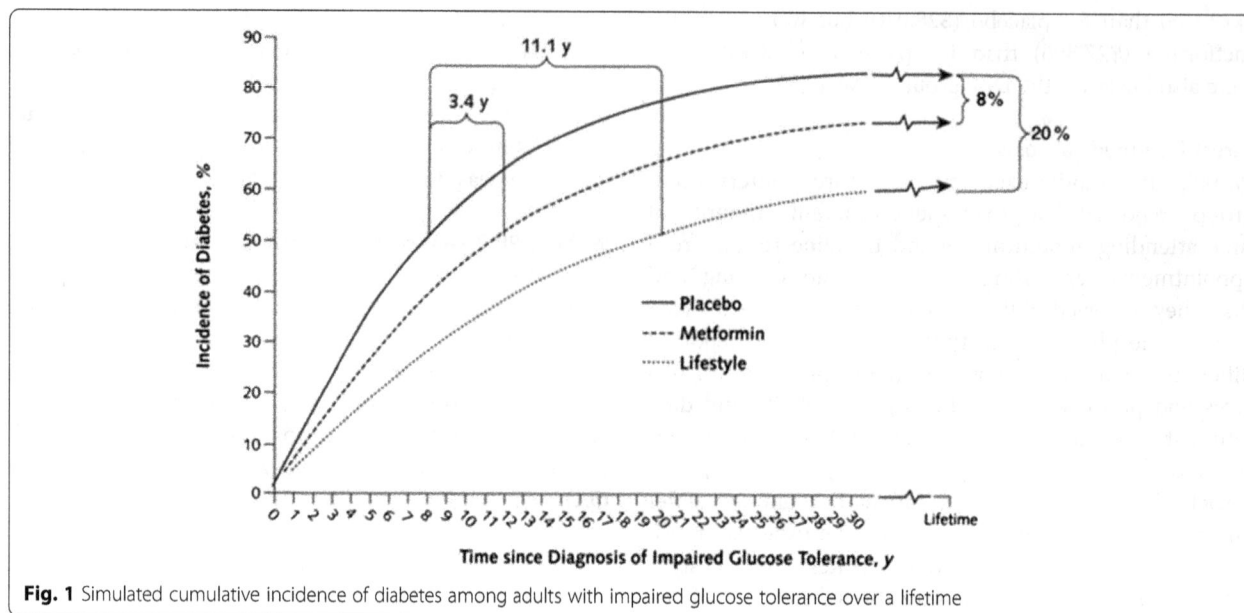

Fig. 1 Simulated cumulative incidence of diabetes among adults with impaired glucose tolerance over a lifetime

the placebo intervention, the metformin intervention cost approximately $31,300 per QALY-gained [7].

In sensitivity analyses, we found that compared to the placebo intervention, the lifestyle intervention was cost-saving in participants younger than 45 years of age and cost-effective in all age groups (Table 4). In contrast, the metformin intervention was cost-effective in the younger age groups but cost more than $100,000 per QALY-gained in participants 65 years of age and older. The lifestyle intervention was cost-effective in all age groups because it was effective in all age groups. The reduced cost-effectiveness of the metformin intervention in the older age groups was largely related to its reduced effectiveness in older participants.

If the lifestyle intervention were implemented in a closed group of 10 patients and costs were reduced accordingly, and if the metformin intervention used generic metformin at 25 % the cost of Glucophage, the lifestyle intervention would be cost-saving relative to the placebo intervention and the metformin intervention would cost approximately $1800 per QALY-gained (Table 4). If future adherence were less than that observed in the DPP and the effectiveness of the lifestyle and metformin interventions were 20 % or even 50 % less than that observed in the DPP, the lifestyle intervention would cost $3100 to $7900 per QALY compared with the placebo intervention, and the metformin intervention would cost $38,000 to $52,600 per QALY (Table 4). If both the lifestyle and metformin interventions were implemented at lower costs, reflecting group lifestyle classes and generic metformin pricing, and effectiveness was reduced by 20 % or 50 % relative to that observed in the DPP, the lifestyle intervention would be cost-saving relative to the placebo intervention and the metformin intervention would cost approximately $6600 to $21,000 per QALY (Table 4).

10-year within DPP/DPPOS cost-effectiveness analysis

Figure 2 illustrates the effectiveness of the DPP/DPPOS interventions as assessed over 10 years of follow-up. After the conclusion of DPP, when all participants were offered a group lifestyle intervention, the relative difference in the effectiveness of the interventions decreased but the beneficial effects of the lifestyle and metformin interventions relative to the placebo intervention persisted.

Table 5 summarizes the differences in total costs and QALYs and the incremental cost-effectiveness ratios of the lifestyle and metformin interventions compared to placebo over the combined 10 years of DPP/DPPOS. The incremental cost-effectiveness ratio is also shown for DPP group lifestyle intervention compared to placebo. From the health system perspective and from the societal perspective, lifestyle cost more than placebo but was also

Table 3 Simulated economic outcomes in the Diabetes Prevention Program intervention groups over a lifetime[a]

Outcome	Lifestyle intervention	Metformin intervention	Placebo Intervention
Lifetime intervention costs, $	9,718	8,801	2,907
Lifetime outcome costs, $	42,256	46,460	48,432
Total lifetime direct medical costs, $	51,974	55,261	51,339
Lifetime QALYs	10.89	10.45	10.32
Δ Cost vs. placebo, $	635	3,922	—
Δ QALY vs. placebo	0.57	0.13	—
Δ Cost / Δ QALY, $	1,124	31,286	—

QALY quality-adjusted life-year
[a]Costs and QALYs discounted at 3 % per year

Table 4 Simulated economic outcomes in the Diabetes Prevention Program intervention groups over a lifetime: Sensitivity analyses

Variable	Lifestyle Intervention vs. Placebo Intervention			Metformin Intervention vs. Placebo Intervention		
	Δ Cost, $	Δ QALY[a]	Δ Cost/Δ QALY, $	Δ Cost, $	Δ QALY[a]	Δ Cost/Δ QALY,$
Base-case analysis	635	0.57	1,124	3,922	0.13	31,286
Age 25–44 y	−395	0.63	Cost-saving	2,574	0.27	9,573
Age 45–54 y	489	0.63	781	4,024	0.13	30,013
Age 55–64 y	1,807	0.53	3,409	4,413	0.07	64,904
Age 65–74 y	2,617	0.39	6,646	4,119	0.02	173,593
Age ≥ 75 y	2,508	0.21	11,700	3,255	0.01	273,207
Reduced cost[b]	-3,696	0.57	Cost-saving	220	0.13	1,755
20 % reduced effectiveness	1,417	0.46	3,102	4,084	0.11	38,145
50 % reduced effectiveness	2,371	0.30	7,886	4,307	0.80	52,562
Reduced cost[b] and 20 % reduced effectiveness	-2,181	0.41	Cost-saving	635	0.10	6,576
Reduced cost[b] and 50 % reduced effectiveness	-348	0.23	Cost-saving	1,198	0.06	20,994

[a]*QALY* quality-adjusted life-year
[b]Assumes that lifestyle intervention is implemented in a closed group of 10 patients and that metformin intervention is implemented with generic metformin

more effective as assessed by QALYs-gained. From a health system perspective, with both costs and health outcomes discounted at 3 % per year, the cost of the lifestyle intervention compared to the placebo intervention was approximately $12,900 per QALY-gained. In contrast, from a health system and societal perspective, metformin had slightly lower costs and nearly the same outcome (as assessed by QALYs) as placebo. The DPP group lifestyle intervention cost approximately $1500 per QALY-gained from a health system perspective and $8400 per QALY-gained from a societal perspective after discounting.

Conclusions

When a new treatment is cost-saving - that is, more effective and less costly than usual care, it should be widely adopted and used. Unfortunately, fewer than 1 in 5 new treatments in health and medicine is cost-saving compared to usual care [15]. Published cost-effectiveness ratios, that is the cost in dollars per QALY-gained for prevention and

treatment range from less than $10,000 per QALY-gained to greater than $1 million per QALY-gained with most falling between $10,000 and $50,000 per QALY-gained [15]. While influenza immunization has been demonstrated to be cost-saving in the Medicare population, interventions such as mammography, antihypertensive treatment, and cholesterol treatment for secondary prevention of cardiovascular disease have been estimated to cost between $10,000 and $60,000 per QALY [16]. Widely implemented interventions such as dialysis for end-stage renal disease ($50,000 to $100,000 per QALY) and left ventricular assist devices ($500,000 to $1.4 million per QALY) are substantially more expensive [15, 16].

From the perspective of a health system or society, what is the value of delaying or preventing the development of type 2 diabetes? From a health system perspective, it delays or prevents the direct medical costs of diabetes including the costs of diabetes education and nutritional counseling, glucose monitoring, antihyperglycemic

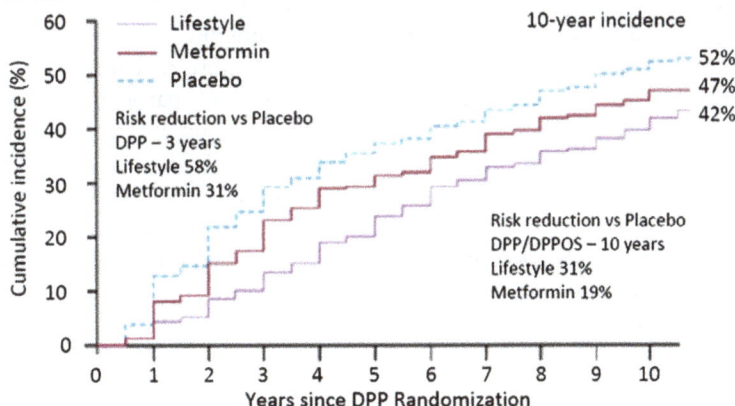

Fig. 2 Observed cumulative incidence of diabetes among adults with impaired glucose tolerance over the combined 10-years of DPP/DPPOS

Table 5 Differences in total costs and QALYs and incremental cost-effectiveness ratios for lifestyle and metformin vs placebo over 10 years

Differences in costs (Δ cost)	Lifestyle vs placebo	Metformin vs placebo	DPP group lifestyle vs placebo[a]
Health system perspective[b]			
Undiscounted	1,656	−251	$81
Discounted[b]	1,748	−205	$201
Societal perspective[d]			
Undiscounted	2,572	−3,644	$996
Discounted[b]	2,688	−3,021	$1,141
Differences in QALYs (Δ QALY)			
Undiscounted	0.15	0.01	0.15
Discounted[c]	0.14	0.01	0.14
Health system perspective[b]			
Undiscounted	10,759	Cost-saving	$528
Discounted[c]	12,878	Cost-saving	$1,478
Societal perspective[d]			
Undiscounted	16,699	Cost-saving	$6,468
Discounted	19,812	Cost-saving	$8,412

[a]Sensitivity analysis. Assumes that the core curriculum and follow-up visits were conducted as group session with ten participants during the 3 years of DPP

[b]Includes total direct medical costs

[c]Both costs and QALYs discounted at 3 %

[d]Includes direct medical costs, direct nonmedical costs including participant time, and indirect costs

treatments, and surveillance and treatment of complications and comorbidities. From a societal perspective, diabetes prevention also reduces costs to the individual not reimbursed by the health system and time lost from work and usual activities. It also improves quality of life.

The direct medical costs of diabetes are enormous. The American Diabetes Association estimated that total per capita healthcare expenditures for people with diabetes are approximately $13,700 per year, of which, $7900 is attributable to diabetes [17]. This estimate likely overstates the costs of diabetes in DPP participants with diabetes since they were actively diagnosed, very early in their clinical course, and had few complications or comorbidities. In 2000, using data from a single managed care health plan, we estimated that the median, annual, direct medical cost of care for a man with diet-controlled type 2 diabetes with no microvascular, neuropathic, or cardiovascular risk factors or complications was approximately $1700 [13]. More recently, using data from approximately 7100 type 2 diabetic patients enrolled in 8 managed care health plans participating across the United States, we estimated that the mean, annual, per capita, direct medical costs of care would be approximately $2500 for a man with recent onset diabetes without complications or comorbidities [18]. These

costs of uncomplicated type 2 diabetes are quite consistent with those observed during DPP/DPPOS. Compared to the substantial costs of diabetes, the costs of the lifestyle, metformin and DPP group lifestyle interventions were quite small.

During DPP and DPPOS, the costs of the lifestyle and metformin interventions were greater than the cost of the placebo intervention, but the cumulative, undiscounted, per capita costs of the lifestyle and metformin interventions were small in comparison to the cost of nonintervention-related medical care (medical care received outside the DPP/DPPOS). Indeed, within 3 years, the cumulative undiscounted costs of nonintervention-related medical care exceeded the 10-year cumulative direct medical costs of the lifestyle and metformin interventions. Within 10 years, the total, cumulative, undiscounted costs of the interventions and nonintervention-related medical care were only slightly higher for lifestyle than placebo and lower for metformin than placebo.

With respect to the cost-effectiveness of diabetes prevention, it is now clear that our use of a 3-year time horizon in our within-trial economic analysis [6] resulted in a higher cost per QALY-gained than the analyses which used a lifetime or a 10-year time horizon. With a three-year time horizon, treatment costs were higher and the benefits of the lifestyle and metformin interventions were less. The costs of both the lifestyle and metformin interventions were greatest in year 1, decreased substantially in years 2 and 3 and decreased further during years 4 through 10. In contrast, much of the benefit of the lifestyle and metformin interventions, as assessed by both cumulative, non-intervention-related direct medical costs and quality-of-life, occurred after three years of follow-up. The results highlight the importance of adopting a longer time horizon when assessing the impact of an intervention for a chronic disease.

The results of the 10-year within trial economic analysis of DPP/DPPOS support the results of our lifetime simulation. In the lifetime simulation, from the perspective of a health system, both the lifestyle intervention and the metformin intervention were cost-effective, and the results were robust to plausible changes in intervention cost and participant adherence. In the 10-year within trial economic analysis, lifestyle was cost-effective and metformin was marginally cost-saving or at least cost neutral compared to placebo.

There are at least two limitations to the 10-year within-trial analysis which might, in part, explain the difference between it and the results of our lifetime simulation. First, DPPOS was an observational follow-up of DPP, a randomized controlled clinical trial. It is likely that during DPPOS, when 57 % of placebo participants attended at least one group lifestyle intervention session, the placebo intervention was more effective than "usual care". Thus, if real-world usual care were used for comparison, the difference in effectiveness between the lifestyle and placebo interventions might have been greater. Second, in our analysis of the DPP group lifestyle intervention, we assumed that lifestyle could be implemented in a group rather than individual format at one-third lower cost and achieve the same outcomes. Although group-implemented lifestyle interventions have been shown to be at least as effective as individual programs for weight loss, there has not been a direct comparison of individual and group lifestyle interventions for diabetes prevention.

Taken together, these analyses demonstrate that although more expensive, lifestyle intervention, when compared to placebo, is cost-effective, and generic metformin when compared to placebo is cost-effective or even cost-saving from a health system and societal perspective. If a DPP group lifestyle intervention could be delivered at 1/3 lower cost than the DPP lifestyle intervention and achieve the same outcomes, it might also be cost-saving compared to placebo.

The challenges associated with motivating a racially and ethnically diverse population to take up and maintain the weight loss and physical activity goals of the DPP over the long term should not be underestimated. Nevertheless, flexible interventions delivered by skilled lifestyle coaches that accommodate individual preferences and reflect local community and cultural contexts may achieve these goals [19–21]. In conclusion, these economic analyses should assist health plans and policy makers in comparing the benefit of diabetes prevention to other preventive and palliative interventions. The adoption of diabetes prevention programs by health plans and society will result in important health benefits and represents a good value for money.

Abbreviations
DPP: Diabetes Prevention Program; DPPOS: Diabetes Prevention Program Outcomes Study.

Competing interests
Conflict of Interest Statement: This work was supported by George Washington University Subaward No. 21049-31-CCLS40010F; George Washington University U01-DK-048489-18; Grant Number P60DK020572 (MDRTC) from the National Institute of Diabetes and Digestive and Kidney Diseases; and Grant Number P30DK092926 (MCDTR) from the National Institute of Diabetes and Digestive and Kidney Diseases. The author declares that he has no competing interests.

Author's contributions
WH is the sole author responsible for the concept, design, analysis, and drafting of this manuscript.

Acknowledgement
The Research Group gratefully acknowledges the commitment and dedication of the participants of the DPP and DPPOS. During the DPPOS, the National Institute of Diabetes and Digestive and Kidney Diseases (NIDDK) of the National Institutes of Health provided funding to the clinical centers and the Coordinating Center for the design and conduct of the study, and collection, management, analysis, and interpretation of the data (U01 DK048489). The Southwestern American Indian Centers were supported directly by the NIDDK, including its Intramural Research Program, and the Indian Health Service. The General Clinical Research Center Program, National Center for Research Resources, and the Department of Veterans Affairs supported data collection at many of the clinical centers. Funding was also provided by the National Institute of Child Health and Human Development, the National Institute on Aging, the National Eye Institute, the National Heart Lung and Blood Institute, the Office of Research on Women's Health, the National Institute on Minority Health and Health Disparities, the Centers for Disease Control and Prevention, and the American Diabetes Association. Bristol-Myers Squibb and Parke-Davis provided additional funding and material support during the DPP, Lipha (Merck-Sante) provided medication and LifeScan Inc. donated materials during the DPP and DPPOS. The opinions expressed are those of the investigators and do not necessarily reflect the views of the funding agencies. A complete list of Centers, investigators, and staff can be found in the Additional file 1.

References
1. The Diabetes Prevention Program Research Group. Reduction in the incidence of type 2 diabetes with lifestyle modification or metformin. N Engl J Med. 2002;346:393–403.
2. Diabetes Prevention Program Research Group. The Diabetes Prevention Program (DPP): description of lifestyle intervention. Diabetes Care. 2002;25:2165–71.
3. Diabetes Prevention Program Research Group. The diabetes prevention program. Design and methods for a clinical trial in the prevention of type 2 diabetes. Diabetes Care. 1999;22:623–34.
4. The Diabetes Prevention Program Research Group. 10-year follow-up of diabetes incidence and weight loss in the Diabetes Prevention Program Outcomes Study. Lancet. 2009;374:1677–86.
5. The Diabetes Prevention Program Research Group. Costs associated with the primary prevention of type 2 diabetes mellitus in the Diabetes Prevention Program. Diabetes Care. 2003;26:36–47.
6. The Diabetes Prevention Program Research Group. Within-trial cost-effectiveness of lifestyle intervention or metformin for the primary prevention of type 2 diabetes. Diabetes Care. 2003;26:2518–23.
7. Herman WH, Hoerger TJ, Brandle M, Hicks K, Sorensen S, Zhang P, et al. The cost-effectiveness of lifestyle modification or metformin in preventing type 2 diabetes in adults with impaired glucose tolerance. Ann Intern Med. 2005;142:323–32.
8. Palmer AJ, Roze S, Valentine WJ, Spinas GA, Shaw JE, Zimmet PZ. Intensive lifestyle changes or metformin in patients with impaired glucose tolerance: modeling the long-term health economic implications of the diabetes prevention program in Australia, France, Germany, Switzerland, and the United Kingdom. Clin Ther. 2004;26:304–21.
9. Caro JJ, Getsios D, Caro I, Klittich WS, O'Brien JA. Economic evaluation of therapeutic interventions to prevent Type 2 diabetes in Canada. Diab Med. 2004;21:1229–36.
10. Eddy DM, Schlessinger L, Kahn R. Clinical outcomes and cost-effectiveness of strategies for managing people at high risk for diabetes. Ann Intern Med. 2005;143:251–64.
11. The Diabetes Prevention Program Research Group. The 10-year cost-effectiveness of lifestyle intervention or metformin for diabetes prevention: An intent-to-treat analysis of the DPP/DPPOS. Diabetes Care. 2012;35:723–30.
12. Hoerger TJ, Segel JE, Zhang P, Sorensen SW: Validation of the CDC-RTI diabetes cost-effectiveness model. RTI Press publication No. MR-0013-0909. Research Triangle Park, N.C: RTI International, 2009.
13. Brandle M, Zhou H, Smith BR, Marriott D, Burke R, Tabaei BP, et al. The direct medical cost of type 2 diabetes. Diabetes Care. 2003;26:2300–4.

14. Coffey JT, Brandle M, Zhou H, Marriott D, Burke R, Tabaei BP, et al. Valuing health-related quality of life in diabetes. Diabetes Care. 2002;25:2238–43.
15. Cohen JT, Neumann PJ, Weinstein MC. Does preventive care save money? Health economics and the presidential candidates. N Engl J Med. 2008;358:661–3.
16. Neumann PJ, Rosen AB, Weinstein MC. Medicare and cost-effectiveness analysis. N Engl J Med. 2005;353:1516–22.
17. American Diabetes Association. Economic costs of diabetes in the U.S. in 2012. Diabetes Care. 2013;36:1033–46.
18. Li R, Bilik D, Brown MB, Zhang P, Ettner SL, Ackermann RT, et al. Medical costs associated with type 2 diabetes complications and comorbidities. Am J Manag Care. 2013;19:421–30.
19. Davis NJ, Ma Y, Delahanty LM, Hoffman HJ, Mayer-Davis E, Franks PW, et al. Predictors of sustained reduction in energy and fat intake in the Diabetes Prevention Program Outcomes Study intensive lifestyle intervention. J Acad Nutr Diet. 2013;113:1455–64.
20. Venditti EM, Wylie-Rosett J, Delahanty LM, Mele L, Hoskin MA, Edelstein SL, et al. Short and long-term lifestyle coaching approaches used to address diverse participant barriers to weight loss and physical activity adherence. Int J Behav Nutr Phys Act. 2014;11:16.
21. Jaacks LM, Ma Y, Davis N, Delahanty LM, Mayer-Davis EJ, Franks PW, et al. Long-term changes in dietary and food intake behaviour in the Diabetes Prevention Program Outcomes Study. Diabet Med. 2014;31:1631–42.

12

A clinician's guide to understanding resistance to thyroid hormone due to receptor mutations in the TRα and TRβ isoforms

Brijesh K. Singh and Paul M. Yen*

Abstract

There are two genes that express the major thyroid hormone receptor isoforms. Mutations in both these genes have given rise to Resistance to Thyroid Hormone (RTH) syndromes (RTHβ, RTHα) that can have variable phenotypes for mutations of the same receptor isoform as well as between the two receptor isoforms. In general, the relative tissue-specific distribution of TRβ and TRα determine RTH in different tissues for each form of RTH. These differences highlight some of the isoform-specific roles of each TR isoform. The diagnosis of RTH is challenging for the clinician but should be considered whenever a patient presents with unexplained elevated serum free T_4 (fT_4) and unsuppressed TSH levels, as well as decreased serum free T_4/T_3 ratio. Here we provide a guide for the clinician to diagnose and treat both types of RTH.

Keywords: Resistance to thyroid hormone, Thyroid hormone receptors, Dominant negative activity, Thyroid stimulating hormone, Human mutation

Background

Fuller Albright first showed that pseudohypoparathyroidism represented a form of hormone resistance syndrome 75 years ago [1]. Since then, others have used clinical, biochemical, and molecular studies to identify many examples of hormone resistance with mutations in their corresponding receptors [18]. Indeed, hormone resistance due to mutations in many nuclear hormone receptors (NRs) such as the estrogen, glucocorticoid, peroxisome proliferator activator, and vitamin D receptors have been identified in affected individuals [53]. Similarly, numerous cases of resistance to thyroid hormone (RTH) and the corresponding mutations in the genes encoding human thyroid hormone receptors (TRs) have been reported.

In this current review, we will focus on a brief description of TRs and thyroid hormone (TH) action, as well as new clinical, biochemical, and molecular insights into RTH obtained from patients harboring mutations in the two TR isoforms, TRβ and TRα. After the recent identification of RTH in patients with mutations in the *THRA* gene, a new nomenclature was adopted to distinguish between types of RTH due to specific TR isoforms (please see below) [34]. The RTH syndromes due to TRβ and TRα are now called RTHβ and RTHα, respectively. Since RTHβ was identified and studied almost 50 years before the identification of RTHα (even though the precise mechanism for the former was not known at the time) [35], we will discuss RTHβ first. Mutations in the TH transporter, MCT8, and selenoprotein mutations that affect intracellular TH concentration but do not affect the function of TRs also have been identified. For more details on these syndromes, the reader is referred to several excellent recent reviews [15, 47]. New insights on the two forms of RTH have led to better understanding of the roles of the two TR isoforms on the function of different tissues as well as the regulation of the hypothalamic, pituitary, and thyroid (HPT) axis. Considering RTHβ and RTHα as potential diagnoses for abnormal thyroid function tests requires a rational approach for

* Correspondence: paul.yen@duke-nus.edu.sg
Laboratory of Hormonal Regulation, Cardiovascular and Metabolic Disorders Program, Duke-NUS Graduate Medical School, 8 College Road, Singapore 169857, Singapore

distinguishing these syndromes from other causes of inappropriate TSH secretion and low serum T_4/T_3 ratio, respectively, and will be discussed in more detail later in this article.

Thyroid hormone action

THs are involved in the regulation of metabolism, proliferation, and growth of most tissues [5, 12, 28]. Serum TH levels are tightly controlled by the HPT axis to deliver appropriate amounts of TH to target tissues. The two major THs (T_3 and T_4) are iodothyrosines synthesized by the thyroid gland under the control of thyrotropin/thyroid stimulating hormone (TSH), a glycoprotein heterodimer that is produced by the pituitary gland. TSH, in turn, is regulated by thyrotropin releasing hormone (TRH), a tripeptide generated by the hypothalamus that is released into its own portal system to reach the pituitary. Both the production of TRH and TSH are under negative feedback control determined by the circulating free TH concentrations. Circulating THs, particularly T_4, are mostly bound to transport proteins such as thyroxine-binding globulin (TBG), transthyretin (TTR), and albumin (HSA, human serum albumin). TBG binds 75% of serum T_4 whereas TTR and HSA bind approximately 20% and 5%, respectively.

Although T_4 is the major secreted form, T_3 is significantly more potent than T_4 and binds to TRs with 10-fold higher affinity [21, 25]. Thus, T_3 is considered the active form of the hormone whereas T_4 serves primarily as a less active precursor. After delivery to target tissues, THs utilize transporters (e.g., MCT8, MCT10, and OATP1C1) to cross the cell membrane and enter the cell [9]. THs then are metabolized by the iodothyronine deiodinases (Dio1, Dio2, and Dio3), a subfamily of selenoproteins [8]. The deiodinases serve as additional control points for TH action by regulating serum and intracellular TH concentrations. In particular, activation of TH is mediated by Dio1 and Dio2 conversion of T_4 to

T_3 whereas inactivation of TH is regulated by Dio3 conversion to metabolites such as reverse triiodothyronine (rT_3) and diiodothyronine (T_2) [44].

Thyroid hormone receptors

TRs belong to the nuclear receptor (NR) family that includes the steroid hormone, vitamin D, peroxisome proliferator activator, and retinoic acid receptors. Unlike peptide- or protein-binding receptors that are located on the cellular membrane, NRs are intracellular and bind to their cognate hormones either in the cytoplasm (steroid hormones) or nucleus (TH, vitamin D, retinoic acid) [53]. After binding to hormone, they have the ability to bind to hormone response elements (HREs) located in the promoter regions of target genes. As such, NRs can be considered hormone-inducible transcription factors. There are two major THR genes, THRA and THRB, that are expressed in a tissue-specific manner [12]. Two major THRA receptor splice variants (TRα1 and TRα2) are encoded by the THRA gene (Fig. 1a) and two major THRB isoforms (TRβ1 and TRβ2) are generated by alternate promoter choice on the THRB gene (Fig. 1b). TRα1 is highly expressed in the heart, bone, and skeletal muscle whereas TRα2 is widely expressed throughout the whole body. The alternative splicing of the THRA mRNA transcript leads to changes in the carboxy-terminus sequence of TRα2 that renders it incapable of binding to TH. It is possible that TRα2 may regulate alternative splicing of the THRA gene or may interfere with TRα1 action at the protein level. TRβ1 is predominately expressed in brain, liver and kidney whereas TRβ2 is found in the pituitary, retina, and cochlea. TRα1, TRβ1, and TRβ2 bind T_3 with similar affinity.

TRs have a modular structure, with a central DNA-binding domain and a C-terminal ligand-binding domain [5, 12, 28]. They typically will bind to DNA as heterodimers with another nuclear hormone receptor family member, retinoid X receptors (RXRs) (Fig. 2). These

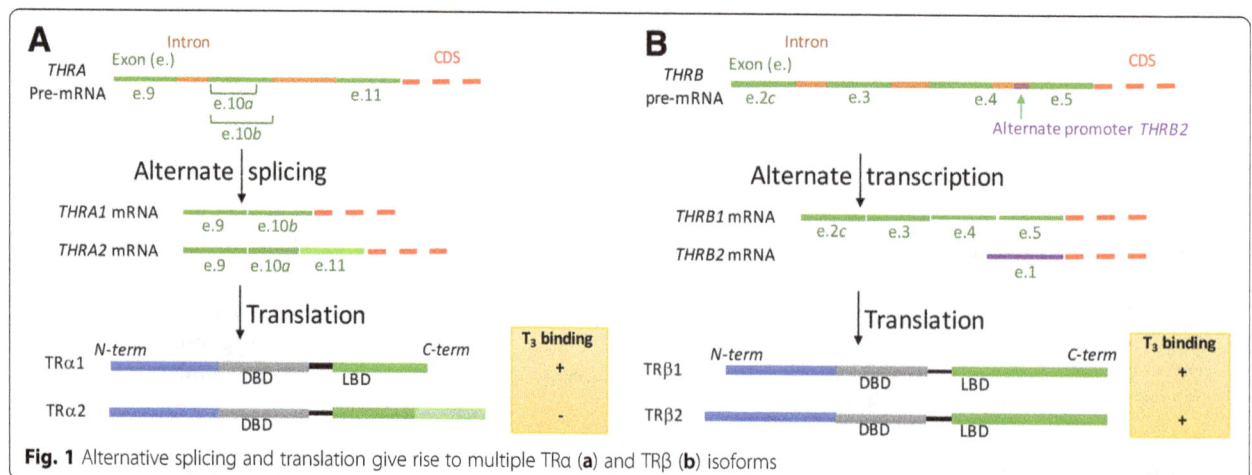

Fig. 1 Alternative splicing and translation give rise to multiple TRα (**a**) and TRβ (**b**) isoforms

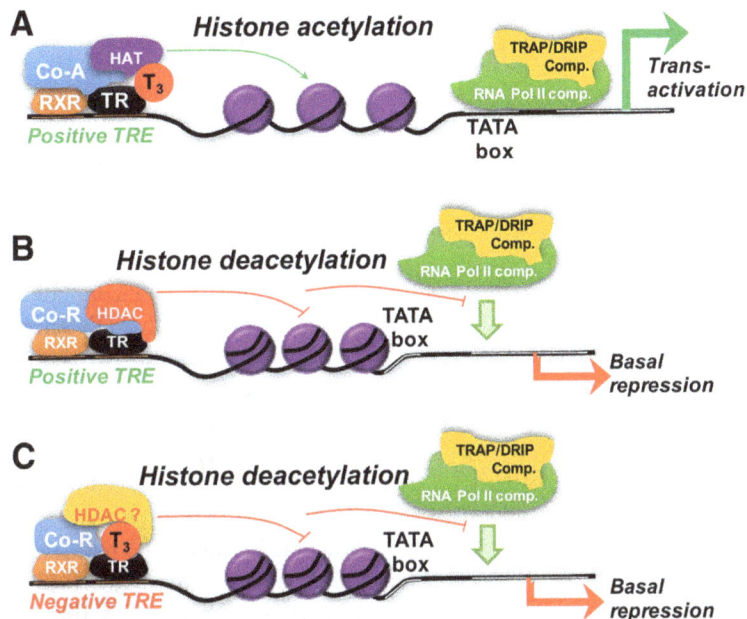

Fig. 2 Role of co-activator and co-repressor recruitment in positively-regulated target genes. **a** For positively-regulated target genes, in the presence of T_3, co-activators (Co-A) and histone acetyl transferases (HAT) are recruited by the T_3-bound TR/RXR heterodimer sitting on the thyroid hormone response element (TRE). This leads to histone acetylation and chromatin nearby changes to a more open conformation to facilitate recruitment of RNA pol II to the TATA box region. Subsequently another co-activator complex, TH receptor-associated protein/vitamin D receptor interacting protein complex (TRAP/DRIP comp), is recruited by ligand-bound TR/RXR and RNA polymerase II complex to activate transcription. **b** For positively-regulated target genes in the absence of T_3, TR/RXR has a different conformation than its T_3-bound state, and has poor affinity for co-activator complexes. Instead, it recruits a co-repressor complex (Co-R) with histone deacetylase activity (HDAC). This leads to histone deacetylation and formation of a more closed chromatin conformation that does not allow RNA pol II binding to the promoter and thus "represses" transcription. **c** In some negatively-regulated target genes, in the presence of ligand, co-repressor and HDAC are recruited by TR/RXR sitting on the TRE. This leads to decreased histone acetylation and a more closed chromatin conformation that prevents RNA pol II binding to the promoter of the target gene, and thus negatively regulates transcription in the presence of T_3. Please see text for more details

heterodimers can recognize specific DNA sequences, thyroid hormone response elements (TREs), located in the promoter regions of target genes. TREs typically are composed of two-half sites, most often organized as direct repeats, separated by 4 nucleotides (consensus DR4: 5′(A/G)GG(A/T)CANNNN(A/G)GG(A/T)CA 3′). TRs bind in a head to tail orientation with the upstream 5′ half site of DR4 bound by RXR and the downstream 3′ half site by TR. Interestingly, both unliganded and liganded TRs can bind to TREs; however, ligand binding to TRs induces conformational changes in the receptor that facilitate the recruitment of co-activators with histone acetyltransferase (HAT) and methyltransferase activity to induce conformational changes at specific chromatin sites in the promoters of positively-regulated target genes. These changes generate a permissive local chromatin environment that enables the binding and recruitment of the general transcriptional machinery (Fig. 2a) to the transcriptional start site and initiate transcription. In the absence of TH, TRs also can bind to TREs but they recruit co-repressors with histone deacetylase (HDAC) activity instead of co-activators/ HATs owing to their

different conformation in the unliganded state. The co-repressor complex alters its surrounding chromatin structure by removing acetyl groups from histones to induce a conformational change in the histone structure that inhibits the binding of RNA polymerase II, and results in a decrease in target gene transcription (Fig. 2b). TREs can be located near or far from transcriptional start sites. The co-activator or co-repressor transcriptional complexes bound to them can interact co-operatively with multiple TR/TRE complexes in the promoter region to further regulate transcription. Taken together, this model suggests that TR/RXR heterodimer binding to the TRE and its recruitment of co-activators/corepressors play important roles in TH-mediated gene transcription (see below). Recently, using a method to examine TR binding throughout the whole genome, chromatin immunoprecipitation sequencing (ChIP-Seq), it was found that TRs can bind to DNA with sequences that do not resemble TREs and in non-promoter regions [4, 33]. Thus, it is likely that TRs interact with other transcription factors or chromatin via protein-protein interactions at these sites. There also is evidence that TH also may bind with low affinity to other non-TR proteins in the cell to mediate novel actions; but so far, these mechanisms are poorly understood [12].

The transcription of approximately half of all target genes is negatively regulated either indirectly (through the activation/increased expression of repressor transcription factors) or directly by TRs (Fig. 1c) [29]. Currently, the mechanism for negative regulation by TRs still is not well understood. *TSHβ* and the *CGA* are two negatively-regulated target genes that are expressed in pituitary thyrotrophs. They generate two proteins, thyroid stimulating hormone β (TSHβ) and the common glycoprotein hormone α-subunit protein (α-GSU), that dimerize with each other to form TSH. Studies in pituitary-specific TR knockout mice suggest that the TRβ2 is the major isoform that controls the TH-mediated negative regulation of these target genes in the pituitary [51].

Resistance to thyroid hormone β
Clinical features
RTHβ is a rare disorder characterized by elevated levels of circulating free thyroid hormones, inappropriately normal or elevated TSH secretion, and decreased peripheral tissue responses to iodothyronine action (Fig. 3a) [7, 30, 36]. The incidence of RTHβ is estimated to be 1

case per 50,000 live births with affected individuals identified in Europe, Asia, and North and South America. So far, over 160 different mutations in TRβ have been found in RTHβ patients from more than 350 families. RTHβ follows an autosomal dominant inheritance pattern in families (80%) but also can be found sporadically in affected individuals with no other family history of RTHβ (20%) [36]. Patients with RTHβ typically have a heterozygous mutation in the *THRB* allele leading to the expression of a defective TRβ that has dominant negative activity on the transcriptional activities of the TRs encoded by the other normal *THRB* allele and the two normal *THRA* alleles [7, 36]. Major exceptions to this pattern were the first reported RTHβ kindred in which an autosomal recessive pattern of inheritance was observed [35]. The affected patients later were shown to harbor homozygous mutations in both *THRB* alleles that generated a severely truncated, nonfunctional form of TRβ [36].

In the clinical setting, RTHβ often is detected at childbirth during neonatal screening for congenital thyroid dysfunction when abnormal levels of T4, TSH, or both are identified, and further diagnostic testing undertaken. However, RTHβ also can go undetected due to its heterogenous presentation and variable symptoms [7, 36]. Goiter frequently is the main clinical finding that prompts the physician to order thyroid function tests and further investigations. In many cases, the high TH levels can compensate for tissue resistance; thus, affected individuals may appear to be clinically euthyroid. However, upon closer inspection, the compensation may be incomplete, and hypothyroidism is found in tissues that express predominantly TRβ (see below) such as the liver, kidney, and lung. Additionally, high endogenous TH levels sometimes can produce hyperthyroid effects, particularly in tissues that express predominantly TRα such as the heart and bone [7, 36]. These tissues do not express much mutant TRβ so it is likely that they are responding to the high circulating concentrations of TH [56].

In addition to goiter, the most common presenting signs and symptoms in patients with RTHβ are short stature, attention deficit disorder, and resting tachycardia although some patients may be entirely asymptomatic (Table 1). Moreover, the phenotypes and severity of TH dysfunction frequently vary among affected individuals expressing the same *THRB* mutation. Importantly, this variability in clinical phenotype may even occur among different affected family members with the same *THRB* mutation [7, 36]. These observations suggest that other genetic and epigenetic modifiers may affect the expression/penetrance of the RTHβ phenotype.

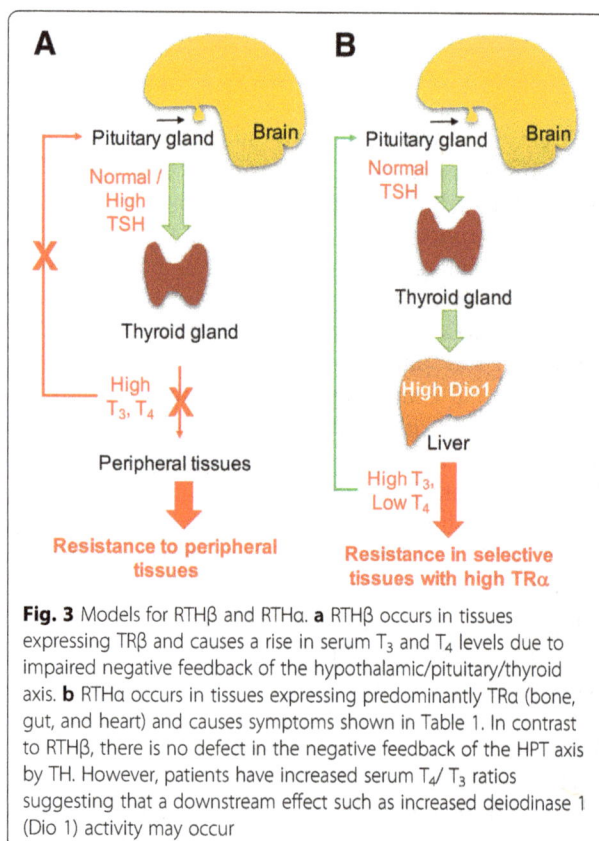

Fig. 3 Models for RTHβ and RTHα. **a** RTHβ occurs in tissues expressing TRβ and causes a rise in serum T_3 and T_4 levels due to impaired negative feedback of the hypothalamic/pituitary/thyroid axis. **b** RTHα occurs in tissues expressing predominantly TRα (bone, gut, and heart) and causes symptoms shown in Table 1. In contrast to RTHβ, there is no defect in the negative feedback of the HPT axis by TH. However, patients have increased serum T_4/T_3 ratios suggesting that a downstream effect such as increased deiodinase 1 (Dio 1) activity may occur

Differential diagnosis
There are other clinical conditions of inappropriate TSH expression with increased serum T_4, and they should be

Table 1 Clinical features and diagnostic tests for RTHβ and RTHα

RTHβ	RTHα
Typical Clinical Features	
-Goiter	-Bradycardia
-Resting tachycardia	-Neurodevelopmental delay
-Osteoporosis	-Anaemia
-Short stature	-Skeletal dysplasia
-Attention deficit disorder	-Dysmorphia
-Family history (80%)	-Constipation
Diagnostic Tests	
-Increased fT$_3$, fT$_4$ (Rule out antibody interference)	-Decreased T$_4$/T$_3$ ratio
-Normal/Elevated TSH	-Normal TSH
-Normal dialyzed free T$_4$	-Exon sequencing of TRα
-Rule out autoimmune thyroiditis (anti-thyroid peroxidase, thyroglobulin, and TSH receptor antibodies)	
-Check serum markers TH hyperfunction (increased SHBG, ferritin, pro-collagen-1-N-terminal peptide (PINP) and decreased cholesterol in hyperthyroidism but normal in RTH)	
-Check serum a-GSU and compare with TSH (a-GSU (µg/l)/TSH (mU/l)] × 10 > 1.0 (suggests TSHoma)	
-Consider pituitary MRI (rule out TSHoma)	
-Exon sequencing of TRβ	

considered when attempting to make the diagnosis of RTHβ in a particular patient [36, 48]. First, there are several conditions or situations that can cause an *apparent* increase in serum T$_4$ with detectable TSH levels. These include: increased serum binding proteins (e.g., thyroxine binding globulin), abnormal serum binding proteins with altered binding affinity for THs (e.g., familial dysalbuminemic hyperthyroxinemia (FDH) and transthyretin variant), and anti-TSH or T$_4$ antibodies. Measurement of serum free T$_4$ levels, particularly by equilibrium dialysis and pre-clearance of anti-TSH/T$_4$ autoantibodies before hormone measurements usually can distinguish these possiblities from RTHβ. Serum fT$_3$ also should be normal in these cases. Additionally, it is important to evaluate family members for symptoms associated with RTHβ. Uncovering similar abnormalities in thyroid function tests among siblings and parents will provide important clues for the diagnosis of RTHβ since 80–90% case of RTHβ are familial.

Next, it is important to consider *transient* causes for elevated serum T$_4$ and detectable TSH levels such as: systemic illness (sick euthyroid syndrome), acute psychiatric disorders, the neonatal period when there is a sudden burst of T$_4$ release post-natally before full equilibration of the HPT axis, and early thyroxine replacement therapy in hypothyroid patients. Additionally, certain drugs can cause abnormal thyroid function tests that resemble those seen in RTHβ. Amiodarone, oral contrast agents, and β-blockers interfere with the conversion of T$_4$ to T$_3$ by inhibiting the enzymatic activity of Dio1. Serum TSH may be in the normal range in these patients. Amphetamines stimulate TRH release acutely leading to increased serum TSH and TH levels. Heparin induces lipoprotein lipase activity to increase serum free fatty levels that can interfere with TH binding to serum transport proteins.

The remaining other major cause for « inappropriate »TSH secretion with elevated serum T$_4$ levels is TSH-secreting pituitary adenoma (TSHoma). Several important diagnostic tests are helpful for distinguishing between RTHβ and this condition: pituitary MRI (abnormal in TSHoma) and the common glycoprotein α-subunit hormone subunit (α-GSU) /TSH ratio. In the latter diagnostic measurement, there can be an inappropriately elevated secretion of common α-GSU in TSHomas such that the α-GSU /TSH ratio is elevated relative to TSH (α-GSU (µg/l)/TSH (mU/l)] × 10 > 1.0 in TSHomas) due to dysregulated over-secretion of α-GSU. However, this ratio may need to considered with caution when the circulating levels of other pituitary glycoproteins, particularly luteinizing hormone and follicle stimulating hormone, are elevated in post-menopausal women and can give a spuriously high ratio. Although not routinely used in the U.S. outside the academic setting, approximately 90% patients with RTHβ had normal or increased (similar to hypothyroid) TSH responses to TRH stimulation (200 µg bolus intravenously, sampling at 0, 20, 60, 90 and 120 min) whereas patients with TSHomas typically had high basal levels and only 39% responded to TRH [36, 41]. The reason for the occurrence of normal vs. increased TSH responses to TRH in patients with RTHβ may be that some patients have « compensated » pituitary response to the higher circulating TH levels whereas some patients do not, and thus have relative pituitary hypothyroidism. When TRH stimulation tests were performed after 3 days of T$_3$ suppression at 50, 100, and 200 µg/days, euthyroid patients had suppressed TSH levels at 50 µg T$_3$/day and almost all RTHβ patients also had some degree of TSH level suppression at 200 µg T$_3$/day, albeit to a lesser degree than euthyroid patients since most still had some residual TSH response at that dose of T$_3$. In contrast, only 25% patients with TSHomas had any significant suppression of TSH levels after high dose T_3 treatment [36, 41].

Measurement of metabolic markers of thyroid hormone action such as serum SGOT, SGPT, cholesterol, triglycerides, ferritin, osteocalcin, creatine phosphokinase (CPK), and sex hormone binding globulin (SHBG), also can be helpful in determining peripheral resistance. Serum prolactin can be elevated in patients with hypothyroidism and is increased in some patients with RTHβ, particularly those who previously were treated with ablative therapy. However, most RTHβ patients had normal basal prolactin levels (i.e., without TRH stimulation). [36, 40] Among these markers, serum SHBG appears to be the one that is most reliably affected by decreased TH action. Serum SHBG levels in RTH patients are similar to those found in euthyroid patients but is significantly decreased when compared to thyrotoxic patients. Thus, a normal SHBG level in conjunction with elevated TH levels and unsuppressed TSH would be suggestive of RTH. Ferritin and osteocalcin levels are typically elevated in hyperthyroidism; thus, normal levels also would be supportive of RTH. SGOT, SGPT, cholesterol, and triglyceride levels are responsive to TH but are nonspecific for hyperthyroidism, and thus may have limited utility. Additionally, TH effects on the neuromuscular system also can be assessed by measuring serum CPK concentration (elevated in RTH), and performing careful neurological examination looking for signs of hypothyroidism. Finally, if clinical and laboratory evidence support the diagnosis of RTHβ, a direct sequencing of the *THRB* gene exons, particularly those sequences that encode the LBD should be considered (see below). Identification of the mutation may be useful for future prenatal diagnosis of RTHβ. Specific TRβ mutation testing is available commercially from Quest Diagnostics (Madison, NJ) and several companies offer whole exome sequencing (e.g., Macrogen (Rockville, MD), Otogenetics (Atlanta, GA), and GATC (Constance, Germany)). Finally, a letter with a clear explanation of the diagnosis should be provided to the patient and be presented to any physican taking care of the patient in order to prevent inappropriate treatment for elevated serum T_3 or T_4.

TRβ Mutations and mechanism

In both familial and sporadic cases of RTHβ, TRβ point mutations cluster in the 3 major "hot spots" of the LBD [13, 17, 38]. In familial RTHβ, affected members have one normal and one abnormal *THRB* allele, consistent with the autosomal dominant pattern of inheritance seen in these families. In sporadic RTHβ mutations, similar findings in the *THRB* alleles also are observed. Since TRβ mutations occur in the LBD, they often lead to decreased T_3-binding affinity. So far, no germ line

mutations have been identified in the DBD or N-terminal regions of TRβ. In patients with RTHβ, most mutations are nucleotide substitutions that result in single amino acid changes. However, nucleotide deletions or insertions that cause single amino acid deletions and frameshift mutations, and premature stop codons also have been reported. Interestingly, the first described case of RTHβ occurred was inherited in a recessive pattern, and later shown to be due to complete from the exoncoding region resulting in absence of TRβ [42]. Since DNA-binding is required for the autosomal dominant inheritance in RTH, it is possible that mutations in the amino-terminus or DNA-binding may have a recessive phenotype. The inability to find mutations in these regions, suggests that if they exist, they may have little or no distinctive phenotype suggesting TH dysfunction. It is noteworthy that so far, no LBD mutations have been found that increase T_3-binding affinity or its transcriptional activity.

At the molecular level, mutant TRβs have decreased transcriptional activity due to their reduced ligand-binding affinity. They also can competitively block normal TRs from binding to TREs since they generally retain their DNA-binding capability [54]. This interference of normal TR function by the mutant TRβ (so called "dominant negative effect") leads to decreased overall transcriptional activity in target genes (Fig. 4) [30, 52]. Further support for this model comes from studies showing loss of dominant negative activity by mutant TRβs in which a second mutation was introduced into the DBD to abrogate DNA binding [27]. Moreover, it is likely that unliganded TR/co-repressor complex needs to leave the TREs in the presence of TH before liganded TR/co-activator complex can bind to the TREs and activate transcription. In this connection, constitutive binding of mutant TRs to TREs, combined with decreased corepressor dissociation and coactivator recruitment prevent normal T_3-bound TRs from binding to TREs and activate transcription of target genes [26, 39]. Together, these effects likely are the main contributors for the dominant negative inhibition on transcription of target genes by mutant TRs. In general, the severity of T_3 binding impairment by mutant TRs correlates with the severity of clinical phenotype, although there are some exceptions [7].

Treatment

In most patients, RTHβ appears to be adequately compensated by the increased endogenous supply of TH reflected by the increased serum fT_3 and fT_4 levels and normal or near normal TSH levels. These patients appear clinically euthyroid and eumetabolic [50]. Special care must be made not to misdiagnose and inappropriately treat these RTHβ patients for "hyperthyroidism"

A Wild type TR in normal subject or RTH patients

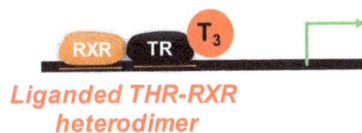

*Liganded THR-RXR
heterodimer*

B Mutant TR in RTH patients

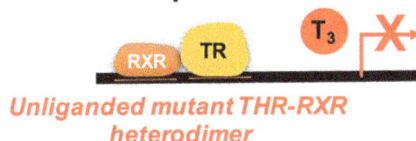

*Unliganded mutant THR-RXR
heterodimer*

Fig. 4 Model for resistance to thyroid hormone in RTHβ patients. **a** In both normal and RTH patients, wild-type TRβ and TRα isoforms derived from normal *THRB* and *THRA* alleles bind as TR/RXR heterodimers to the TRE and are able to activate transcription. **b** The mutant TRβ encoded by the abnormal *THRB* allele in RTH patients bind to the TRE constitutively in both the presence and absence of T_3. Since it has decreased ligand-binding affinity, its ability to recruit co-activators and activate transcription is impaired. The unliganded mutant TR/RXR heterodimer thus competes with T_3-bound wild type TR/RXR heterodimer for binding to the TRE

because of the high serum TH levels [49]. Unfortunately, some patients with RTHβ have undergone unnecessary radioactive iodine ablation, thyroid surgery, or anti-thyroidal medical treatment (e.g., propylthiouracil, carbimazole) based upon the presumption of hyperthyroidism. These inappropriate treatments led to worsened symptoms, as patients were rendered more hypothyroid in resistant tissues despite normalization of serum TSH and T_4 levels. Likewise, patients with compensated RTHβ do not require additional thyroxine treatment despite their RTHβ. Such treatment should only be considered in uncompensated RTHβ patients that have undergone thyroid ablation or surgery and have limited or no thyroid reserve or have decreased thyroid function due to autoimmune disease. Previous thyroid function test results when the patient was in the "compensated" baseline state before surgery or thyroid injury can be extremely useful for determining the optimal replacement dose in these RTHβ patients level, and can be used to follow patients' responses to treatment.

The possibility of uncompensated RTHβ in de novo cases should be suspected if patients have TSH levels higher than normal levels, together with elevated serum fT_3 and fT_4 levels. Thus, elevated TSH levels without any signs or symptoms of hypothyroidism should raise the suspicion of possible RTHβ, and serum fT_3 and fT_4 levels obtained if they were not measured during an initial screening. In patients with previous thyroid surgery or Hashimoto's thyroiditis, uncompensated RTHβ might be suspected if unusually high replacement doses of levothyroxine are necessary to reduce the elevated TSH levels. Finally, in some cases of uncompensated RTHβ, patients may be asymptomatic or have complaints suggestive of hypothyroidism while exhibiting paradoxically high

serum fT_3 and fT_4 levels and a TSH level that is above the normal range.

The assessment of uncompensated RTHβ also is made clinically, in conjunction with laboratory tests that suggest peripheral resistance (e.g., decreased serum SHBG). However, RTHβ may manifest itself in children by decreased and/or delayed growth or failure to gain weight. When RTHβ is not compensated, thyroxine can be given in incremental doses with simultaneous monitoring of parameters linked to TH action such as liver function tests, CPK, SHBG, PRL, and TSH until normal levels are achieved. In children, levothyroxine has been used under close supervision to improve growth and school performance; however, the results, have been variable. The presence of tachycardia should not be a reason to withhold treatment for uncompensated RTHβ as it can be managed by concomitant administration of a β-adrenergic blocker such as atenolol.

Recently, TRβ-specific analogs that have higher affinity for TRβ than TRα have been developed [6]. These drugs primarily are aimed as potential therapies for hypercholesterolemia, obesity, and diabetes. However, it is possible that these drugs may also be useful in patients with RTHβ. In this connection triiodothyroacetic acid (TRIAC) has been used to treat patients with RTHβ; however, there have been no studies thus far comparing the effectiveness of TRIAC vs. levothyroxine for the treatment of uncompensated RTHβ [32].

Resistance to thyroid hormone α (RTHα)
Clinical features
Previous studies in genetic models of RTHα such as TRα knockout mice that do not express TRα and mutant TRα knock-in mice that express a TRα mutation in the *THRA* gene locus, suggested that lack of TRα or

expression of an inactive TRα were not lethal [16]. Surprisingly, these genetic perturbations caused only relatively mild hypothyroid-like symptoms, particularly in the heart and bone. The prevalence of RTHα in man is not known but it is possible that this disorder has not been adequately recognized clinically since it lacks a distinctive phenotype and also may be associated with unusual phenotypes such as autism spectrum disorder. An examination of large databases showed approximately 100 non-synonymous variants in *THRA* in 60,000 exomes; however, only a small number of these variants were mutated at homologous TRα sites and would be expected to give a distinct phenotype [24].

RTHα in man was first described in a 6-year-old girl with skeletal dysplasia, bradycardia, growth retardation, neurodevelopmental delay, and constipation. Interestingly, the patient harbored a TRα mutation (Glu403X) that led to a frameshift mutation as well as loss of helix 12 in the LBD due to the introduction of a premature stop codon. This mutation decreased both its ligand binding affinity for TH and its transcriptional activity similar to the TRβ mutations found in RTHβ [10, 24]. This individual had borderline low or normal T_4, borderline high or normal T_3, and normal TSH concentrations in her serum. Shortly afterwards, several adult male and female individuals were identified that harbored frameshift/premature stop mutations within the TRα1 LBD [14, 45]. These patients also had additional features in their phenotypes such as macrocephaly, anemia, and dysmorphic facies. Based upon the reports of nearly 30 patients with RTHα [14, 23, 24, 43], clinical features that are most commonly found among RTHα patients include bradycardia, constipation, reduced and delayed bone growth, delayed psychomotor development, decreased metabolic rate, as well as skeletal abnormalities manifested by delayed fusion of epiphyses and reduced bone growth (Table 1). Additionally, dysmorphic features have been reported in some affected individuals from several kindreds, and they include: macrocephaly, late fontanelle closure, dysmorphic and broad facies, flattened nose, enlarged tongue, and thickened lips. Of note, many of these features can resemble those found in congenital and primary hypothyroidism. Additionally, the tissues associated with these features contain mostly TRα, and thus would be expected to be "hypothyroid" with respect to TH action due to the dominant negative effect by mutant TRα. Interestingly, several cases of RTHα also were identified after screening for abnormal thyroid function in patients with dysmorphic features [24]. On the other hand, there can be large variation in the severity of the phenotypes in RTHα as some patients can have mild phenotypes with minimal symptoms [14]. When RTHα patients are compared with RTHβ, it appears that they can present with a wider repertoire of phenotypes than RTHβ as well as exhibit phenotypes that are distinct from RTHβ.

RTHα patients typically have increased/high-normal T_3 and decreased/low-normal serum T_4 levels, resulting in a markedly reduced T_4/T_3 ratio (Fig. 4a). Low serum rT_3 levels also have been reported in some cases. Of note, serum TSH levels are usually normal. The reason for the low T_4/T_3 ratio in affected individuals is not known; however, it is noteworthy that increased hepatic DIO1 expression was observed in a dominant negative TRα knockin mouse model [55] so it is possible that increased conversion of T_4 to T_3 may be involved in generating this serum TH profile. Additionally, TRα is highly expressed in the skin so RTHα in that tissue could lead to decreased DIO3 expression and activity, and thus lead to accumulation of serum T_3 [11].

Differential diagnosis

Although rare, RTHα should be considered in the differential for children with decreased growth rate, dysmorphic features, and delayed psychomotor development. It also should be considered in adults with a similar previous history as well as in patients with unexplained constipation, megacolon, and bradycardia [24, 46]. The low serum T_4/T_3 level is a distinctive and consistent feature in RTHα that can help identify potential cases. Of note, this biochemical abnormality also can be seen in disorders involving decreased TH synthesis since T_4 is the major form of TH that is synthesized and released by the thyroid gland. Thus, congenital hypothyroidism or environmental causes of hypothyroidism (e.g., iodine deficiency) can exhibit this serum TH profile. Additionally, patients with Allan–Herndon–Dudley syndrome, a condition in which patients harbor a mutation in one of the major TH transporters, MCT8, can present with a similar TH profile [15]. However, these patients have severe mental retardation and progressive spastic paralysis as well as an x-linked inheritance pattern so it is relatively easy to distinguish them from patients with RTHα based upon their clinical features.

Mechanism

In patients with RTHα, TRα mutations in the LBD due to nucleotide substitutions that cause missense amino acid changes, deletions, or insertions, as well as frameshift/premature stop mutations have been described [14, 24, 43]. Of note, none of the *THRA* mutations described so far involve the exon regions or the expression of the *REV-ERBα*, a gene that is transcribed from the opposite strand of the *THRA* locus. Heterozygous *THRA* mutations are found in both sporadic and familial RTHα. Thus, the molecular mechanism for RTHα is similar to RTHα, by virtue of the expression of the mutant TRα from one *THRA* allele and a normal TRα from the other *THRA* allele, and normal TRβs from the two *THRB* alleles [24]. The mutant TRα has "dominant negative activity" on normal TRs expressed within the cell. The degree of dominant activity depends upon the relative amount of mutant TRα expressed within a particular cell as well as the residual ligand-binding and DNA-binding affinities of the mutant TRα.

Mutant TRαs bind to T_3 with decreased affinity or fail to bind ligand; and thus lead to decreased or no transcriptional activity, respectively. Similar to TRβ mutations in RTHβ, TRα1 mutants inhibit the function of normal TRs in a dominant negative manner when they are co-expressed in transfected cells. In support of this mechanism in affected individuals, expression of TH-responsive target genes are blunted in peripheral blood mononuclear cells of a patient with RTHα [24], suggesting that mutant TRαs can exert dominant negative activity in vivo (Fig. 4). Additionally, studies have shown that many of the naturally occurring TRα mutations have decreased release of NCoR due to lower T_3 binding affinity by mutant TRαs.

Treatment

In adults with RTHα, titrating the appropriate levothyroxine dose is difficult. Heart rate and cardiac contractility can remain blunted despite thyroxine therapy. Excessive thyroxine treatment to correct cardiac parameters also may lead to undesirable toxicities in tissues that express predominantly TRβ such as the liver. Interestingly, thyroxine therapy does not ameliorate the anaemia observed in RTHα patients. In children, the treatment of RTHβ is challenging [24, 46]. TH induces the expression of insulin-like growth factor 1 (IGF1) and sex hormone binding globulin (SHBG) and decreases the production of cholesterol and triglycerides. Thus, thyroxine therapy can improve overall height and bone growth in RTHα [23, 24]. Of note, growth hormone in combination with thyroxine to increase IGF1 has not led to significant improvement in height and growth [24]. Thyroxine therapy also can improve the constipation symptoms commonly found in children with RTHα.

Thyroxine therapy suppresses serum TSH levels and increases fT_3 above normal levels. Serum SHBG, which is induced by TH in the liver, as well as bone turnover markers also can increase above normal levels, most likely due to increased TH activity in tissues and cell types that express mostly TRβ Just as in the case for RTHβ, development of TRα1-selective thyromimetics may be helpful to selectively activate normal TRα1 and/or mutant TRα1 with weak binding affinity for T_3 to overcome TH resistance in tissues that express predominantly TRα. Another potential therapeutic strategy is to develop drugs that enable nuclear receptor co-repressor

(NCoR) to dissociate from unliganded TR or to abrogate the activity of histone deacetylases recruited by NCoR. In this connection, an inhibitor of histone deacetylase, suberoylanilide hydroxamic acid improved some of the phenotypic abnormalities of RTHα such as delayed and decreased growth and bone development in a mouse model of RTHα [20].

RTH in patients without TRβ mutations

Several patients with RTH have been identified who do not have TRβ or TRα mutations [31, 37]. Additionally, no mutations in various candidate co-factors involved in TR-mediated transcription were found. It is likely that epigenetic effects that alter the expression of various genes involved in transcription may be involved, although it has not been investigated in these patients so far.

Somatic TR mutations

Somatic TRα and TRβ mutations have been identified in human hepatic, thyroid, and renal cell cancers [19, 22] in addition to TSH-secreting pituitary adenomas [2, 3]. These findings suggest that TR mutations likely contribute to RTH in these tumors; however, they are not sufficient to cause oncogenesis since RTH patients with germline TRβ mutations do not appear to have an increased risk for cancer.

Conclusion

Although RTHβ and RTHα are rare genetic disorders that cause RTH, they need to be considered when patients present with enigmatic thyroid function tests. In particular, when patients present with high free T_3 and T_4 with non-suppressed TSH levels (RTHβ) or reduced free T_4/ free T_3 ratio with normal TSH level in the serum (RTHα). Associated with each condition are some characteristic features in their phenotype that also highlight the isoform-specific expression and particular roles of TRβ and TRα. The clinical spectrum for both RTHβ and RTHα is wide and heterogenous; moreover, there can be variable phenotypes in patients with the same mutations. These observations suggest that genetic and epigenetic modifiers likely play important roles in the phenotypes of affected individuals. The identification of TR mutations as causes for the two forms RTH, elucidation of their mechanism for causing resistance, correlation of genotype with phenotype, and the development of criteria for clinical diagnosis and treatment of RTH provide elegant examples of the convergence of basic, translational, and clinical research to improve the understanding and management of a genetic endocrine disorder.

Abbbreviations
ChIP-Seq: chromatin immunoprecipitation sequencing; FDH: familial dysalbuminemic hyperthyroxinemia; fT₃: serum free T₃ concentration;

fT$_4$: serum free T$_4$ concentration; HAS: human serum albumin; HAT: histone acetyltransferase HREs hormone response elements; HPT: hypothalamic, pituitary, and thyroid; IGF1: insulin-like growth factor 1; NCoR: nuclear receptor co-repressor; NR: nuclear receptor; rT$_3$: serum reverse triiodothyronine concentration; RTH: resistance to thyroid hormone; RTHα: resistance to thyroid hormone receptor α; RTHβ: resistance to thyroid hormone β; RXRs: retinoid X receptors; SHBG: sex hormone binding globulin; TBG: thyroxine-binding globulin; TH: thyroid hormone; *THRA*: thyroid hormone receptor β gene; *THRB*: thyroid hormone receptor β gene; TR: thyroid hormone receptor; TREs: thyroid hormone response elements; TRH: thyrotropin releasing hormone; TRIAC: triiodothyroacetic acid; TRα: thyroid hormone receptor α; TRβ: thyroid hormone receptor β; TSH: thyrotropin/thyroid stimulating hormone; TSHoma: TSH-secreting pituitary adenoma; TSHβ: thyroid stimulating hormone β subunit; TTR: transthyretin; α-GSU: common glycoprotein hormone α-subunit protein

Acknowledgements
n/a

Funding
NMRC Singapore.

Authors' contributions
Writing PMY Figures and writing BKS. Both authors read and approved the final manuscript.

References
1. Albright F, Burnett CH, Smith PH, Parson W. Pseudohypopara-thyroidism — an example of Seabright's bantam syndrome. Endocrinology. 1942;30:922.
2. Ando S, Sarlis NJ, Krishnan J, Feng X, Refetoff S, Zhang MQ, Oldfield EH, Yen PM. Aberrant alternative splicing of thyroid hormone receptor in a TSH-secreting pituitary tumor is a mechanism for hormone resistance. Mol Endocrinol. 2001a;15:1529–38.
3. Ando S, Sarlis NJ, Oldfield EH, Yen PM. Somatic mutation of TRbeta can cause a defect in negative regulation of TSH in a TSH-secreting pituitary tumor. J Clin Endocrinol Metab. 2001b;86:5572–6.
4. Ayers S, Switnicki MP, Angajala A, Lammel J, Arumanayagam AS, Webb P. Genome-wide binding patterns of thyroid hormone receptor beta. PLoS One. 2014;9:e81186.
5. Bassett JH, Harvey CB, Williams GR. Mechanisms of thyroid hormone receptor-specific nuclear and extra nuclear actions. Mol Cell Endocrinol. 2003;213:1–11.
6. Baxter JD, Webb P. Thyroid hormone mimetics: potential applications in atherosclerosis, obesity and type 2 diabetes. Nat Rev Drug Discov. 2009;8:308–20.
7. Beck-Peccoz P, Chatterjee VK. The variable clinical phenotype in thyroid hormone resistance syndrome. Thyroid. 1994;4:225–32.
8. Bernal, J. (2000). Thyroid hormones in brain development and function. In Endotext, L.J. De Groot, P. Beck-Peccoz, G. Chrousos, K. Dungan, A. Grossman, J.M. Hershman, C. Koch, R. McLachlan, M. New, R. Rebar, et al., eds. (South Dartmouth (MA)).
9. Bernal J, Guadano-Ferraz A, Morte B. Thyroid hormone transporters–functions and clinical implications. Nat Rev Endocrinol. 2015;11:406–17.
10. Bochukova E, Schoenmakers N, Agostini M, Schoenmakers E, Rajanayagam O, Keogh JM, Henning E, Reinemund J, Gevers E, Sarri M, et al. A mutation in the thyroid hormone receptor alpha gene. N Engl J Med. 2012;366:243–9.
11. Cheng SY. Isoform-dependent actions of thyroid hormone nuclear receptors: lessons from knockin mutant mice. Steroids. 2005;70:450–4.
12. Cheng SY, Leonard JL, Davis PJ. Molecular aspects of thyroid hormone actions. Endocr Rev. 2010;31:139–70.
13. Collingwood TN, Wagner R, Matthews CH, Clifton-Bligh RJ, Gurnell M, Rajanayagam O, Agostini M, Fletterick RJ, Beck-Peccoz P, Reinhardt W, et al. A role for helix 3 of the TRbeta ligand-binding domain in coactivator recruitment identified by characterization of a third cluster of mutations in resistance to thyroid hormone. EMBO J. 1998;17:4760–70.
14. Demir K, van Gucht AL, Buyukinan M, Catli G, Ayhan Y, Bas VN, Dundar B, Ozkan B, Meima ME, Visser WE, et al. Diverse genotypes and phenotypes of three novel thyroid hormone receptor-alpha mutations. J Clin Endocrinol Metab. 2016;101:2945–54.
15. Dumitrescu, A.M., and Refetoff, S. (2000). Impaired sensitivity to thyroid hormone: defects of transport, metabolism and action. In Endotext, L.J. De Groot, G. Chrousos, K. Dungan, K.R. Feingold, A. Grossman, J.M.

Hershman, C. Koch, M. Korbonits, R. McLachlan, M. New, et al., eds. (South Dartmouth (MA)).
16. Flamant F, Samarut J. Thyroid hormone receptors: lessons from knockout and knock-in mutant mice. Trends Endocrinol Metab. 2003;14:85–90.
17. Hayashi Y, Sunthornthepvarakul T, Refetoff S. Mutations of CpG dinucleotides located in the triiodothyronine (T3)-binding domain of the thyroid hormone receptor (TR) beta gene that appears to be devoid of natural mutations may not be detected because they are unlikely to produce the clinical phenotype of resistance to thyroid hormone. J Clin Invest. 1994;94:607–15.
18. Jameson, J.L. (2004). Molecular mechanisms of end-organ resistance. Growth Horm IGF res *14 Suppl A*, S45-50.
19. Kamiya Y, Puzianowska-Kuznicka M, McPhie P, Nauman J, Cheng SY, Nauman A. Expression of mutant thyroid hormone nuclear receptors is associated with human renal clear cell carcinoma. Carcinogenesis. 2002;23:25–33.
20. Kim DW, Park JW, Willingham MC, Cheng SY. A histone deacetylase inhibitor improves hypothyroidism caused by a TRalpha1 mutant. Hum Mol Genet. 2014;23:2651–64.
21. Lin KH, Fukuda T, Cheng SY. Hormone and DNA binding activity of a purified human thyroid hormone nuclear receptor expressed in Escherichia Coli. J Biol Chem. 1990;265:5161–5.
22. Lin KH, Shieh HY, Chen SL, Hsu HC. Expression of mutant thyroid hormone nuclear receptors in human hepatocellular carcinoma cells. Mol Carcinog. 1999;26:53–61.
23. Moran C, Agostini M, Visser WE, Schoenmakers E, Schoenmakers N, Offiah AC, Poole K, Rajanayagam O, Lyons G, Halsall D, et al. Resistance to thyroid hormone caused by a mutation in thyroid hormone receptor (TR)alpha1 and TRalpha2: clinical, biochemical, and genetic analyses of three related patients. Lancet Diabetes Endocrinol. 2014;2:619–26.
24. Moran C, Chatterjee K. Resistance to thyroid hormone due to defective thyroid receptor alpha. Best Pract Res Clin Endocrinol Metab. 2015;29:647–57.
25. Mukku VR, Kirkland JL, Hardy M, Stancel GM. Evidence for thyroid hormone receptors in uterine nuclei. Metabolism. 1983;32:142–5.
26. Nagaya T, Jameson JL. Thyroid hormone receptor dimerization is required for dominant negative inhibition by mutations that cause thyroid hormone resistance. J Biol Chem. 1993;268:15766–71.
27. Nagaya T, Madison LD, Jameson JL. Thyroid hormone receptor mutants that cause resistance to thyroid hormone. Evidence for receptor competition for DNA sequences in target genes J Biol Chem. 1992;267:13014–9.
28. Oetting A, Yen PM. New insights into thyroid hormone action. Best Pract Res Clin Endocrinol Metab. 2007;21:193–208.
29. Ohba K, Leow MK, Singh BK, Sinha RA, Lesmana R, Liao XH, Ghosh S, Refetoff S, Sng JC, Yen PM. Desensitization and incomplete recovery of hepatic target genes after chronic thyroid hormone treatment and withdrawal in male adult mice. Endocrinology. 2016;157:1660–72.
30. Ortiga-Carvalho TM, Sidhaye AR, Wondisford FE. Thyroid hormone receptors and resistance to thyroid hormone disorders. Nat Rev Endocrinol. 2014;10:582–91.
31. Parikh S, Ando S, Schneider A, Skarulis MC, Sarlis NJ, Yen PM. Resistance to thyroid hormone in a patient without thyroid hormone receptor mutations. Thyroid. 2002;12:81–6.
32. Radetti G, Persani L, Molinaro G, Mannavola D, Cortelazzi D, Chatterjee VK, Beck-Peccoz P. Clinical and hormonal outcome after two years of triiodothyroacetic acid treatment in a child with thyroid hormone resistance. Thyroid. 1997;7:775–8.
33. Ramadoss P, Abraham BJ, Tsai L, Zhou Y, Costa-e-Sousa RH, Ye F, Bilban M, Zhao K, Hollenberg AN. Novel mechanism of positive versus negative regulation by thyroid hormone receptor beta1 (TRbeta1) identified by genome-wide profiling of binding sites in mouse liver. J Biol Chem. 2014;289:1313–28.
34. Refetoff S, Bassett JH, Beck-Peccoz P, Bernal J, Brent G, Chatterjee K, De Groot LJ, Dumitrescu AM, Jameson JL, Kopp PA, et al. Classification and proposed nomenclature for inherited defects of thyroid hormone action, cell transport, and metabolism. J Clin Endocrinol Metab. 2014;99:768–70.
35. Refetoff S, DeWind LT, DeGroot LJ. Familial syndrome combining deaf-mutism, stuppled epiphyses, goiter and abnormally high PBI: possible target organ refractoriness to thyroid hormone. J Clin Endocrinol Metab. 1967;27:279–94.
36. Refetoff S, Weiss RE, Usala SJ. The syndromes of resistance to thyroid hormone. Endocr Rev. 1993;14:348–99.
37. Reutrakul S, Sadow PM, Pannain S, Pohlenz J, Carvalho GA, Macchia PE, Weiss RE, Refetoff S. Search for abnormalities of nuclear corepressors, coactivators, and a coregulator in families with resistance to thyroid

hormone without mutations in thyroid hormone receptor beta or alpha genes. J Clin Endocrinol Metab. 2000;85:3609–17.

38. Ribeiro RC, Apriletti JW, Wagner RL, West BL, Feng W, Huber R, Kushner PJ, Nilsson S, Scanlan T, Fletterick RJ, et al. Mechanisms of thyroid hormone action: insights from X-ray crystallographic and functional studies. Recent Prog Horm Res. 1998;53:351–92. discussion 392-354

39. Safer JD, Cohen RN, Hollenberg AN, Wondisford FE. Defective release of corepressor by hinge mutants of the thyroid hormone receptor found in patients with resistance to thyroid hormone. J Biol Chem. 1998;273:30175–82.

40. Sarne, D.H., Refetoff, S,, Rosenfield, R.L, Farriaux, J.P. (1988) Sex hormone-binding globulin in the diagnosis of peripheral tissue resistance to thyroid hormone: the value of changes after short term triiodothyronine administration. J Clin Endocrinol Metab 66:740–746.

41. Sarne DH, Sobieszczyk S, Ain KB, Refetoff S. Serum thyrotropin and prolactin in the syndrome of generalized resistance to thyroid hormone: responses to thyrotropin-releasing hormone stimulation and short term triiodothyronine suppression. J Clin Endocrinol Metab. 1990;70:1305–11.

42. Takeda K, Sakurai A, DeGroot LJ, Refetoff S. Recessive inheritance of thyroid hormone resistance caused by complete deletion of the protein-coding region of the thyroid hormone receptor-beta gene. J Clin Endocrinol Metab. 1992;74:49–55.

43. Tang Y, Yu M, Lian X. Resistance to thyroid hormone alpha, revelation of basic study to clinical consequences. J Pediatr Endocrinol Metab. 2016;29: 511–22.

44. Taylor PN, Peeters R, Dayan CM. Genetic abnormalities in thyroid hormone deiodinases. Curr Opin Endocrinol Diabetes Obes. 2015;22:402–6.

45. van Mullem A, van Heerebeek R, Chrysis D, Visser E, Medici M, Andrikoula M, Tsatsoulis A, Peeters R, Visser TJ. Clinical phenotype and mutant TRalpha1. N Engl J Med. 2012;366:1451–3.

46. van Mullem AA, Visser TJ, Peeters RP. Clinical consequences of mutations in thyroid hormone receptor-alpha1. Eur Thyroid J. 2014;3:17–24.

47. Visser TJ. Thyroid hormone transporters and resistance. Endocr Dev. 2013;24:1–10.

48. Weintraub BD, Menezes-Ferreira MM, Petrick PA. Inappropriate secretion of TSH. Endocr Res. 1989;15:601–17.

49. Weiss RE, Refetoff S. Treatment of resistance to thyroid hormone–primum non nocere. J Clin Endocrinol Metab. 1999;84:401–4.

50. Weiss RE, Refetoff S. Resistance to thyroid hormone. Rev Endocr Metab Disord. 2000;1:97–108.

51. Wondisford FE. Thyroid hormone action: insight from transgenic mouse models. J Investig Med. 2003;51:215–20.

52. Yen PM. Molecular basis of resistance to thyroid hormone. Trends Endocrinol Metab. 2003;14:327–33.

53. Yen PM. Classical nuclear hormone receptor activity as a mediator of complex biological responses: a look at health and disease. Best Pract Res Clin Endocrinol Metab. 2015;29:517–28.

54. Yen PM, Sugawara A, Refetoff S, Chin WW. New insights on the mechanism(s) of the dominant negative effect of mutant thyroid hormone receptor in generalized resistance to thyroid hormone. J Clin Invest. 1992;90:1825–31.

55. Zavacki AM, Ying H, Christoffolete MA, Aerts G, So E, Harney JW, Cheng SY, Larsen PR, Bianco AC. Type 1 iodothyronine deiodinase is a sensitive marker of peripheral thyroid status in the mouse. Endocrinology. 2005;146:1568–75.

56. Zhang XY, Kaneshige M, Kamiya Y, Kaneshige K, McPhie P, Cheng SY. Differential expression of thyroid hormone receptor isoforms dictates the dominant negative activity of mutant Beta receptor. Mol Endocrinol. 2002;16:2077–92.

13

Brief review: cell replacement therapies to treat type 1 diabetes mellitus

Alberto Hayek[1] and Charles C. King[2*]

Abstract

Human embryonic stem cells (hESCs) and induced pluripotent cells (iPSCs) have the potential to differentiate into any somatic cell, making them ideal candidates for cell replacement therapies to treat a number of human diseases and regenerate damaged or non-functional tissues and organs. Key to the promise of regenerative medicine is developing standardized protocols that can safely be applied in patients. Progress towards this goal has occurred in a number of fields, including type 1 diabetes mellitus (T1D). During the past 10 years, significant technological advances in hESC/iPSC biochemistry have provided a roadmap to generate sufficient quantities of glucose-responsive, insulin-producing cells capable of eliminating diabetes in rodents. Although many of the molecular mechanisms underlying the genesis of these cells remain to be elucidated, the field of cell-based therapeutics to treat T1D has advanced to the point where the first Phase I/II trials in humans have begun. Here, we provide a concise review of the history of cell replacement therapies to treat T1D from islet transplantations and xenotranplantation, to current work in hESC/iPSC. We also highlight the latest advances in efforts to employ insulin-producing, glucose-responsive β-like cells derived from hESC as therapeutics.

Background

There remains an urgent and critical need for new treatments for type 1 diabetes (T1D). A current prevailing hypothesis is that cell replacement for pancreatic β-cells destroyed by autoimmune attack will optimally restore euglycemia. While efforts to augment endogenous populations of a patient's residual β-cells or pancreatic specific stem cells remains an active avenue of research, efforts to enhance proliferation of these populations of cells without further autoimmune damage has had limited success. Conversely, the development of in vitro generated populations of insulin-producing, glucose-responsive cells has overcome many significant challenges, including generation of chemically defined conditions for reproducibly differentiating hESCs into endocrine precursors (EPs) and, the development of strategies to purify these precursor cells to avoid the development of benign tumors such as teratomas. With the basic protocols in place other pressing issues will move to the forefront, including prevention of cell destruction following transplantation,

encapsulation, and the application of newer anti–rejection therapies.

Islet transplantation as a treatment for T1D – a historical perspective

The modern age of islet transplantation was ushered in by pioneering studies of Lacy and Kostianovsky who developed a method to isolate and purify islets from rat pancreas [1]. Building upon this work, Kemp and colleagues demonstrated that direct injection of freshly isolated pancreatic islets into the portal vein of rats with streptozotocin-induced diabetes was able to restore normoglycemia [2]. Subsequently, the same protocol was found to be effective in diabetic rhesus monkeys [3]. In 1990, the first successful human clinical islet transplantations were performed [4]. However, only a small number of patients were able to maintain long term euglycemia. Until the publication of the "Edmonton protocol" [5] in the year 2000, the prognosis for maintaining insulin independence was less than 10 % at 1-year post procedure. The Edmonton group brought about hope that their results –100 % in 7 patients-would last more than 1 year. Further follow up showed that after 5 years the rate of insulin-independence was down to 10 %. In the last 5 years, refinements in islet isolation and newer

* Correspondence: chking@ucsd.edu
[2]Pediatric Diabetes Research Center, University of California, San Diego, La Jolla, CA 92093, USA
Full list of author information is available at the end of the article

immunosuppressive agents offer a 50 % possibilities of success for up to 5 years post-transplant [6]. More recently, Moassesfar and colleagues have compared results from islet vs. pancreas transplantation and found that, in terms of insulin independence after 3 years post-transplantation, both approaches were approximately 70 % efficient [7]. Although significant hurdles remain with immunosuppression and the availability of donated pancreases to treat patients with T1D, recent advances in the field are encouraging for overcoming these two problems. Patients who received combinatorial treatment with both T-cell depleting anti-thymocyte globulin (ATG) and the TNF inhibitor etanercept had dramatically higher rates of insulin independence at 3 and 5 years after final infusion compared with patients treated with T-cell depleting antibodies alone or with the traditional standard IL2 receptor antibodies [8]. Recently, application of the Clinical Islet Transplantation 07 (CIT07) protocol demonstrated improvedβ-cell secretory capacity, indicating an increased functional islet β-cell mass. The CIT07 protocol incorporates T-cell depletion and TNF inhibition described above with inhibitor maintenance therapies described in the original Edmonton protocol [9].

Alternate sources for islet transplantation
Expanded populations of human β-cells and human fetal pancreatic cells
Over 20 years ago, our laboratory identified the combination of hepatocyte growth factor/scatter factor (HGF/SF) and the HTB-9 extracelluar matrix from human bladder carcinoma cells, as potent stimuli for β cell replication [10]. Cells could remain in culture over 15 doublings, but with time, both insulin mRNA and protein levels dropped precipitously. Although PDX1 expression was maintained, significant production of insulin was not observed after transplantation. Loss of β cell phenotype was found to be associated with epithelial-to-mesenchymal transition (EMT) [11]. In the past few years, exciting work has focused on the ability to reverse EMT by mesenchymal-to-epithelial transition (MET) through modulation of TGFβ and NOTCH signaling in low passage β-cells [12–14]. miR-375, a microRNA previously implicated in both definitive endoderm formation and islet function [15, 16], was identified as critical regulator of MET and β-cell dedifferentiation [17]. Viral expression of miR-375 in expanded β-cells increased expression of the epithelial marker E-cadherin, as well as the islet/β-cell transcription factors PDX1, MAFA, and NEUROD1. In cells treated with a miR-375 virus, expression of the mesenchymal markers N-cadherin and vimentin decreased. Together, these studies represent significant strides in understanding the underlying biochemistry that regulates β-cell expansion and temporal gene expression.

Investigations using human fetal pancreatic cells from the mid 1980s to the 1990s first provided evidence that human fetal tissues could be manipulated in vitro to advance differentiation to β-cells from endocrine precursors previously identified in experiments performed during pancreas development in rodents. Full appropriate response to glucose in terms of insulin release was not obtained until the cells were transplanted into immune-deficient mice for periods of 10 to 12 weeks [18–21]. These observations proved valuable to the understanding of the new cell supply derived from human stem cells as discussed below.

Although much has been published about the potential for β-cell regeneration through replication of existing β-cells and/or differentiation from putative precursors, clinical protocols for their use are not available since the positive results reported in small animals models have not been possible to translate to humans.

Pancreatic exocrine cell reprogramming
Abnormalities of the exocrine pancreas in T1D have been described since 1940 but still scant attention has focused on research in this area. A recent review describes subclinical exocrine dysfunction associated with the characteristic findings in the islets of T1D subjects, but it remains unclear whether the two are related to the autoimmune response after the onset of T1D [22]. Because the pancreatic exocrine cells share a similar microenvironment and lineage with endocrine pancreatic cells, they are prime targets for reprogramming and therapeutic use in humans. In 2000, Bonner-Weir and colleagues reported that in vitro human adult ductal tissue cultured on Matrigel for 4 weeks increased insulin content by 10–15 fold. Upon glucose challenge, the cells secreted insulin [23]. In follow-up studies, adenoviral infection of pancreatic endocrine cells with the transcription factors (PDX1, NGN3, NEUROD, or PAX4) was found to induce insulin transcription [24]. In vivo reprogramming of pancreatic exocrine cells in mice using PDX1, NGN3, and MAFA were found to be functionally equivalent to β-cells and able to ameliorate hyperglycemia [25]. Recent work from Lemper and colleagues found that human pancreatic exocrine cells, when transduced with MAPK and STAT3, activated expression of NGN3. Expression of insulin was limited to cells grown under the initial conditions [26]. Advances in reprogramming of mouse and human pancreatic exocrine cells in the absence of genetic manipulation were reported by Baeyens and Klein [27, 28]. In the first study, mouse ascinar cells were converted to β-like cells upon incubation with EGF (epidermal growth factor) and CNTF (ciliary neurotrophic factor). These cells were functional, glucose responsive, and restored normal glycemia for extended periods. Similar to the work of

Lemper, this study identified STAT3 as a critical regulator of this process. In the second study, BMP-7 (bone morphogenic protein 7) was found to induce conversion of human adult pancreatic nonendocrine pancreatic tissue into endocrine-like cells with elevated insulin content and that were glucose responsive in vitro and after transplantation. The recent successes in these systems and the abundance of exocrine cells suggest a potentially therapeutic relevant cell population to treat T1D patients. However, clinical use of these cells is hampered by safe and effective targeting of reprogramming transcription factors and control of their activity once in selected cells.

Xenotransplantation

Xenotransplantation provides another alternative for the limited supply issue faced from the too few human islets available from donated human pancreases. In 2006, two groups reported long-term survival of porcine islets in non-human primates [29, 30]. Recently, Shin et al. demonstrated that pig islet grafts survived for greater than 6 months and were able to maintain normoglycemia for >6 months in four immunosuppressed non-human primates [31]. Given issues of supply and demand, porcine islet xenotransplantation for T1D now appears to be a therapeutic consideration following extensive preclinical investigations, suggesting that clinical trials may be now justified. Two current reviews provide in-depth insight into the advances and shortcomings in this field [32, 33].

hESCs

An effective cell-based therapeutic for T1D requires cells that sense glucose fluctuations and respond with appropriate insulin secretion. While islet transplantation has shown promise as a treatment for type T1D, a major obstacle to this approach is the shortage of the islets containing insulin-producing cells. Over the past decade, hESCs/iPSCs have emerged as promising sources for the pancreatic β-cells lost in T1D. hESCs are characterized by their capacity for self-renewal and differentiation to almost any specific cell type in the human body. The first study demonstrating functional and meaningful secretion of insulin after transplantation into mice of β-cells generated from hESC was published in 2008 [34], less than 10 years after the initial reports on spontaneous in vitro differentiation of hESC into insulin producing cells [35]. The advent of iPSCs in 2007 by Takahashi and Yamanaka [36, 37] opened the possibility of reprogramming a patient's own fibroblasts into β-cells for use in clinical situations, including T1D. Since the initial publications, this patient-specific approach towards treatment of various diseases has allowed researchers to address the effect of point mutations, gene deletions, or translocations on the function of a cell in culture or in a model animal system.

Although critical gaps in the understanding of the molecular mechanisms that drive the genesis of insulin producing cells from hESCs/iPSCs exist, many of the essential growth factors and inhibitors have been identified. Below, we briefly highlight the various steps in hESC differentiation toward glucose-responsive, insulin secreting cells.

Maintenance of pluripotency and definitive endoderm formation (DE) Pluripotency of hESCs initially required co-culture with a fibroblast feeder layer that secreted unidentified soluble factors that helped maintain pluripotency. Unlike mouse ES cells, hESC were unable to maintain pluripotency by incubation with leukemia inhibitor factor (LIF) [38]. In 2005, Beattie et al. identified low levels of activin A as critical factor secreted by feeder layers that maintained pluripotency [39]. Later, it was determined that elevated activin A levels, combined with inhibition of PI 3-kinase signaling was required for efficient DE formation [40, 41].

Glucose-responsive, insulin producing cells from DE Over the past decade many different groups have contributed to generate differentiation protocols that mimic pancreas development (reviewed by van Hoof, et al. [42]). From the seminal studies on DE formation, several protocols were published for the generation of insulin producing cells, mimicking the extensive knowledge acquired on pancreatic development in *Xenopus* and rodents [34, 43, 44]. Large populations of cells were obtained expressing transcription factors present in pancreatic endoderm, including PDX1 and NGN3. However, a large percentage of the cells were poly-hormonal, simultaneously expressing somatostatin, glucagon and/or insulin. Expression of multiple hormone markers within a single cell and findings indicating poor response to glucose in terms of insulin release, suggested that the protocols required further refinements. Hrvatin et al. employed mRNA profiling to demonstrate that insulin-expressing cells derived from hESCs are more similar to human fetal pancreatic cells than mature β-cells [45]. ViaCyte, a biotechnology company in San Diego, CA was instrumental in the development of protocols to generate glucose-responsive, insulin secreting cells from hESC, circumvented these issues by transplanting pancreatic progenitor cells into mice which subsequently matured into functional β-like cells in vivo capable of protecting against streptozotocin-induced hyperglycemia [34]. In more recent work form the same group, the pancreatic progenitor cells were further differentiated into islet-like cells that contained a high percentage (~80 %) endocrine cells, of which about half expressed insulin [46]. Recently, three refined protocols for generating glucose-responsive, insulin-producing cells have been published by Pagliuca et al. [47], Rezania et al. [48], and Russ et al. [49]. In all protocols, cells are cultured in suspension (3D culture) which better mimics the conditions for in vivo growth and differentiation. Although there is considerable variance between the protocols during formation of definitive endoderm, primitive gut tube, and posterior foregut formation, the culture conditions to drive cells from pancreatic endocrine precursors to immature β-cells and finally to mature β-cells is remarkably similar between the last 3 reports (Rezania, Pagliuca, and Russ). Specifically, each protocol requires retinoic acid to dampen the sonic hedgehog signaling pathway, a known inhibitor of pancreas development [50]. Additionally, each protocol uses the ATP competitive Alk5 inhibitor II to signaling through TGFβ RI signaling and LDN193189/Noggin to block signaling through BMP Type I receptors. Finally, both the Rezania and Pagliuca protocols require the thyroid hormone triiodothyronine (T3), which has previously been shown to be required for liver development [51]. Sixteen to twenty weeks post engraftment, the CyT49/VC-01 cells from the ViaCyte protocol had matured in vivo to become pancreatic endoderm cells that were able to protect against streptozotocin (STZ)-induced hyperglycemia [52]. Similarly, diabetes was reversed approximately 6 weeks after transplantation using the Rezania protocol [48]. hESCs differentiated using the Pagliuca protocol were found to secrete human insulin in response to a glucose challenge after transplantation in a manner that prevented hyperglycemia in the Akita mouse [47]. β-like cells derived from the Russ protocol were able to reduce blood glucose levels, after short-term transplantation under the kidney capsule of nude mice [49].

Careful examination of the similarities and differences between the four protocols reveals limitations between the different methods to generate glucose-responsive, insulin-producing cells from hESCs. Rezania and Pagliuca relied upon previously established protocols for generation of primitive gut tube and posterior foregut and primarily focused on optimization of the later stages of hESC differentiation. Russ found that elimination of Noggin during posterior foregut formation (high retinoic acid levels) followed by combined treatment with EGF/ KGF enhanced PDX1/NKX6.1 expression and reduced the number of polyhormonal cells. This work emphasizes the importance of temporal activation of signaling pathways during hESC differentiation.

Encapsulation of hESC for transplantation Reproducible protocols to generate cells that can ablate diabetes in mice have led to questions about how these cells can be used therapeutically. Similar to the situation with islets, transplanted stem cells also face the problem of rejection. Cell encapsulation has been actively pursued as

a means of abrogating rejection by protecting the encapsulated cells from the immune system while allowing adequate oxygenation, nutrient delivery, and glucose and insulin transport across the barrier. Although no successful and reproducible human islet encapsulation lasting more than a few weeks has been reported in patients with T1D (See review [53]), ViaCyte has reported that insulin-producing cells derived from hESC can function in vivo in their proprietary macro-encapsulation devices [46].

Clinical trials ViaCyte has obtained FDA approval and initiated a phase I/II clinical trial for the implantation of encapsulated endocrine progenitor cells derived from hESCs from their VC-01cell line. (see https://clinicaltrials.gov/show/NCT02239354).

Unresolved issues in hESC biology While the general differentiation protocol to generate pancreatic endoderm cells has been elucidated, a detailed molecular roadmap of the signal transduction, transcription factor, and epigenetic networks does not yet exist. It is critical to understand the interplay between growth factors and inhibitors during specific stages of differentiation. We have observed considerable heterogeneity between different hESC lines in their ability to generate insulin positive cells from pluripotent cells (King unpublished data). Preliminary data suggests that significant differences in expression of receptor tyrosine kinases and G-protein coupled receptors exist on the different cell lines that significantly alter signaling, proliferation, apoptosis, expression of transcription factors and epigenetic modifications. These biochemical differences in cell lines could have multiple repercussions in the interpretation of results with clinical trials. ViaCyte has demonstrated a reproducible in vitro hESC expansion and banking method for their VC-01 cell line that achieves 50–100 fold expansion per week [52]. Scalability was also demonstrated in the differentiation protocols described by Pagliuca and Russ [47, 49]. However, to date, these are the only three hESC systems for which this has been demonstrated. Whether this same expansion without loss of insulin expression can be demonstrated for other hESC lines or iPSCs remains to be determined as well as the number of hESCs derived β-cells to effectively ameliorate type 1 diabetes in humans.

iPSCs

Like hESCs, iPSCs have infinite self-renewal capacity and the ability to differentiate into any cell type, providing the hope of patient-specific cells for therapeutic use. iPSCs can be generated from virtually any adult somatic and peripheral blood cell through reprogramming by the addition of integrating retroviral vectors containing four pluripotency transcription factors, OCT4, SOX2, KLF4, and c-MYC [36]. iPSCs behave similarly to hESCs expressing multiple markers of pluripotency, have unlimited potential for self-renewal, and can be differentiated into cells from all three germ layers. Studies utilizing mouse reprogrammed iPSCs to generate β-cells used a considerably different protocol from hESCs. However the differentiated cells, upon transplantation, secreted insulin in response to glucose and normalized blood glucose levels [54]. To date, iPSCs generated from patients with T1Dhave used integrating retroviral vectors. Recently, Kudva reported using nonintegrating Sendai viral vector to reprogram cells from patients with T1D [55], raising the hope that problems of viral integration into the host genome could eliminate the risk for development of neoplasias.

Barriers to the clinical translation of iPSCs Redifferentiation of iPSCs from diabetic patients into pancreatic islets has the potential to allow for patient-specific cell replacement therapy. This field has been recently reviewed by Neofytou et al. [56], pointing out the challenges that a research setting would face by embarking on clinical trials. Briefly summarized, a GMP facility is required with capacity for characterization assays including cell line stability, karyotyping, and differentiation capacity, expression of pluripotency antigens, purity assays and cell type heterogeneity. These efforts represent a significant monetary allocation that few research institutions are capable of sustaining. Once the cells have undergone directed differentiation, following transplantation the possibilities of benign (teratoma) or malignant (carcinomas) are a safety concern to be dealt with after rigorous safety and toxicity studies are performed. As is the case with hESCs, iPSCs may also become immunogenic following differentiation protocols, a situation requiring careful studies aimed at creating immune tolerance before human trials are considered. It has been calculated that the generation of iPSC-derived tissue product for clinical use approaches one million dollars [57]. In their review, Neofytoy at al, also discuss the implications for the use of iPSC HLA-match allogeneic cell lines banking for commercialization vs. autologous cell lines that may required FDA regulatory standards even more difficult to fulfill.

Conclusions

This review has focused upon current state of cell replacement therapeutics in T1D. These cells are designed to function when transplanted into humans without eliciting an immune response. While considerable headway is being made in this respect, other factors that may influence the progression of type 1 diabetes cannot be ignored. For example, loss of β-cell function has been observed in NOD mice before the onset of hyperglycemia [58],

possibly as a response to the combination of autoimmunity and endoplasmic reticulum stress [59]. Whether these factors play a role in the human system remains to be elucidated. In conclusion, the prospects for a cell based therapy-using ESC or iPSC in T1D still requires extensive research for the application of clinical protocols that satisfies scientific scrutiny and the FDA.

Abbreviations
DE: definitive endoderm; EMT: epithelial-to-mesenchymal transition; EPs: endocrine precursors; hESCs: human embryonic stem cells; iPSCs: induced pluripotent stem cells; NGN3: neurogenin 3; PDX1: pancreatic and duodenal homeobox factor 1; T1D: type 1 diabetes mellitus.

Authors' contributions
AH and CK both contributed equaly to the design and writing of this manuscript. Both authors read and approved the final manuscript.

Acknowledgements
This work was supported by the Larry L. Hillblom Foundation (CCK).

Author details
[1]Scripps Whittier Diabetes Institute, La Jolla, CA 92037, USA. [2]Pediatric Diabetes Research Center, University of California, San Diego, La Jolla, CA 92093, USA.

References
1. Lacy PE, Kostianovsky M. Method for the isolation of intact islets of Langerhans from the rat pancreas. Diabetes. 1967;16:35–9.
2. Kemp CB, Knight MJ, Scharp DW, Lacy PE, Ballinger WF. Transplantation of isolated pancreatic islets into the portal vein of diabetic rats. Nature. 1973; 244:447.
3. Scharp DW, Murphy JJ, Newton WT, Ballinger WF, Lacy PE. Transplantation of islets of Langerhans in diabetic rhesus monkeys. Surgery. 1975;77:100–5.
4. Tzakis AG, Ricordi C, Alejandro R, Zeng Y, Fung JJ, et al. Pancreatic islet transplantation after upper abdominal exenteration and liver replacement. Lancet. 1990;336:402–5.
5. Shapiro AM, Lakey JR, Ryan EA, Korbutt GS, Toth E, et al. Islet transplantation in seven patients with type 1 diabetes mellitus using a glucocorticoid-free immunosuppressive regimen. N Engl J Med. 2000;343:230–8.
6. Barton FB, Rickels MR, Alejandro R, Hering BJ, Wease S, et al. Improvement in outcomes of clinical islet transplantation: 1999–2010. Diabetes Care. 2012; 35:1436–45.
7. Moassesfar S, Masharani U, Frassetto LA, Szot GL, Tavakol M, et al. A Comparative Analysis of the Safety, Efficacy, and Cost of Islet Versus Pancreas Transplantation in Nonuremic Patients With Type 1 Diabetes. Am J Transplant. 2016;16(2):518–26.
8. Bellin MD, Barton FB, Heitman A, Harmon JV, Kandaswamy R, et al. Potent induction immunotherapy promotes long-term insulin independence after islet transplantation in type 1 diabetes. Am J Transplant. 2012;12:1576–83.
9. Rickels MR, Liu C, Shlansky-Goldberg RD, Soleimanpour SA, Vivek K, et al. Improvement in beta-cell secretory capacity after human islet transplantation according to the CIT07 protocol. Diabetes. 2013;62:2890–7.
10. Otonkoski T, Beattie GM, Rubin JS, Lopez AD, Baird A, et al. Hepatocyte growth factor/scatter factor has insulinotropic activity in human fetal pancreatic cells. Diabetes. 1994;43:947–53.
11. Gershengorn MC, Hardikar AA, Wei C, Geras-Raaka E, Marcus-Samuels B, et al. Epithelial-to-mesenchymal transition generates proliferative human islet precursor cells. Science. 2004;306:2261–4.
12. Bar Y, Russ HA, Sintov E, Anker-Kitai L, Knoller S, et al. Redifferentiation of expanded human pancreatic beta-cell-derived cells by inhibition of the NOTCH pathway. J Biol Chem. 2012;287:17269–80.

13. Russ HA, Ravassard P, Kerr-Conte J, Pattou F, Efrat S. Epithelial-mesenchymal transition in cells expanded in vitro from lineage-traced adult human pancreatic beta cells. PLoS One. 2009;4:e6417.

14. Toren-Haritan G, Efrat S. TGFbeta pathway inhibition redifferentiates human pancreatic islet beta cells expanded in vitro. PLoS One. 2015;10:e0139168.

15. El Ouaamari A, Baroukh N, Martens GA, Lebrun P, Pipeleers D, et al. miR-375 targets 3'-phosphoinositide-dependent protein kinase-1 and regulates glucose-induced biological responses in pancreatic beta-cells. Diabetes. 2008;57:2708–17.

16. Joglekar MV, Joglekar VM, Hardikar AA. Expression of islet-specific microRNAs during human pancreatic development. Gene Expr Patterns. 2009;9:109–13.

17. Nathan G, Kredo-Russo S, Geiger T, Lenz A, Kaspi H, et al. MiR-375 promotes redifferentiation of adult human beta cells expanded in vitro. PLoS One. 2015;10:e0122108.

18. Beattie GM, Butler C, Hayek A. Morphology and function of cultured human fetal pancreatic cells transplanted into athymic mice: a longitudinal study. Cell Transplant. 1994;3:421–5.

19. Beattie GM, Lopez AD, Hayek A. In vivo maturation and growth potential of human fetal pancreases: fresh versus cultured tissue. Transplant Proc. 1995; 27:3343.

20. Beattie GM, Lopez AD, Otonkoski T, Hayek A. Transplantation of human fetal pancreas: fresh vs. cultured fetal islets or ICCS. J Mol Med. 1999;77:70–3.

21. Beattie GM, Otonkoski T, Lopez AD, Hayek A. Functional beta-cell mass after transplantation of human fetal pancreatic cells: differentiation or proliferation? Diabetes. 1997;46:244–8.

22. Campbell-Thompson M, Rodriguez-Calvo T, Battaglia M. Abnormalities of the exocrine pancreas in type 1 diabetes. Curr Diab Rep. 2015;15:79.

23. Bonner-Weir S, Taneja M, Weir GC, Tatarkiewicz K, Song KH, et al. In vitro cultivation of human islets from expanded ductal tissue. Proc Natl Acad Sci U S A. 2000;97:7999–8004.

24. Noguchi H, Xu G, Matsumoto S, Kaneto H, Kobayashi N, et al. Induction of pancreatic stem/progenitor cells into insulin-producing cells by adenoviral-mediated gene transfer technology. Cell Transplant. 2006;15:929–38.

25. Zhou Q, Brown J, Kanarek A, Rajagopal J, Melton DA. In vivo reprogramming of adult pancreatic exocrine cells to beta-cells. Nature. 2008;455:627–32.

26. Lemper M, Leuckx G, Heremans Y, German MS, Heimberg H, et al. Reprogramming of human pancreatic exocrine cells to beta-like cells. Cell Death Differ. 2015;22:1117–30.

27. Baeyens L, Lemper M, Leuckx G, De Groef S, Bonfanti P, et al. Transient cytokine treatment induces acinar cell reprogramming and regenerates functional beta cell mass in diabetic mice. Nat Biotechnol. 2014;32:76–83.

28. Klein D, Alvarez-Cubela S, Lanzoni G, Vargas N, Prabakar KR, et al. BMP-7 induces adult human pancreatic exocrine-to-endocrine conversion. Diabetes. 2015;64:4123–34.

29. Cardona K, Korbutt GS, Milas Z, Lyon J, Cano J, et al. Long-term survival of neonatal porcine islets in nonhuman primates by targeting costimulation pathways. Nat Med. 2006;12:304–6.

30. Hering BJ, Wijkstrom M, Graham ML, Hardstedt M, Aasheim TC, et al. Prolonged diabetes reversal after intraportal xenotransplantation of wild-type porcine islets in immunosuppressed nonhuman primates. Nat Med. 2006;12:301–3.

31. Shin JS, Kim JM, Kim JS, Min BH, Kim YH, et al. Long-term control of diabetes in immunosuppressed nonhuman primates (NHP) by the transplantation of adult porcine islets. Am J Transplant. 2015;15:2837–50.

32. Ellis CE, Korbutt GS. Justifying clinical trials for porcine islet xenotransplantation. Xenotransplantation. 2015;22:336–44.

33. Park CG, Bottino R, Hawthorne WJ. Current status of islet xenotransplantation. Int J Surg. 2015;23:261–6.

34. Kroon E, Martinson LA, Kadoya K, Bang AG, Kelly OG, et al. Pancreatic endoderm derived from human embryonic stem cells generates glucose-responsive insulin-secreting cells in vivo. Nat Biotechnol. 2008;26:443–52.

35. Assady S, Maor G, Amit M, Itskovitz-Eldor J, Skorecki KL, et al. Insulin production by human embryonic stem cells. Diabetes. 2001;50:1691–7.

36. Takahashi K, Tanabe K, Ohnuki M, Narita M, Ichisaka T, et al. Induction of pluripotent stem cells from adult human fibroblasts by defined factors. Cell. 2007;131:861–72.

37. Takahashi K, Okita K, Nakagawa M, Yamanaka S. Induction of pluripotent stem cells from fibroblast cultures. Nat Protoc. 2007;2:3081–9.

38. Humphrey RK, Beattie GM, Lopez AD, Bucay N, King CC, et al. Maintenance of pluripotency in human embryonic stem cells is STAT3 independent. Stem Cells. 2004;22:522–30.

39. Beattie GM, Lopez AD, Bucay N, Hinton A, Firpo MT, et al. Activin A maintains pluripotency of human embryonic stem cells in the absence of feeder layers. Stem Cells. 2005;23:489–95.

40. D'Amour KA, Agulnick AD, Eliazer S, Kelly OG, Kroon E, et al. Efficient differentiation of human embryonic stem cells to definitive endoderm. Nat Biotechnol. 2005;23:1534–41.

41. McLean AB, D'Amour KA, Jones KL, Krishnamoorthy M, Kulik MJ, et al. Activin a efficiently specifies definitive endoderm from human embryonic stem cells only when phosphatidylinositol 3-kinase signaling is suppressed. Stem Cells. 2007;25:29–38.

42. Van Hoof D, D'Amour KA, German MS. Derivation of insulin-producing cells from human embryonic stem cells. Stem Cell Res. 2009;3:73–87.

43. D'Amour KA, Bang AG, Eliazer S, Kelly OG, Agulnick AD, et al. Production of pancreatic hormone-expressing endocrine cells from human embryonic stem cells. Nat Biotechnol. 2006;24:1392–401.

44. Rezania A, Bruin JE, Riedel MJ, Mojibian M, Asadi A, et al. Maturation of human embryonic stem cell-derived pancreatic progenitors into functional islets capable of treating pre-existing diabetes in mice. Diabetes. 2012;61: 2016–29.

45. Hrvatin S, O'Donnell CW, Deng F, Millman JR, Pagliuca FW, et al. Differentiated human stem cells resemble fetal, not adult, beta cells. Proc Natl Acad Sci U S A. 2014;111:3038–43.

46. Agulnick AD, Ambruzs DM, Moorman MA, Bhoumik A, Cesario RM, et al. Insulin-producing endocrine cells differentiated in vitro from human embryonic stem cells function in macroencapsulation devices in vivo. Stem Cells Transl Med. 2015;4:1214–22.

47. Pagliuca FW, Millman JR, Gurtler M, Segel M, Van Dervort A, et al. Generation of functional human pancreatic beta cells in vitro. Cell. 2014;159:428–39.

48. Rezania A, Bruin JE, Arora P, Rubin A, Batushansky I, et al. Reversal of diabetes with insulin-producing cells derived in vitro from human pluripotent stem cells. Nat Biotechnol. 2014;32:1121–33.

49. Russ HA, Parent AV, Ringler JJ, Hennings TG, Nair GG, et al. Controlled induction of human pancreatic progenitors produces functional beta-like cells in vitro. EMBO J. 2015;34:1759–72.

50. Chen Y, Pan FC, Brandes N, Afelik S, Solter M, et al. Retinoic acid signaling is essential for pancreas development and promotes endocrine at the expense of exocrine cell differentiation in Xenopus. Dev Biol. 2004;271:144–60.

51. Gomes LF, Lorente S, Simon-Giavarotti KA, Areco KN, Araujo-Peres C, et al. Tri-iodothyronine differentially induces Kupffer cell ED1/ED2 subpopulations. Mol Aspects Med. 2004;25:183–90.

52. Schulz TC, Young HY, Agulnick AD, Babin MJ, Baetge EE, et al. A scalable system for production of functional pancreatic progenitors from human embryonic stem cells. PLoS One. 2012;7:e37004.

53. Tomei AA, Villa C, Ricordi C. Development of an encapsulated stem cell-based therapy for diabetes. Expert Opin Biol Ther. 2015;15:1321–36.

54. Jeon K, Lim H, Kim JH, Thuan NV, Park SH, et al. Differentiation and transplantation of functional pancreatic beta cells generated from induced pluripotent stem cells derived from a type 1 diabetes mouse model. Stem Cells Dev. 2012;21:2642–55.

55. Kudva YC, Ohmine S, Greder LV, Dutton JR, Armstrong A, et al. Transgene-free disease-specific induced pluripotent stem cells from patients with type 1 and type 2 diabetes. Stem Cells Transl Med. 2012;1:451–61.

56. Neofytou E, O'Brien CG, Couture LA, Wu JC. Hurdles to clinical translation of human induced pluripotent stem cells. J Clin Invest. 2015;125:2551–7.

57. Bravery CA. Do human leukocyte antigen-typed cellular therapeutics based on induced pluripotent stem cells make commercial sense? Stem Cells Dev. 2015;24:1–10.

58. Ize-Ludlow D, Lightfoot YL, Parker M, Xue S, Wasserfall C, et al. Progressive erosion of beta-cell function precedes the onset of hyperglycemia in the NOD mouse model of type 1 diabetes. Diabetes. 2011;60:2086–91.

59. Tersey SA, Nishiki Y, Templin AT, Cabrera SM, Stull ND, et al. Islet beta-cell endoplasmic reticulum stress precedes the onset of type 1 diabetes in the nonobese diabetic mouse model. Diabetes. 2012;61:818–27.

14

Determinants of nurse satisfaction using insulin pen devices with safety needles: an exploratory factor analysis

Giovanni Veronesi[1], Carmine S. Poerio[2], Alessandra Braus[3], Maurizio Destro[4], Lavinia Gilberti[3], Giovanni Meroni[5], Estella M. Davis[6] and Antonio C. Bossi[2*]

Abstract

Background: A paucity of data exists to examine nurses' satisfaction with the use of insulin pens with safety needles in hospitalized patients with diabetes. We investigated major determinants of nurses' preference of the method of insulin administration in the context of a General Hospital in Northern Italy.

Methods: Consecutive patients admitted to three hospital units of different care intensity requiring insulin received insulin therapy through either the vial/syringe method (October to December 2012) or pen/safety needles with dual-ended protection method (January to March 2013). Before the implementation of insulin pens, floor nurses received a specific training program for proper insulin pen injection technique including individual testing of the devices (pen/safety needles). At the end of the study, nurses completed the Nursing Satisfaction Survey Questionnaire. Cronbach's alpha was used to determine the internal consistency and reliability of the questionnaire. Major determinants of satisfaction were investigated through an exploratory factor analysis. The association between each retained factor and time spent to teach patients how to self-inject insulin with pen devices was also investigated.

Results: Fifty-three out of 60 nurses (mean age ± SD 36.2 ± 8.5 years, 85 % women, 57 % with 10+ years of working experience) returned the questionnaire. Internal consistency of the questionnaire was satisfactory (Cronbach's alpha > 0.9). Three months after their introduction, about 92 % of nurses considered pen devices an "improvement" over the vial/syringe method. Two factors explained 85 % of nurses' satisfaction, one related to convenience and ease of use, and the other to satisfaction/time spent for dose preparation and administration. The latter factor was inversely correlated with time spent on patients' training tasks.

Conclusions: Nurses' satisfaction with pen devices was higher than previously reported, possibly reinforced by safety needles with dual-ended protection. Perceived workload was a major determinant of nurse satisfaction using pen devices with safety needles. To facilitate the introduction of insulin pens in the hospital setting, it should be specifically addressed during training programs in the switch-over period.

Keywords: Nurse satisfaction, Insulin therapy, Insulin pens, Safety needles, Inpatient care

* Correspondence: antonio_bossi@ospedale.treviglio.bg.it
[2]Metabolic Diseases and Diabetes Unit, A.O. Ospedale Treviglio-Caravaggio, P.le Ospedale, 1 – 24047 Treviglio, BG, Italy
Full list of author information is available at the end of the article

Background

The prevalence of insulin pens worldwide has been recently estimated to be 60 % of insulin users; the figure being higher in Europe than in the US, and about 75 % in Italy [1]. Studies evaluating patient preference comparing self-administration of insulin using pen devices compared to traditional vial and syringe method found patients preferred insulin pens with respect to several items including ease of use, convenience, less injection pain, ease in handling, and ease of dosing [2]. Conversely, whether insulin pen devices should replace traditional vial and syringe in hospitalized patients is still a controversial subject [3]. Together with patients' satisfaction [4, 5], economic evaluation [4–6] and safety issues related to the potential risk of biological contaminations for both nurses and patients [5–7], nurses' satisfaction constitutes a key perspective for the management of hospitalized patients with diabetes requiring insulin injections. However, information on this topic is scarce, with the only data coming from the US, where 70 % of nurses considered insulin pens an "improvement" over conventional vial and syringe method 11 months after their introduction in two floors of one hospital [8]. The safety needles in this study differed from ours because they did not have a dual-ended protection. In addition, a limitation of this study was that nurses' satisfaction was measured using a survey questionnaire developed by the authors that was not formally validated [8]. There are a variety of validated tools for patient's satisfaction with self-administration of insulin [9–11], one of them specifically comparing pen devices with vial/syringe [11], but to the best of our knowledge, no validated questionnaire exists to assess nurses' satisfaction with insulin administration method to hospitalized patients. The existence of a validated tool is important to be able to compare findings from different populations using a standardized measure, to understand the determinants of nurses' satisfaction and utilize survey findings to adequately promote and enhance implementation of insulin pens in the hospital setting. In this paper, we report on nurse satisfaction, as assessed in Davis et al. [8], in the context of a pilot study aimed at implementing the use of insulin pens in hospitalized patients with diabetes at the Treviglio General Hospital in northern Italy. In addition, we performed an exploratory factor analysis, to investigate the latent structure behind nurses' satisfaction.

Methods

Study setting

The SANITHY (SAfety Needles and Insulin pens at Treviglio Hospital – ItalY) study is a pilot study designed to implement the use of insulin pens in the hospital setting at the Treviglio General Hospital, northern Italy. From October to the end of December 2012, consecutive patients requiring multi-injection insulin therapy and admitted to three hospital units of different intensity of care (Cardiology and Coronary Care Unit; Neurology and Stroke Unit; Medicine and Urgency Unit) received the traditional vial and syringe method. Insulin pens and safety needles were adopted in the same hospital units the next successive three months from January to the end of March 2013 in consecutive patients requiring insulin therapy. The following insulin and prefilled insulin pens were utilized: Humalog© and Humalog Kwikpen© (Eli Lilly and Company, Indianapolis, USA) as rapid acting insulin; Lantus© and Lantus SoloSTAR© (Sanofi, Paris, France) as long-acting basal insulin. Together with pen devices, pen needles with a dual-ended protection safety system Autoshield Duo© (Becton, Dickinson and Company, Franklin Lakes, NJ, USA) were utilized. The dual-ended protection covers both the portion of the needle in contact with the patient, and the back-end which penetrates into the rubber tip of the pen. Prior to the study, nurses received a specific training program on insulin pens consisting of small-group sessions and hands-on training, with individual testing to insure competence in using the insulin pen devices and safety needles properly. Thereafter, study nurses administered prescribed insulin therapy with pens and safety needles to inpatients, under an expert's supervision, to demonstrate the acquired technical skill. Moreover, slides and a short explicative movie were available on our hospital Local Area Network portal (e-learning) and a 24 h, 7 day a week, toll-free phone number was active during the study period to interact with expert consultants. The pilot study was approved by the Independent Ethical Committee of the Treviglio Hospital.

The nursing satisfaction survey questionnaire

The Nursing Satisfaction Survey Questionnaire (NSSQ) was proposed by Davis et al. to evaluate nurse satisfaction using pen devices as compared to vials/syringes in a sample of US nurses [8], in a study setting very similar to ours. The first section of the NSSQ collects information on the number of years practiced as a nurse, as well as on the previous experience with insulin administration and with study pen devices. Nurses' satisfaction with insulin pen devices as compared to vial/syringes is then investigated through 8 items, each on a 5-point Likert scale ranging from "strongly disagree" to "strongly agree", addressing different aspects such as insulin preparation and administration, convenience and ease of use, confidence and comfort in insulin administration, and time spent in dose preparation and administration. Items are reported in Table 2. Finally, the questionnaire attempts to quantify the time spent by the nurses to teach study patients how to self-inject insulin with each device, categorized as "<5 min", "<15 min", "<30 min", "<60 min", "60+ min". One question is dedicated to naïve insulin patients, and another one to experienced insulin patients. The Italian version of the questionnaire is available upon request to the corresponding author.

Study population and data collection

With the author's permission, the NSSQ was translated to Italian and first administered to $n = 44$ nurses (questionnaire test sample) working in units not involved in the pilot study, but of the same Medical Sciences Department. The internal consistency was found to be satisfactory (Cronbach's alpha = 0.91), thus, the questionnaire was administered to study nurses ($n = 60$, with characteristics comparable to the first group) at the end of the study period. The responses to the questionnaire were anonymous and completed independently.

Statistical analysis

Study sample characteristics were summarized using standard statistics including mean, standard deviation and proportions. Responses to each of the 8 items assessing satisfaction with pen devices compared to vial/syringes were attributed a score ranging from 1 ("strongly disagree") to 5 ("strongly agree"); the sum of the item responses could range between 8 and 40. We reported the mean score and standard deviation for each item, as well as the prevalence of a positive response defined as "agree" or "strongly agree", as suggested by the authors [8]; and tested the null hypothesis of prevalence of positive answer equal to 50 % (i.e., no preference) using a two-sided exact binomial proportion test. To identify the latent structure of nurses' satisfaction, we performed an exploratory factor analysis, given that the original NSSQ was not validated. The Kaiser-Meyer-Olkin measure of sampling adequacy value of 0.85 and the Bartlett test of sphericity (p-value: <.0001) supported the use of factor analysis. We fixed in 80 % the minimum proportion of cumulative variance to be explained by the factors as a general rule to decide the factors number; a scree plot was also used. Since the analysis made on the questionnaire test sample revealed a strong correlation between the 8 items, we considered an oblique factor rotation (promax), to allow for a non-zero correlation between the factors [12]. Internal validation for each retained factor was assessed through Cronbach's alpha [13]. Finally, we assessed the relationship between each retained factor and time spent to teach patients how to self-inject insulin with pen devices. We reported the median (25°–75° percentile) of each factor score (as the sum of the responses to the items included in the factor) by categories of time, and formally tested

the null hypothesis of no difference in factors score by time through a Kruskal-Wallis non parametric test [14]. All the statistical analyses were performed using the SAS software, version 9.3.2.

Results

Out of the 60 study nurses, 53 returned the questionnaire, corresponding to a participation rate of 88 %. The study population of nurse respondents was on average 36 years old, 85 % women, 66 % had a nursing degree, and 57 % worked for 10 years or more as nurses (Table 1). Self-reported experience with insulin administration was extensive (50 patients or more) for 71 %, and 94 % had experience using insulin pens (mainly in outpatients settings) prior to the study. The BD AutoShield Duo©, new to the Italian market, had never been used by any of the nurses in the study. Most questionnaires were completed fully. Only 2 had questions that were left blank and were excluded from the analysis. Table 2 reports the mean score and the standard deviation, as well as the prevalence of response, to each question assessing nurses' satisfaction with insulin pens over vial/syringes. On average, the total score for the sum of the 8 items was 34.6 ± 6.3, with a median of 38. Considering single items, the lower mean score was 4.0 for the item on dose accuracy ("Felt more confident I was giving the correct dose using pens"). This item was also the one with the lowest prevalence of positive answers (76.5 %, summing up 39.2 % of "agree" and 37.3 % of "strongly agree"). For the remaining items, the

Table 1 Characteristics of the study population at the end of the study

N of responders	53
Mean age (SD)	36.2 (8.5)
Women (%)	85.4
Nursing degree (%)	65.9
Time practicing as a nurse (%)	
Less than 1 year	0.0
1 to 3 years	18.9
3 to 5 years	9.4
5 to 10 years	15.1
10+ years	56.6
Experience with insulin administration (%)	
None	0.0
Limited (up to 5 pts)	3.9
Average (up to 20 pts)	15.7
Substantial (up to 50 pts)	9.8
Extensive (50+ pts)	70.6
Experience using insulin pens (%)	94.3

SD standard deviation

Table 2 Mean score (standard deviation) and prevalence of response for each item assessing nurses' satisfaction of insulin pens compared with traditional vial/syringe method. Responders with complete questionnaire ($n = 51$)

#	Item description	Mean[a] (SD)	% of nurses answering[b]				
			Strongly disagree	Disagree	Unsure	Agree	Strongly agree
1	More satisfied with preparing insulin using pens	4.4 (1.1)	5.9	2.0	3.9	25.5	62.8
2	More satisfied with administering insulin using pens	4.5 (0.9)	2.0	3.9	3.9	27.5	62.8
3	Pens are more convenient	4.5 (0.8)	0.0	3.9	3.9	31.4	60.8
4	Pens are more simple & easy to use	4.3 (0.8)	0.0	3.9	7.8	41.2	47.1
5	Felt more confident I was giving the correct dose using pens	4.0 (1.1)	3.9	9.8	9.8	39.2	37.3
6	Felt more comfortable administering insulin to patients using pens	4.4 (0.8)	2.0	2.0	3.9	39.2	52.9
7	Took less time to prepare and give insulin using pens	4.1 (1.0)	2.0	9.8	3.9	43.1	41.2
8	Pens are an improvement over conventional	4.5 (0.7)	0.0	2.0	5.9	31.4	60.8
	Total score	34.6 (6.3)	-	-	-	-	-

[a]:Scoring: 1 = strongly disagree; 5 = strongly agree
[b]:response as in Davis et al. [8]

prevalence of positive answers was above 80 %, ranging from 84.3 % (item 7, time spent for insulin preparation and administration) to 92 % (items 3, convenience, 6, feeling comfortable, and 8, improvement). The p-values of the exact binomial test for positive answers different from 50 % were <0.0001 for all the items. The exploratory factor analysis suggested the existence of two factors to explain 85.3 % of total variance; the standardized regression coefficients identifying each factor are reported in Table 3. The first factor (items 6, 3, 8 and 4) was related to general aspects such as feeling comfortable with using pen devices, convenience, ease of use, and improvement over traditional method; this factor explained 77 % of variance. The second factor (items 5, 1, 2, 7) specifically focused on satisfaction in dose preparation and administration, including dose accuracy, and total time required for insulin injection; this factor explained 8.3 % of variance. The inter-factor correlation was positive and equal to 0.65; the

Cronbach's alpha assessing internal consistency for these two factors was above 0.90.

During the study period, 38 and 47 nurses instructed patients how to use an insulin pen device to naïve or to experienced insulin users with diabetes, respectively. In Table 4 we report the median score (25°–75° percentile) for the two retained factors by time spent teaching patients, stratified by patient's experience. When the number of patients was low (below 5), the original time categories were further collapsed to increase the size. In naïve insulin users, the factor score did not differ according to the different amount of time spent (Kruskal-Wallis p-values >0.05). Considering experienced insulin patients, the median scores for both factors decreased for increasing time spent. In particular, the median of the second factor decreased by 5.5 points from 19.5 to 14, as time spent ranged from below 5 min to above 16 min (Kruskal-Wallis p-value 0.04).

Table 3 Standardized Regression Coefficients, proportion of variance explained and internal consistency, for the first two factors explaining 80 % or more of variance of nurses' satisfaction. Exploratory factor analysis with oblique rotation; responders with complete questionnaire ($n = 51$)

#	Item description	Factor 1	Factor 2
6	Felt more comfortable administering insulin to patients using pens	1.019	−0.123
3	Pens are more convenient	0.877	0.121
8	Pens are an improvement over conventional	0.803	0.185
4	Pens are more simple & easy to use	0.701	0.241
5	Felt more confident I was giving the correct dose using pens	−0.139	1.015
1	More satisfied with preparing insulin using pens	0.317	0.659
2	More satisfied with administering insulin using pens	0.415	0.597
7	Took less time to prepare and give insulin using pens	0.430	0.579
	Proportion of variance explained by each factor	77.0	8.3
	Factor's internal consistency (Cronbach's alpha)	0.94	0.92

Table 4 Median score (25°–75° percentile) for the two factors retained from factor analysis according to different levels of time spent teaching a patient how to self-inject insulin with insulin pens, according to patient's experience with insulin injection

	Naïve insulin user patients			Experienced insulin user patients		
	n	Factor 1[a]	Factor 2[b]	n	Factor 1[a]	Factor 2[b]
Time spent to teach how to use insulin pens						
<5 min	4	20 (16.5; 20)	18.5 (16; 20)	20	20 (17; 20)	19.5 (17; 20)
<15 min	24			20	19 (16; 20)	18 (16; 19)
<30 min	9	19 (16; 20)	19 (16; 19)	2	17 (14; 19)	14 (8; 19)
31+ min	1			5		
Kruskal-Wallis test p-value	-	0.6	0.3	-	0.09	0.04

When the number of patients was low (below 5), the original time categories were further collapsed to increase the size
[a]:sum of responses to the following items: feeling comfortable, convenience, improvement, ease of use (item 6, 3, 8, 4). 1 = strongly disagree; 5 = strongly agree
[b]:sum of responses to the following items: satisfaction in dose preparation and administration (item 5, 1, 2, 7). 1 = strongly disagree; 5 = strongly agree

Discussion

In this study population of 53 hospital nurses completing a pilot study on insulin administration using prefilled pens and BD Autoshield Duo©, about 92 % of nurses considered these devices an improvement over traditional vial/syringe method. Two factors explain 85 % of nurses' satisfaction, one related to feeling comfortable, convenience, ease of use and improvement; while the other focused on satisfaction in dose preparation and administration, including time spent, and confidence in dose accuracy. The latter factor only was inversely associated with time spent teaching patients how to self-inject insulin using a pen device. A growing body of evidence shows several benefits of insulin pens for inpatient care, both from the hospital's and the patient's perspectives. Insulin pens have being suggested to be cost-effective and to improve patients' quality of life during the hospital stay as well [4, 5, 15]. However, information on nurses' satisfaction using insulin pens in hospitalized patients is sparse, with the only data coming from the US [8]. The nurse level of satisfaction with insulin pens, measured with the same questionnaire, from our study was generally higher than in Davis and colleagues [8], who reported a positive answer for the item "improvement" in 70 % of nurses (92 % in our population). Two reasons may explain these differences. First, we assessed satisfaction at 3 months while Davis et al. after 11 months of insulin pen use, suggesting that satisfaction may wane over time if not adequately supported and promoted. Second, although both studies utilized insulin pen safety needles to reduce the risk of needlestick injuries [16], the BD Autoshield Duo©, used in our study only, had a dual ended protection. Thus, it is possible that the consciousness of a complete protection from needle-stick injuries played a major role in reinforcing nurses' satisfaction. Training alone, in fact, can reduce, but not eliminate, the risk of injuries related to pen use [6]. The population of nurses caring for patients with diabetes is subject to a relatively high risk of needle-stick injuries, with a significant amount of post-injury emotional distress [17]. Study nurses experienced 2 needle-stick injuries during the 3 month-period with standard syringe/vial for insulin administration, and no injury in the experimental period with pen devices and double-safety needles (data not shown). Strengths of this study include that study participants represented nurses from three hospital units with different care intensities in a general hospital (Cardiology and Coronary Care Unit; Neurology and Stroke Unit; Medicine and Urgency Unit), a high survey response rate (88 %), and the very satisfactory internal consistency in the questionnaire's compilation (Cronbach's alpha >0.90). A study limitation was the short time period of insulin pen and safety needle use (3 months) from which to evaluate nurses' satisfaction with the new insulin administration method. Other factors may contribute to lower nurse satisfaction with insulin pen devices over a longer time period. For instance, to minimize the risk of contamination related to sharing the pen device among multiple users [7], study nurses performed a "sure self-identification" by asking name, surname, and date of birth to every patient. A more sophisticated electronic "code-number" system of identification could be more suitable over the long-term period [18]. We also recommend caution when generalizing our findings to nurses working in non-medical hospital units such as surgery or emergency departments. Finally, although our sample size meets some minimum requisite for exploratory factor analysis (cases/item ratio > 5), it is desirable that our findings should be replicated by larger confirmatory studies. To the best of our knowledge, our exploratory factor analysis is the first attempt to identify major determinants of nurses' satisfaction using insulin pen devices with safety needles. The first factor to a great extent matches patients' preference for pen devices over the traditional vial/syringes in terms of ease and convenience of use [2]. The second factor instead could be interpreted as nurses' perception of work load, as it referred to several aspects of dose preparation and administration, including perceived time spent, and confidence in dose accuracy. This factor was also inversely related to time spent teaching patients how to self-inject insulin using pen devices. Nurses' training programs for the implementation of pen devices in the hospital setting are mainly focused on reducing risk to the patient and personnel [6, 18, 19]. Our findings imply that nurses' satisfaction can be strengthened during the training program by targeting all aspects related to nurses' perceived workload. The proposed educational program for instance included several supervised interactive sessions, with individual competency testing of insulin pens with dual-ended safety needles with additional instructional material available on-line (e-learning). Moreover, familiarization with insulin pens in the hospital could reduce future costs in the outpatient setting [3]. Appropriate discharge education should be provided to patients who transition to insulin pen devices from the vial/syringe method.

Conclusions

In conclusion, this study confirmed nurses' preference for pen/safety needles over the traditional vial/syringes method for insulin administration in the setting of a General Hospital in Northern Italy. The recent introduction of a safety needle with a dual-ended protection may have strengthened satisfaction compared to previously published data. Nurses' workload perception was a determinant of satisfaction, and should be targeted during an interchange training program for successful implementation of insulin pens in the hospital setting.

Competing interests
GV obtained sponsorship from Eli Lilly. ACB received research grants from Eli Lilly, Novo Nordisk, and consultant/advisor honoraria from Johnson & Johnson, Boehringer Ingelheim.

Authors' contributions
GV, CSP, and ACB planned the study design, wrote and edited the manuscript; CSP and ACB in addition were responsible for data collection while GV is the responsible for the statistical analyses. CSP, AB, EGG, and MD were investigators and participated in the interpretation of data, and critically reviewed the manuscript. GM, LG, and EMD critically reviewed and participated in the manuscript editing. All authors read and approved the final manuscript.

Acknowledgments
The Authors would like to thank the nurses involved in the study, as well as Colleagues and healthcare professionals of the Department of Medical Science, Treviglio Hospital; Dr. Anna Cremaschi (Risk Manager), Arch. Genny Baiettini (Security Manager), Dr. Roberto Sacchi (Occupational Health Physician), Dr. Emilio G. Galli (Head, Nephrology and Dialysis Unit), Dr. Bruno Ferraro (Head, Neurology and Stroke Unit), and Dr. Paolo Sganzerla (Head, Cardiology and Coronary Care Unit), Treviglio Hospital.

Funding
The SANITHY study was funded by the Treviglio Hospital Management.

Author details
[1]Department of Clinical and Experimental Medicine, Research Centre in Epidemiology and Preventive Medicine, University of Insubria, Varese, Italy. [2]Metabolic Diseases and Diabetes Unit, A.O. Ospedale Treviglio-Caravaggio, P.le Ospedale, 1 – 24047 Treviglio, BG, Italy. [3]Pharmacy Unit, A.O. Ospedale Treviglio-Caravaggio, Treviglio, BG, Italy. [4]Medical Science Department, A.O. Ospedale Treviglio-Caravaggio, Treviglio, BG, Italy. [5]Hospital Health Management Direction, A.O. Ospedale Treviglio-Caravaggio, Treviglio, BG, Italy. [6]Creighton University School of Pharmacy and Health Professions, Omaha, NE, USA.

References
1. IMS Health: IMS Midas™. Insulin sales volume. 2009.
2. Molife C, Lee LJ, Shi L, Sawhney M, Lenox SM. Assessment of patient-reported outcomes of insulin pen devices versus conventional vial and syringe. Diabetes Technol Ther. 2009;11(8):529–38.
3. Perfetti R. Reusable and disposable insulin pens for the treatment of diabetes: understanding the global differences in user preference and an evaluation of inpatient insulin pen use. Diabetes Technol Ther. 2010;12 Suppl 1:S79–85.
4. Cornell S. Managing diabetes-related costs and quality of life issues: Value of insulin analogs and pens for inpatient use. Health Policy. 2010;96(3):191–9.
5. Davis EM, Christensen CM, Nystrom KK, Foral PA, Destache C. Patient satisfaction and costs associated with insulin administered by pen device or syringe during hospitalization. Am J Health Syst Pharm. 2008;65(14):1347–57.
6. Ward LG, Aton SS. Impact of an interchange program to support use of insulin pens. Am J Health Syst Pharm. 2011;68(14):1349–52.
7. Herdman ML, Larck C, Schliesser SH, Jelic TM. Biological contamination of insulin pens in a hospital setting. Am J Health Syst Pharm. 2013;70(14):1244–8.
8. Davis EM, Bebee A, Crawford LA, Destache C. Nurse satisfaction using insulin pens in hospitalized patients. Diabetes Educ. 2009;35(5):799–809.
9. Bradley C. The diabetes treatment satisfaction questionnaire: guide to psychological measurement in diabetes research and practice. Chur, Switzerland: Harwood Academic Publishers; 1994. p. 111–32.
10. Cappelleri JC, Gerber RA, Kourides IA, Gelfand RA. Development and factor analysis of a questionnaire to measure patient satisfaction with injected and inhaled insulin for type I diabetes. Diabetes Care. 2000;23:1799–803.
11. Szeinbach SL, Barnes JH, Summers KH, Lenox SM. Development of an instrument to assess expectations of and preference for an insulin injection pen compared with the vial and syringe. Clin Ther. 2004;26:590–7.
12. Tabachnisk BG, Fidell LS, editors. Using multivariate statistics. 4th ed. Needham Heights, MA: Allyn & Bacon, 2001.
13. Cronbach LJ. Coefficient alpha and the internal structure of tests. Psychometrika. 1951;16:297–334.
14. Siegel S, Castellan NJ. Non parametric statistics for the behavioral sciences. 2nd ed. New York: McGraw-Hill; 1992.
15. Davis EM, Foral PA, Dull RB, Smith AN. Review of insulin therapy and pen use in hospitalized patients. Hosp Pharm. 2013;48:396–405.
16. Pellissier G, Migueres B, Tarantola A, Abiteboul D, Lolom I, Bouvet E, et al. Risk of needlestick inkuries by injection pens. J Hosp Infect. 2006;63(1):60–4.
17. Lee JM, Botteman MF, Nicklasson L, Cobden D, Pashos CL. Needlestick injury in acute care nurses caring for patients with diabetes mellitus: a retrospective study. Curr Med Res Opin. 2005;21:741–7.
18. Schaefer MK, Kossover RA, Perz JF. Sharing insulin pens: are you putting patients at risk? Diabetes Care. 2013;36(11):e188–9.
19. Institute for Safe Medication Practices. Considering insulin pens for routine hospital use? Consider this. www.ismp.org/Newsletters/acutecare/articles/20080508.asp (accessed 2015 Aug 27).

15

Thyroid nodule update on diagnosis and management

Shrikant Tamhane[1,2]* (iD) and Hossein Gharib[1,2]

Abstract

Thyroid nodules are common. The clinical importance of thyroid nodules is related to excluding malignancy (4.0 to 6.5% of all thyroid nodules), evaluate their functional status and assess for the presence of pressure symptoms. Incidental thyroid nodules are being diagnosed with increasing frequency in the recent years with the use of newer and highly sensitive imaging techniques. The high prevalence of thyroid nodules necessitates that the clinicians use evidence-based approaches for their assessment and management. New molecular tests have been developed to help with evaluation of malignancy in thyroid nodules. This review addresses advances in thyroid nodule evaluation, and their management considering the current guidelines and supporting evidence.

Keywords: Thyroid, Thyroid nodules, Molecular markers, Benign, Malignant, FNA, Management, Ultrasonography

Background

Thyroid nodule is a discrete lesion in the thyroid gland that is radiologically distinct from the surrounding thyroid parenchyma [1]. Thyroid nodules are common; their prevalence in the general population is high, the percentages vary depending on the mode of discovery: 2–6 % (palpation), 19–35 % (ultrasound) and 8–65 % (autopsy data) [2–4]. They are discovered either clinically on self-palpation by a patient, or during a physical examination by the clinician or incidentally during a radiologic procedure such as ultrasonography (US) imaging, computed tomography (CT) or magnetic resonance imaging (MRI) of the neck, or fluorodeoxyglucose (FDG) positron emission tomography; with the increased use of sensitive imaging techniques, thyroid nodules are being diagnosed incidentally with increasing frequency in the recent years [5, 6]. Though thyroid nodules are common, their clinical significance is mainly related to excluding malignancy (4.0 to 6.5% of all thyroid nodules) [3, 7–9], evaluating their functional status and if they cause pressure symptoms.

Diagnosis and evaluation of thyroid nodules

Thyroid nodules can be caused by many disorders: benign (colloid nodule, Hashimoto's thyroiditis, simple or hemorrhagic cyst, follicular adenoma and subacute thyroiditis) and malignant (Papillary Cancer, Follicular Cancer, Hurthle Cell (oncocytic) Cancer, Anaplastic Cancer, Medullary Cancer, Thyroid Lymphoma and metastases –3 most common primaries are renal, lung & head-neck) [3, 10, 11].

Initial assessment of a patient found to have a thyroid nodule either clinically or incidentally should include a detailed and relevant history plus physical examination. Laboratory tests should begin with measurement of serum thyroid-stimulating hormone (TSH). Thyroid scintigraphy/radionuclide thyroid scan should be performed in patients presenting with a low serum TSH [1]. Thyroid ultrasound should be performed in all those suspected or known to have a nodule to confirm the presence of a nodule, evaluate for additional nodules and cervical lymph nodes and assess for suspicious sonographic features. The next step in the evaluation of a thyroid nodule, if they meet the criteria as discussed later, is a fine needle aspiration (FNA) biopsy [12].

*Algorithm of thyroid nodule work up is presented at the end of the review (Fig. 1).

---

* Correspondence: Tamhane.Shrikant@Mayo.edu
[1]Mayo Clinic College of Medicine, Rochester, MN 55905, USA
[2]Division of Endocrinology, Diabetes, Metabolism, and Nutrition, Mayo Clinic, 200 First Street SW, Rochester, MN 55905, USA

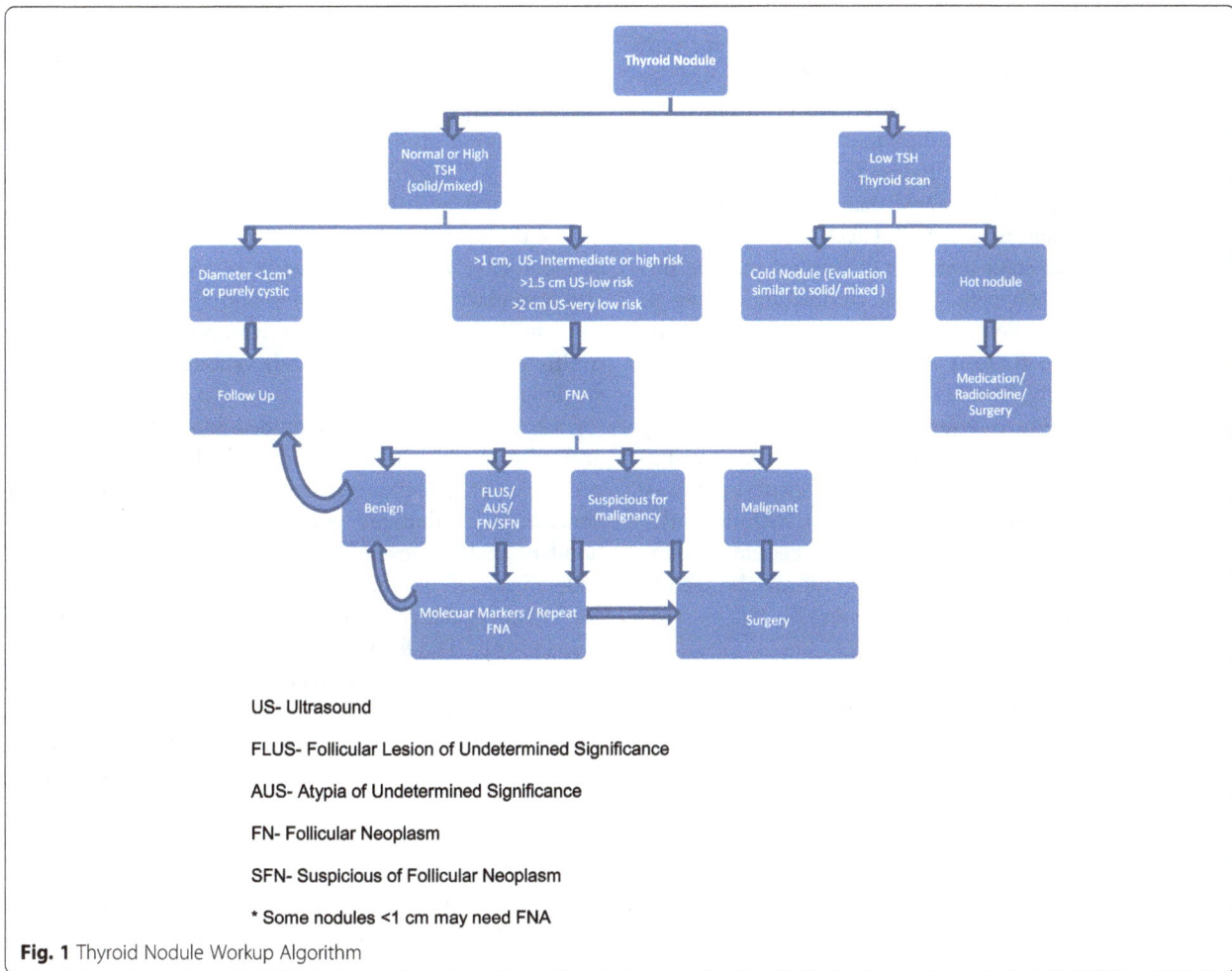

Fig. 1 Thyroid Nodule Workup Algorithm

US- Ultrasound

FLUS- Follicular Lesion of Undetermined Significance

AUS- Atypia of Undetermined Significance

FN- Follicular Neoplasm

SFN- Suspicious of Follicular Neoplasm

* Some nodules <1 cm may need FNA

History and physical examination

Comprehensive history with focus on risk factors predicting malignancy (Table 1 [1, 3, 13]) should be part of the initial evaluation of a patient with thyroid nodule. Symptoms of hypothyroidism or hyperthyroidism should be assessed. Patients should be questioned about local pressure symptoms such as difficulty in swallowing or breathing, cough and change in voice.

Physical examination focusing on the thyroid gland assessing the volume and consistency and the nodular features such as size, number, location and consistency should be performed. Thyroid nodules that are smaller, usually < 1 cm and those located posteriorly or substernally will be difficult to palpate [14, 15]. Cervical lymph nodes should be assessed. Examination of signs of hypo or hyperthyroidism should be done.

Table 1 Increased risk of malignancy in thyroid nodule on history and physical exam [1, 3, 13]

- History of childhood head/neck irradiation [113]
- Total body irradiation for bone marrow transplantation [114]
- Exposure to ionizing radiation from fallout in childhood or adolescence [115, 116]
- Family history of PTC, MTC, or thyroid cancer syndrome (e.g., Cowden's syndrome, familial polyposis, Carney complex, multiple endocrine neoplasia [MEN] 2, Werner syndrome) [117]
- Enlarging nodule/rapid nodule growth
- Cervical lymphadenopathy
- Fixed nodule to surrounding tissue
- Vocal cord paralysis/hoarseness

Laboratory tests

Serum TSH

Serum TSH should be measured in all patients with thyroid nodules. In patients with low TSH levels, radionuclide thyroid scan should be performed next to assess the functional status of the nodule. In a patient with a thyroid nodule, an increased serum TSH or TSH even in the upper limit of normal is associated with increased risk and an advanced stage of malignancy [16, 17].

Serum calcitonin

In patients with thyroid nodules, the routine assessment of serum calcitonin is controversial and there are no definite recommendations for or against it [1, 18, 19]. Many prospective, non-randomized studies, mostly from outside US have assessed the value of measuring serum calcitonin [20–22]. The studies which show that use of serum calcitonin for screening may detect C-cell hyperplasia and MTC at an earlier stage and overall survival may be improved, are based on pentagastrin stimulation testing to increase specificity. Pentagastrin is not available in the United States, and there is still an ambiguity about the sensitivity/specificity, threshold cut off values and cost-effectiveness [22–24]. False-positive calcitonin results may be obtained in patients with hypercalcemia, hypergastrinemia, neuroendocrine tumors, renal insufficiency, papillary and follicular thyroid carcinomas, goiter, chronic autoimmune thyroiditis and prolonged use of certain medications [12, 25, 26]. False negative test result may be seen in rare MTCs that do not secrete calcitonin [27, 28].

Serum thyroglobulin (Tg)

In patients with thyroid nodules, routine measurement of serum thyroglobulin is not recommended as it can be elevated in many thyroid diseases and is neither specific nor sensitive for thyroid cancer [29, 30].

Serum TPO antibodies

Routine measurement of serum anti-thyroid peroxidase (TPO) antibodies is not necessary for thyroid nodule evaluation [31].

Imaging studies

Radionuclide thyroid scan/scintigraphy

In patients with thyroid nodule and a low serum TSH, suggesting overt or subclinical hyperthyroidism, the next step is to determine if the nodule is autonomously functioning. Thyroid scintigraphy is useful to determine the functional status of a nodule.

Scintigraphy, a diagnostic test used in nuclear medicine, utilizing iodine radioisotopes (more commonly used; usually ^{123}I) or technetium pertechnetate (^{99}Tc), measures timed radioisotope uptake by the thyroid gland. The uptake of the radioisotopes will be greater in hyperfunctioning nodule and will be lower in most benign and virtually all malignant thyroid nodules than adjacent normal thyroid tissue [32–34].

Nodules may appear 'hot', 'warm' or 'cold' depending on whether the tracer uptake is greater than, equal to or less than the surrounding normal thyroid tissue respectively [11]. Autonomous nodules may appear hot or indeterminate and account for 5 to 10 % of palpable nodules. FNA evaluation of a hyperfunctioning nodule is not necessary as most hyperfunctioning nodules are benign [1].

Thyroid sonography/ultrasound

Thyroid Ultrasound (US) is a noninvasive imaging technique that should be performed on all patients with nodules suspected clinically or incidentally noted on other imaging studies such as carotid ultrasound, CT, MRI, or 18-FDG-PET scan.

Ultrasound will help confirm the thyroid nodule/s, assess the size, location and evaluate the composition, echogenicity, margins, presence of calcification, shape and vascularity of the nodules and the adjacent structures in the neck including the lymph nodes. If there are multiple nodules, all the nodules should be assessed for suspicious US characteristics.

FNA decision making is guided by both nodule size and ultrasound characteristics, the latter being more predictive of malignancy than size [35, 36]. The nodular characteristics that are associated with a higher likelihood of malignancy include a shape that is taller than wide measured in the transverse dimension, hypoechogenicity, irregular margins, microcalcifications, and absent halo [35–41]. The feature with the highest diagnostic odds ratio for malignancy was suggested to be the nodule being taller than wider [42]. The more suspicious characteristics that the nodule has, it increases the likelihood of malignancy. In contrast, benign nodule predicting US characteristics include purely cystic nodule (< 2 % risk of malignancy) [39], spongiform appearance (99.7 % specific for benign thyroid nodule) [40, 42–44].

The recent ATA guidelines classify nodules into 5 risk groups based on US results [1]. However, the current AACE guidelines suggest a more practical, 3-tier risk classification: low risk, intermediate risk and high risk thyroid lesions, based on their US characteristics [13].

In patients with thyroid nodules and low TSH who have undergone thyroid scintigraphy, ultrasound is useful to check for concordance of the nodule and hyperfunctioning area on the scan, which do not need FNA and to evaluate other nonfunctional or intermediate nodules, which may require FNA based on sonographic criteria [1].

Fine needle aspiration biopsy (FNA)

FNA is considered the gold standard test for evaluating thyroid nodules. It is an office procedure, done under no or local anesthesia with 23 to 27 gauge needle, to obtain tissue samples for cytological examination. It is a safe, accurate and cost-effective way for evaluating thyroid nodules [45–54].

FNA can be done using palpation or with ultrasound guidance. US machines (7.5 to 10 MHz transducers), provide clear and continuous visualization of thyroid gland and allow for real time visualization of the needle tip to ensure accurate sampling. Ultrasound guided technique has lower nondiagnostic and false negative cytology rates compared to palpation technique [48, 55]. US guided FNA is preferred for difficult to palpate nodules, predominantly cystic or posteriorly located nodules [1]. In practice more clinicians are using ultrasound guided FNA (either free hand technique or with the help of a needle guide) over palpation guided technique for all thyroid FNA.

Indications for FNA

Over the years there has been a change in guidelines with regards to judiciously selecting the thyroid nodules for further evaluation with FNA. The approach has been toward a conservative direction. The changes are reflected in the recently published ATA guidelines [1] (Table 2).

FNA should not be performed on thyroid nodules < 1 cm in diameter with some exceptions discussed later in this section. For nodules > 1 cm, FNA is recommended to further evaluate the thyroid nodule with some exceptions [1].

FNA biopsy is recommended for nodules > 1 cm with high suspicion features (solid hypoechoic nodule or solid hypoechoic component of a partially cystic nodule with either one or more of features: irregular margin or microcalcification or taller than wide shape or rim calcification or evidence of extra thyroidal extension; estimated malignancy risk of 70–90 %) or > 1 cm with intermediate suspicion features (hypoechoic solid nodule with smooth margins without microcalcification, extra thyroidal extension or taller than wide shape; estimated malignancy risk 10–20 %). Low suspicion features include isoechoic or hyperechoic solid nodule or partially cystic nodules with eccentric solid areas without the features of highly suspicious nodule (estimated malignancy risk of 5–10 %). Cyst drainage may also be performed, especially in symptomatic patients. Very low suspicion features include spongiform (aggregation of multiple microcystic components in more than 50 % of the nodule volume [40, 52]) or partially cystic nodules without the features of the above mentioned suspicious category features (estimated malignancy risk of < 3 %).

Cervical lymph node assessment (anterior, central and lateral compartment) should be performed in all patients

with thyroid nodule. Suspicious lymph nodes (microcalcification, cystic, peripheral vascularity, hyperechogenicity, round shape [56]) should have FNA evaluation for cytology and washout Tg measurement. This is one of the scenarios where a subcentimeter thyroid nodule associated with these abnormal cervical lymph nodes should undergo FNA. Also in patients with the clinical risk factors mentioned in Table 1 and with the high pretest likelihood for thyroid cancer associated with these features, FNA at sizes lower than those recommended can be considered [1, 13]. PET positive nodules have a higher incidence of malignancy ~40–45 % and FNA is recommended in nodules > 1 cm [1, 57, 58].

The US features of each nodule should be assessed independently to determine the need for FNA biopsy. The nodules that are not biopsied should be monitored with periodic US with follow up duration and frequency based on factors including sonographic features and risk factors. Also conservative approach of active surveillance without FNA may be reasonable approach for patients who meet the above FNA criteria but are at high surgical risk and those with relatively short life expectancy [1].

Cytological diagnosis

FNA cytology of the thyroid nodule is reported using various classification systems. In US, the Bethesda System for Reporting Thyroid Cytopathology is the most commonly used. The diagnostic groups suggested are [59, 60]:

Benign – This includes macrofollicular or adenomatoid/hyperplastic nodules, colloid adenomas (most common), nodular goiter, lymphocytic and granulomatous thyroiditis. 0–3 % predicted risk of malignancy.

Follicular lesion or atypia of undetermined significance (FLUS or AUS) – This includes lesions with atypical cells, or mixed macro- and microfollicular nodules. 5–15 % predicted risk of malignancy.

Follicular neoplasm or suspicious for a follicular neoplasm (FN/SFN) – This includes microfollicular nodules, including Hurthle cell lesions/ suspicious for Hurthle cell neoplasm. 15–30 % predicted risk of malignancy.

Suspicious for malignancy. 60–75 % predicted risk of malignancy.

Malignant. This includes PTC (most common), MTC, anaplastic carcinoma, and high-grade metastatic cancers. 97–99 % predicted risk for malignancy.

Nondiagnostic or Unsatisfactory. 1–4 % predicted risk of malignancy.

Other classification systems such as UK-RCPath (Royal College of Pathology) or Italian AME Consensus and modifications of these systems are also used to report

Table 2 Recommendations for diagnostic FNA based on size and US features [1, 35–37, 85, 86, 118–120]

A. Nodules ≥ 1 cm with intermediate or high suspicion US pattern

B. Nodules ≥ 1.5 cm with low suspicion US pattern

C. Nodules ≥ 2 cm with very low suspicion US pattern (e.g., spongiform). Observation an alternate option.

D. For nodules that do not meet the above criteria, FNA is not required, including nodules < 1 cm (with some exceptions) and purely cystic nodules.

ATA Guidelines 2015

cytology results [13]. The interpretation of the FNA smears is influenced by the expertise of the cytopathologist and there is inherent limitation to the reproducibility of the cytopathological results [45, 46, 61, 62]. Accuracy of the results is also influenced by the skill of the operator, FNA technique and specimen preparation. FNA results are categorized as either diagnostic/satisfactory, if it contains at least six groups, each containing of at least 10 well-preserved thyroid epithelial cells, else nondiagnostic/unsatisfactory [11, 13]. FNA results are crucial in guiding the further steps in the management of thyroid nodule.

Benign cytology (~70 % of all FNAs) is the most common finding on FNA [13, 45, 48]. Indeterminate results (~10–15 % of all FNAs), which are without a distinct cytological diagnosis [45, 46, 63], include the diagnostic groups of FLUS/AUS and FN/SFN. This diagnostic group possesses a challenge in terms of next steps for management. In practice, although the majority of these patients undergo surgery, the majority of the nodules are found benign. Molecular tests have been developed in an attempt to determine whether an indeterminate nodule is benign or malignant.

Nondiagnostic or unsatisfactory smears (~15 % of all FNAs) have inadequate number of cells to make a diagnosis and result from cystic fluid without cells, bloody smears, or improper techniques in preparing slides [11, 64–67].

Molecular markers

The use of molecular markers in thyroid nodules has been suggested for diagnostic purpose in case of indeterminate cytological diagnosis, to assist with decision making about management option (surgical treatment). These tests are performed using samples from needle washings collected during fine needle aspiration biopsy. The molecular tests which have the most available data are: Afirma Gene-expression Classifier [68], seven-gene panel of genetic mutations and rearrangements [69] and galectin-3 immunohistochemistry [70].

The Afirma gene-expression classifier (167 GEC; mRNA expression of 167 genes) evaluates for the presence of benign gene expression profile. It has a high sensitivity (92 %) and negative predictive (93 %) value but low positive predictive value and specificity (48–53 %) [68, 71]. It is used as a rule out test to identify benign nodules. A benign GEC result predicts low risk of malignancy but the nodules classified as benign still have ~5 % risk of malignancy [71, 72].

The seven gene mutation and rearrangement analysis panel evaluates for BRAF, NRAS, HRAS and KRAS point mutations and common rearrangements of RET/PTC and PAX8/PPARγ. It has a high specificity (86–100 %) and positive predictive value (84–100 %) but poor sensitivity

(reported from 44 to 100 %) [69, 73–75]. It is being used as a rule in test for thyroid malignancy.

This field is evolving and many other molecular tests are being developed (mRNA markers, miRNA markers, etc.) [70, 76–80]. None of the available tests can decisively confirm the presence or absence of malignancy in all indeterminate thyroid nodules. Long term data are needed to confirm its utility in clinical practice. Most of the assays are trained on classic papillary cancers and have limited data in follicular cancers. One has to consider performance of a diagnostic test based on prevalence of the disease (cancer); at high cancer prevalence rate, NPV falls dramatically. Tests are expensive and in deciding their use in management of indeterminate nodules, one should also consider the pretest probability of malignancy with clinical risk features, sonographic characteristics and the size of the nodule, the degree of patient concern and patient preferences, and if the patient would be able to come back for a follow up. In the current settings, molecular testing should only be used to supplement cytopathologic evaluation or clinical and imaging assessment [81]. Patients should be counselled regarding the current clinical utility and limitations of these tests. The AACE Guidelines recommend neither for nor against their use in clinical practice [13]. This field is new and evolving, the recommendations of the use of these molecular tests can be expected to change in the future.

Management

Various factors including serum TSH, clinical risk factor assessment, size of the nodule, ultrasound characteristics, patient preferences and results of the FNA biopsy should be considered in management of thyroid nodule. FNA biopsy cytological diagnosis is the most crucial determinant in decision making.

For autonomous or hyperfunctioning nodules, if the patient has hyperthyroidism, management options include radioiodine therapy or surgery. If the patient has subclinical hyperthyroidism (low TSH with normal FT4), management depends on clinical risk of complications (atrial fibrillation in patients over the age of 60 to 65 years and osteoporosis in postmenopausal women) and the degree of TSH suppression [82–84].

Nodules less than 1 cm with some exceptions should not be biopsied and followed up closely [1]. Also for these patients the frequency and duration of follow up will depend on the additional risk factors present.

For nodules selected for FNA, management primarily depends on cytologic results. According to the Bethesda Classification scheme, FNA of the nodules yields six major results with subsequent different management for each category. However the management of indeterminate nodules (FLUS/AUS and FN/SFN) has similar principles and will be discussed together.

Nodules with benign cytology

The risk of malignancy in nodules reported as benign is 0–3 % [85–88]. Patients with benign nodules are usually managed conservatively without surgery; immediate further diagnostic studies are not required [1]. Though there is a risk of false negative results associated with cytology reporting, initial benign FNA has negligible mortality risk in long term follow up [89].

The frequency and duration of follow up of the benign nodules have been variable in clinical practice. In the nodules that have suddenly enlarged, hemorrhage and cystic degeneration is the most common cause; malignancy is rare even in nodules that have grown [90, 91]. There is no clear evidence to suggest that nodules with larger size (> 3 or 4 cm) with benign cytology should be managed differently than smaller nodules [62, 92]. The follow up of the benign cytological diagnosis should be decided on the sonographic characteristic of the nodule rather than growth [93, 94].

Per the 2015 ATA guidelines, nodules with high suspicious US pattern should have repeat US and FNA within 12 months; while those with low to intermediate suspicious US pattern should have repeat US in 12–24 months. The decision to repeat FNA or observe with repeat US is based on > 20 % growth in at least 2 nodule dimensions or > 50 % increase in nodule volume or the appearance of new suspicious US pattern. Nodules with very low suspicious patterns should have US repeated at 24 months or more. Continued surveillance for a nodule with repeat second benign cytology is not needed [1, 95].

Surgical removal may be needed for benign nodules if they are causing pressure or structural symptoms. TSH suppressive therapy has no role in the management of benign nodule. Percutaneous ethanol ablation can be considered for thyroid cysts and certain complex thyroid nodules [13].

Indeterminate nodules (FLUS/ AUS or FN/SFN)

FLUS/AUS and FN/SFN have 5–15 % and 15–30 % predicted risk of malignancy, respectively. Practice pattern vary considerably in management of indeterminate nodules [96]. Molecular tests have impacted the management strategies in this category. The clinical risk factors, US characteristics (Elastography in addition can be considered in these cases), patient preference and availability/feasibility of the molecular tests should be considered in the decision making process. Some scores such as Mcgill thyroid nodule scores have been tried in pre-operative decision making in thyroid nodules [97].

FLUS/AUS category includes lesions with focal architecture or nuclear atypia whose significance cannot be further determined and specimens that are limited because of poor fixation or obscuring blood [98]. The interpretation of the features which comprise this category is based entirely on the observer which results in poor reproducibility and a second review by experienced high volume cytopathologist can be considered [99, 100]. Repeat FNA or molecular testing (extra sample can be collected at the time of initial testing) can be considered to supplement the malignancy risk assessment [68, 69, 101, 102]. If either of them is not performed or inconclusive, based on clinical and US risk factors and patient preference, either surveillance with repeat US or diagnostic surgery can be chosen [1]. With the new developments in molecular testing, the approach to this category may change in the future.

For FN/SFN, surgical excision for diagnosis had been an established practice. With the molecular testing being available, it can be used to supplement the malignancy risk assessment again after considering the clinical and US risk factors and patient preference [68, 103]. If the molecular testing is not available/performed or inconclusive, diagnostic surgical excision can be considered. Patients with surgical histology specimens showing benign follicular adenoma (absence of capsular or vascular invasion) do not require further treatment. However, patients whose surgical histology shows follicular thyroid cancer might need to have a completion thyroidectomy [1, 13, 69].

Suspicious for malignancy

This category includes specimens strongly suspicious for malignancy, but lacking diagnostic criteria [60]. Diagnostic surgery and histologic exam would be needed in most of the cases. For nodules with the cytology reported as suspicious for malignancy, after consideration of clinical and US risk factors and patient preference, molecular tests (seven-gene mutation and rearrangement panel) can be considered if it would alter the surgical decision making, which is the recommended modality of management [1, 69, 104].

As more data become available on the molecular tests, the management of this category may potentially change in the future.

Malignant

This category includes papillary cancer, follicular carcinoma, Hurthle cell (oncocytic) carcinoma, medullary cancer, thyroid lymphoma, anaplastic cancer, and cancer metastatic to the thyroid. Surgery is generally recommended for these patients [1, 13, 105, 106]. Circumstances in which active surveillance may be considered include low risk papillary microcarcinoma (< 1 cm), patients with high surgical risk, short life expectancy and if concurrent surgical or medical issues need to be addressed first. For cancer due to metastasis, further investigations to find the primary lesion should be undertaken.

Nondiagnostic

This category includes cytologically inadequate specimen. If no or scant follicular tissue is obtained, the absence of malignant cells does not mean a negative biopsy in patients with nondiagnostic FNA. In such cases, FNA using US-guidance should be repeated and if possible with onsite cytological assessment [1, 13, 107]. If the results are still nondiagnostic, core needle biopsy or close observation or diagnostic surgical excision can be considered depending on the suspicious pattern on sonography, clinical risk factors and growth of the nodule during active surveillance [1, 108, 109].

Pregnancy

The evaluation of a thyroid nodule in a pregnant woman should be done in same way as one would in nonpregnant state. However, for the pregnant women with nodule and suppressed TSH that persists after first trimester, further evaluation can be delayed after pregnancy and cessation of lactation when the radionuclide scan can be performed. For a nodule with FNA suggesting PTC, if it is discovered early in pregnancy and if it grows substantially (20 % growth in at least 2 dimensions or 50 % increase in volume or new suspicious US pattern) by 24 weeks gestation or if suspicious cervical lymph nodes are noted on US, surgery should be considered during the second trimester of pregnancy. However, if it is diagnosed in the latter half of the pregnancy or if it is diagnosed early in the pregnancy and remains stable by midgestation, surgery may be performed after delivery. Consideration could be given to administration of levothyroxine therapy to keep the TSH in the range of 0.1–1 mU/L [1, 13, 110–112].

Conclusions

Thyroid nodules are common and carry a 4–6.5 % risk of malignancy. The initial evaluation in all patients with a thyroid nodule includes a detailed history and physical examination assessing risk factors, measurement of serum TSH and neck ultrasonography to assess the size and suspicious characteristics. Fine needle aspiration (FNA) biopsy is an accurate and cost effective way to evaluate thyroid nodules. Nodules with diameter < 1 cm with some exceptions require no FNA and can be observed with a follow up US. Patients with benign nodules are usually followed without surgery. Where available, mRNA classifier system or mutational analysis can be used for further evaluating FNA aspirates with cytology of follicular neoplasm or follicular lesion/atypia of undetermined significance. Patients with cytology suggesting cancer should be referred for surgery.

The high prevalence and increasing diagnosis of incidental thyroid nodules requires clinicians to adopt evidence-based approaches to evaluate, risk stratify and provide appropriate treatment. As more evidence becomes available, active surveillance may become possible for selected cases of thyroid cancer patients.

Acknowledgements

Not applicable.

Authors' contributions

ST was involved in literature search/review and formulation and writing the manuscript. HG provided guidance regarding the literature. HG also assisted with manuscript writing/review. All authors read and approved the final manuscript.

References

1. Haugen BR, Alexander EK, Bible KC, et al. 2015 American Thyroid Association Management Guidelines for Adult Patients with Thyroid Nodules and Differentiated Thyroid Cancer: The American Thyroid Association Guidelines Task Force on Thyroid Nodules and Differentiated Thyroid Cancer. Thyroid. 2016;26(1):1–133.
2. Tunbridge WM, Evered DC, Hall R, et al. The spectrum of thyroid disease in a community: the Whickham survey. Clin Endocrinol (Oxf). 1977;7(6):481–93.
3. Hegedus L. Clinical practice. The thyroid nodule. N Engl J Med. 2004; 351(17):1764–71.
4. Dean DS, Gharib H. Epidemiology of thyroid nodules. Best Pract Res Clin Endocrinol Metab. 2008;22(6):901–11.
5. Davies L, Welch HG. Current thyroid cancer trends in the United States. JAMA Otolaryngol Head Neck Surg. 2014;140(4):317–22.
6. Li N, Du XL, Reitzel LR, Xu L, Sturgis EM. Impact of enhanced detection on the increase in thyroid cancer incidence in the United States: review of incidence trends by socioeconomic status within the surveillance, epidemiology, and end results registry, 1980–2008. Thyroid. 2013;23(1):103–10.
7. Werk Jr EE, Vernon BM, Gonzalez JJ, Ungaro PC, McCoy RC. Cancer in thyroid nodules. A community hospital survey. Arch Intern Med. 1984;144(3):474–6.
8. Belfiore A, Giuffrida D, La Rosa GL, et al. High frequency of cancer in cold thyroid nodules occurring at young age. Acta Endocrinol (Copenh). 1989;121(2):197–202.
9. Lin JD, Chao TC, Huang BY, Chen ST, Chang HY, Hsueh C. Thyroid cancer in the thyroid nodules evaluated by ultrasonography and fine-needle aspiration cytology. Thyroid. 2005;15(7):708–17.
10. Tan GH, Gharib H. Thyroid incidentalomas: management approaches to nonpalpable nodules discovered incidentally on thyroid imaging. Ann Intern Med. 1997;126(3):226–31.
11. Gharib H, Papini E. Thyroid nodules: clinical importance, assessment, and treatment. Endocrinol Metab Clin North Am. 2007;36(3):707–35. vi.
12. Castro MR, Gharib H. Continuing controversies in the management of thyroid nodules. Ann Intern Med. 2005;142(11):926–31.
13. Gharib H, Papini E, Garber JR, et al. American Association of Clinical Endocrinologists, American College of Endocrinology, and Associazione Medici Endocrinologi Medical Guidelines for Clinical Practice for the Diagnosis and Management of Thyroid Nodules - 2016 Update. Endocr Pract. 2016;22(5):622–39.
14. Tan GH, Gharib H, Reading CC. Solitary thyroid nodule. Comparison between palpation and ultrasonography. Arch Intern Med. 1995;155(22):2418–23.

15. Singh S, Singh A, Khanna AK. Thyroid incidentaloma. Indian J Surg Oncol. 2012;3(3):173–81.

16. Boelaert K, Horacek J, Holder RL, Watkinson JC, Sheppard MC, Franklyn JA. Serum thyrotropin concentration as a novel predictor of malignancy in thyroid nodules investigated by fine-needle aspiration. J Clin Endocrinol Metab. 2006;91(11):4295–301.

17. Haymart MR, Repplinger DJ, Leverson GE, et al. Higher serum thyroid stimulating hormone level in thyroid nodule patients is associated with greater risks of differentiated thyroid cancer and advanced tumor stage. J Clin Endocrinol Metab. 2008;93(3):809–14.

18. Costante G, Filetti S. Early diagnosis of medullary thyroid carcinoma: is systematic calcitonin screening appropriate in patients with nodular thyroid disease? Oncologist. 2011;16(1):49–52.

19. Gharib H, Papini E, Paschke R. Thyroid nodules: a review of current guidelines, practices, and prospects. Eur J Endocrinol. 2008;159(5):493–505.

20. Elisei R, Bottici V, Luchetti F, et al. Impact of routine measurement of serum calcitonin on the diagnosis and outcome of medullary thyroid cancer: experience in 10,864 patients with nodular thyroid disorders. J Clin Endocrinol Metab. 2004;89(1):163–8.

21. Niccoli P, Wion-Barbot N, Caron P, et al. Interest of routine measurement of serum calcitonin: study in a large series of thyroidectomized patients. The French Medullary Study Group. J Clin Endocrinol Metab. 1997;82(2):338–41.

22. Costante G, Meringolo D, Durante C, et al. Predictive value of serum calcitonin levels for preoperative diagnosis of medullary thyroid carcinoma in a cohort of 5817 consecutive patients with thyroid nodules. J Clin Endocrinol Metab. 2007;92(2):450–5.

23. Machens A, Hoffmann F, Sekulla C, Dralle H. Importance of gender-specific calcitonin thresholds in screening for occult sporadic medullary thyroid cancer. Endocr Relat Cancer. 2009;16(4):1291–8.

24. Chambon G, Alovisetti C, Idoux-Louche C, et al. The use of preoperative routine measurement of basal serum thyrocalcitonin in candidates for thyroidectomy due to nodular thyroid disorders: results from 2733 consecutive patients. J Clin Endocrinol Metab. 2011;96(1):75–81.

25. Toledo SP, Lourenco Jr DM, Santos MA, Tavares MR, Toledo RA, Correia-Deur JE. Hypercalcitoninemia is not pathognomonic of medullary thyroid carcinoma. Clinics (Sao Paulo). 2009;64(7):699–706.

26. Erdogan MF, Gursoy A, Kulaksizoglu M. Long-term effects of elevated gastrin levels on calcitonin secretion. J Endocrinol Invest. 2006;29(9):771–5.

27. Wang TS, Ocal IT, Sosa JA, Cox H, Roman S. Medullary thyroid carcinoma without marked elevation of calcitonin: a diagnostic and surveillance dilemma. Thyroid. 2008;18(8):889–94.

28. Dora JM, Canalli MH, Capp C, Punales MK, Vieira JG, Maia AL. Normal perioperative serum calcitonin levels in patients with advanced medullary thyroid carcinoma: case report and review of the literature. Thyroid. 2008;18(8):895–9.

29. Suh I, Vriens MR, Guerrero MA, et al. Serum thyroglobulin is a poor diagnostic biomarker of malignancy in follicular and Hurthle-cell neoplasms of the thyroid. Am J Surg. 2010;200(1):41–6.

30. Lee EK, Chung KW, Min HS, et al. Preoperative serum thyroglobulin as a useful predictive marker to differentiate follicular thyroid cancer from benign nodules in indeterminate nodules. J Korean Med Sci. 2012;27(9):1014–8.

31. Repplinger D, Bargren A, Zhang YW, Adler JT, Haymart M, Chen H. Is Hashimoto's thyroiditis a risk factor for papillary thyroid cancer? J Surg Res. 2008;150(1):49–52.

32. Shambaugh 3rd GE, Quinn JL, Oyasu R, Freinkel N. Disparate thyroid imaging. Combined studies with sodium pertechnetate Tc 99 m and radioactive iodine. Jama. 1974;228(7):866–9.

33. Blum M, Goldman AB. Improved diagnosis of "nondelineated" thyroid nodules by oblique scintillation scanning and echography. J Nucl Med. 1975;16(8):713–5.

34. Reschini E, Ferrari C, Castellani M, et al. The trapping-only nodules of the thyroid gland: prevalence study. Thyroid. 2006;16(8):757–62.

35. Leenhardt L, Hejblum G, Franc B, et al. Indications and limits of ultrasound-guided cytology in the management of nonpalpable thyroid nodules. J Clin Endocrinol Metab. 1999;84(1):24–8.

36. Papini E, Guglielmi R, Bianchini A, et al. Risk of malignancy in nonpalpable thyroid nodules: predictive value of ultrasound and color-Doppler features. J Clin Endocrinol Metab. 2002;87(5):1941–6.

37. Nam-Goong IS, Kim HY, Gong G, et al. Ultrasonography-guided fine-needle aspiration of thyroid incidentaloma: correlation with pathological findings. Clin Endocrinol (Oxf). 2004;60(1):21–8.

38. Cappelli C, Castellano M, Pirola I, et al. The predictive value of ultrasound findings in the management of thyroid nodules. QJM. 2007;100(1):29–35.

39. Frates MC, Benson CB, Doubilet PM, et al. Prevalence and distribution of carcinoma in patients with solitary and multiple thyroid nodules on sonography. J Clin Endocrinol Metab. 2006;91(9):3411–7.

40. Moon WJ, Jung SL, Lee JH, et al. Benign and malignant thyroid nodules: US differentiation–multicenter retrospective study. Radiology. 2008;247(3):762–70.

41. Remonti LR, Kramer CK, Leitao CB, Pinto LC, Gross JL. Thyroid ultrasound features and risk of carcinoma: a systematic review and meta-analysis of observational studies. Thyroid. 2015;25(5):538–50.

42. Brito JP, Gionfriddo MR, Al Nofal A, et al. The accuracy of thyroid nodule ultrasound to predict thyroid cancer: systematic review and meta-analysis. J Clin Endocrinol Metab. 2014;99(4):1253–63.

43. Bonavita JA, Mayo J, Babb J, et al. Pattern recognition of benign nodules at ultrasound of the thyroid: which nodules can be left alone? AJR Am J Roentgenol. 2009;193(1):207–13.

44. Moon WJ, Kwag HJ, Na DG. Are there any specific ultrasound findings of nodular hyperplasia ("leave me alone" lesion) to differentiate it from follicular adenoma? Acta Radiol. 2009;50(4):383–8.

45. Gharib H. Fine-needle aspiration biopsy of thyroid nodules: advantages, limitations, and effect. Mayo Clin Proc. 1994;69(1):44–9.

46. Gharib H, Goellner JR. Fine-needle aspiration biopsy of thyroid nodules. Endocr Pract. 1995;1(6):410–7.

47. Bomeli SR, LeBeau SO, Ferris RL. Evaluation of a thyroid nodule. Otolaryngol Clin North Am. 2010;43(2):229–38. vii.

48. Castro MR, Gharib H. Thyroid fine-needle aspiration biopsy: progress, practice, and pitfalls. Endocr Pract. 2003;9(2):128–36.

49. Jeffrey PB, Miller TR. Fine-needle aspiration cytology of the thyroid. Pathology (Phila). 1996;4(2):319–35.

50. Hamberger B, Gharib H, Melton 3rd LJ, Goellner JR, Zinsmeister AR. Fine-needle aspiration biopsy of thyroid nodules. Impact on thyroid practice and cost of care. Am J Med. 1982;73(3):381–4.

51. Hamburger JI, Hamburger SW. Fine needle biopsy of thyroid nodules: avoiding the pitfalls. N Y State J Med. 1986;86(5):241–9.

52. Sakorafas GH. Thyroid nodules; interpretation and importance of fine-needle aspiration (FNA) for the clinician - practical considerations. Surg Oncol. 2010;19(4):e130–9.

53. Can AS. Cost-effectiveness comparison between palpation- and ultrasound-guided thyroid fine-needle aspiration biopsies. BMC Endocr Disord. 2009;9:14.

54. Singh Ospina N, Brito JP, Maraka S, et al. Diagnostic accuracy of ultrasound-guided fine needle aspiration biopsy for thyroid malignancy: systematic review and meta-analysis. Endocrine. 2016;53:651–61.

55. Danese D, Sciacchitano S, Farsetti A, Andreoli M, Pontecorvi A. Diagnostic accuracy of conventional versus sonography-guided fine-needle aspiration biopsy of thyroid nodules. Thyroid. 1998;8(1):15–21.

56. Leenhardt L, Erdogan MF, Hegedus L, et al. 2013 European thyroid association guidelines for cervical ultrasound scan and ultrasound-guided techniques in the postoperative management of patients with thyroid cancer. Eur Thyroid J. 2013;2(3):147–59.

57. Yoon JH, Cho A, Lee HS, Kim EK, Moon HJ, Kwak JY. Thyroid incidentalomas detected on 18 F-fluorodeoxyglucose-positron emission tomography/computed tomography: Thyroid Imaging Reporting and Data System (TIRADS) in the diagnosis and management of patients. Surgery. 2015; 158(5):1314–22.

58. Flukes S, Lenzo N, Moschilla G, Sader C. Positron emission tomography-positive thyroid nodules: rate of malignancy and histological features. ANZ J Surg. 2016;86(6):487–91.

59. Baloch ZW, LiVolsi VA, Asa SL, et al. Diagnostic terminology and morphologic criteria for cytologic diagnosis of thyroid lesions: a synopsis of the National Cancer Institute Thyroid Fine-Needle Aspiration State of the Science Conference. Diagn Cytopathol. 2008;36(6):425–37.

60. Cibas ES, Ali SZ. The Bethesda System for Reporting Thyroid Cytopathology. Thyroid. 2009;19(11):1159–65.

61. Gharib H, Goellner JR. Fine-needle aspiration biopsy of the thyroid: an appraisal. Ann Intern Med. 1993;118(4):282–9.

62. Pinchot SN, Al-Wagih H, Schaefer S, Sippel R, Chen H. Accuracy of fine-needle aspiration biopsy for predicting neoplasm or carcinoma in thyroid nodules 4 cm or larger. Arch Surg. 2009;144(7):649–55.

63. Cersosimo E, Gharib H, Suman VJ, Goellner JR. "Suspicious" thyroid cytologic findings: outcome in patients without immediate surgical treatment. Mayo Clin Proc. 1993;68(4):343–8.

64. Gharib H, Goellner JR, Zinsmeister AR, Grant CS, Van Heerden JA. Fine-needle aspiration biopsy of the thyroid. The problem of suspicious cytologic findings. Ann Intern Med. 1984;101(1):25–8.

65. Chow LS, Gharib H, Goellner JR, van Heerden JA. Nondiagnostic thyroid fine-needle aspiration cytology: management dilemmas. Thyroid. 2001; 11(12):1147–51.

66. Schmidt T, Riggs MW, Speights Jr VO. Significance of nondiagnostic fine-needle aspiration of the thyroid. South Med J. 1997;90(12):1183–6.

67. McHenry CR, Walfish PG, Rosen IB. Non-diagnostic fine needle aspiration biopsy: a dilemma in management of nodular thyroid disease. Am Surg. 1993;59(7):415–9.

68. Alexander EK, Kennedy GC, Baloch ZW, et al. Preoperative diagnosis of benign thyroid nodules with indeterminate cytology. N Engl J Med. 2012;367(8):705–15.

69. Nikiforov YE, Ohori NP, Hodak SP, et al. Impact of mutational testing on the diagnosis and management of patients with cytologically indeterminate thyroid nodules: a prospective analysis of 1056 FNA samples. J Clin Endocrinol Metab. 2011;96(11):3390–7.

70. Bartolazzi A, Orlandi F, Saggiorato E, et al. Galectin-3-expression analysis in the surgical selection of follicular thyroid nodules with indeterminate fine-needle aspiration cytology: a prospective multicentre study. Lancet Oncol. 2008;9(6):543–9.

71. Alexander EK, Schorr M, Klopper J, et al. Multicenter clinical experience with the Afirma gene expression classifier. J Clin Endocrinol Metab. 2014;99(1):119–25.

72. Marti JL, Avadhani V, Donatelli LA, et al. Wide Inter-institutional Variation in Performance of a Molecular Classifier for Indeterminate Thyroid Nodules. Ann Surg Oncol. 2015;22(12):3996–4001.

73. Cantara S, Capezzone M, Marchisotta S, et al. Impact of proto-oncogene mutation detection in cytological specimens from thyroid nodules improves the diagnostic accuracy of cytology. J Clin Endocrinol Metab. 2010;95(3):1365–9.

74. Nikiforov YE, Steward DL, Robinson-Smith TM, et al. Molecular testing for mutations in improving the fine-needle aspiration diagnosis of thyroid nodules. J Clin Endocrinol Metab. 2009;94(6):2092–8.

75. Beaudenon-Huibregtse S, Alexander EK, Guttler RB, et al. Centralized molecular testing for oncogenic gene mutations complements the local cytopathologic diagnosis of thyroid nodules. Thyroid. 2014;24(10):1479–87.

76. Franco C, Martinez V, Allamand JP, et al. Molecular markers in thyroid fine-needle aspiration biopsy: a prospective study. Appl Immunohistochem Mol Morphol. 2009;17(3):211–5.

77. Fadda G, Rossi ED, Raffaelli M, et al. Follicular thyroid neoplasms can be classified as low- and high-risk according to HBME-1 and Galectin-3 expression on liquid-based fine-needle cytology. Eur J Endocrinol. 2011;165(3):447–53.

78. Prasad NB, Somervell H, Tufano RP, et al. Identification of genes differentially expressed in benign versus malignant thyroid tumors. Clin Cancer Res. 2008;14(11):3327–37.

79. Nikiforova MN, Tseng GC, Steward D, Diorio D, Nikiforov YE. MicroRNA expression profiling of thyroid tumors: biological significance and diagnostic utility. J Clin Endocrinol Metab. 2008;93(5):1600–8.

80. Agretti P, Ferrarini E, Rago T, et al. MicroRNA expression profile helps to distinguish benign nodules from papillary thyroid carcinomas starting from cells of fine-needle aspiration. Eur J Endocrinol. 2012;167(3):393–400.

81. Bernet V, Hupart KH, Parangi S, Woeber KA. AACE/ACE disease state commentary: molecular diagnostic testing of thyroid nodules with indeterminate cytopathology. Endocr Pract. 2014;20(4):360–3.

82. Bauer DC, Rodondi N, Stone KL, Hillier TA. Thyroid hormone use, hyperthyroidism and mortality in older women. Am J Med. 2007;120(4):343–9.

83. Auer J, Scheibner P, Mische T, Langsteger W, Eber O, Eber B. Subclinical hyperthyroidism as a risk factor for atrial fibrillation. Am Heart J. 2001; 142(5):838–42.

84. Biondi B, Cooper DS. The clinical significance of subclinical thyroid dysfunction. Endocr Rev. 2008;29(1):76–131.

85. Orlandi A, Puscar A, Capriata E, Fideleff H. Repeated fine-needle aspiration of the thyroid in benign nodular thyroid disease: critical evaluation of long-term follow-up. Thyroid. 2005;15(3):274–8.

86. Illouz F, Rodien P, Saint-Andre JP, et al. Usefulness of repeated fine-needle cytology in the follow-up of non-operated thyroid nodules. Eur J Endocrinol. 2007;156(3):303–8.

87. Oertel YC, Miyahara-Felipe L, Mendoza MG, Yu K. Value of repeated fine needle aspirations of the thyroid: an analysis of over ten thousand FNAs. Thyroid. 2007;17(11):1061–6.

88. Tee YY, Lowe AJ, Brand CA, Judson RT. Fine-needle aspiration may miss a third of all malignancy in palpable thyroid nodules: a comprehensive literature review. Ann Surg. 2007;246(5):714–20.

89. Nou E, Kwong N, Alexander LK, Cibas ES, Marqusee E, Alexander EK. Determination of the optimal time interval for repeat evaluation after a benign thyroid nodule aspiration. J Clin Endocrinol Metab. 2014; 99(2):510–6.

90. Kim SY, Han KH, Moon HJ, Kwak JY, Chung WY, Kim EK. Thyroid nodules with benign findings at cytologic examination: results of long-term follow-up with US. Radiology. 2014;271(1):272–81.

91. Ashcraft MW, Van Herle AJ. Management of thyroid nodules. II: Scanning techniques, thyroid suppressive therapy, and fine needle aspiration. Head Neck Surg. 1981;3(4):297–322.

92. Yoon JH, Kwak JY, Moon HJ, Kim MJ, Kim EK. The diagnostic accuracy of ultrasound-guided fine-needle aspiration biopsy and the sonographic differences between benign and malignant thyroid nodules 3 cm or larger. Thyroid. 2011;21(9):993–1000.

93. Kwak JY, Koo H, Youk JH, et al. Value of US correlation of a thyroid nodule with initially benign cytologic results. Radiology. 2010;254(1):292–300.

94. Rosario PW, Purisch S. Ultrasonographic characteristics as a criterion for repeat cytology in benign thyroid nodules. Arq Bras Endocrinol Metabol. 2010;54(1):52–5.

95. Durante C, Costante G, Lucisano G, et al. The natural history of benign thyroid nodules. Jama. 2015;313(9):926–35.

96. Burch HB, Burman KD, Cooper DS, Hennessey JV, Vietor NO. A 2015 Survey of Clinical Practice Patterns in the Management of Thyroid Nodules. J Clin Endocrinol Metab. 2016;101(7):2853–62. jc20161155.

97. Varshney R, Forest VI, Mascarella MA, et al. The Mcgill thyroid nodule score - does it help with indeterminate thyroid nodules? J Otolaryngol Head Neck Surg. 2015;44:2.

98. Shi Y, Ding X, Klein M, et al. Thyroid fine-needle aspiration with atypia of undetermined significance: a necessary or optional category? Cancer. 2009; 117(5):298–304.

99. Davidov T, Trooskin SZ, Shanker BA, et al. Routine second-opinion cytopathology review of thyroid fine needle aspiration biopsies reduces diagnostic thyroidectomy. Surgery. 2010;148(6):1294–9. discussion 9–301.

100. Cibas ES, Baloch ZW, Fellegara G, et al. A prospective assessment defining the limitations of thyroid nodule pathologic evaluation. Ann Intern Med. 2013;159(5):325–32.

101. Baloch Z, LiVolsi VA, Jain P, et al. Role of repeat fine-needle aspiration biopsy (FNAB) in the management of thyroid nodules. Diagn Cytopathol. 2003;29(4):203–6.

102. Yang J, Schnadig V, Logrono R, Wasserman PG. Fine-needle aspiration of thyroid nodules: a study of 4703 patients with histologic and clinical correlations. Cancer. 2007;111(5):306–15.

103. Nikiforov YE, Carty SE, Chiosea SI, et al. Highly accurate diagnosis of cancer in thyroid nodules with follicular neoplasm/suspicious for a follicular neoplasm cytology by ThyroSeq v2 next-generation sequencing assay. Cancer. 2014;120(23):3627–34.

104. Moon HJ, Kwak JY, Kim EK, et al. The role of BRAFV600E mutation and ultrasonography for the surgical management of a thyroid nodule suspicious for papillary thyroid carcinoma on cytology. Ann Surg Oncol. 2009;16(11):3125–31.

105. Gharib H, Papini E, Paschke R, et al. American Association of Clinical Endocrinologists, Associazione Medici Endocrinologi, and EuropeanThyroid Association Medical Guidelines for Clinical Practice for the Diagnosis and Management of Thyroid Nodules. Endocr Pract. 2010;16 Suppl 1:1–43.

106. Cobin RH, Gharib H, Bergman DA, et al. AACE/AAES medical/surgical guidelines for clinical practice: management of thyroid carcinoma. American Association of Clinical Endocrinologists. American College of Endocrinology. Endocr Pract. 2001;7(3):202–20.

107. Orija IB, Pineyro M, Biscotti C, Reddy SS, Hamrahian AH. Value of repeating a nondiagnostic thyroid fine-needle aspiration biopsy. Endocr Pract. 2007; 13(7):735–42.

108. Suh CH, Baek JH, Kim KW, et al. The Role of Core-Needle Biopsy for Thyroid Nodules with Initially Nondiagnostic Fine-Needle Aspiration Results: A Systematic Review and Meta-Analysis. Endocr Pract. 2016; 22(6):679–88.

109. Moon HJ, Kwak JY, Choi YS, Kim EK. How to manage thyroid nodules with two consecutive non-diagnostic results on ultrasonography-guided fine-needle aspiration. World J Surg. 2012;36(3):586–92.

110. Moosa M, Mazzaferri EL. Outcome of differentiated thyroid cancer diagnosed in pregnant women. J Clin Endocrinol Metab. 1997;82(9):2862–6.

111. Uruno T, Shibuya H, Kitagawa W, Nagahama M, Sugino K, Ito K. Optimal timing of surgery for differentiated thyroid cancer in pregnant women. World J Surg. 2014;38(3):704–8.

112. Messuti I, Corvisieri S, Bardesono F, et al. Impact of pregnancy on prognosis of differentiated thyroid cancer: clinical and molecular features. Eur J Endocrinol. 2014;170(5):659–66.

113. Schneider AB, Ron E, Lubin J, Stovall M, Gierlowski TC. Dose–response relationships for radiation-induced thyroid cancer and thyroid nodules: evidence for the prolonged effects of radiation on the thyroid. J Clin Endocrinol Metab. 1993;77(2):362–9.

114. Curtis RE, Rowlings PA, Deeg HJ, et al. Solid cancers after bone marrow transplantation. N Engl J Med. 1997;336(13):897–904.

115. Pacini F, Vorontsova T, Demidchik EP, et al. Post-Chernobyl thyroid carcinoma in Belarus children and adolescents: comparison with naturally occurring thyroid carcinoma in Italy and France. J Clin Endocrinol Metab. 1997;82(11):3563–9.

116. Shibata Y, Yamashita S, Masyakin VB, Panasyuk GD, Nagataki S. 15 years after Chernobyl: new evidence of thyroid cancer. Lancet. 2001;358(9297):1965–6.

117. Hemminki K, Eng C, Chen B. Familial risks for nonmedullary thyroid cancer. J Clin Endocrinol Metab. 2005;90(10):5747–53.

118. McCartney CR, Stukenborg GJ. Decision analysis of discordant thyroid nodule biopsy guideline criteria. J Clin Endocrinol Metab. 2008;93(8):3037–44.

119. Cooper DS, Doherty GM, Haugen BR, et al. Revised American Thyroid Association management guidelines for patients with thyroid nodules and differentiated thyroid cancer. Thyroid. 2009;19(11):1167–214.

120. Moon WJ, Baek JH, Jung SL, et al. Ultrasonography and the ultrasound-based management of thyroid nodules: consensus statement and recommendations. Korean J Radiol. 2011;12(1):1–14.

16

Managing diabetes in the digital age

Viral N. Shah[1,2] and Satish K. Garg[1,2,3]*

Abstract

The prevalence of diabetes is rising globally. Poor glucose control results in higher rates of diabetes-related complications and an increase in health care expenditure. Diabetes self-management education (DSME) training has shown to improve glucose control, and thus may reduce long-term complications. Implementation of diabetes self-management education programs may not be feasible for all the institutions or in developing countries due to lack of resources and higher costs associated with DSME training. With the increasing use of smartphones and Internet, there is an opportunity to use digital tools for training people with diabetes to self-manage their disease. A number of mobile applications, Internet portal, and websites are available to help patients to improve their diabetes care. However, the studies are limited to show its effectiveness and cost-benefits in diabetes self-management. In addition, there are many challenges ahead for the digital health industry. In this review, we assess the use of newer technologies and digital health in diabetes self-management with a focus on future directions and potential challenges.

Keywords: Diabetes, Digital health, Artificial pancreas, Closed-loop system, Electronic health records, Mobile health, mHealth, Diabetes self-management, Mobile applications

Introduction

The International Diabetes Federation (IDF) estimates a global epidemic of diabetes. In 2014, 387 million people had diabetes, and it will increase to 592 million by 2035 [1].

Poor glucose control leads to long-term diabetes, micro- and macro-vascular complications resulting in higher morbidity, and mortality that accounts for 4.9 million deaths in 2014 and $612 billion in health care expenditure [1]. Therefore, American Diabetes Association (ADA) recommends glycosylated hemoglobin (A1c) goal of 7 or less to prevent diabetes complications [2]. To achieve this goal, diabetes self-management education (DSME) is crucial [2, 3]. As expected, DSME is associated with a higher cost as $4.8 million were reimbursed by the Center for Medicare and Medicaid (CMS) in 2010 for DSME training for the Medicaid population [4]. In addition, about 77 % of people with diabetes live in low- and middle-income countries [1] that do not have adequate resources to provide such training to patients. Even in the USA, only about 20 % of adults with diabetes are cared for by an endocrinologist/diabetologist [5, 6].

The wireless broadband and smartphone market totals 1.5 billion globally as of 2013 which is expected to rise to 6.5 billion by 2018 [7]. With increasing numbers of smartphone users, it is possible to apply mobile app technology to empower patients to better manage their diabetes. As the number of people with diabetes rises, and with an inadequate number of specialists and lack of resources in developing countries, there is an opportunity and growing need to develop cost-effective supporting tools for DSME to improve overall diabetes outcomes.

In this manuscript, we review the use of newer technologies and digital health in diabetes self-management with a focus on future directions and potential challenges.

Review
Diabetes self-management goes digital

DSME and training is a collaborative process through which people with, or at risk for, diabetes gain the knowledge and skills needed to modify their behavior and successfully self-manage the disease to improve health outcomes [8]. The components of DSME are

* Correspondence: Satish.Garg@ucdenver.edu
[1]Barbara Davis Center for Diabetes, University of Colorado Denver, 1775 Aurora Court, A140, Aurora, CO 80045, USA
[2]School of Medicine, University of Colorado Denver, Aurora, CO, USA
Full list of author information is available at the end of the article

healthy eating, self-monitoring of blood sugar (SMBG), medication adherence, and diabetes complications risk reduction behavior. Table 1 summarizes the available mobile applications (apps) to help patients with diabetes to self-manage the disease. Management of diabetes is generally self-directed, and individuals need to make day-to-day decisions related to controlling their disease [8]. Effective management requires patients to understand and use appropriate technologies for glucose monitoring and medication compliance as well as complex treatment strategies; therefore, DSME is recognized as a crucial component in diabetes care and in limited pilot studies. It has been shown to be cost-effective and efficacious in lowering A1c and blood pressure [9–11].

Online diabetes education

The conventional education for diabetes self-management has been supplemented with several web portals, blogs, and structured online educational materials. The online portals and apps may be cost-effective, convenient, easy to use and learn anywhere at anytime to understand diabetes, its complications, and how to individualize and self-manage. Government organizations such as the National Institute of Diabetes and Digestive and Kidney Diseases (http://www.niddk.nih.gov/health-information/health-topics/Diabetes/Pages/default.aspx), professional diabetes organizations such as the ADA (http://www.diabetes.org) and the American Association of Clinical Endocrinologists (http://empoweryourhealth.org/endocrine-conditions/diabetes) and many pharmaceutical industries and other non-profit organizations provides online information on diabetes, diabetes-related health problems and education. A number of apps such as Diabetes EDC, Point of Care Diabetes, Diabetes journal, Prognosis Diabetes, Diabetes Forecast, Diabetes Forum and Diabetes FAQ also provide basic diabetes education. In addition, researchers have also designed digital virtual environment [e.g. SLIDES (Second Life Impacts Diabetes Education and Self-management by Duke University, Durham, NC, USA] by creating virtual 3D community to provide DSME training based on social cognitive theory [12].

Healthy eating

Counting carbohydrates is useful for people with insulin-requiring diabetes to administer appropriate prandial insulin doses to maintain euglycemia [13, 14]. Pilot studies show that taking fat and protein into account for insulin dose calculations result in significant A1C reductions compared with only carbohydrate counting [15]. Similarly, counting calories and making healthy choices are equally important for weight management [16]. Several books on carbohydrate and calorie counting are available for the patients to use; however, it is inconvenient to carry books all the time. Therefore, apps help patients improve their nutritional choices and monitor their food and caloric intake. Many apps include a feature that allows users to search food databases by typing or scanning bar codes. For example, GoMeal, My Fitness pal, Calorie Counter by MyNetDiary, and Glucose Buddy offer extensive databases, allowing users to quickly look up nutritional information including carbohydrate content and calories. In addition, these apps offer target planning and goal setting to help users manage their weight and caloric intake. Above all, apps are in development to analyze food content based on images of the food [17].

Table 1 Mobile apps to support diabetes management[ab]

Diet	Physical activity	Blood glucose e-log book
Healthy out	Track 3	Diabetic
Foodily	My Fitness pal	Diabetes in check
Whole food market recipe	Moves	Diabetes companion
CarbControl	Nike + running	My sugar Junior
Lose it	Strava	Go meal
Weight watchers	UP by jawbone	Glooko
Daily burn	Endomondo	Glucose buddy
Calorie counter PRO	GymPact	DiabetesApp lite
iCookbook diabetic	FitnessFast	My net diary
Fooducate	Pacer	Glucose companion
EatLocal		
Calorie king		
HEALTHeDiabetes		
Glucose monitoring	**Insulin dose calculators**	**Relaxation and meditation**
iBGStar	Insulin calculator	Calm
Telcare	iBolus calc	Sleep cycle
	Insulin dose calculator pro	Equanimity
	Diabetes personal calculator	
Diabetes education	Rapid calc diabetes manager	**Medication adherence**
WebMD	PredictBGL	MyMedSchedule
Diabetes insight	EZ insulin calculator	MyMeds
Up to date	Insulin units	MedSimple
Managing type 1 Diabetes		Pillmanager
Diabetes EDC		Pill reminder
Diabetes @point of care		RxmindMe Prescription
		Pillboxie

[a]Most apps have more than one feature. [b]the list is not comprehensive, there are number of apps available in each category

Insulin dose calculators

Accurate bolus insulin doses require calculations based on factors such as current and target blood glucose, carbohydrate-to-insulin ratios, total grams of carbohydrate in meals, insulin sensitivity factors, and insulin on board [18]. It is difficult for insulin requiring patients to account for all these factors for their insulin dosing. Introduction of automatic bolus calculators integrated in the insulin pump (bolus wizard) have shown to help patients to more accurately meet prandial insulin dosage requirements, improve postprandial glycemic excursions, and achieve optimal glycemic control [18–20]. However, it was estimated that of 13.2 million people with diabetes, only 162,000 were insulin pump users in 2002 [21, 22]. The majority of people with diabetes do not use insulin pumps due to cost, lack of insurance coverage, or other unrelated issues. Apps such as Insulin Calculator, Bolus Calc, Insulin Dose Calculator Pro, and Diabetes Personal Calculator for non-pump users are available to help patients in insulin dosing. The Food and Drug Administration (FDA) has not approved most of the available apps.

Physical activity

The Surgeon General's Report on Physical Activity and Health in 1996 highlighted the pivotal role of physical activity in health promotion and disease prevention [23]. Modest weight loss has been shown to improve insulin resistance in overweight and obese people with diabetes [24]. ADA recommends moderate weight loss (7 % of body weight) for overweight individuals with diabetes [2]. Key components of weight loss management are self-monitoring of physical activity by means of recording frequency, intensity, time, type of activity, and a healthy diet [25, 26]. However, recording physical activity puts an additional burden on participants. Therefore, many developers have created digital tools for physical activity monitoring such as pedometers, wristband sensors, and personal digital assistants. Examples of few mobile apps for monitoring steps and physical activities are; pacer, Steps pedometer and step counter activity tracker, Map My Walk, Stepz, Walker-Pedometer Lite, Footsteps, iRunner and Runtastic Pedometer. Fitbit, the Jawbone Up24 and the Nike Fuelband are examples of wristband sensor that tracks person's physical activity. These apps allow users to track their activity, count calories, and provide ways for weight management. In addition, many apps help people change their physical activity by providing instruction to perform such activities, modeling/demonstrating, feedback on performance, planning social support/change, prompting review of goals, facilitating social comparison, setting graded tasks, and goal setting for a behavioral outcome [27].

Studies have shown that the use of apps results in greater weight loss compared to conventional physical activities without the help of tracking apps [28]. The Task Force for Community Preventive Services noted that health promotion activities tailored to an individual's specific needs increase the likelihood of beginning an exercise program and increase the frequency of exercise [29]. It has also been noted that employee education programs for physical activity at the work place improved health outcomes [30]. Considering this, many organizations (e.g. Be Colorado Move program by the University of Colorado, http://becolorado.org/programs/be-colorado-move and EHP Wellness Program by Cleveland Clinic http://www.clevelandclinic.org/healthplan/wellness.htm) have initiated incentives for their employees to use tracking apps and record their daily physical activities. Studies have shown that financial incentives are more effective than usual care or no intervention for encouraging healthy behavior change [30–32].

Self-monitoring of blood glucose

Self-monitoring of blood glucose (SMBG) is recognized as an important tool for decision-making for both patients and health care providers [33]. ADA recommends that patients whose medication regimen includes multiple daily insulin injections or insulin pumps should test their blood glucose three times or more per day [2]. However, not all patients with diabetes test blood glucose three times or more a day. Hurdles in poor adherence to SMBG include a) inaccurate meters b) big and bulkier devices c) need to poke a finger multiple times d) need to carry an additional device all the time and e) paper log book entry [34, 35]. This results in poor compliance and inadequate glucose control with wide glucose excursions. With the advances in blood glucose meters and mobile technology, it has become possible to address several of these issues. For example, iBGStar is an external device that fits easily to an iPhone and functions as a glucose meter that helps patients carry their glucose meter along with a smartphone (http://www.ibgstar.us/). Studies have shown that iBGstar use is associated with higher patient satisfaction and better glycemic outcomes in adults with type 1 diabetes [36]. Most manufacturers have designed clinical decision supporting websites to download blood glucose meter to analyze the glycemic pattern and trends to help patients and clinicians with treatment decision. Example of such decision supporting tools are CareLink, LibreView and Accu-chek connect. A number of apps such as GoMeal, Diabetes Net Diary, and Glooko provide an e-Log book where blood glucose data can be saved and printed later or can be emailed to health care providers. In addition, these apps have graphical displays to see and interpret blood glucose entries and thus motivate patients to improve blood glucose testing frequency resulting in better glucose control. Most glucose meter manufacturers are now planning to integrate insulin calculators with traditional blood glucose meters to help patients on multiple daily injections take their bolus insulin dose. Recently, FDA approved Accu-Check Aviva Expert glucose meter with built-in insulin advisor as it has shown to improve glycemic control and treatment satisfaction without increasing severe hypoglycemia in insulin requiring patients with diabetes [37].

Medication adherence

Medication non-adherence remains a common health problem resulting in about 50 % of medication related hospitalization and accounts for about $100 billion in health care costs [38]. Medication non-adherence is very common in people with diabetes resulting in poor glycemic control [39, 40]. Studies have shown that short message service (SMS) results in better medication adherence and have opened avenues for apps development [41, 42]. The advantages of using the adherence apps are simple to use and navigate, data storage, medication instruction, and features to download and print a medication chart [41, 42]. Most of the medication adherence apps like MyMedSchedule, My Meds, MedSimple, Medagenda, Pillmanager, Pill reminder, and RxmindMe Prescription cost little.

Digital health care information

The health care system is shifting to a value-based model. CMS launched the "electronic health record (EHR) financial incentive" program that mandates physicians to use EHR to document meaningful use [43]. With the increasing use of HER, which is Health Insurance Portability and Accountability Act (HIPAA) compliant, it has become possible to allow the patients to access their health records and communicate with the providers easily. It has been shown that patient access to personal health records has the potential to improve self-care and influence clinical decision-making. The large EHR systems in the USA: Kaiser Permanente (My Health manager), EPIC (My Chart), and VistA (U.S. Department of Veterans Affairs) have introduced an internet portal as well as apps to share health information with patients. Patient access of such systems has significantly reduced primary care office visits and telephone contacts [44]. Similarly, EMIS Access and Renal Patient View in the UK have been shown to reduce administration overload and secondary care [45].

Outcomes with the use of digital tools for diabetes self-management

The use of digital health tools has increased. Almost one third of U.S. smartphone owners were using health apps in 2014, and half of them were using fitness-related apps [46]. Despite an increase in the use of health-related apps, data is lacking on its benefits and cost-effectiveness. Small studies have shown better glucose control, improved SMBG frequencies, better patient satisfaction, moderate weight loss, and medication adherence with the use of digital tools [17, 20, 28, 36, 41, 47]. A recent review of a major electronic database for clinical trials including 16 randomized controlled trials with 3,578 adult participants with type 2 diabetes mellitus by Pal and colleagues showed small benefits on glycemic control (pooled effect on HbA1c: −0.2 %) with the use of computer-based diabetes self-management interventions. In a subgroup analysis on mobile phone–based interventions, they found a larger effect on A1c reduction (pooled effect on HbA1c was −0.50 %). Nevertheless, they did not find benefits of computer- or mobile-based interventions on improving depression, quality of life, or weight. In addition, the authors highlighted deficiencies such as selection bias and inadequate randomization procedure [48].

In addition, studies from developing countries are promising for the use of mobile or internet technologies for diabetes management [49–51]. A large randomized control trial showed that type 2 diabetes could be prevented by changing lifestyles with frequent short messages (SMS) tailored to change subject's behavior [49].

However, most of these studies are underpowered and of short duration. A recent large clinical trial randomized 151 patients with type 2 diabetes into a) the mobile phone-based self-management system [Few Touch Application (FTA); consists of blood glucose-measuring system with automatic wireless data transfer, diet manual, physical activity registration, and management of personal goals] b) FTA plus health counseling based on behavior change theory by a diabetes specialist nurse and c) control. The authors did not find a difference in HbA1c levels, self-management, health-related quality of life, depressive symptoms, or lifestyle changes between groups after the 1-year intervention [52]. In a review of 21 published studies from 2000 to 2010 by Holtz et al. that used mobile intervention for diabetes self-management, the authors concluded that most of these studies lacked a sufficient sample size or intervention length to determine whether the results are clinically meaningful. In addition, they also noted that the majority (95 %) of studies examined the use of mobile phones from a patient perspective [53]. Similarly, Baron and colleagues reviewed 20 published studies from 2002 to 2011 that investigated the clinical effectiveness of interventions requiring patients to transmit blood glucose (BG) readings to an online server via a mobile device. They concluded that evidences for effectiveness of mobile or online interventions for diabetes remains weak due to high variability between studies and methodological weaknesses [54].

Barriers to use digital tools for diabetes management

1) *Cost:* A potential barrier to any new medical technology is the cost. In addition, the use of apps requires the person to use an expensive smartphone and an internet data plan. Most payers do not cover the cost of having these devices or apps due to lack of conclusive data. Though diabetes is a major problem in developing countries, these technologies have not been used due to the higher cost of smartphone devices and Internet services. In addition, internet access may be another big problem in certain rural part of developing countries as well as developed countries such as USA [55].

2) *Insufficient scientific evidences:* Despite increased enthusiasm with the use of digital tools for diabetes self-management, the evidence for safety, efficacy, and cost-effectiveness of these tools are largely unknown. As described earlier, most of the studies on effectiveness of apps or internet-based tools for diabetes self-management were underpowered to see a meaningful and statistical difference and were of short duration [48, 49]. In addition, source information available on the blogs or through social media that are not regulated may not be scientific and may mislead patients. Similarly, most of the nutrition and physical activity related mobile apps have not been evaluated for the accuracy of information or measures. Large randomized controlled trials of long duration are necessary to establish the safety, efficacy, and cost-effectiveness of apps in diabetes self-management.

3) *Not useful in certain populations:* Most available apps may not be useful for the elderly, non-English speakers, physically challenged, and subjects from a lower socio-economical status.

4) *Data protection:* With the increasing use of EHR, digital tools, smart watches, and apps, we generate a large amount of data that is stored on servers. There are a few problems with sensitive data storage by the institutions or governments wanting to store health records or national records. If the data is collected in one country and stored on the server in other country, a whole different set of legal rules might be enforced. In addition, there is a growing controversy on who owns the data: patients or the device or software owner?

5) *Data security:* Certain devices such as an artificial pancreas (e.g. insulin pump, CGM and blood glucose meter) are connected via Bluetooth. Wireless communication can be intercepted by electromagnetic devices or hacked by cyber attackers [56]. This poses significant risks to a person using such devices for diabetes management.

6) *Regulatory barriers:* Although the use of digital tools is helpful in the self-management of diabetes, improper use of digital tools or technical issues with the algorithms or software can lead to undesirable side effects. For example, insulin dose calculator software is helpful for patients with diabetes to determine bolus insulin doses. The technical problem can result in higher insulin dose calculation and can result in severe hypoglycemia. Considering the increasing use of digital health and its potential harms, the FDA issued a guideline for app and health software developers [57]. As recommended by the FDA, any computer- or software-based devices (including apps) intended to be used for the electronic transfer, storage, display, and/or format conversion of medical device data is considered a Medical Device Data Systems (MDDS) and they are classified in three different classes [Class III being high-risk to Class I being low-risk] based on the potential risks of using the software or a digital tool [57]. It has been recommended for the software or device developer to follow the regulatory requirements such as Establishment registration, Medical Device listing, Quality System (QS) regulation, Labeling requirements, Medical Device Reporting, and Reporting Corrections and Removals depending on the device or software risk [57]. Similarly, the European Union has also issued regulatory framework for the mHealh [58].

Future of digital health for diabetes

Despite many barriers to overcome, the digital industry is growing at a fast pace. A $60 billion investment in digital health globally was made in 2013, and it is expected to reach $233 billion by 2020 [59]. Greater focus on digital health resulted in the U.S. government removing additional barriers for digital innovations (e.g. the introduction of the Healthcare Innovation and Marketplace Technologies Act [60]). Similarly, the FDA has also launched a "patient preference initiative" program to identify and develop methods for assessing patients' benefits and risks related to specific conditions providing further boosts to the digital health industry [61].

Currently, EHR systems are not interconnected. However, in future, all EHR systems will hopefully be integrated using a common platform. Similarly, the developers of the mobile apps or digital devices are interested in interconnecting their devices with other platforms. For example, Fitbit integrates with various apps.

Recent attempts have been made to develop mobile software that can calculate nutritional information for the patients based on their food intake. Frøisland developed and tested a mobile-phone-based tool to capture (DiaMob) and visualize adolescents' food intake aimed at understanding carbohydrate counting and to facilitate communication to daily treatment changes [17]. Implementing a visualization tool is an important contribution for young people to understand the basics of diabetes and to empower young people to define their treatment challenges. It empowers patients' independence and management of their disease.

Insulin pumps and continuous glucose monitors have significantly changed the treatment outcomes in insulin-requiring diabetic patients. Studies have shown that insulin pump and CGM (sensor augmented therapy) result in better glucose control, less hypoglycemia, and reduce glucose excursion [62]. Two controllers or receivers overwhelm many patients; therefore, Medtronic and Animas insulin pumps have integrated CGM data on insulin pumps. Nevertheless, patients still have to wear CGM and insulin pumps separately. The research is under way to a) to prolong life of continuous glucose monitors b) integrate CGM with an infusion set (Pod Talk and Medtronic in-Duo) and c) replace finger stick blood glucose monitoring to non invasive ways of glucose monitoring. Similarly, artificial pancreas development is going to integrate algorithms in apps so that patients will be able to operate an insulin pump and CGM via mobile devices to have better patient acceptance and experience.

Recently, a growing interest in developing videogames to change health behaviors has arisen due to their increased popularity among adults and youth. Such games can change health behaviors by providing information on healthy food and physical activity [63].

Research is underway to develop apps to remotely monitor a patient's health. For example, iExaminer is a small device that can be attached to an iPhone and take pictures of the retina, which can be transferred to the provider (http://www.welchallyn.com/en/microsites/iexaminer.html). Studies have shown that teleophthalmology is an effective model for improving eye care in underserved areas of developing countries [64].

Conclusion
There is much enthusiasm amongst industry and patients to use digital tools for diabetes self-management. Large randomized control trials are needed to establish the effectiveness and cost-benefits of digital tools in improving diabetes-related outcomes. Despite many challenges to overcome, the future of the digital health industry is promising.

Competing interests
The authors declare that they have no competing interests.

Authors' contributions
VNS, SKG conceived idea. VNS wrote first draft and SKG edited. Both authors contributed equally. Both authors read and approved the final manuscript.

Author details
[1]Barbara Davis Center for Diabetes, University of Colorado Denver, 1775 Aurora Court, A140, Aurora, CO 80045, USA. [2]School of Medicine, University of Colorado Denver, Aurora, CO, USA. [3]Diabetes Technology and Therapeutics, New Rochelle, USA.

References
1. IDF Diabetes Atlas Sixth Edition Poster Update 2014. Available at http://www.idf.org/diabetesatlas/update-2014. Accessed on April 27, 2015.
2. American Diabetes Association. Standards of medical care in diabetes—2015. Diabetes Care. 2015;38:S1–S90.
3. Nicoll KG, Ramser KL, Campbell JD, Suda KJ, Lee MD, Wood GC, et al. Sustainability of improved glycemic control after diabetes self-management education. Diabetes Spectrum. 2014;27(3):207–11.
4. Jornsay D L, Garnett E D. Diabetes Champions: Culture Change Through Education. Diabetes Spectrum 2014; 27:188-192.
5. Stewart AF. The United States endocrinology workforce: a supply–demand mismatch. J Clin Endocrinol Metab. 2008;93:1164–6.
6. Beck RW, Tamborlane WV, Bergenstal RM, Miller KM, DuBose SN, Hall CA. T1D Exchange Clinic Network The T1D Exchange clinic registry. J Clin Endocrinol Metab. 2012;97:4383–9.
7. Klonof DC. The current status of mHealth for diabetes: will it be next big thing? J Diabetes Sci Technol. 2013;7:749–58.
8. American Association of Diabetes Educators. AADE7 self-care behaviours. Diabetes Educ. 2008;34:445–9.
9. Brunisholz KD, Briot P, Hamilton S, Joy EA, Lomax M, Barton N, et al. Diabetes self-management education improves quality of care and clinical outcomes determined by a diabetes bundle measure. J Multidiscip Healthc. 2014;7:533–42.
10. Yuan C, Lai CW, Chan LW, Chow M, Law HK, Ying M. The effect of diabetes self-management education on body weight, glycemic control, and other metabolic markers in patients with type 2 diabetes mellitus. J Diabetes Res. 2014;2014:789761.
11. Tshiananga JK, Kocher S, Weber C, Erny-Albrecht K, Berndt K, Neeser K. The effect of nurse-led diabetes self-management education on glycosylated hemoglobin and cardiovascular risk factors: a meta-analysis. Diabetes Educ. 2012;38:108–23.
12. Johnson C, Feinglos M, Pereira K, Hassell N, Blascovich J, Nicollerat J, et al. Feasibility and preliminary effects of a virtual environment for adults with type 2 diabetes: pilot study. JMIR Res Protoc. 2014;3(2):e23.
13. Bell KJ, Barclay AW, Petocz P, Colagiuri S, Brand-Miller JC. Efficacy of carbohydrate counting in type 1 diabetes: a systematic review and meta-analysis. Lancet Diabetes Endocrinol. 2014;2:133–40.
14. Bergenstal RM1, Johnson M, Powers MA, Wynne A, Vlajnic A, Hollander P, et al. Adjust to target in type 2 diabetes: comparison of a simple algorithm with carbohydrate counting for adjustment of mealtime insulin glulisine. Diabetes Care. 2008;31:1305–10.
15. Pan'kowska E, Blazik M, Groele L. Does the fat-protein meal increase postprandial glucose level in type 1 diabetes patients on insulin pump: the conclusion of a randomized study. Diabetes Technol Ther. 2012;14:16–22.
16. Hartmann-Boyce J, Johns DJ, Jebb SA, Aveyard P, Behavioural Weight Management Review Group. Effect of behavioural techniques and delivery mode on effectiveness of weight management: systematic review, meta-analysis and meta-regression. Obes Rev. 2014;15:598–609.
17. Frøisland DH, Årsand E. Integrating visual dietary documentation in mobile-phone-based self-management application for adolescents with type 1 diabetes. J Diabetes Sci Technol. 2015;9:541–8.
18. Gross TM, Kayne D, King A, Rother C, Juth S. A Bolus Calculator Is an Effective Means of Controlling Postprandial Glycemia in Patients on Insulin Pump Therapy. Diabetes Technol Ther. 2003;5:365–9.
19. Schmidt S, Nørgaard K. Bolus calculators. J Diabetes Sci Technol. 2014;8:1035–41.
20. Rossi MC, Nicolucci A, Lucisano G, Pellegrini F, Di Bartolo P, Miselli V, et al. DID Study Group. Impact of the "Diabetes Interactive Diary" telemedicine system on metabolic control, risk of hypoglycemia, and quality of life: a randomized clinical trial in type 1 diabetes. Diabetes Technol Ther. 2013;15:670–9.
21. Kanakis SJ, Watts C, Leichter SB. The business of insulin pumps in diabetes care: clinical and economic considerations. Clinical Diabetes. 2002;20:214–6.
22. Centers for Disease Control and Prevention. Number (in Millions) of Civilian, Noninstitutionalized Persons with Diagnosed Diabetes, United States, 1980–2011. Available at http://www.cdc.gov/diabetes/statistics/prev/national/figpersons.htm Accessed on May 5, 2015.
23. U.S. Department of Health and Human Services. Physical Activity and Health: A Report of the Surgeon General. Centers for Disease Control and Prevention,

National Center for Chronic Disease Prevention and Health Promotion. Washington, DC: U.S. Govt. Printing Office; 1996.

24. Dengel DR, Kelly AS, Olson TP, Kaiser DR, Dengel JL, Bank AJ. Effects of weight loss on insulin sensitivity and arterial stiffness in overweight adults. Metabolism. 2006;55:907–11.

25. Burke LE, Warziski M, Starrett T, et al. Self-monitoring dietary intake: current and future practices. J Ren Nutr. 2005;15:281–90.

26. Jakicic JM. The role of physical activity in prevention and treatment of body weight gain in adults. J Nutr. 2002;132:3826S–29S.

27. Conroy DE, Yang CH, Maher JP. Behavior change techniques in top-ranked mobile apps for physical activity. Am J Prev Med. 2014;46:649–52.

28. Turner-McGrievy GM, Beets MW, Moore JB, Kaczynski AT, Barr-Anderson DJ, Tate DF. Comparison of traditional versus mobile app self-monitoring of physical activity and dietary intake among overweight adults participating in an mHealth weight loss program. J Am Med Inform Assoc. 2013;20:513–8.

29. Centers for Disease Control and Prevention. Increasing physical activity: a report on recommendations of the Task Force on Community Preventive Services. Morb Mortal Wkly Rep. 2001;50(RR18):1–14.

30. VanWormer JJ, Pronk NP. Rewarding change: principles for implementing worksite incentive programs. In: Pronk NP, editor. ACSM's worksite health handbook. 2nd ed. Champaign, IL: Human Kinetics; 2009. p. 239–47.

31. Giles EL, Robalino S, McColl E, Sniehotta FF, Adams J. The effectiveness of financial incentives for health behaviour change: systematic review and meta-analysis. PLoS One. 2014;9:e90347.

32. Sutherland K, Christianson JB, Leatherman S. Impact of targeted financial incentives on personal health behavior: a review of the literature. Med Care Res Rev. 2008;65(6 Suppl):36S–78S.

33. Garg SK, Hirsch IB. Self-monitoring of blood glucose. Diabetes Technol Ther. 2015;17 Suppl 1:S3–S11.

34. Spollett GR. Self-Monitoring of Blood Glucose: An Underutilized Tool. Clinical Diabetes. 2010;28:127–9.

35. Moser EG, Morris AA, Garg SK. Emerging diabetes therapies and technologies. Diabetes Res Clin Pract. 2012;97:16–26.

36. ShahV HW, Gottlieb P, Beatson C, Snell-Bergeon J, Garg S. Role Of Mobile Technology To Improve Diabetes Care In Adults With Type 1 Diabetes: The Remote-T1d Study. Diabetes Technol Ther. 2015;17:A25–6.

37. Ziegler R, Cavan DA, Cranston I, Barnard K, Ryder J, Vogel C, et al. Use of an insulin bolus advisor improves glycemic control in multiple daily insulin injection (MDI) therapy patients with suboptimal glycemic control: first results from the ABACUS trial. Diabetes Care. 2013;36:3613–9.

38. Osterberg L, Blaschke T. Adherence to medication. N Engl J Med. 2005;353:487–97.

39. Krass I, Schieback P, Dhippayom T. Adherence to diabetes medication: A systematic review. Diabetic Medicine 2014. doi:10.1111/dme.12651.

40. Egede LE, Gebregziabher M, Echols C, Lynch CP. Longitudinal effects of medication nonadherence on glycemic control. Ann Pharmacother. 2014;48:562–70.

41. Vervloet M, Linn AJ, van Weert JC, de Bakker DH, Bouvy ML, van Dijk L. The effectiveness of interventions using electronic reminders to improve adherence to chronic medication: a systematic review of the literature. J Am Med Inform Assoc. 2012;19:696–704.

42. Dayer L, Heldenbrand S, Anderson P, Gubbins PO, Martin BC. Smartphone medication adherence apps: potential benefits to patients and providers: response to Aungst. J Am Pharm Assoc. 2013;53:345.

43. Centers for Medicare, Medicaid Services (CMS), Office of the National Coordinator for Health Information Technology (ONC), HHS. Medicare and Medicaid programs; modifications to the Medicare and Medicaid Electronic Health Record (EHR) Incentive Program for 2014 and other changes to EHR Incentive Program; and health information technology: revision to the certified EHR technology definition and EHR certification changes related to standards. Final rule. Fed Regist. 2014;79(171):52909–33.

44. Zhou YY, Garrido T, Chin HL, et al. Patient access to an electronic health record with secure messaging: impact on primary care utilization. Am J Manag Care. 2007;13:418–24.

45. Wake DJ, Cunningham SG. Digital diabetes. British Journal of Diabetes and Vascular Disease. 2013;13:13–20.

46. Mobi health news. http://mobihealthnews.com/32183/nielsen-46-million-people-used-fitness-apps-in-january/. Accessed on May15,2015.

47. Overland J, Abousleiman J, Chronopoulos A, Leader N, Molyneaux L, Gilfillan C. Improving Self-Monitoring of Blood Glucose among Adults

with Type 1 Diabetes: Results of the Mobile™ Study. Diabetes Ther. 2014;5:557–65.

48. Pal K, Eastwood SV, Michie S, Farmer A, Barnard ML, Peacock R, et al. Computer-based interventions to improve self-management in adults with type 2 diabetes: a systematic review and meta-analysis. Diabetes Care. 2014;37:1759–66.

49. Ramachandran A, Snehalatha C, Ram J, Selvam S, Simon M, Nanditha A, et al. Effectiveness of mobile phone messaging in prevention of type 2 diabetes by lifestyle modification in men in India: a prospective, parallel-group, randomised controlled trial. Lancet Diabetes Endocrinol. 2013;1:191–8.

50. Bin Abbas B, Al Fares A, Jabbari M, El Dali A, Al OF. Effect of mobile phone short text messages on glycemic control in type 2 diabetes. Int J Endocrinol Metab. 2015;13:e18791.

51. Shariful Islam SM, Lechner A, Ferrari U, Seissler J, Holle R, Niessen LW. Mobile phone use and willingness to pay for SMS for diabetes in Bangladesh. J Public Health (Oxf). 2015 Feb 16. pii: fdv009. [Epub ahead of print]

52. Holmen H, Torbjørnsen A, Wahl AK, Jenum AK, Småstuen MC, Arsand E, et al. A Mobile Health Intervention for Self-Management and Lifestyle Change for Persons With Type 2 Diabetes, Part 2: One-Year Results From the Norwegian Randomized Controlled Trial; RENEWING HEALTH. JMIR Mhealth Uhealth. 2014;2:e57.

53. Holtz B, Lauckner C. Diabetes management via mobile phones: a systematic review. Telemed J E Health. 2012;18:175–84.

54. Baron J, McBain H, Newman S. The impact of mobile monitoring technologies on glycosylated hemoglobin in diabetes: a systematic review. J Diabetes Sci Technol. 2012;6:1185–96.

55. Smith A. Smartphone Ownership-2013 update. Washington DC. Pew Research Center; available at http://www.pewinternet.org/2013/06/05/smartphone-ownership-2013/ [accessed on August 21,2015]

56. O'Keeffe DT, Maraka S, Basu A, Keith-Hynes P, Kudva YC. Cybersecurity in Artificial Pancreas Experiments. Diabetes Technol Ther. 2015;17(9):664–6 [Epub ahead of print].

57. U.S. Food and Drug Administration. Draft guidance for industry and Food and Drug Administration staff, mobile medical applications. Available from http://www.fda.gov/downloads/MedicalDevices/DeviceRegulationandGuidance/GuidanceDocuments/UCM263366.pdf. Accessed May 5, 2015

58. European Commission. Green paper on mobile Health (mHealth). Available from http://ec.europa.eu/information_society/newsroom/cf/dae/document.cfm?doc_id=5147. Accessed on May 5, 2015.

59. Statista. http://www.statista.com/statistics/387867/value-of-worldwide-digital-health-market-forecast-by-segment/ Accessed on May 15,2015.

60. H.R.6626 - Health Care Innovation and Marketplace Technologies Act of 2012. https://www.congress.gov/bill/112th-congress/house-bill/6626. Accessed May 15, 2015.

61. FDA Voice. Listening to Patients' Views on New Treatments for Obesity. http://blogs.fda.gov/fdavoice/index.php/tag/patient-preferences-initiative/. Accessed May 15, 2015.

62. Shah VN, Shoskes A, Tawfik B, Garg SK. Closed-loop system in the management of diabetes: past, present, and future. Diabetes Technol Ther. 2014;16:477–90.

63. Kamel Boulos MN, Gammon S, Dixon MC, MacRury SM, Fergusson MJ, Miranda Rodrigues F, et al. Digital games for type 1 and type 2 diabetes: underpinning theory with three illustrative examples. JMIR Serious Games. 2015;3:e3.

64. Prathiba V, Rema M. Teleophthalmology: a model for eye care delivery in rural and underserved areas of India. Int J Family Med. 2011;2011:683267.

Diabetic retinopathy: research to clinical practice

Anjali R. Shah[1*] and Thomas W. Gardner[1,2]

Abstract

Background: Diabetic Retinopathy (DR) is a leading cause of visual impairment in the United States. The CDC estimates that the prevalence of DR will triple from 2005 to 2050.

Main body: The report summarizes major past advances in diabetes research and their impact on clinical practice. Current paradigms and future directions are also discussed.

Conclusions: DR is a leading cause of visual impairment in the US. Significant progress has been made in the understanding and treatment of DR, but rising prevalence demands innovative approaches to management in the future.

Keywords: Diabetic retinopathy

Background

Diabetic retinopathy (DR) is the ocular manifestation of end-organ damage in diabetes mellitus. Eduard Jaeger first described the visible retinal changes of DR in 1856, but the causal relationship between retinal exam findings and diabetes mellitus was controversial until 1875 when Leber confirmed the findings [1]. Today, DR is a leading cause of visual impairment in the United States. In 2005, 5.5 million people had diabetic retinopathy, and 1.2 million people had vision-threatening DR. Due, in large part, to the projected increase in prevalence of diabetes mellitus, the CDC projects that by 2050 those numbers will triple, to 16.0 million and 3.4 million, respectively (https://www.cdc.gov/visionhealth/publications/diabetic_retinopathy.htm). Fortunately, a better understanding of the risk factors contributing to the development of DR, the pathology of the disease, and its functional manifestations have allowed for significant advances in the prevention and treatment of diabetic retinopathy. This review presents the contributions of research to the clinical management of the disease in the past, discuss current paradigms on DR treatment and prevention, and demonstrate how today's research will contribute to improved outcomes in the future.

* Correspondence: arshah@med.umich.edu
[1]Departments of Ophthalmology and Visual Sciences, University of Michigan Medical Schoo, W.K. Kellogg Eye Center, 1000 Wall St, Ann Arbor, MI 48105, USA
Full list of author information is available at the end of the article

Diabetic retinopathy: Research to clinical practice—Past

Since the earliest description of DR, the vascular features of the disease have been predominant. Early drawings show intraretinal hemorrhages, vascular sheathing and lipid exudates throughout the retina. These findings were confirmed with histopathological specimens, such as the work of Arthur Ballantyne, who, in 1945, showed that capillary wall changes contributed to the development of DR [1]. Laboratory research on endothelial cell dysfunction and clinical observations using fluorescein angiography solidified the paradigm of DR as a vascular disease, and led to early suggestions of using light photocoagulation, or laser therapy, to treat retinopathy in the 1960s [2]. In 1968, the Airlie House Symposium brought prominent ophthalmologists and researchers in diabetic retinopathy together. It was during this meeting that a standard classification system for diabetic retinopathy was created, and the foundation was set for future large clinical trials.

The Diabetic Retinopathy Study (DRS) and Early Treatment of Diabetic Retinopathy Study (ETDRS), conducted in the 1970s and 1980s, respectively, demonstrated the considerable effects of laser treatment in eyes with proliferative retinopathy and macular edema. The DRS found that pan-retinal photocoagulation (PRP) inhibited the progression of retinopathy in patients with proliferative (neovascular) changes [3]. ETDRS defined

Diabetic Retinopathy

Timeline of Major Advances

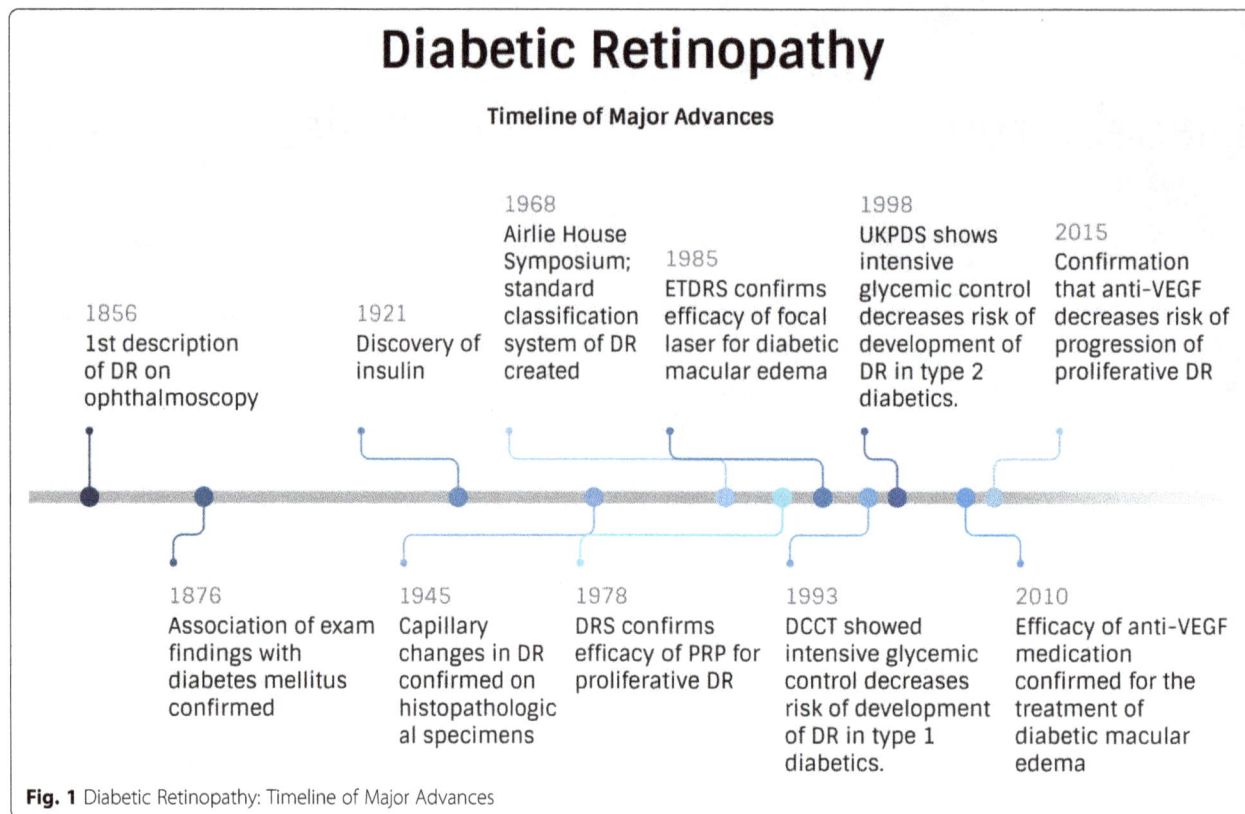

1856
1st description of DR on ophthalmoscopy

1921
Discovery of insulin

1968
Airlie House Symposium; standard classification system of DR created

1985
ETDRS confirms efficacy of focal laser for diabetic macular edema

1998
UKPDS shows intensive glycemic control decreases risk of development of DR in type 2 diabetics.

2015
Confirmation that anti-VEGF decreases risk of progression of proliferative DR

1876
Association of exam findings with diabetes mellitus confirmed

1945
Capillary changes in DR confirmed on histopathological specimens

1978
DRS confirms efficacy of PRP for proliferative DR

1993
DCCT showed intensive glycemic control decreases risk of development of DR in type 1 diabetics.

2010
Efficacy of anti-VEGF medication confirmed for the treatment of diabetic macular edema

Fig. 1 Diabetic Retinopathy: Timeline of Major Advances

"clinically significant macular edema" and demonstrated that focal photocoagulation significantly reduces the risk of vision loss from diabetic macular edema [4]. As a result of these landmark trials, PRP and focal laser became standard care for patients with advanced diabetic retinal disease in the 1980's, and, despite the success of intravitreal injection therapy, continue to be frequently performed procedures today. These studies also led to the development of guidelines and screening programs to allow timely detection and treatment of DR.

In addition to making strides in the treatment of diabetic retinopathy, the latter half of the twentieth century saw major advances in understanding the risk factors leading to development and progression of disease. The importance of tight metabolic control wasn't unequivocally demonstrated until 1993 when the Diabetes Control and Complications Trial (DCCT) followed type 1 diabetic patients with mild or no retinopathy for a mean of 6.5 years, and found that intensive insulin therapy reduced the adjusted mean risk for development of retinopathy by as much as 76% [5]. Similar results were noted in persons with type 2 diabetes by the United Kingdom Prospective Diabetes Study (UKPDS) Group; intensive control of blood sugar led to a significant 25% reduction in the risk of any microvascular complications, including retinopathy, nephropathy and neuropathy. Most of this decrease in risk, however, was attributed to

decreased need for laser in proliferative retinopathy. Overall, there was a 21% reduction in the risk of progression of DR [6].

The role of hypertension in the development and progression of diabetic complications was also demonstrated initially in 1998 by UKPDS [7]. Tight blood pressure control (defined as <150/85 mmHg) achieved a 34% reduction in the rate of progression of DR, independent of glycemic control after 7.5 years. These findings were subsequently supported by several studies showing that blood pressure management significantly reduces the risk of progression of DR [8, 9]. As a result of better systemic management of diabetes mellitus and hypertension, as well as the development of screening programs and improved, more timely treatment, the incidence of proliferative DR and/or diabetic macular has decreased significantly, especially in type 1 diabetics. From 1980 to 2007, the Wisconsin Epidemiologic Study of Diabetic Retinopathy (WESDR) showed a 77% decrease in the estimated annual incidence of proliferative DR among persons with type 1 diabetes, and the incidence of visual impairment due to diabetic retinopathy decreased by 57% in that same time period [10, 11]. The prevalence of DR in persons with type 2 diabetes aged 40 or older in WESDR (1980–1982) was 50%, and 35% in the Beaver Dam Eye Study (1988–1990), suggesting a substantial decrease in prevalence of DR during the interval 8 year period. This reduction may be attributed to better overall medical care of patients with diabetes [12].

The translation of research to clinical practice in the twentieth century is a story of great achievement—both for individuals suffering from diabetes and its complications, and on the public health front. In 1992, it was estimated that the Diabetic Retinopathy Study alone, which cost $10.5 million to conduct, generated a net savings of $2.89 billion to society in the first decade after the trial was completed [13].

Diabetic retinopathy: Research to clinical practice—Present

The success of clinical and epidemiological research of the 1970s, 80s and 90s encouraged further research into risk factors for development and progression of disease. In addition to hyperglycemia and hypertension, large randomized clinical trials showed the efficacy of lowering serum lipid levels. Notably, fenofibrate was shown to reduce the need for laser photocoagulation [9, 14]. In conjunction with simvastatin, fenofibrate reduced the risk of progression of non-proliferative retinopathy by one-third [9], though fenofibrate did not reduce cardiovascular risk [15]. Despite this sizable effect, fenofibrate therapy for DR has not become standard practice. Reasons for deferred incorporation of fenofibrate into routine clinical practice are unclear and likely multifactorial. In addition to a lack of clarity on when and how to use the medication, the lack of a commercial sponsor may also play a role. Additional risk factors for progression of DR discovered were the presence of nephropathy [16] and pregnancy [17]. Thus, comprehensive systemic care of persons with diabetes is required to achieve optimal vision.

Though focal laser and PRP reduce the risk of vision loss and DR progression, there are several limitations to photocoagulation. Laser is primarily a destructive procedure, such that PRP may impair peripheral vision, and decrease night vision [18]. In addition, focal laser seldom actually improves visual acuity [19]. Thus, more effective treatments for the early and late stages of DR are needed.

The paradigm of DR as a primarily vascular disease was pursued further. Several studies confirmed that neuro-inflammation plays a prominent role in the pathogenesis of DR [20–22]. Steroids, delivered intravitreally, are effective in improving vision in patients with diabetic macular edema, though they cause cataract development and increased intraocular pressure leading to glaucoma [23, 24]. Intravitreal steroids have also been suggested to reduce the rate of progression of DR to proliferative disease as well [25, 26].

Increased levels of inflammatory mediators ultimately lead to breakdown of the blood-retinal-barrier, increased vascular permeability, and angiogenesis via the release of cytokines and growth factors, including vascular endothelial growth factor (VEGF) [27–29]. The resulting new pharmacotherapeutic targets led to significant changes in the management of patients with DR, and the development of a new standard of care.

Several clinical trials showed the efficacy of intravitreal anti-VEGF medication in the treatment of diabetic macular edema [30–32]. These studies confirmed that administration of repeated monthly intravitreal ranibizumab injections (an anti-VEGF medication) plus prompt or deferred laser yielded a modestly greater improvement in visual acuity from baseline than laser alone with minimal side effects, leading to the adoption of a new standard of care in the treatment of diabetic macular edema. In addition, progression of DR can also be slowed in 25–30% of eyes treated for 2 years with the use of anti-VEGF medications [33]. It is interesting to note that despite the decrease in progression noted in 25–30% of treated eyes, the majority of patients did not demonstrate such positive effects. These results suggest that there are factors in addition to VEGF that likely mediate DR progression. A large randomized clinical trial showed that an average of nine intravitreal injections of ranibizumab was non-inferior to PRP at 2 years, with fewer patients who received ranibizumab requiring vitrectomy surgery over the study period [34].

Research on the role of inflammation in DR, and the subsequent increase in vascular permeability led to significant changes in the way patients have been managed in the past decade. Anti-VEGF therapy for diabetic macular edema has been shown in multiple randomized clinical trials to be more effective at improving vision than laser, and several cost-effectiveness analyses have confirmed the value of these treatments to patients and society [35, 36]. The efficacy of anti-VEGF treatment has also been proven in the treatment of proliferative DR and use of these medications in the management of this condition has increased, often as a first line treatment for complications of proliferative DR, such as vitreous hemorrhage. Other factors, however, have prevented wide-spread adoption of the practice as standard of care. For optimum results, anti-VEGF medications demand frequent administration—potentially indefinitely—resulting in concerns about the overall cost of treatment and the increased burden placed on physicians and patients by the need for frequent, consistent follow up to maintain treatment gains. Intravitreal anti-VEGF therapy does offer, though, a viable adjuvant or alternative treatment in many cases of proliferative disease [37]. Thus, we now have surgical (laser) and pharmacologic (anti-VEGF) options to treat DR and patients and many physicians tailor these approaches, using them separately or together, to optimize benefits and convenience. Figure 1 depicts the timeline of major advances in diabetic retinopathy research to date.

This significant progress in management of diabetic retinopathy was coupled with, and made possible by, important developments in ocular imaging [38]. Optical coherence tomography (OCT) is a non-invasive diagnostic test that is performed in the office, providing detailed cross-sectional anatomic images of the retina. In its widest application, OCT allows for early detection of anatomical changes in the macula, such as the development of thickening and cystic spaces noted in diabetic macular edema. OCT testing is routinely used to clinically diagnose and manage patients with diabetic macular edema, and data on central retinal thickness from the OCT is used as an end-point in large clinical trials [39]. Additional imaging techniques such as ultra-wide-field fundus photography and angiography allow better visualization of the peripheral retina than conventional cameras, and better identification of areas of poor vascular perfusion [40]. These imaging modalities help with clinical management of patients, and provide further insight into structural changes in every stage of DR.

Diabetic retinopathy: Research to clinical practice-future

The progress of the late 20th and early 21st centuries has been significant, allowing improved ability to delay development of DR, and to administer treatment that significantly reduces the risk of vision loss. However, the large projected increase in prevalence of DR, coupled with the need for frequent administration of intravitreal injections clearly indicates a need for alternative options in the future. In addition, current management strategies are either preventative (intensive glycemic and blood pressure control), or targeted towards advanced disease (diabetic macular edema, or proliferative DR). Yet, a growing body of literature suggests functional decline and associated health-related quality of life reductions in earlier stages of DR [41]. Visual dysfunction in the form of decreased sensitivity on visual field testing and diminished photoreceptor function as measured by electroretinogram have been reported prior to the development of vascular lesions [42, 43].

Thus, the paradigm on DR has changed. Alterations in the neurosensory retina, undetectable by ophthalmoscopy, are recognized as important early contributors to visual decline, and it is now established that neurosensory degeneration may precede visible vascular changes, or occur alongside them [44]. That is, the entire neurovascular unit, comprised of vascular, glial, microglial and neuronal cells, is compromised by diabetes [45]. When the neurovascular unit is no longer intact and adaptive processes fail after years of uncontrolled diabetes, the states of diabetic macular edema and proliferative retinopathy represent "retinal failure," equivalent to renal failure [46]. Current treatments of anti-VEGF and lasers address these late stages of disease, but only fenofibrate,

blood pressure and metabolic control have shown demonstrable effects in the pre-failure stages.

Laboratory research confirms that metabolic pathways triggered by hyperglycemia, insulin deficiency [47] and dyslipidemia [48] lead to abnormalities in both the neural retina as well as the retinal capillary bed. A better understanding of all the molecular players in these pathways has produced several potential pharmacotherapeutic targets for DR, which includes both the inhibition of mediators of neural damage, and enhancement of agents that may be neuroprotective. Hernández et al. [49] recently provided a thorough review of potential new therapeutics based on pathogenic mechanisms of DR, much of which is summarized in Table 1.

In addition to finding new targets to treat earlier stages of DR, research is being conducted using nanoparticles to allow for sustained delivery of drug, as well as alternative (topical) drug delivery systems. Nanotechnology is currently being applied to anti-VEGF medications, and several other new mediators of inflammation and angiogenesis. Nanoparticles are particularly designed to cross the blood-retinal barrier, thereby allowing for better penetration into the retina [50]. These methods remain under development and clinical application appears to remain in the future for DR.

If treating DR in earlier stages is to truly become a common clinical practice, though, new diagnostic techniques are needed to identify changes before they are visible on exam and to track response to treatment. Circulating biomarkers and new imaging modalities are being investigated to use as clinical indicators and new endpoints for clinical trials. Inflammatory cytokines are most often reported as circulating biomarkers associated with early DR. Three inflammatory mediators in particular: interleukin 6 (IL-6), tumor necrosis factor α (TNF-α), and C-reactive protein (CRP), when combined in a z-score, are associated with development of retinopathy, nephropathy and cardiovascular disease in diabetics [51]. Inflammatory and vasoactive mediators produced and measured locally, in intraocular fluids, have also been identified. An increase in glial fibrillary acidic protein (GFAP), for example, is noted in the aqueous humor of patients with diabetes and no signs of DR or with non-proliferative DR compared to age-matched healthy controls [52]. Challenges remain, however, in finding biomarkers specific to DR that are also easily/non-invasively measured. As such, new imaging techniques combined with a better understanding of biomarkers is promising for developing better diagnostic tools for early disease. Frimmel et al. recently reported a technique in which imaging probes were developed to target a specific endothelial surface molecule known to participate in breakdown of the blood-retinal barrier in DR (ICAM-1). This probe

Table 1 Potential Therapeutics for Diabetic Retinopathy

Target	Role	Current Status	Concerns
Somatostatin	Neuroprotective, antiangiogenic. Downregulated in retinas of diabetics, associated with retinal neurodegeneration [54].	Recently completed multi-center phase II-III trial (EUROCONDOR) to assess the safety of topically administered somatostatin. (EudraCT Number: 2012–001200-38) Results have yet to be published.	
Glucagon-like peptide (GLP-1)	Neuroprotective [55]	Intravitreal injections of exedin-4 (a GLP-1 analogue) prevent ERG abnormalities in rats with streptozotoin-induced diabetes [56]. Topical administration of GLP-1R agonists prevents retinal neurodegeneration in mice with diabetes [57].	2 large clinical trials of GLP-1 analogues in type 2 diabetics with high cardiovascular risk (LEADER and SUSTAIN-6) have shown neutral benefit [58] or even worsening of DR compared to placebo [59]. However, these studies were not designed to assess progression of DR.
Doxycycline	Anti-inflammatory and neuroprotective [60]	Low-dose oral doxycycline improves inner retinal function in DR compared to placebo [61].	Although statistical significance was achieved at multiple time points, it was a small, proof-of-concept trial.
Interleukin 1β (IL-1β)	Inflammatory cytokine	Systemic IL-1β inhibition has been shown to stabilize retinal neovascular changes in proliferative DR and reduce macular edema [62].	Open-label, small, prospective pilot study. Reduction in macular edema was not statistically significant.
Tumor necrosis factor α (TNF-α)	Inflammatory, induces vascular changes	Intravitreal injection of TNF-α inhibitor decreased capillary degeneration in diabetic rats [63].	Very small study in rats, with other primary endpoints.

allowed for visualization of the expression of ICAM-1 on the endothelial surface in vivo in rats. Increased visibility of the probe was noted on imaging from diabetic animals compared to controls [53], suggesting that synergistic development of biomarkers and imaging technology will allow for detection of early DR in the future.

A projected tripling in the prevalence of DR in the next several decades, however, cannot be effectively managed with new diagnostic and treatment options alone. Changes in health care delivery paradigms will also be required. Similar to the recent shift towards team-based approaches for cancer, diabetes will need to be approached in a more comprehensive manner. Close collaboration between ophthalmologists, endocrinologists, nephrologists, nutritionists, social workers, and all others involved in the care of a diabetic patient will be imperative for an efficient use of community and health system resources, and to optimize outcomes for individual patients.

Conclusion

The immense improvements in the care of patients with diabetes and DR over the past 50 years are an example of the significant impact laboratory and clinical research can make on the management of chronic systemic illness. Despite great advances, though, the projected increase in the number of patients with DR in the coming decades reminds us that there is still progress to be made. Current research leading to a better understanding of molecular pathways, development of novel therapeutic targets, and use of nanotechnology, coupled with constantly improving diagnostic and imaging technology and collaborative health care delivery systems, promises to further our ability to enhance and maintain vision in diabetic patients.

Abbreviations
CRP: C-reactive protein; DCCT: Diabetes Control and Complications Trial; DR: Diabetic retinopathy; GFAP: Glial fibrillary acidic protein; GLP-1: Glucagon-like peptide; IL-1β: Interleukin 1β; IL-6: Interleukin 6 (IL-6); OCT: Optical coherence tomography; PRP: Pan-retinal photocoagulation; TNF-α: Tumor necrosis factor α; UKPDS: United Kingdom Prospective Diabetes Study; VEGF: Vascular endothelial growth factor; WESDR: Wisconsin Epidemiologic Study of Diabetic Retinopathy

Funding
R01EY20582, R24DK082841, The Taubman Institute and Research to Prevent Blindness.

Authors' contributions
AS and TG both contributed to authorship of this manuscript. All authors read and approved the final manuscript.

Competing interests
The authors declare no competing interests.

Author details
[1]Departments of Ophthalmology and Visual Sciences, University of Michigan Medical Schoo, W.K. Kellogg Eye Center, 1000 Wall St, Ann Arbor, MI 48105, USA. [2]Molecular and Integrative Physiology, University of Michigan Medical School, W.K. Kellogg Eye Center, 1000 Wall St, Ann Arbor, MI 48105, USA.

References
1. Wolfensberger TJ, Hamilton AM. Diabetic retinopathy—an historical review. Semin Ophthalmol. 2001;17:2–7.
2. Wetzig PC, Worlton JT. Treatment of diabetic retinopathy by light coagulation. Br J Ophthalmol. 1963;47(9):539–41.

3. Photocoagulation treatment of proliferative diabetic retinopathy. The second report of the diabetic retinopathy study findings. Ophthalmology. 1978;85:82–105.

4. Photocoagulation for diabetic macular edema. Early treatment of diabetic retinopathy study report number 1. Arch Ophthalmol. 1985;103:1796–806.

5. The Diabetes Control and Complications Trial Research Group. The effect of intensive treatment of diabetes on the development and progression of long-term complications in insulin-dependent diabetes mellitus. N Engl J Med. 1993;329:977–86.

6. UK Prospective Diabetes Study (UKPDS) Group. Intensive blood-glucose control with sulphonylureas or insulin compared with conventional treatment and risk of complications in patients with type 2 diabetes (UKPDS 33). Lancet. 1998;352:837–53. (Erratum Lancet 1999; 354:602)

7. UK Prospective Diabetes Study Group. Tight blood pressure control and risk of macrovascular and microvascular complications in type 2 diabetes: UKPDS 38. BMJ. 1998;317(7160):703–13. (Erratum BMJ 1999: 318(7175): 29)

8. Leske MC, Wu S-Y, Hennis A, Hyman L, et al. Barbados eye study group hyperglycemia, blood pressure, and the 9-year incidence of diabetic retinopathy: the Barbados eye studies. Ophthalmology. 2005;112:799–805.

9. ACCORD Study Group, ACCORD Eye Study Group. Effects of medical therapies on retinopathy progression in type 2 diabetes. N Engl J Med. 2010;363:233–44.

10. Klein R, Klein BE. Are individuals with diabetes seeing better? A long term epidemiological perspective. Diabetes. 2010;59:1853–60.

11. Klein R, Lee KE, Gangnon RE, Klein BE. The 25-year incidence of visual impairment in type 1 diabetes mellitus: the Wisconsin epidemiologic study of diabetic retinopathy. Ophthalmology. 2010;117:63–70.

12. The Eye Diseases Prevalence Research Group. The prevalence of diabetic retinopathy among adults in the United States. Arch Ophthalmol. 2004; 122(4):552–63.

13. Drummond MF, Davies LM, Frederick III. FL; assessing the costs and benefits of medical research: the diabetic retinopathy study. Soc Sci Med. 1992;34(9): 973–81.

14. FIELD Study Investigators. Effect of fenofibrate on the need for laser treatment for diabetic retinopathy (FIELD study); a randomized controlled trial. Lancet. 2007;370:1687–97.

15. Mitka M. Aggressive lipid, hypertension targeting yields no benefit for some with diabetes. JAMA. 2010;303(17):1681–3.

16. Estacio RO, McGarling E, Biggerstaff S, Jeffers BW, et al. Overt albuminuria predicts diabetic retinopathy in Hispanics with NIDDM. Am J Kidney Dis. 1998;31:947–53.

17. Diabetes Control and Complications Trial Research Group. Effect of pregnancy on microvascular complications in the diabetes control and complications trial. Diabetes Care. 2000;23:1084–91.

18. Writing Committee for the Diabetic Retinopathy Clinical Research Network, Gross JG, Glassman AR, et al. Panretinal photocoagulation vs intravitreous ranibizumab for proliferative diabetic retinopathy: a randomized clinical trial. JAMA. 2015;314:2137–46.

19. Diabetic Retinopathy Clinical Research Network, Elman MJ, Aiello LP, Beck RW, et al. Randomized trial evaluating ranibizumab plus prompt or deferred laser for diabetic macular edema. Ophthalmology. 2010;117:1064–77.

20. Adamis AP. Is diabetic retinopathy an inflammatory disease? Br J Ophthalmol. 2002;86:363–5.

21. Kern TS. Contributions of inflammatory processes to the development of the early stages of diabetic retinopathy. Exp Diabetes Res. 2007;2007:95103.

22. Tang J, Kern TS. Inflammation in diabetic retinopathy. Prog Retin Eye Res. 2011;30(5):343–58.

23. Diabetic Retinopathy Clinical Research Network. A randomized trial comparing intravitreal triamcinolone acetonide and focal/grid photocoagulation for diabetic macular edema. Ophthalmology. 2008;115(9): 1447–9.

24. Haller JA, Kuppermann BD, Blumenkranz MS, Williams GA, Weinberg DV, Chou C, Whitcup SM. Randomized controlled trial of an Intravitreous Dexamethasone drug delivery system in patients with diabetic macular edema. Arch Ophthalmol. 2010;128(3):289–96.

25. Bressler NM, Edwards AR, Beck RW, Flaxel CJ, Glassman AR, Ip MS, Kollman C, Kuppermann BD, Stone TW. Diabetic retinopathy clinical research network. Exploratory analysis of diabetic retinopathy progression through 3 years in a randomized clinical trial that compares Intravitreal Triamcinolone

Acetonide with focal/grid photocoagulation. Arch Ophthalmol. 2009; 127(12):1566–71.

26. Wykoff CC, Chakravarthy U, Camochiaro PA, et al. Long term effects of intravitreal 0.19 mg fluocinolone acetonide implant on progression and regression of diabetic retinopathy. Ophthalmology. 2017;124(4):440–9.

27. Rangasamy S, McGuire PG, Franco Nitta C, Monickaraj F, Oruganti SR, Das A. Chemokine mediated monocyte trafficking in to the retina, role of inflammation in alteration of the blood-retinal barrier in diabetic retinopathy. PLoS One. 2014;9(10):e10858.

28. Vujosevic S, Simó R. Local and systemic inflammatory biomarkers of diabetic retinopathy: an integrative approach. Invest Ophthalmol Vis Sci. 2017;58(6): BIO68–75.

29. Abcouwer SF. Angiogenic factors and cytokines in diabetic retinopathy. Journal of clinical & cellular immunology. 2013;1(11):1–12.

30. Diabetic Retinopathy Clinical Research Network, Elman MJ, Aiello LP, et al. Randomized trial evaluating ranibizumab plus prompt or deferred laser or triamcinolone plus prompt laser for diabetic macular edema. Ophthalmology. 2010;117:1064–7.

31. Mitchell P, Bandello F, Schmidt-Erfurth U, RESTORE Study Group, et al. The RESTORE study: ranibizumab monotherapy or combined with laser versus laser monotherapy for diabetic macular edema. Ophthalmology. 2011;118:618–25.

32. Nguyen QD, Brown DM, Marcus DM, RISE and RIDE Research Group, et al. Ranibizumab for diabetic macular edema: results from 2 phase III randomized trials: RISE and RIDE. Ophthalmology. 2012;119:789–801.

33. Bressler SB, Liu D, Glassman AR, Blodi BA, Castellarin AA, Jampol LM, Kaufman PL, Melia M, Singh H, Wells JA. For the diabetic retinopathy clinical research network. Change in diabetic retinopathy through 2 YearsSecondary analysis of a randomized clinical trial comparing Aflibercept, Bevacizumab, and Ranibizumab. JAMA Ophthalmol. 2017;135(6):558–68.

34. Writing Committee for the Diabetic Retinopathy Clinical Research Network. Panretinal photocoagulation vs Intravitreous Ranibizumab for proliferative diabetic retinopathy. A randomized clinical trial. JAMA. 2015;314(20):2137–46.

35. Haig J, Barbeau M, Ferreira A. Cost-effectiveness of ranibizumab in the treatment of visual impairment due to diabetic macular edema. J Med Econ. 2016;19:663–71.

36. Brown GC, Brown MM, Turpcu A, Rajput Y. The cost-effectiveness of ranibizumab for the treatment of diabetic macular edema. Ophthalmology. 2015;122:1416–25.

37. Solomon SD, Chew E, Duh EJ, Sobrin L, Sun JK, Vanderbeek BL, Wykoff CC, Gardner TW. Diabetic retinopathy: a position statement by the American Diabetes Association. Diabetes Care. 2017;40:412–8.

38. Cohen SR, Gardner TW. Diabetic retinopathy and diabetic macular edema. Dev Ophthalmol. 2016;55:137–46.

39. Virgili G, Menchini F, Murro V, Peluso E, Rosa F, Casazza G. Optical coherence tomography (OCT) for detection of macular oedema in patients with diabetic retinopathy. Cochrane Database Syst Rev. 2011;2011(7): CD008081.

40. Silva PS, Cavallerano JD, NMN H, Tolls D, Thakore K, Patel B, Sehizadeh M, Tolson AM, Sun JK, Aiello LP. Comparison of nondiabetic retinal findings identified with Nonmydriatic Fundus photography vs Ultrawide field imaging in an ocular Telehealth program. JAMA Ophthalmol. 2016;134(3): 330–4.

41. Mazhar K, Varma R, Choudhury F, Los Angeles Latino Eye Study Group, et al. Severity of diabetic retinopathy and health-related quality of life: the Los Angeles Latino eye study. Ophthalmology. 2011;118:649–55.

42. Jackson GR, Barber AJ. Visual dysfunction associated with diabetic retinopathy. Curr Diab Rep. 2010;10:380.

43. Jackson JR, Scott IU, Quillen DA WL, Hershey ME, Gardner TW. Inner retinal visual dysfunction is a sensitive marker of nonproliferative diabetic retinopathy. Br J Ophthalmol. 2012;96(5):699–703.

44. Sohn EH, van Dijk HW, Jiao C, et al. Retinal neurodegeneration may precede microvascular changes characteristic of diabetic retinopathy in diabetes mellitus. Proc Natl Acad Sci U S A. 2016;113(19):E2655–64. doi:10.1073/pnas. 1522014113.

45. Gardner TW, Davila JR. The neurovascular unit and the pathophysiologic basis of diabetic retinopathy. Graefes Arch Clin Exp Ophthalmol. 2017;255:1–6.

46. Gray EJ, Gardner TW. Retinal Failure in Diabetes: a Feature of Retinal Sensory Neuropathy. Curr Diab Rep. 2015;15:107.

47. Fort PE, Losiewicz MK, Reiter CEN, et al. Differential roles of hyperglycemia and Hypoinsulinemia in diabetes induced retinal cell death: evidence for retinal insulin resistance. Lo ACY, ed. PLoS One. 2011;6(10):e26498. 10.1371/journal.pone.0026498.

48. Sas KM, Kayampilly P, Byun J, et al. Tissue-specific metabolic reprogramming drives nutrient flux in diabetic complications. JCI Insight. 2016;1(15):e86976.

49. Hernández C, Simó-Servat A, Bogdanov P, et al. Diabetic retinopathy: new therapeutic perspectives based on pathogenic mechanisms. J Endocrinol Investig. 2017). ePub ahead of print; doi:10.1007/s40618-017-0648-4.

50. Campos EJ, Campos A, Martins J, Ambrósio AF. Opening eyes to nanomedicine: where we are, challenges and expectations on nanotherapy for diabetic retinopathy. Nanomedicine. 2017;13(6):2101–13.

51. Schram MT, Chaturvedi N, Schalkwijk CG, et al. Diabetologia. 2005;48:370–8.

52. Vujosevic S, Micera A, Bini S, Berton M, Esposito G, Midena E. Aqueous humor biomarkers of Müller cell activation in diabetic eyes. Invest Ophthalmol Vis Sci. 2015;56:3913–8.

53. Frimmel S, Zandi S, Sun D, et al. Molecular imaging of retinal endothelial injury in diabetic animals. Journal of Ophthalmic & Vision Research. 2017; 12(2):175–82.

54. Carrasco E, Hernández C, Miralles A, Huguet P, Farrés J, Simó R. Lower somatostatin expression is an early event in diabetic retinopathy and is associated with retinal neurodegeneration. Diabetes Care. 2007;30(100):2902–8.

55. Hölscher C. Potential role of glucagon-like peptide (GLP-1) in neuroprotection. CNS Drugs. 2012;26:871–82.

56. Zhang Y, Zhang J, Wang Q, Lei X, Chu Q, Xu GT, Ye W. Intravitreal injection of Exendin-4 analogue protects retinal cells in early diabetic rats. Invest Ophthalmol Vis Sci. 2011;52(1):278–85.

57. Hernández C, Bogdanov P, Corraliza L, García-Ramírez M, Solà-Adell C, Arranz JA, Arroba AI, Valverde A, Simó R. Topical administration of GLP-1 receptor agonists revents retinal neurodegeneration in experimental diabetes. Diabetes. 2016;65:172–87.

58. Marso SP, Daniels GH, Brown-Frandsen K, Kristensen P, Mann JF, Nauck MA, et al. LEADER steering committee, LEADER trial investigators. N Engl J Med. 2016;375(4):311–22.

59. Marso SP, Bain SC, Consoli A, Eliaschewitz FG, Jódar E, Leiter LA, et al. SUSTAIN-6 investigators. Semaglutide and cardiovascular outcomes in patients with type 2 diabetes. N Engl J Med. 2016;375:1834–44.

60. Federici TJ. The non-antibiotic properties of tetracyclines: clinical potential in ophthalmic disease. Pharmacol Res. 2011;64:614–23.

61. Scott IU, Jackson GR, Quillen DA, Klein R, Liao J, Gardner TW. Effect of Doxycycline vs placebo on retinal function and diabetic retinopathy progression in mild to moderate nonproliferative diabetic RetinopathyA randomized proof-of-concept clinical trial. JAMA Ophthalmol. 2014;132(9): 1137–42.

62. Stahel M, Becker M, Graf N, Michaels S. Systemic interleukin 1β inhibition in proliferative diabetic retinopathy: a prospective open-label study using Canakinumab. Retina. 2016;36(2):385–91.

63. Behl Y, Krothapalli P, Desta T, Roy S, Graves DT. FOXO1 plays an important role in enhanced microvascular cell apoptosis and micovascular cell loss in type 1 and type 2 diabetic rats. Diabetes. 2009;58:917–25.

18

Weight loss and bone mineral density in obese adults: a longitudinal analysis of the influence of very low energy diets

Palak Choksi[1]* ⓘ, Amy Rothberg[1,4], Andrew Kraftson[1], Nicole Miller[1], Katherine Zurales[1], Charles Burant[1,2,4], Catherine Van Poznak[1] and Mark Peterson[3]

Abstract

Background: The long-term effect of weight reduction on skeletal health is not well understood. The purpose of this study was to examine the impact of an intensive medical weight loss intervention using very low energy diet (VLED) (~ 800 cal/day) that result in significant changes in body weight, on total body bone mineral density (BMD) over 2 years.

Methods: We examined the impact of VLED-induced weight loss on BMD and FFM (Fat-free Mass) after 3–6 months and again while in weight maintenance at 2 years in 49 subjects. The effects of absolute and relative rate of weight reduction assessed by change in weight in kilograms were assessed using general linear modeling, with baseline BMD (or FFM) as a covariate, and age, sex and changes in body weight as primary model predictors.

Results: At the end of 2 years, the average weight loss was greater for men (weight: 23.51 ± 12.5 kg) than women (weight: 16.8 ± 19.2 kg) and BMD loss was greater among women (0.03 ± 0.04 g/cm^2 vs 0.01 ± 0.04 g/cm^2) (all $p < 0.05$). After adjusting for baseline BMD, age, and sex, there was a small but significant association between total weight loss and 2-year BMD (β = − 0.001 g/cm^2; $p = 0.01$). Similarly, there was a significant independent association between total weight loss and 2-year FFM (β = − 116.5 g; $p < 0.01$).

Conclusions: Despite significant weight loss with VLED, there was only a small loss is BMD.

Keywords: Bone density, DXA, Weight loss, Obesity, Very low energy diets

Background

Among Americans aged 20 years and older, the prevalence of obesity is approximately 35%. Obesity contributes to morbidity and mortality [1]. By 2030, the total healthcare costs attributed to obesity may reach as much as $957 billion [2]. Despite addressing many of the associated co-morbid conditions of obesity, little attention has been paid to the potentially long-term effects of weight change on bone health. Although bone loss is known to occur following bariatric surgeries, little is known about the effects of diet-induced weight loss, and specifically weight loss achieved by a very-low energy diets (VLED).

Bone strength adapts to meet demands of musculoskeletal loading, and therefore, body weight is one of the strongest predictors of bone mineral density (BMD) [3]. Mechanical stimulation of bone leads to osteoblast proliferation, and conversely, reduction in mechanical loading can cause an increase in bone turnover [4]. Lean body mass and fat mass are both independent positive determinants of bone mass, and although BMD may be higher among obese individuals, BMD per unit of BMI is lower and not necessarily protective from the risk of fractures [5, 6]. Excess weight due to adiposity is detrimental to bone, and therefore, obesity itself may predict fractures [7]. Clinical opinions and research pertaining to the impact of weight loss on the bone has been inconclusive. Short-term, longitudinal studies have shown that weight loss achieved through energy restriction can result in an increase in bone turnover that is sustained

* Correspondence: palak@med.umich.edu
[1]Department of Internal Medicine, University of Michigan, 24 Frank Lloyd Wright Dr, Ann Arbor, MI 48106, USA
Full list of author information is available at the end of the article

even during weight maintenance [8, 9]. In addition to BMD, bone turnover markers are thought to predict fracture risk [10]. The long-term effects of VLED on BMD and bone turnover markers following weight loss are yet to be identified.

Very-low energy diets are those that contain ≤800 cal per day, and provide essential daily nutritional requirements. VLEDs have become increasing popular in medically-supervised weight reduction programs for short durations (e.g., 8–12 weeks), with typical weight losses of 1.5–2.5 kg/week, or 18–20% after 8–12 weeks [11, 12]. When incorporated as part of an intensive, behavioral lifestyle program, the majority of VLED induced weight loss can be sustained long-term [11]. This approach offers a less costly, less invasive and practical alternative to endoluminal and surgical approaches.

Due to the growing obesity prevalence, dietary strategies that restrict calories have shown utility for improving metabolic health and health-related quality-of-life [13]. However, the long-term effect of weight reduction on skeletal health is not well understood. The primary objective of our study was to determine the longitudinal association between VLED-induced weight loss on whole body BMD. In addition, we examined whether weight loss influenced an important bone turnover marker.

Methods

Design

We included adults who were enrolled in and completed a 2-year weight management program. All participants provided written informed consent and the study protocol was reviewed and approved by the University of Michigan Institutional Review Board. The trial is registered at Clinicaltrials.gov (NCT02043457). The University of Michigan Weight Management Program (MWMP) is a 2-year, multidisciplinary, multicomponent, obesity management program, and has been previously described in detail [13]. Briefly, participants consume a VLED in the form of total meal replacements and are asked to increase physical activity from low to moderate intensity for 40 min per day. Each meal replacement shake contained 160 kcal, 14 g of protein, 23 g of carbohydrates and were fortified with calcium, multiple vitamins including vitamin D. In addition, all participants were prescribed a multivitamin and Vitamin D3 2000 IU daily. After 3 to 6 months, participants were transitioned to regular foods and asked to increase physical activity to moderate-vigorous for 40–60 min per day. Thereafter, the intervention was focused on behavioral and pharmacologic strategies to prevent weight regain. An individualized diet plan comprised of approximately 1200–1800 kcal/day was designed, implemented and titrated to maintain the individual's reduced weight. A registered dietitian evaluated participants weekly for one month

and then monthly for the remainder of the two years. The physician saw participants monthly for three months and then every three months for the rest of the two years. Participants underwent whole body DXA scanning on a (GE Lunar prodigy Advance; Control serial number 070401531487; control model number 7635) by a trained research technician at baseline, after transition to weight maintenance at approximately 6 months, and at the end of the 2-year program. In addition, serum for bone turnover markers was collected to assess the impact of weight loss on bone resorption.

Study participants

The program was designed for obese (BMI ≥30 kg/m^2 [or ≥27 kg/m^2 in Asian Americans]) adults ≥18 years of age. Participants in the program were representative of the demographic of southeastern Michigan, primarily Non-Hispanic whites, educated and employed. The clinic was founded on the principles of the National Heart Lung and Blood Institute (NHLBI) report that addressed long-term weight management for obese individuals (available at https://www.ncbi.nlm.nih.gov/pubmed/24961824) [14]. Participants were excluded if they had unstable psychiatric disorders requiring frequent changes in medications, cancer within the last 5 years (other than non-melanomatous skin cancers), active gallbladder or chronic kidney disease with eGFR ≤35 ml/min, and/or prior bariatric surgery.

Demographic, clinical and metabolic data were collected and entered into a database. This data included participant's anthropometric, co-morbid health conditions, medications, laboratory, biopsychosocial and imaging data that was updated after each visit.

Primary outcomes

Morphological Assessment: Whole body BMD, total adiposity assessed as total fat mass (FM) and percent body fat (%BF) were measured by dual-energy X-ray absorptiometry in the Michigan Clinical Research Unit. Determination of FFM was performed for the whole body as a part of the DXA scan. DXA allows for precise assessment of FFM, comprised of fat-free soft tissue and BMD.

Biochemical analyses: Serum cross-linked C-telopeptide (CTX) was collected at baseline, after weight loss between 3 and 6 months, and at the end of the 2-year program for n = 25 subjects (selected based on available fasting samples). All blood samples were collected into (2 ml tubes containing EDTA following a 12 h overnight fast to reduce variation associated with circadian rhythms and feeding [15]. The tests were analyzed at the University of Michigan, Michigan Diabetes Research Center (MDRC) Chemistry laboratory. Serum CTX levels were measured by enzyme-linked immunosorbent assay (ELISA). CTX assessments were done in duplicate and all assays were performed in a single run to eliminate interassay variability. The detection limits of this assay were 25–800 ng/ml, and inter and intraassay precision (Coefficients of variation) for CTX assays were < 15%).

Statistical analysis

Descriptive statistics were used to explore the distribution, central tendency, and variation of each measurement, with an emphasis on graphical methods such as histograms, scatterplots, and boxplots. Descriptive statistics for all demographic and morphologic characteristics were reported at baseline, after short-term weight loss, and at the 2-year time point, as change from baseline. Multiple linear regression analyses with post-intervention outcomes as the dependent variable were used to assess the role of weight loss on change in total body BMD and FFM. All models included baseline morphologic characteristics for muscle, BMD and FFM. For the primary aim, age and weight loss were included as continuous predictors of 2-year BMD and FFM. Several interaction terms were tested to determine the mediating effect of age and sex, on changes in muscle, BMD and FFM. Regression assumptions were checked and appropriate transformations (e.g., log) performed if necessary.

For the sub-analysis, we used a multiple linear regression approach to evaluate the association between changes in body weight, BMD, FFM and changes in serum CTX. Due to the smaller sample of adults with complete morphological and serum data ($n = 25$), models included only age as a covariate, and a change score for body weight, BMD, FFM as predictors of change in serum CTX.

Results

Forty-nine participants completed both the induction and maintenance phase and had complete DXA scans available at baseline, at 3–6 months and at the end of 2 years. At the end of two years, all participants had significant changes in body weight, mean (-20.8 ± 11.2 kg), %FM (-6.7 ± 6.0%), FFM (-3.45 ± 3.41 kg,), and BMD (-0.02 ± 0.04 g/cm^2) (all $p < 0.05$) Descriptive characteristics of participants stratified by sex are presented in Table 1. The decline in BMD was similar for both men and women; however, a statistically significant loss occurred in BMD among women only.

At two years, the mean weight reduction was greater for men than women; however, change in absolute BMD was greater among women ($p < 0.05$). In multivariable analyses shown in Table 2, after adjusting for age, sex, and baseline BMD, we found that the total weight lost at the end of 2 years was associated with a small but statistically significant loss in BMD at 2-years. There was a 0.001 g/cm^2 decrease in 2-year BMD per kilogram weight loss. While men lost more FM, women lost significantly more %FFM

than men. Figure 1 shows the changes in % body weight, body fat, BMD and FFM from baseline to 2 years in men and women. In addition, there was a significant independent association between total weight lost and 2-year FFM ($\beta = -116.5$ g; $p < 0.01$). Figure 2 includes partial residual scatter plot revealing the correlations between relative changes in body weight and relative changes in BMD (a) and FFM (b), controlling for age and sex.

In addition, we evaluated the changes in BMD at the end of the intensive phase of weight loss (i.e. after 15% weight loss). There was a small but statistically significant loss in BMD among women only (0.02 ± 0.01 g/cm^2; $p < 0.001$). In both men and women, the loss in BMD at the end of the intensive phase was significantly correlated to bone loss at 2 years ($r = 0.77$; $p < 0.01$) and ($r = 0.33$, $p < 0.05$) respectively.

In the sub-analyses we evaluated changes in the bone resorption marker, serum CTX and its independent association with changes in body weight, BMD, FFM and %BF. After adjusting for age, change in %BF was the only significant predictor of changes in serum CTX ($\beta = 23.56$ pg/mL; $p = 0.04$).

Discussion

In our study, participants were involved in a two-year weight management program that included a three-month active weight loss phase utilizing an 800-kcal/day standard VLED. Our results show that VLED-induced weight loss can result in a small reduction in total body BMD and FFM at 2-years. Specifically, we found that for every kilogram of weight loss there was a 0.001 g/cm^2 reduction in BMD and 0.1 kg decrease in FFM at 2-years, after adjusting for age, sex, and baseline BMD. However, it is important to note that this loss of BMD and FFM may also arise from natural consequences of the aging process, as previously described in numerous studies [16]. Indeed, BMD declined substantially in the late peri-menopause, with an average loss of 0.018–0.010 g/cm^2/yr. from the spine and hip ($P < 0.001$ for both). In post menopause, rates of loss from the spine and hip were 0.022 and 0.013 g/cm^2/yr. ($P < 0.001$) [17]. Serum CTX levels increased following the intensive phase and remained stable in the maintenance phase. Neither baseline serum CTX nor changes in CTX levels following weight loss were associated with bone loss.

The effect of weight loss on the bone has been controversial with inconsistent clinical opinions and research findings. In the Dubbo Osteoporosis Epidemiologic study, weight change was found to be an independent predictor of rate of bone loss [18]. Moderate weight reduction (greater than 5%) can negatively influence BMD especially if achieved purely through calorie restriction [19, 20]. This was also observed in the LOOK AHEAD study, and while intensive lifestyle interventions resulted in better glycemic control and weight loss, a statistically

Table 1 Morphological characteristics for men and women at baseline and at 2-years

	Men (n = 29)			Women (n = 20)		
	Baseline	Year 2	Mean Δ	Baseline	Year 2	Mean Δ
Age (years)	51.59 (6.91)	53.58 (6.89)	–	49.30 (7.69)	51.28 (7.70)	–
Body Weight (kg)	123.68 (13.58)	102.56 (15.16)	23.51 (12.45)[†‡]	104.47 (16.78)[*]	89.45 (14.10)	16.80 (7.60)[†]
Body Mass Index (kg·m^{-2})	38.58 (3.86)	31.94 (3.92)	7.39 (3.99)[†]	39.17 (4.62)	33.53 (3.92)	6.32 (2.74)[†]
Body Fat (%)	41.79 (4.41)	32.95 (7.22)	8.84 (6.53)[†‡]	51.45 (4.39)[*]	47.88 (5.59)	3.57 (3.29)[†]
Fat Free Mass (kg)	72.72 (6.95)	69.45 (7.55)	3.27 (4.01)[†]	51.26 (5.72)[*]	47.54 (6.07)	3.72 (2.38)[†]
Bone Mineral Density (g/cm^2)	1.37 (0.06)	1.36 (0.09)	0.01 (0.04)	1.27 (0.07)[*]	1.24 (0.08)	0.03 (0.04)[†‡]
T-score	1.88 (0.77)	1.72 (1.07)	0.16 (0.56)	1.79 (0.84)	1.47 (0.99)	0.32 (0.53)[†]

[*]Significant difference between men and women at baseline ($p < 0.05$)
[†]Significant difference within sex from baseline to 2 years ($p < 0.05$)
[‡]Significant difference between men and women for absolute changes from baseline to 2 years ($p < 0.05$)

significant loss in BMD was noted at the total hip and femoral neck [21]. The impact of calorie restriction on BMD is seen in younger individuals as well as premenopausal women therefore suggesting that the mechanism is not solely related to age and the effects of sex steroids [22, 23]. In middle-aged individuals, weight variability has been shown to increase the risk of hip fractures [24]. However, the long-term impact of calorie restriction on fractures is not known [23, 25]. In recently published data from the LOOK AHEAD study, long term weight loss in overweight and obese adults with type 2 diabetes mellitus was not associated with an increase in overall risk of fractures but maybe associated with an increased risk of frailty fractures [26]. A few other studies evaluating the long-term effects of > 5% weight reduction did not use severe calorie restricted diets [18, 27, 28]. Due to significant energy restriction, VLEDs induce greater weight loss than moderate calorie restricted diets. Citing the need for further research, a meta-analysis performed by Zibellini et al., found that low calorie or VLED's did not cause a reduction in BMD; however, the majority of

studies evaluating the impact of VLEDs on bone loss have been limited to one year [25]. In addition, low energy diets that are supplemented with calcium or high proteins are known to mitigate the rise in bone turnover [29]. In our study, although the changes were statistically significant, the change in BMD was small, and thus may not necessarily be clinically relevant in the short term, or with respect to future fracture risk. We postulate that the loss in BMD was likely attenuated by the macro/micro-nutrient composition of the meal replacement and adequate vitamin D and mineral intake and less sedentary behavior.

Bariatric surgery remains the most effective form of treatment for severe obesity and historically, Roux-en-Y gastric bypass (RYGB) procedure was the most commonly performed procedure. Though these surgeries are very effective, the risk of bone loss associated with gastric bypass surgery is well documented [30–33]. Surgical procedures are associated with decreases in bone mass and increases in bone turnover markers [34]. Prospective studies have shown that bone loss following gastric

Table 2 Multiple regression showing the associations between changes in body weight (primary predictor) and BMD and FFM at 2-years (dependent variable), after adjustment for age, sex, and baseline values (ANCOVA)

	Model Predictor(s)	β	SE	t	Pr > | t |	Adjusted R^2
BMD at 2 Years						0.88
	Intercept	−0.084	0.120	−0.680	0.500	
	Age	−0.002	0.001	−2.980	0.005	
	Sex	−0.015	0.014	−1.080	0.285	
	Baseline BMD	1.155	0.082	14.010	< 0.001	
	Change in Body Weight	−0.001	0.001	−2.460	0.017	
FFM at 2 Years						0.94
	Intercept	5.790	6.780	0.860	0.397	
	Age	−0.052	0.066	−0.790	0.435	
	Sex	−2.420	1.880	−1.290	0.205	
	Baseline FFM	0.950	0.074	12.770	< 0.001	
	Change in Body Weight	−0.117	0.045	−2.620	0.012	

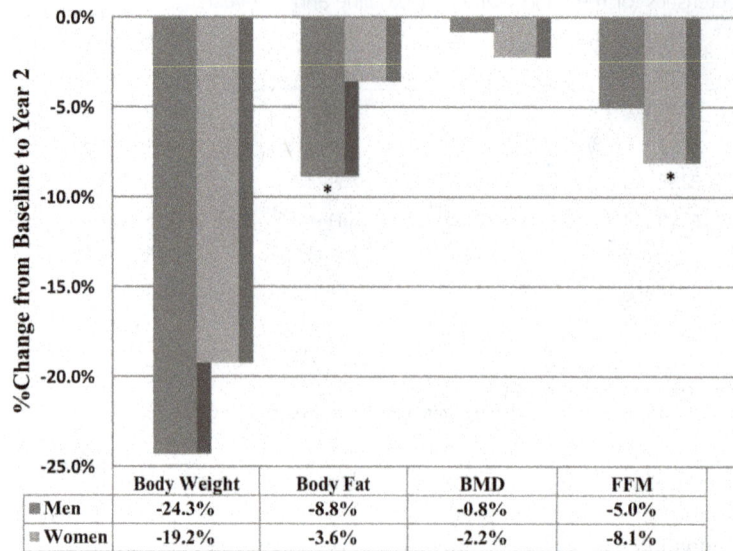

Fig. 1 Relative change in body weight, body fat, BMD and fat free mass from baseline to 2 years in men and women

	Body Weight	Body Fat	BMD	FFM
■ Men	-24.3%	-8.8%	-0.8%	-5.0%
■ Women	-19.2%	-3.6%	-2.2%	-8.1%

bypass preferentially affects the hip [32, 35]. Of the various bariatric procedures, sleeve gastrectomy is likely associated with less bone loss than RYGB although the studies are small and more data are needed [36]. We postulate that the derangements in calcium and Vitamin D absorption are likely to play a greater role in bone loss after surgical procedures. VLEDs may therefore represent a safer, non-invasive alternative to weight loss without the negative impact on bone.

Evidence pertaining to the long-term impact of weight loss on bone turnover is lacking. Some studies have shown low bone turnover in obesity while others have contrary findings [37, 38]. Following bariatric surgery,

Balsa et al. showed an increase in bone turnover markers [39]. In our study, we did not find a correlation between serum CTX and BMD.

Limitations

In this study, DXA imaging at one year was not available. With this information, we would have been able to assess the sequential changes in BMD in individuals whose weight remained stable and those who experienced weight cycling. In addition, we looked at the total body BMD rather than routinely used sites to assess fragility such as the lumbar spine, femoral neck or hip, and this may result in under diagnosis of osteoporosis [40].

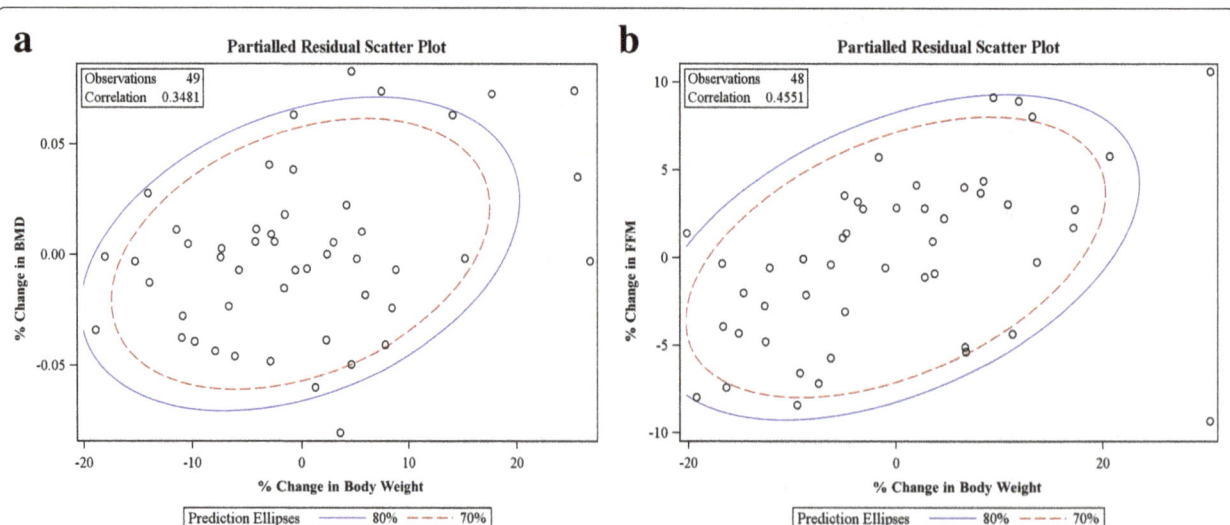

Fig. 2 Partial residual scatter plot revealing the correlations between relative changes in body weight and relative changes in BMD (**a**) and FFM (**b**), controlling for age and sex

Although the utility of DXA in obese individuals is debatable, DXA remains the gold standard and the only available test for measuring BMD in clinical practice [41]. In addition, whether changes in total body water with these diets affects fat and fat-free mass assessments via DXA remains unclear. Our sample size for subgroup analyses on bone markers was small, and thus we had to combine men and women. Future larger studies should aim to determine the longitudinal, dimorphic patterns of weight loss and BMD changes, taking into consideration the mediating influence of serum BTM changes. Lastly, although moderate intensity and regular physical activity was prescribed as part of the program, physical activity and participation was self-reported. Since physical activity and exercise are linked with bone health, future efforts are certainly needed to determine if objectively measured exercise during VLED interventions can ameliorate changes in BMD and FFM. Our future studies will prospectively evaluate key variable such as gonadal status, use of bone altering medications and physical activity.

Conclusion

Obesity has negative effects on bone metabolism and is associated with a number of cardio-metabolic conditions that pose threats to bone health. We have shown absolute weight loss that can impact BMD. Although VLED can promote significant weight loss the decline in BMD is minor with unclear clinical applicability and must be weighed against the myriad of other benefits resulting from weight loss.

Abbreviations
BMD: Bone Mineral Density; BMI: Body Mass Index; CTX: Serum cross-linked C-Telopeptide; DXA: Dual X-Ray Absorptiometry; FFM: Fat-Free Mass; FM: Fat Mass; VLED: Very Low Energy Diets

Acknowledgements
The authors would also like to thank Dr. Henry Bone for his useful feedback on the manuscript.

Funding
The authors would like to acknowledge the University of Michigan Nutrition Obesity Research Center (MNORC: Grant Number DK089503) and the Michigan Center for Diabetes Translational Research (MCDTR: Grant Number P30DK092926) from the National Institute of Diabetes and Digestive and Kidney Diseases, National Institutes of Health.
Additional support was provided by the A. Alfred Taubman Medical Institute and the Robert C. and Veronica Atkins Foundation.
Dr. Choksi was supported by the Michigan Institute for Clinical & Health Research (MICHR: Port Grant 2UL1TR000433).
Dr. Peterson is funded by the National Institutes of Health (1KO1 HD074706). The funders had no role in the design and conduct of the study; the collection, analysis, and interpretation of the data; or the preparation, review, or approval of the manuscript.

Authors' contributions
PC: participated in study concept, design, statistical analysis and drafting the manuscript. AR: participated in study concept, design, statistical analysis and drafting the manuscript. AK: Helped in drafting the manuscript. NM and KZ: participated with data collection and reviewed the manuscript. CB and CVP: participated in its design and coordination and helped to draft the manuscript. MP: participated in study concept, design, statistical analysis and drafting the manuscript. All authors read and approved the final manuscript.

Ethics approval and consent to participate
All participants provided written informed consent and the study protocol was reviewed and approved by the University of Michigan Institutional Review Board. The trial is registered at Clinicaltrials.gov (NCT02043457).

Competing interests
The authors declare that they have no competing interests.

Author details
[1]Department of Internal Medicine, University of Michigan, 24 Frank Lloyd Wright Dr, Ann Arbor, MI 48106, USA. [2]Molecular and Integrative Physiology, University of Michigan, Ann Arbor, USA. [3]Department of Physical Medicine and Rehabilitation, University of Michigan, Ann Arbor, USA. [4]Department of Nutritional Sciences, University of Michigan, Ann Arbor, USA.

References
1. Flegal KM, Carroll MD, Kit BK, Ogden CL. Prevalence of obesity and trends in the distribution of body mass index among US adults, 1999-2010. JAMA. 2012;307:491–7.
2. Wang CY, McPherson K, Marsh T, Gortmaker SL, Brown M. Health and economic burden of the projected obesity trends in the USA and the UK. Lancet. 2011;378:815–25.
3. Heaney RPAS, Dawson-Highes B. Peak Bone mass. Ost Int. 2000;11:985–1009.
4. Iqbal J, Zaidi M. Molecular regulation of mechanotransduction. Biochem Biophys Res Commun. 2005;328:751–5.
5. Zaidi M, Buettner C, Sun L, Iqbal J. Minireview: the link between fat and bone: does mass beget mass? Endocrinology. 2012;153(5):2070–5.
6. Zhu K, Hunter M, James A, Lim EM, Walsh JP. Associations between body mass index, lean and fat body mass and bone mineral density in middle-aged Australians: the Busselton healthy ageing study. Bone. 2015;74:146–52.
7. Nielson CM, Srikanth P, Orwoll ES. Obesity and fracture in men and women: an epidemiologic perspective. J Bone Miner Res. 2012;27:1–10.
8. Hinton PS, LeCheminant JD, Smith BK, Rector RS, Donnelly JE. Weight loss-induced alterations in serum markers of bone turnover persist during weight maintenance in obese men and women. J Am Coll Nutr. 2009;28: 565–73.
9. Rector RS, Loethen J, Ruebel M, Thomas TR, Hinton PS. Serum markers of bone turnover are increased by modest weight loss with or without weight-bearing exercise in overweight premenopausal women. Appl Physiol Nutr Metab. 2009;34:933–41.
10. Garnero P, Delmas PD. Contribution of bone mineral density and bone turnover markers to the estimation of risk of osteoporotic fracture in postmenopausal women. J Musculoskelet Neuronal Interact. 2004;4:50–63.
11. Anderson JW, Grant L, Gotthelf L, Stifler LT. Weight loss and long-term follow-up of severely obese individuals treated with an intense behavioral program. Int J Obes. 2007;31:488–93.
12. Rothberg AE, McEwen LN, Kraftson AT, Neshewat GM, Fowler CE, Burant CF, Herman WH. The impact of weight loss on health-related quality-of-life: implications for cost-effectiveness analyses. Qual Life Res. 2014;23:1371–6.
13. Rothberg AE, McEwen LN, Kraftson AT, Fowler CE, Herman WH. Very-low-energy diet for type 2 diabetes: an underutilized therapy? J Diabetes Complicat. 2014;28:506–10.
14. Guidelines (2013) for managing overweight and obesity in adults. Preface to the expert panel report (comprehensive version which includes systematic

evidence review, evidence statements, and recommendations). Obesity (Silver Spring). 2014;22(Suppl 2):S40.

15. Seibel MJ. Biochemical markers of bone turnover: part I: biochemistry and variability. Clin Biochem Rev. 2005;26:97–122.

16. Cauley JA, Danielson ME, Greendale GA, Finkelstein JS, Chang YF, Lo JC, Crandall CJ, Neer RM, Ruppert K, Meyn L, Prairie BA, Sowers MR. Bone resorption and fracture across the menopausal transition. the Study of Women's Health Across the Nation Menopause. 2012;19:1200–7.

17. Finkelstein JS, Brockwell SE, Mehta V, Greendale GA, Sowers MR, Ettinger B, Lo JC, Johnston JM, Cauley JA, Danielson ME, Neer RM. Bone mineral density changes during the menopause transition in a multiethnic cohort of women. J Clin Endocrinol Metab. 2008;93:861–8.

18. Nguyen TV, Seibel MJ, Eisman JA. Bone loss, physical activity, and weight change in elderly women: the Dubbo osteoporosis epidemiology study. J Bone Miner Res. 1998;13:1458–67.

19. Jensen LB, Kollerup G, Quaade F, Sorensen OH. Bone minerals changes in obese women during a moderate weight loss with and without calcium supplementation. J Bone Miner Res. 2001;16:141–7.

20. Villareal DT, Fontana L, Weiss EP, Racette SB, Steger-May K, et al. Bone mineral density response to caloric restriction-induced weight loss or exercise-induced weight loss: a randomized controlled trial. Arch Intern Med. 2006;166:2502–10.

21. Schwartz AV, Johnson KC, Kahn SE, Shepherd JA, Nevitt MC, Peters AL, Walkup MP, Hodges A, Williams CC, Bray GA. Effect of 1 year of an intentional weight loss intervention on bone mineral density in type 2 diabetes: results from the Look AHEAD randomized trial. J Bone Miner Res. 2012;27:619–27.

22. Hamilton KC, Fisher G, Roy JL, Gower BA, Hunter GR. The effects of weight loss on relative bone mineral density in premenopausal women. Obesity (Silver Spring). 2013;21:441–8.

23. Villareal DT, Fontana L, Das SK, Redman L, Smith SR, Saltzman E, Bales C, Rochon J, Pieper C, Huang M, Lewis M, Schwartz AV, Group CS. Effect of two-year caloric restriction on bone metabolism and bone mineral density in non-obese younger adults: a randomized clinical trial. J Bone Miner Res. 2016;31:40–51.

24. Meyer HE, Tverdal A, Selmer R. Weight variability, weight change and the incidence of hip fracture: a prospective study of 39,000 middle-aged Norwegians. Osteoporos Int. 1998;8:373–8.

25. Zibellini J, Seimon RV, Lee CM, Gibson AA, Hsu MS, Shapses SA, Nguyen TV, Sainsbury A. Does diet-induced weight loss lead to bone loss in overweight or obese adults? A systematic review and meta-analysis of clinical trials. J Bone Miner Res. 2015;30(12):2168–78.

26. Johnson KC, Bray GA, Cheskin LJ, Clark JM, Egan CM, Foreyt JP, Garcia KR, Glasser S, Greenway FL, Gregg EW, Hazuda HP, Hergenroeder A, Hill JO, Horton ES, Jakicic JM, Jeffery RW, Kahn SE, Knowler WC, Lewis CE, Miller M, Montez MG, Nathan DM, Patricio JL, Peters AL, Pi-Sunyer X, Pownall HJ, Reboussin D, Redmon JB, Steinberg H, Wadden TA, Wagenknecht LE, Wing RR, Womack CR, Yanovski SZ, Zhang P, Schwartz AV. The effect of intentional weight loss on fracture risk in persons with diabetes: results from the Look AHEAD randomized clinical trial. J Bone Miner Res. 2017; 32(11):2278–87.

27. Ensrud KE, Ewing SK, Stone KL, Cauley JA, Bowman PJ, Cummings SR. Intentional and unintentional weight loss increase bone loss and hip fracture risk in older women. J Am Geriatr Soc. 2003;51:1740–7.

28. Sogaard AJ, Meyer HE, Ahmed LA, Jorgensen L, Bjornerem A, Joakimsen RM, Emaus N. Does recalled dieting increase the risk of non-vertebral osteoporotic fractures? The Tromso study. Osteoporos Int. 2012;23:2835–45.

29. Redman LM, Rood J, Anton SD, Champagne C, Smith SR, Ravussin E. Calorie restriction and bone health in young, overweight individuals. Arch Intern Med. 2008;168:1859–66.

30. Carrasco F, Ruz M, Rojas P, et al. Changes in bone mineral density, body composition and adiponectin levels in morbidly obese patients after bariatric surgery. Obese Surg 2009:41–46.

31. Coates PS, Fernstrom JD, Fernstrom MH, Schauer PR, Greenspan SL. Gastric bypass surgery for morbid obesity leads to an increase in bone turnover and a decrease in bone mass. J Clin Endocrinol Metab. 2004;89:1061–5.

32. Vilarrasa N, San José P, Garcia I, et al. Evaluation of bone mineral density loss in morbidly obese women after gastric bypass: 3-year follow-up. Obes Surg. 2011;21:465–72.

33. von Mach MA, Stoeckli R, Bilz S, Kraenzlin M, Langer I, Keller U. Changes in bone mineral content after surgical treatment of morbid obesity. Metabolism. 2004;53:918–21.

34. Rodríguez-Carmona Y, López-Alavez FJ, González-Garay AG, Solís-Galicia C, Meléndez G, Serralde-Zúñiga AE. Bone mineral density after bariatric surgery. A systematic review. Int J Surg. 2014;12:976–82.

35. Fleischer J, Stein EM, Bessler M, Della Badia M, Restuccia N, Olivero-Rivera L, McMahon DJ, Silverberg SJ. The decline in hip bone density after gastric bypass surgery is associated with extent of weight loss. J Clin Endocrinol Metab. 2008;93:3735–40.

36. Nogues X, Goday A, Pena MJ, Benaiges D, de Ramon M, Crous X, Vial M, Pera M, Grande L, Diez-Perez A, Ramon JM. Bone mass loss after sleeve gastrectomy: a prospective comparative study with gastric bypass. Cir Esp. 2010;88:103–9.

37. Cifuentes M, López-Alavez FJ, Lewis RD et al. Bone turnover and body weight relationships differ in normal-weight compared to heavier postmenopausal women. Osteoporos Int. 2003;14(2):116–22.

38. Ostrowska Z, Zwirska-Korczala K, Bunter B et al. Assessment of bone metabolism in obese women. Endocr Regul 1998; 32.

39. Balsa JA, Botella-Carretero JI, Peromingo R, Caballero C, Munoz-Malo T, Villafruela JJ, Arrieta F, Zamarron I, Vazquez C. Chronic increase of bone turnover markers after biliopancreatic diversion is related to secondary hyperparathyroidism and weight loss. Relation with bone mineral density. Obes Surg. 2010;20:468–73.

40. Graat-Verboom L, Spruit MA, van den Borne BE, Smeenk FW, Wouters EF. Whole-body versus local DXA-scan for the diagnosis of osteoporosis in COPD patients. J Osteoporos. 2010;2010:640878.

41. Yu EW, Thomas BJ, Brown JK, Finkelstein JS. Simulated increases in body fat and errors in bone mineral density measurements by DXA and QCT. J Bone Miner Res. 2012;27:119–24.

19

Perspectives on the impact of painful diabetic peripheral neuropathy in a multicultural population

Martin Eichholz[1], Andrea H. Alexander[2], Joseph C. Cappelleri[3], Patrick Hlavacek[2], Bruce Parsons[2], Alesia Sadosky[2*] and Michael M. Tuchman[4]

Abstract

Background: Since few studies have characterized painful diabetic peripheral neuropathy (pDPN) symptoms in multicultural populations, this study fielded a survey to better understand pDPN and its impact in African-American, Caucasian, and Hispanic populations.

Methods: Kelton fielded a survey by phone or Internet, in English or Spanish, among adults with pDPN symptoms in the United States between August and October 2015; African-Americans and Hispanics were oversampled to achieve at least 500 subjects for each group. Patients were required to have been diagnosed with pDPN or score $\geq$ 3 on ID Pain validated screening tool. The survey elicited information on pDPN symptoms and interactions with healthcare providers (HCPs), and included the Brief Pain Inventory and pain-specific Work Productivity and Assessment Questionnaire (WPAI:SHP).

Results: Respondents included 823 Caucasians, 525 African-Americans, and 537 Hispanics; approximately half of African-Americans and Hispanics were <40 years of age, vs 12% of Caucasians. Pain was less likely to be rated moderate or severe by African-Americans (65%) and Hispanics (49%) relative to Caucasians (87%; $p < 0.05$). African-Americans and Hispanics were less likely than Caucasians to report experiencing specific pDPN sensory symptoms. Significantly fewer African-Americans and Hispanics reported receiving a pDPN diagnosis relative to Caucasians ($p < 0.05$), and higher proportions of African-Americans and Hispanics reported difficulty communicating with their HCP ($p < 0.05$). WPAI:SHP activity impairment was lower in Hispanics (43%) relative to African-Americans (53%) and Caucasian (56%; $p < 0.05$).

Conclusions: Multicultural patients reported differences in pDPN symptoms and pain relative to Caucasians, and fewer received a pDPN diagnosis. While further evaluation is needed to understand these differences, these data suggest a need to broaden pDPN educational initiatives to improve patient-HCP dialogue and encourage discussion of pDPN symptoms and their impact in a multicultural setting.

Keywords: Painful diabetic peripheral neuropathy, Race, Ethnicity, Pain, Productivity

* Correspondence: Alesia.sadosky@pfizer.com
[2]Pfizer Inc., 235 East 42nd Street, New York, NY 10017, USA
Full list of author information is available at the end of the article

Background

Diabetic peripheral neuropathy (DPN) is a common complication of Type 1 and Type 2 diabetes that is characterized by nerve damage. When DPN presents with painful symptoms the condition is known as painful diabetic peripheral neuropathy (pDPN). While the epidemiology of pDPN has not been well-characterized, an overall prevalence of 15% has been estimated in the diabetic population [1]. However, prevalence rates exceeding 30% in patients with diabetes have been reported in more recent regional studies [2, 3], and a systematic review of neuropathic pain in the general population reported a pDPN prevalence of 0.8% that represents approximately 26% of individuals with Type 2 diabetes [4].

The substantial patient and economic burdens associated with pDPN are well-recognized and include reductions in patient function, quality of life, and productivity [5, 6], as well as greater healthcare resource utilization and costs relative to patients with diabetes and with DPN without pain [7].

Despite studies evaluating quality of life and other patient-reported outcomes in pDPN, there are limited data on the severity and impact of painful pDPN symptoms from the patient's perspective. A survey in patients and clinicians who treat patients with diabetes not only showed that misperceptions on the cause and management of pDPN were common in both stakeholder groups but also indicated additional disparities between patient and clinician perspectives regarding communication, severity, and treatment [8]. However, less is known about the patient perceptions of pDPN and interactions between these patients and their healthcare providers (HCPs) in a multicultural population. Therefore, the objective of this study was to characterize the impact of pDPN and identify barriers to its management in a multicultural US population with a focus on African-Americans and Hispanics relative to Caucasians.

Methods

Design and populations

Kelton fielded a survey among pDPN patients in the United States between August and October 2015. For inclusion, patients were required to be adults (≥ 18 years old) who self-reported being diagnosed with either Type 1 or Type 2 diabetes *and* either self-reported having received a diagnosis of pDPN by an HCP *or* had a score ≥ 3 on ID Pain [9] (i.e., experienced ≥3 of the following symptoms within the past week: pins and needles, hot/burning, numbness, electrical shocks, or pain that is made worse with the touch of clothing or bed sheets). ID Pain is a validated measure that is used to screen patients for the presence of neuropathic pain based on its demonstrated ability to discriminate between nociceptive and neuropathic pain [9].

The survey, which was developed without patient input but in collaboration with experts in the field, including clinicians, was administered by Internet among Caucasians, and by either Internet or phone among African-Americans and Hispanics, with Internet respondents recruited from a national research panel and phone respondents recruited from purchased phone lists. Oversampling via phone was performed to achieve a goal of at least 500 Hispanic patients and 500 African-American patients. The survey could be completed in English or Spanish, with the Spanish version back-translated by native Spanish-speakers to ensure accuracy of the questionnaire.

The survey (Additional file 1) consisted of batteries of questions that were in part derived from a previous, similar survey [8]. The goal was to capture perspectives on pDPN symptoms (numbness; pins and needles; pain or discomfort at night; tingling or prickling sensation; sensitivity to touch; burning pain or sensation; shooting pain; radiating pain; stinging; stabbing pain; electric shock-like symptoms or sudden pain attacks; throbbing pain), perceptions of pain associated with the symptoms, and how patients discuss these symptoms with their physician.

Additionally, the survey included the Brief Pain Inventory (BPI) [10] and the Work Productivity and Assessment Questionnaire disease-specific version (WPAI:SHP) adapted for pain [11], both of which demonstrate sound psychometric measurement properties and have been used as outcomes across a wide variety of disease states. The BPI rates worst, least, and average pain in the past 24 h and the average pain subscale was used to categorize pain as mild, moderate, and severe based on established cut points for the average pain scale of 0–3 for mild, 4–6 for moderate, and 7–10 for severe [12]. The WPAI:SHP measures impact of the disease on productivity at work due to absenteeism (work time missed), presenteeism (impairment while at work), overall work impairment, and activity impairment outside of work during the past 7 days.

Statistical analysis

Survey results reflect an unweighted sample. The margin of error was ±3.1% for the total patient sample and 4.0% for the oversampled groups. Analyses for categorical data and continuous data were conducted using chi-square tests and t-tests, respectively. The impact of ethnicity was explored based on the combined main sample and oversample and controlled for effects of age, education, and household income using layered cross-tabulations (chi-square tests) and stepwise linear regression [13]. The cross-tabulations were conducted using 16 demographic strata: 3 age groups (18–34 years, 35–54 years, and ≥55 years), 6 education levels, and 7 income levels shown in the demographics table (Table 1).

Table 1 Demographic characteristics of the patient populations

Variable	Value		
	Caucasians (n = 823)	African-Americans (n = 525)	Hispanics (n = 537)
Sex, %			
Male	43	48	42
Female	57	52	58
Age, years, mean	55.7[ab]	41.0	37.0
Age distribution, %			
18–29 years	3[ab]	25[b]	21
30–39 years	9[ab]	24	38
40–49 years	16[b]	20	24
50–59 year	30[ab]	18[b]	12
60–69 years	30[ab]	10[b]	6
≥ 70 years	12[ab]	3[b]	1
Marital status, %			
Married or living as married	57[ab]	45[b]	72
Living with domestic partner	4[ab]	11	8
Single, never married	14[ab]	30	16
Widowed	5[b]	4[b]	2
Separated	2[b]	3[b]	1
Divorced	18[ab]	7[b]	2
Education, %			
Less than high school	4[b]	6	7
High school	22[b]	25	42[a]
Some college—no degree	31[b]	28	20[a]
Associate's degree	16[b]	15	9[a]
Bachelor's degree	17	18	19
Post-graduate degree	10[b]	8	2[a]
Employment status, %			
Employed	38[ab]	65	69
Retired	31[ab]	12[b]	4
Disabled	19[ab]	10[b]	2
Stay-at-home parent/spouse	9[ab]	5[b]	15
Unemployed, looking for work	2[ab]	4	5
Unemployed, not looking for work	2[b]	2	4
Full time student	< 1[b]	1	2
Annual income, mean	$52,300[b]	$53,700[b]	$58,500
Insurance, %			
Medicare	44[ab]	16[b]	8
Medicaid	14[b]	18	20
Private	33[ab]	47	52
Other	6[ab]	3	2
No insurance	4[ab]	15	18

[a] p < 0.05 vs African-Americans
[b] p < 0.05 vs Hispanics

Stepwise linear regression was also performed among the main sample, using pain severity as the dependent variable and 10 items related to the patients' experience with symptoms as independent variables (numbness; pins and needles; pain or discomfort at night; tingling or prickling sensation; sensitivity to touch; burning pain or sensation; shooting pain; stinging; stabbing pain; electric shock-like symptoms or sudden pain attacks). All analyses were performed using IBM® SPSS® Statistics 23.

Results

Respondent populations

Table 1 presents the demographic characteristics of the multicultural populations, and shows that mean age was significantly higher (p < 0.05) among Caucasians than African-Americans and Hispanics, and differences were also observed in the age distribution. Almost half of the African-Americans (49%) and more than half of the Hispanics (59%) were under 40 years of age, compared with only 12% of Caucasians. Caucasians had the lowest rate of employment and the highest rate of retirees among the three cultural groups, and annual income was highest in Hispanics, lowest among Caucasians. Consistent with the older demographic, a significantly greater proportion of Caucasians relative to the other groups had health insurance through Medicare, and a significantly lower proportion were uninsured (both p < 0.05) (Table 1); private insurance was the primary insurance type among both African-Americans and Hispanics.

While mean time since diabetes diagnosis was slightly but significantly higher among Caucasians (10.9 years) relative to African-Americans (9.4 years) and Hispanics (9.4 years) (both p < 0.05), the medians were similar across ethnicities, 8 years, 8 years, and 9 years, respectively.

Pain and sensory symptoms

African-American and Hispanic patients were less likely than Caucasians to experience a range of sensory symptoms (Fig. 1) that are characteristic of neuropathic pain including some symptoms that appear to drive pain severity such as sensitivity to touch and shooting pain. The layered cross-tabulations of the six symptoms that were significant by ethnicity (electric shock-like pain; pain and discomfort at night; stabbing pain; burning pain sensation; shooting pain; sensitivity to touch) show that these differences by ethnicity generally hold for stabbing pain, with a significant effect of ethnicity for 12 of the 16 strata (p < 0.05); shooting pain, which was significant for 11 strata p < 0.05); and electric shock pain (p < 0.05: for 9 strata) (Table 2). However, significant differences (p < 0.05) by ethnicity were limited for pain and discomfort at night (only 4 strata showed a significant effect of ethnicity), and burning pain and

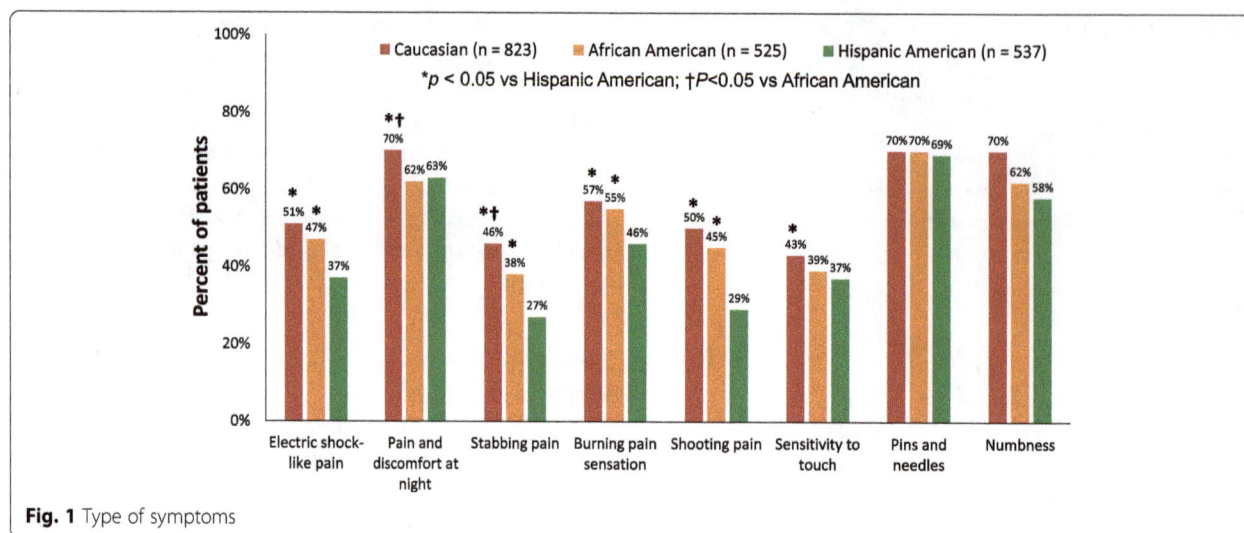

Fig. 1 Type of symptoms

sensitivity to touch (each with 6 strata that showed an ethnicity effect).

A stepwise regression analysis with average pain severity in the past year as dependent variable and the 10 pain symptoms as independent variables showed that sensitivity to touch is the strongest predictor of pain, being responsible for 20% of the total *explained* variance in

overall pain scores. The second strongest predictor was shooting pain (17%), followed by electric shock-like pain (10%). The overall model was significant ($p < 0.05$), with $R^2 = 0.29$ and F = 59.077.

While the average number of reported pDPN symptoms was lower among African-Americans (5.3) and Hispanics (4.7) relative to Caucasians (5.8), the differences were not

Table 2 Layered cross-tabulation for the effect of ethnicity on the percent of respondents who currently experience the pain symptoms that were significant by ethnicity

Strata	p-value					
	Stabbing pain	Shooting pain	Electric shock-like pain	Pain and discomfort at night	Burning pain	Sensitivity to touch
Controlling for age						
18–34 years	< 0.0001	< 0.0001	0.002	NS	0.001	0.004
35–54 years	< 0.0001	< 0.0001	< 0.0001	< 0.001	< 0.0001	0.001
≥ 55 years	NS	NS	NS	NS	NS	NS
Controlling for education						
Less than high school	0.002	0.034	NS	0.021	NS	NS
High school	< 0.0001	< 0.0001	0.006	< 0.0001	<0.0001	NS
Some college – no degree	< 0.0001	0.003	0.007	NS	NS	0.004
Associate's degree	NS	0.024	NS	NS	NS	NS
Bachelor's degree	NS	NS	NS	NS	NS	NS
Post-graduate degree	0.009	0.031	NS	NS	0.024	0.007
Controlling for income						
< $25,000	0.006	NS	NS	NS	NS	NS
$25,000 - $34,999	< 0.0001	< 0.0001	0.002	NS	NS	0.004
$35,000 - $49,999	< 0.0001	< 0.0001	0.009	0.005	0.006	NS
$50,000 - $74,999	0.006	0.014	0.018	NS	NS	NS
$75,000 - $99,999	NS	0.001	0.013	NS	NS	NS
$100,000 - $149,999	0.004	NS	0.028	NS	0.001	0.036
≥ $150,000	0.007	NS	NS	NS	NS	NS

Abbreviations: NS not significant

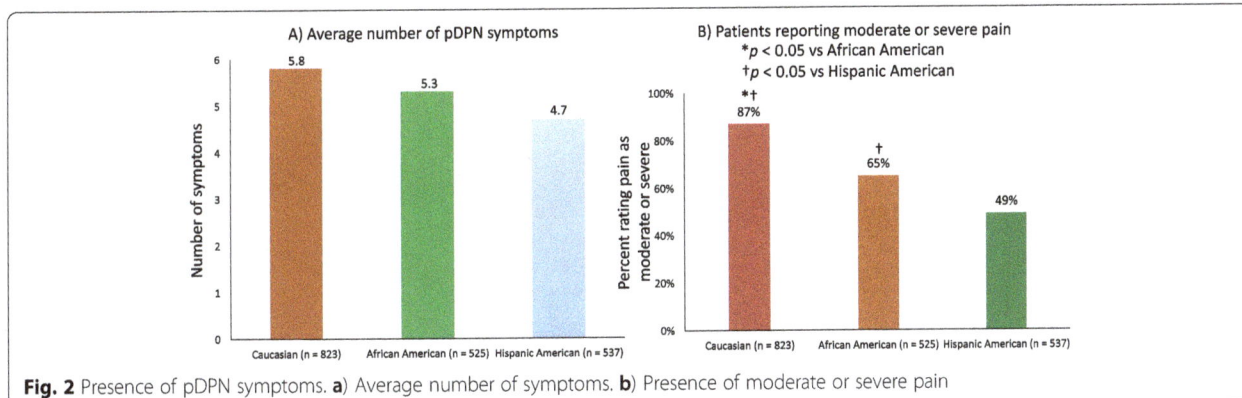

Fig. 2 Presence of pDPN symptoms. **a**) Average number of symptoms. **b**) Presence of moderate or severe pain

significant (Fig. 2a). However, African-Americans and Hispanics were less likely to rate their pain as moderate or severe, 65% and 49%, respectively, relative to Caucasians (87%; both $p < 0.05$) (Fig. 2b). This finding was confirmed through a stepwise linear regression where ethnicity (operationalized as 3 dummy variables, one each for Caucasian, African-American, and Hispanic) as well as age, education, and household income were used as independent variables to predict reported pain levels. The results of the overall significant model show that being Hispanic is the strongest significant predictor of the experienced pain levels (standardized beta coefficient of –0.297), followed by education (beta of 0.211) and being African-American (beta of –0.125). No other independent variable added significant explanatory power.

Patient and healthcare provider dialogue

The proportion of Caucasians who reported receiving a diagnosis of pDPN (87%) was significantly higher than that of African-Americans (51%) and Hispanics (36%) (all $p < 0.05$) (Fig. 3). This significance based on ethnicity was

retained in layered cross-tabulations, with 13 of the 16 strata showing significance ($p \leq 0.001$; only post-graduate degree and income levels of $100,000–$149,999 and $\geq$$150,000 were not significant). Similar patterns were observed when stratified by pain severity; consistently and significantly higher proportions of Caucasians reported a pDPN diagnosis relative to the other two populations across severity levels (all $p < 0.05$), and Hispanics generally reported the lowest rate of diagnosis, although the differences were not significant vs African-Americans.

Significantly lower proportions of African-American and Hispanic patients relative to Caucasians reported discussing their pain symptoms with their healthcare provider across pain severity levels, (all $p < 0.05$) (Fig. 4a). Additionally, among both the African-American and Hispanic populations, there was consistently less comfort with their healthcare providers (Fig. 4b), as indicated by significantly lower proportions of African-Americans and Hispanics who reported that they thought their HCP understood their culture, as well as a harder time communicating.

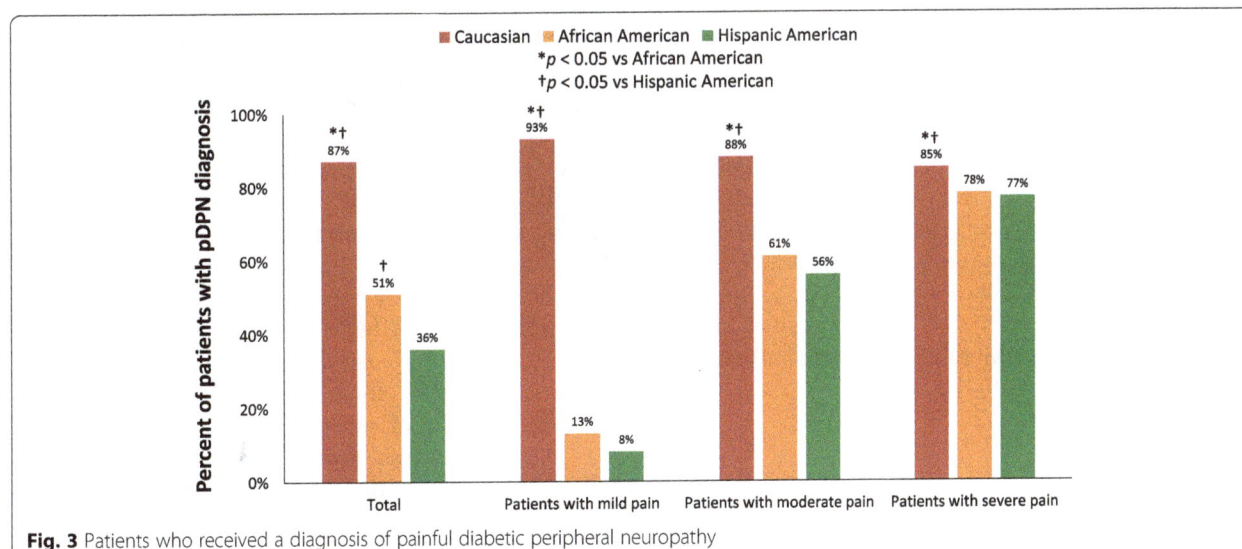

Fig. 3 Patients who received a diagnosis of painful diabetic peripheral neuropathy

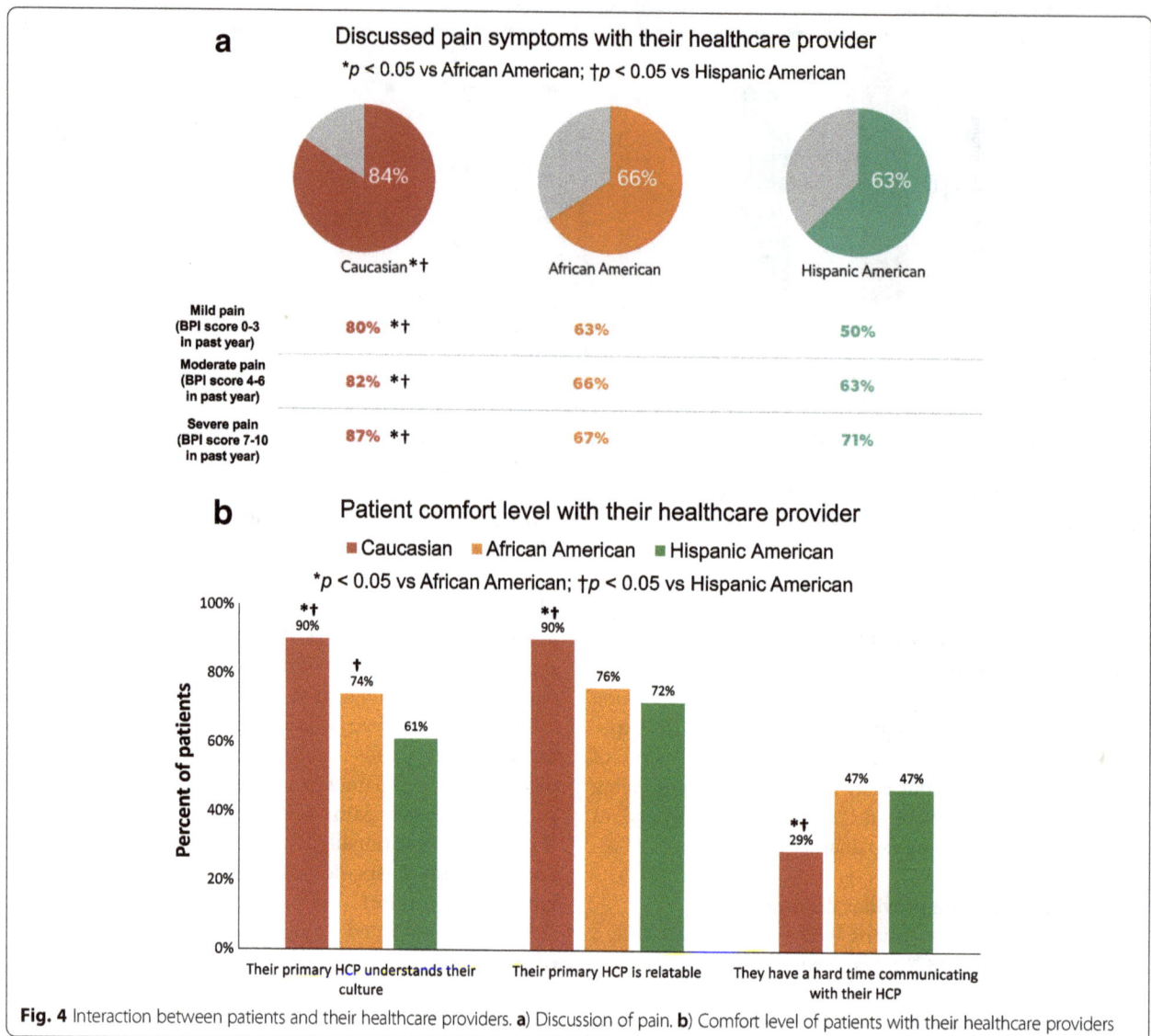

Fig. 4 Interaction between patients and their healthcare providers. **a)** Discussion of pain. **b)** Comfort level of patients with their healthcare providers

Impact of pDPN

Overall work impairment due to pain was substantial among employed patients in the three populations (Fig. 5). While Caucasians reported greater work impairment than African-Americans and Hispanics, none of the differences between groups was significant. Presenteeism was at least three times as high as absenteeism in all populations, and presenteeism among Caucasians was significantly higher relative to Hispanics, 48% and 36%, respectively (*p* < 0.05). Activity impairment was significantly (*p* < 0.05) higher among Caucasians (56%) relative to African-Americans (53%) and Hispanics (43%) (Fig. 5).

Discussion

This study suggests not only that there are significant disparities across cultural groups in their interaction with HCPs regarding pDPN and its symptoms, but that

presentation of pDPN itself is also significantly different across these groups, with lower pain severity and fewer number of pDPN symptoms reported among African-Americans and Hispanics relative to Caucasians. In particular, among the types of symptoms, only for pins and needles was there concordance among all three cultural groups for the percentage of patients reporting this symptom. For the other symptoms, the percent of patients reporting the symptoms was generally lowest among Hispanics and highest among Caucasians.

While it has previously been reported that there are differences in how ethnic groups perceive and report types and severity of experimental pain [14, 15], which may in part result from genetic as well as cultural factors [16, 17], the observations here contrast with a recent review indicating that Hispanics report greater pain sensitivity and experience greater severity relative to non-

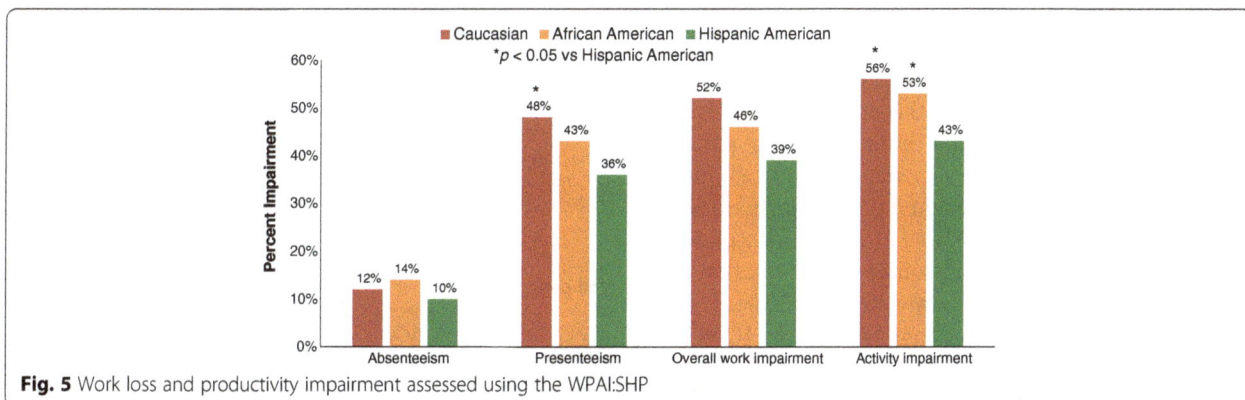

Fig. 5 Work loss and productivity impairment assessed using the WPAI:SHP

Hispanic Whites [15]. However, it is also possible that these perceptions may be dependent on the type of pain, i.e., neuropathic or nociceptive. Whether these differences extend to the clinical setting has not been adequately explored, although the results reported here do suggest potential differences as well as the need for further evaluating pain perceptions in multicultural populations, including sensations related to neuropathic pain such as pDPN.

The robustness of these results was demonstrated by additional analyses that adjusted for demographic and socioeconomic factors, since age, education level, and income may be potential confounding factors that contribute to pain perceptions or HCP interactions. These additional analyses suggest that regardless of socioeconomic status, ethnicity is a general factor in how symptoms associated with pDPN are manifested or perceived.

Additionally, and of potential greater clinical relevance, was the large proportion of African-American and Hispanic populations who were <40 years of age. While it is well-recognized that diabetes disproportionally affects African-Americans and Hispanics [18], to our knowledge this is the first study to suggest that these populations may also have a high prevalence of pDPN symptoms in such a young age group, but a more rigorous epidemiologic study would be needed to corroborate these observations. The overall similarity across ethnicities for time since a diabetes diagnosis further suggests that duration of diabetes is unlikely to meaningfully impact the observed results and their clinical implications.

The differences in symptoms and severity were paralleled by the impact of pain on daily activities on the WPAI:SHP reported by the three populations; the least impairment was consistently reported by Hispanics, and this was significant for Activity impairment vs both other populations, and for Presenteeism vs Caucasians. It should again be noted that the WPAI:SHP responses on work productivity were obtained only from employed respondents, while the activity impairment question was answered by all respondents and was limited to activities

other than employment. These observations on the WPAI:SHP are consistent with a recent review suggesting lower rates of activity limitation among Hispanics with pain relative to other cultural groups despite greater pain sensitivity [15]. Among those employed, presenteeism was three times that of absenteeism in all cultural groups, suggesting that this was the primary driver of work impairment, as has been previously reported among patients with chronic pain conditions [5].

Despite the presence of these symptoms and pain of moderate or severe severity in substantial proportions of African-Americans and Hispanics, fewer of these patients reported receiving a pDPN diagnosis than Caucasians. This lower rate of diagnosis may potentially be due, at least in part, to the observations related to interactions of these populations with their HCPs: Fewer African-American and Hispanic patients reported discussing their pain symptoms with their HCP, and there was consistently less comfort with their HCPs in these groups.

These interactions with HCPs are consistent with the disparities in healthcare resource availability and use that have been reported among minority populations and that contribute to the challenge of diagnosis and management of these patients [19]. In particular, Hispanics have reported language and cultural barriers such as the unavailability of Spanish-speaking healthcare providers or interpreters [15, 20]. While these language and cultural barriers may in part account for the lower comfort level of Hispanics with their HCPs in the current study, it should also be noted that African-Americans reported a similarly hard time communicating with their HCPs as Hispanics did.

Limitations

As with any survey dependent upon respondents, an important limitation is potential selection bias, since patients who agreed to participate may have characteristics and perceptions different from those who refused. A related limitation is that the patient-level data on diagnosis, pain, and symptoms were based on self-report and, as such, may be subject to misunderstanding or mis-interpretation of the questions that may result, at least in part, from cultural differences across the populations.

It should also be noted that this study did not capture other factors that may have contributed to patients' perceptions of their pain experience, such as mood, negative emotions and thoughts, poor pain control, or construals. These factors, as well as others not collected, could be a potential missing source of information that may have contributed to how subjects reported their painful symptoms or interactions with their HCPs, and warrant further evaluation in future studies.

While use of both internet and phone as survey modalities could be criticized, such a design was neces-sary to reach the target populations, and the inability to disentangle the administration modality from the results across the populations represents another limitation. Lastly, the survey results reflect an unweighted sample, and thus may not necessarily be reflective or representa-tive of the entire general population in the United States. However, the findings provide directional insights that can be used to optimize patient care.

Conclusions

Significant differences in patient experiences of pDPN symptoms and pain severity were reported across cul-tural groups including African-Americans, Hispanics, and Caucasians; African-Americans and Hispanics were less likely to experience the same sensations as Cauca-sian patients and reported lower pain ratings. Further evaluation is needed to determine what may account for these observed differences. Differential rates of pDPN diagnosis and comfort levels with HCPs were also reported in this multicultural population, with the differ-ences providing support for barriers that contribute to disparities in healthcare among specific populations.

These results suggest a need to broaden pDPN educa-tional initiatives among both patients and clinicians. While patient intiatives should especially target multicul-tural populations, the goals of clinician initiatives should be to increase attention that symptoms may differ among individuals with different cultural backgrounds and to improve patient-HCP dialogue by encouraging discussion of pDPN symptoms and their impact in multicultural settings.

Abbreviations
BPI: Brief Pain Inventory; HCP: Healthcare provider; pDPN: Painful diabetic peripheral neuropathy; WPAI:SHP: Work Productivity and Assessment Questionnaire disease-specific version

Acknowledgements
Editorial/medical writing support was provided by E. Jay Bienen and was funded by Pfizer.

Funding
This study was conducted by Kelton Global and sponsored by Pfizer Inc.

Authors' contributions
All authors met the International Committee of Medical Journal Editors (ICMJE) recommendations for authorship. AS, AHA, JCC, PT, BP and MMT were involved in conception and design of the study including development of the survey instrument. ME carried out data acquisition. ME and JCC analyzed and interpreted the data with further input from the remaining authors. All authors were involved in drafting the article and revising it critically for important intellectual content. All authors approved the final version to be submitted for publication.

Competing interests
ME is an employee of Kelton Global. AHA was an employee and shareholder of Pfizer at the time of the study and development of the manuscript. BP, JCC, PH, and AS are paid employees and shareholders of Pfizer. MMT is a practicing neurologist and reports no conflicts of interest.

Author details
[1]Kelton Communications, Culver City, CA, USA. [2]Pfizer Inc., 235 East 42nd Street, New York, NY 10017, USA. [3]Pfizer Inc., Groton, CT, USA. [4]Palm Beach Neurological Center, Palm Beach Gardens, FL, USA.

References
1.   Sadosky A, McDermott AM, Brandenburg NA, Strauss M. A review of the epidemiology of painful diabetic peripheral neuropathy, post-herpetic neuralgia, and less commonly studied neuropathic pain conditions. Pain Pract. 2008;8(1):45–56.
2.   Jambart S, Ammache Z, Haddad F, Younes A, Hassoun A, Abdalla K, Selwan CA, Sunna N, Wajsbrot D, Youseif E. Prevalence of painful diabetic peripheral neuropathy among patients with diabetes mellitus in the Middle East region. J Int Med Res. 2011;39(2):366–77.
3.   Alleman CJ, Westerhout KY, Hensen M, Chambers C, Stoker M, Long S, van Nooten FE. Humanistic and economic burden of painful diabetic peripheral neuropathy in Europe: a review of the literature. Diabetes Res Clin Pract. 2015;109(2):215–25.
4.   van Hecke O, Austin SK, Khan RA, Smith BH, Torrance N. Neuropathic pain in the general population: a systematic review of epidemiological studies. Pain. 2014;155(4):654–62.
5.   Stewart WF, Ricci JA, Chee E, Hirsch AG, Brandenburg N. Lost productive time and costs due to diabetes and diabetic neuropathic pain in the US workforce. J Occup Environ Med. 2007;49(6):672–9.
6.   daCosta DiBonaventura M, Cappelleri JC, Joshi AV. A longitudinal assessment of painful diabetic peripheral neuropathy on health status, productivity, and health care utilization and cost. Pain Med. 2011;12(1): 118–26.
7.   Sadosky A, Mardekian J, Parsons B, Hopps M, Bienen EJ, Markman J. Healthcare utilization and costs in diabetes relative to the clinical spectrum of painful diabetic peripheral neuropathy. J Diabetes Complicat. 2015;29(2): 212–7.
8.   Sadosky A, Hopper J, Parsons B. Painful diabetic peripheral neuropathy: results of a survey characterizing the perspectives and misperceptions of patients and healthcare practitioners. Patient. 2014;7(1):107–14.
9.   Portenoy R. Development and testing of a neuropathic pain screening questionnaire: ID pain. Curr Med Res Opin. 2006;22(8):1555–65.
10. Cleeland CS, Ryan KM. Pain assessment: global use of the brief pain inventory. Ann Acad Med Singap. 1994;23(2):129–38.
11. Work Productivity and Activity Impairment Questionnaire: Specific Health Problem V2.0 (WPAI:SHP) [http://www.reillyassociates.net/WPAI_SHP.html].
12. Zelman D, Dukes E, Brandenburg N, Bostrom A, Gore M. Identification of cut-points for mild, moderate and severe pain due to diabetic peripheral neuropathy. Pain. 2005;115(2):29–36.
13. Kleinbaum DG, Kupper LL, Nizam A, Rosenberg ES. Applied regression analysis and other multivariate methods. 5th ed. Boston: Cengage Learning; 2014.
14. Rahim-Williams B, Riley JL 3rd, Williams AK, Fillingim RB. A quantitative review of ethnic group differences in experimental pain response: do biology, psychology, and culture matter? Pain Med. 2012;13(4):522–40.

15. Hollingshead NA, Ashburn-Nardo L, Stewart JC, Hirsh AT. The pain experience of Hispanic Americans: a critical literature review and conceptual model. J Pain. 2016;17(5):513–28.

16. Kim H, Neubert JK, San Miguel A, Xu K, Krishnaraju RK, Iadarola MJ, Goldman D, Dionne RA. Genetic influence on variability in human acute experimental pain sensitivity associated with gender, ethnicity and psychological temperament. Pain. 2004;109(3):488–96.

17. Campbell CM, Edwards RR. Ethnic differences in pain and pain management. Pain Manag. 2012;2(3):219–30.

18. National Diabetes Statistics Report: Estimates of Diabetes and Its Burden in the United States, 2014. Atlanta: U.S. Department of Health and Human Services. http://www.thefdha.org/pdf/diabetes.pdf.

19. National Healthcare Disparities Report, 2013. Publication # 14–0006 [http://www.ahrq.gov/research/findings/nhqrdr/nhdr13/2013nhdr.pdf].

20. Betancourt JR, Corbett J, Bondaryk MR. Addressing disparities and achieving equity: cultural competence, ethics, and health-care transformation. Chest. 2014;145(1):143–8.

20

Graves' hyperthyroidism in pregnancy: a clinical review

Caroline T. Nguyen[1*], Elizabeth B. Sasso[2], Lorayne Barton[3] and Jorge H. Mestman[4]

Abstract

Background: Graves' hyperthyroidism affects 0.2% of pregnant women. Establishing the correct diagnosis and effectively managing Graves' hyperthyroidism in pregnancy remains a challenge for physicians.

Main: The goal of this paper is to review the diagnosis and management of Graves' hyperthyroidism in pregnancy. The paper will discuss preconception counseling, etiologies of hyperthyroidism, thyroid function testing, pregnancy-related complications, maternal management, including thyroid storm, anti-thyroid drugs and the complications for mother and fetus, fetal and neonatal thyroid function, neonatal management, and maternal post-partum management.

Conclusion: Establishing the diagnosis of Graves' hyperthyroidism early, maintaining euthyroidism, and achieving a serum total T4 in the upper limit of normal throughout pregnancy is key to reducing the risk of maternal, fetal, and newborn complications. The key to a successful pregnancy begins with preconception counseling.

Keywords: Hyperthyroidism, Pregnancy, Antithyroid drugs, Methimazole, Propylthiouracil, TRAb, Neonatal hyperthyroidism, Thyroid storm

Background

Graves' Hyperthyroidism (GH) is an autoimmune condition caused by antibodies stimulating the thyroid stimulating hormone receptor (TSHR). GH affects 0.2% of pregnant women [1]. Establishing the correct diagnosis and effectively managing GH in pregnancy is challenging; pregnancy alters thyroid physiology and laboratory testing, antithyroid drugs (ATDs) are associated with teratogenicity, and maternal, fetal, and newborn complications are directly related to control of GH and in a few cases to the levels of serum maternal thyroid-stimulating immunoglobulin (TSI) [2]. Fetal and neonatal hyperthyroidism occurs in 1% to 5% of women with active or a past history of GH and is associated with increased fetal/neonatal morbidity and mortality if not diagnosed and treated [3]. All women of reproductive age with GH or past history of GH should receive preconception counseling.

Preconception counseling

Counseling should take into consideration the woman's desired timeline to conception and include a discussion of the risks and benefits of all treatment options (medical therapy, 131-I radioactive iodine ablation (RAIA), and surgery). Women with GH should be advised to postpone conception and use contraception until GH is controlled. Women with difficult to control GH on high doses of ATD should consider definitive therapy (RAIA or surgery) prior to conception.

In women considering RAIA, a pregnancy test should be done beforehand and conception should be delayed for 6 months until the woman is euthyroid on levothyroxine replacement therapy. TSH Receptor Antibodies (TRAb), measurable in 95% of patients with GH, may increase and stay elevated for months to years after RAIA therapy [4, 5]. Persistently elevated TRAb levels during pregnancy are prognostic of fetal thyroid dysfunction [6]. Consequently, women with very elevated TRAb levels prior to conception may be better candidates for thyroidectomy. After surgery, TRAb levels decrease and normalize within months to one year [4, 5].

In women who continue with ATD treatment, methimazole (MMI) is generally preferred to propylthiouracil (PTU) because MMI is dosed once daily and PTU has

---
* Correspondence: Caroline.Nguyen@med.usc.edu
[1]Division of Endocrinology, Diabetes, & Metabolism, Department of Medicine, Keck School of Medicine, University of Southern California, 1540 Alcazar Street, CHP 204, Los Angeles, Ca 90033, USA
Full list of author information is available at the end of the article

an association with hepatotoxicity. However, PTU is recommended for the first trimester of pregnancy because its teratogenic effects are considered less severe than those of MMI. Switching from MMI to PTU in anticipation of conception should be considered. Alternatively, women may switch to PTU once pregnant.

Patients taking ATDs should use contraception and be counseled to pay close attention to menstrual cycles. A pregnancy test should be done immediately if there is a missed period. The risk of birth defects from ATDs is greatest during weeks 6–10 [7].

Etiologies of hyperthyroidism

While the etiologies of hyperthyroidism are extensive (Table 1), GH and gestational transient thyrotoxicosis (GTT) account for the majority of hyperthyroidism in pregnancy. Distinguishing between GTT and GH is important because GTT is a transient, mild hyperthyroidism that does not require treatment with ATD and is not associated with adverse pregnancy outcomes [8].

Gestational transient thyrotoxicosis (GTT)

GTT affects 1–5% of pregnant women early in pregnancy and is not due to intrinsic thyroid disease [9]. As in GH, patients with GTT may present with palpitations, anxiety,

Table 1 Causes of Hyperthyroidism in Pregnancy [33]

Thyroid Disease
Graves' disease
Chronic thyroiditis
Painless thyroiditis
Subacute thyroiditis
Toxic adenoma
Multinodular goiter
Non-autoimmune hyperthyroidism
Gestational transient thyrotoxicosis
Multiple gestations
Trophoblastic disease
Hyperplacentosis
Hyperreactio luteinalis
TSH receptor mutation
TSH-producing pituitary adenoma
Iatrogenic
Excessive levothyroxine (LT4) intake
Overtreatment
Factitious
Drugs
Iodine
Amiodarone
Lithium

tremors, and heat intolerance. A severe form of GTT is hyperemesis gravidarum, which is characterized by significant nausea, vomiting, and weight loss of up to 5 kg. These symptoms along with negative TRAb and the absence of Graves ophthalmopathy, goiter, and prior history of GH favor the diagnosis of GTT. The clinical course is closely correlated with hCG levels, which begin to rise at week 7 of gestation. Symptoms spontaneously resolve as serum concentration of hCG decreases between weeks 14 and 20 [10].

Women with twin pregnancies, another frequent cause of GTT, have higher levels of human chorionic gonadotropin (hCG) for a more prolonged period of time and consequently may be more symptomatic [11]. Trophoblastic disease (i.e., hydatidiform moles and choriocarcinoma) are also associated with elevated hCG levels and hyperthyroidism. Biochemically, GTT is characterized by a suppressed thyroid-stimulating hormone (TSH) and mildly elevated free thyroxine (FT4). TRAb are typically absent. TSH levels may continue to be suppressed for weeks after resolution of GTT. In very symptomatic patients a trial of beta-blocker may provide relief. In pregnancy, propranolol is preferred as atenolol has been associated with decreased birth weight [12, 13]. Women with a prior history of GTT have a higher likelihood of having a repeat episode [9].

Graves' hyperthyroidism (GH)

As described above, the signs and symptoms of GH in pregnancy are similar to those of a non-pregnant GH patient. The diagnosis of GH should be suspected in a hyperthyroid pregnant woman who 1) was having symptoms prior to pregnancy 2) had a prior diagnosis of hyperthyroidism, and 3) had a previous birth to an infant with thyroid dysfunction.

The small increase in GH incidence and worsening of GH symptoms described in early pregnancy may be from the stimulation of the thyroid gland by hCG or elevation in TRAb levels during the first trimester [14–16]. As pregnancy progresses, changes in the immunologic response lead to improvement in symptoms. Postpartum, a rebound of the immune system can lead to exacerbation of GH [17].

Thyroid function tests

In response to the rising hCG in early pregnancy, TSH concentrations may be below the non-pregnant reference range in up to 10% of normal pregnant women with 0.5–1% of women with completely suppressed TSH levels [18].

In the latter half of pregnancy, increased thyroid-binding globulin (TBG) and decreased serum albumin concentration can affect the widely available FT4 automated immunoassays resulting in significant variability between assays [19–21]. FT4 concentration also continuously declines throughout pregnancy [21]. Consequently, assay and trimester-specific pregnancy reference ranges are necessary if FT4 is used.

During pregnancy, the total thyroxine (TT4) assay is more consistent between assays. An estrogen-driven increase in TBG leads to the steady rise of TT4 from the first trimester until mid-gestation when the TT4 plateaus. After week 16, the non-pregnancy reference range may be adjusted by a factor of 1.5 and used to assess thyroid status (i.e., 4.5–12.5µg/dL becomes 6.75–18.75µg/dL) [21].

In addition, the FT4 index (FT4I) is a reliable marker of free thyroxine status during pregnancy, correcting TT4 for alterations in TBG [21, 22].

Free and total triiodothyronine (FT3/TT3) are rarely useful in the diagnosis and management of GH in pregnancy. One exception is in the diagnosis of an autonomous functioning nodule predominantly secreting T3.

TSH receptor antibodies (TRAb)

TRAb is a general term to define an antibody that binds the TSHR. TRAb can stimulate, block, or be neutral to the TSHR. GH is due to antibodies that stimulate the TSHR. TRAb is useful in confirming the diagnosis of GH [5].

Preconception, the presence of elevated TRAb is prognostic of risk of relapse of GH or failing ATD cessation [23]. During pregnancy, TRAb crosses the placenta and may induce fetal hyperthyroidism. TRAb levels over 3 times the upper limit of normal are associated with hyperthyroidism in the fetus and newborn [5].

TRAb assays can be divided into two categories: 1) TSH-binding inhibiting Ig (TBI)/thyrotropin binding inhibitory immunoglobulin (TBII) are competition-based assays that detect all TRAb (stimulating, blocking, and neutral) in patients' sera by their ability to compete for binding of the TSHR and 2) Thyroid-stimulating Ig (TSI) is a bioassay that detects cyclic adenosine monophosphate (cAMP) production in cells incubated with patients' sera and measures stimulating TRAb [24]. More recently, bioassays now have the ability to differentiate between stimulating and blocking antibodies [25].

TBII has a 97% sensitivity and 99% specificity for GH [26]. While TBII is unable to differentiate between stimulating or blocking antibodies, in a patient who is thyrotoxic an elevated TBI is due to the presence of stimulating TRAb in the majority of cases.

While thyroid peroxidase antibody (TPO-Ab) positivity has been associated with increased risk for pregnancy loss and premature delivery in euthyroid women, it is a nonspecific marker for autoimmune thyroid disease with no prognostic value for the fetus and newborn in Graves' Disease.

Pregnancy-related complications

Poor control of thyrotoxicosis is associated with pregnancy loss, pregnancy-induced hypertension, prematurity, low birth weight, intrauterine growth restriction, stillbirth, thyroid storm, and maternal congestive heart failure [27–29]. Women with uncontrolled GH are 9.2 times more likely to have neonates with low birth weight compared to non-GH women. However, if disease is controlled during pregnancy, they are 2.3 times as likely. Mothers with uncontrolled GH are also 16.5 times more likely to undergo preterm delivery and 4.7 times more likely to develop severe preeclampsia compared with women whose GH was controlled [30]. The rate of fetal demise and stillbirth in mothers with poorly controlled GH is 5.6% [31]. Persistent maternal TBII levels > 5 IU/L (approximately 3× ULN) in the latter half of pregnancy predicted neonatal hyperthyroidism with 100% sensitivity and 43% specificity (Table 2) [32].

Maternal management

ATDs remain the treatment of choice for GH during pregnancy. The lowest dose of ATD needed to maintain TT4 1.5× the upper limit of the non-pregnant reference range or FT4I at the upper limit of the reference range

Table 2 Risk factors for complications associated with hyperthyroidism in pregnancy

Risk factors [27, 28, 30]

- Long-standing GH
- Gestational hypertension
- Twin pregnancies
- Anemia
- Frequent infections (i.e., UTIs)
- Late presentation to obstetric clinic
- Inconsistent use of medications
- Abnormal outcomes in prior pregnancies

Possible complications

- Maternal [28]
  o Miscarriages
  o Gestational hypertension
  o Preeclampsia
  o Congestive heart failure
  o Thyroid storm
- Obstetrical
  o Premature delivery [82]
  o Placental abruption
  o Premature rupture of membrane
  o Gestational Hypertension
- Fetal
  o Congenital malformations [83]
  o Hyperthyroidism
  o Developmental dysplasia of the hip associated with first-trimester maternal hyperthyroidism [84]
  o Intrauterine growth restriction (IUGR)
  o Small for gestational age (SGA) infants
  o Prematurity
  o Stillbirth
- Neonatal
  o Prematurity
  o Hyperthyroidism [32]
  o Neonatal central hypothyroidism [71]
  o Low birth weight [30]

should be used. We have observed that normalization of FT4I can lag behind FT4 during ATD therapy leading to unwarranted larger doses of ATDs [33]. Care must be taken to avoid overtreatment with ATD. TSH may remain suppressed during ATD therapy even when TT4 of FT4I has normalized. The ATD dose should be lowered if TSH becomes detectable [33, 34]. "Block and replace" therapy, which consists of using an ATD in combination with levothyroxine therapy, is not recommended [29].

In the first trimester, PTU can be dosed at 50–150 mg every 8 h depending on the severity of the patient's symptomatology. When switching from MMI to PTU, a ratio of 1:20 is used (i.e., MMI 15 mg = 300 mg of PTU per day dosed as 100 mg PO every 8 h) [2]. After the first trimester, MMI 5-20 mg can be given as a single dose. Occasionally, in very symptomatic patients up to 30-40 mg can be used daily. Propranolol 10-20 mg every 6–8 h can be used to control hyperadrenergic symptoms and tapered and discontinued as tolerated. Long term treatment with ß-blockers has been associated with poor intrauterine growth, fetal bradycardia, and neonatal hypoglycemia [35]. TSH, FT4/FT4I, or TT4 should be checked every 2–4 weeks as clinically indicated and doses of ATDs titrated based on clinical and biochemical response. ATD may be discontinued in women with mild disease requiring low dose of ATD and mildly elevated TRAb. In 30–40% of women, ATD may be discontinued after 30–34 weeks of gestation [34]. Fetal hypothyroidism is an indication to decrease or stop ATD.

Measurement of TRAb in pregnancy

TRAb should be checked in a pregnant woman with a past history of GH or active GH [36, 37]. If TRAb levels are low or undetectable in early pregnancy, no further TRAb testing is recommended [2]. If maternal TRAb is elevated or patient is being treated with ATDs, TRAb should be measured again between weeks 18–22. In those with levels near 3-4× above upper limit of normal (ULN), TRAb should be checked again during weeks 28–34. Maternal TRAb serum concentration greater than 3 times the upper limit of the reference range in the third trimester is a risk factor for neonatal hyperthyroidism [32, 38–40].

The role of thyroidectomy

Thyroidectomy in the second trimester is an effective option if a woman is unable to tolerate ATDs, non-consistent with drug therapy, requiring very high doses of ATDs, has a large goiter, or allergic to ATD. ß-blockade should be used to prepare patients for surgery and continued after surgery. A few days of SSKI or saturated solution of potassium iodide (50-100 mg/day) to help decrease the vascularity of the thyroid gland and control hyperthyroidism can be considered and is safe for the fetus [41].

Thyroid storm (TS) in pregnancy

TS is a rare complication of uncontrolled GH. Given its rarity, the incidence of TS in pregnancy is not clear. Davis et al. described 1 case in 120,000 deliveries over the span of 11 years at a single institution [27]. TS may occur when a chronically hyperthyroid patient encounters an additional stress or precipitating event (i.e., infection, preeclampsia, labor, surgery, or pregnancy) that leads to decompensation. Patients with TS present with tachycardia, thermic dysregulation, and altered mental status. If not adequately treated, TS can lead to multi-organ failure including congestive heart failure. Biochemical testing reveals suppressed TSH and elevated T4. Patients are best served in the ICU as they may require intubation and IV medications. Treatment entails adequate ATD, beta-blockade, and supportive care (Table 3).

Anti-thyroid drugs: Complications for mother and fetus

ATD remains the mainstay treatment of women with GH during pregnancy. 3–5% of these women experience side effects. An allergic reaction is the most common side effect [42]. More severe side effects such as agranulocytosis (0.15%) and liver failure (< 0.1%) are rare [43, 44].

PTU and MMI are equally effective, cross the placenta at comparable rates, and may produce fetal hypothyroidism with or without goiter. Rates of fetal defects have been shown to be similar with both drugs; 2–3% with PTU and 2–4% with MMI [45–47]. Notably, this is similar to the overall 3% rate of major structural or genetic birth defects in the United States [48]. ATD associated defects are most common and severe in those exposed during weeks 6–10 [7, 45, 47, 49, 50]. PTU has traditionally been preferred over MMI in the first trimester because the birth defects associated with PTU are considered less severe and surgically correctable (Table 4) [51, 52]. Recently, a meta-analysis showed an increased risk of neonatal congenital malformations associated with MMI, but not PTU when compared to no ATD exposure [53]. However, other studies have not shown any difference in rates of congenital malformations between those treated with MMI or PTU and the general population [54].

Fetal and neonatal thyroid function

The fetal (f) thyroid gland develops between 5 and 6 weeks gestation [55] and starts secreting thyroxine at 10 weeks of gestation [56]. Fetal thyroid hormone (fTH) production is limited until 18–20 weeks of gestation when fTSH receptors begin to function [57, 58]. fTSH levels will begin to rise until 28 weeks of gestation. fT4 levels will continue to rise until the end of pregnancy [59]. Prior to the onset of fTH production, the fetus relies on TH from the mother via transplacental passage [60].

Immediately after birth there is a rise in TSH, T4, and T3. TSH surges and peaks in the first 24 h of life and

Table 3 Management of Thyroid Storm [34, 63]

ATD management (decreases the synthesis and release of T4 and T3)	• PTU 100-150 mg PO every 8 h (PO, NGT) or • MMI 20 mg PO every 12 h (PO, NGT) or • MMI 40 mg in 200 cm³ water (Per rectum)
Non-selective beta blockade (symptomatic relief) to target: B₁ – Heart rate B₂ – Vasodilation B₃ – Basal metabolic rate and heat production	• Propranolol 1 mg IV bolus followed by 1 mg/h (target heart rate of 90–100 bpm if adequately hydrated)
T4 and T3 release	• SSKI (potassium iodide) 5 drops or Lugol's solution 10 drops every 8 h, 1 h after MMI (PO, NGT)
Generation of T3	• Decadron 4 mg IVPB every 6 h • PTU at above doses decreases peripheral conversion of T4 to T3
Incorporation of T4 and T3 into the nucleus	• L-carnitine 1-2 g twice a day [85]ᵃ
Fever	• Aspirin may increase thyroid hormones and acetaminophen can interfere with steroids. • Should improve with other treatment modalities.
Supportive care	• Antibiotics as infection common precipitating event • IVF –TS patients are at a fluid deficit. Fluid balance should be net positive. • Recommend against active cooling as can lead to peripheral vasoconstriction and hinder release of heat • Avoid aggressive use of diuretics. Intravascular depletion can lead to cardiovascular collapse • Low threshold to intubate

PO per oral, *NGT* nasogastric tube, *PR* per rectum, *IVF* intravenous fluids
ᵃNo studies in pregnant patients

remains elevated for up to 3 to 5 days. T4 and T3 serum concentrations increase up to 6-fold within the first few hours of life, peaking at 24 to 36 h after birth [57, 59].Thyroid function tests gradually decrease to normal levels by 3 to 4 days of age [61].

Monitoring the fetus
Fetal risks in mothers with GH include hyperthyroidism due to inappropriate transplacental passage of maternal TRAb and hypothyroidism due to excessive maternal administration of ATD. During routine OB visits, antepartum surveillance should include assessment of fetal heart rate, typically performed with handheld doppler monitor. Fetal tachycardia is concerning for a thyroid etiology. Other causes of tachycardia such as infection, medications (cocaine, terbutaline), obstetric conditions

Table 4 Birth defect associated with ATD

MMI

• Aplasia cutis
• Choanal atresia
• Esophageal atresia
• Omphalocele
• Urinary tract malformations
• Eye defects
• Ventral septal defects
• Dysmorphic facies
• Athelia
• Developmental delay

PTU

• Pre-auricular sinus/fistula and cysts
• Urinary tract abnormalities in males

(placental abruption, fetal bleeding), and fetal tachyarrhythmias should be ruled out [62].

TRAb titers and the fetus
As discussed previously, maternal serum TRAb titers provide useful prognostic information. TRAbs can cross the placenta and act to stimulate or block fetal thyroid hormone production once the fetal thyroid gland becomes functional [1, 2]. As stated above, persistent maternal TRAb levels greater than 3 times the ULN in the latter half of pregnancy predicted neonatal hyperthyroidism with 100% sensitivity and 43% specificity [32].

Indications for fetal ultrasound (FUS)
Women with a prior fetus or neonate with a thyroid disorder, TRAb greater than 3 times the ULN, fetal tachycardia, and poorly controlled hyperthyroidism should have a FUS. Initial US is generally performed at 18–22 weeks and then every 4 weeks to assess for gestational age, fetal viability, amniotic fluid volume, fetal anatomy, and detection of malformations [2, 63].

US findings of hyperthyroidism
The earliest sonographic sign of fetal thyroid dysfunction is fetal goiter, which appears as a solid neck mass [56, 64]. HR > 160 bpm for over 10 min, intrauterine growth restriction, presence of fetal goiter, advanced bone age, or oligo/polyhydramnios can also be seen in fetal hyperthyroidism [65]. Less commonly, fetal thyrotoxicosis can lead to heart failure, fetal hydrops, and fetal demise [63].

Fetal goiter can cause fetal, obstetric, and neonatal complications including polyhydramnios secondary to reduced swallowing ability, cervical dystocia, and mechanical obstruction of the fetal airway respectively [58, 66, 67]. Cesarean delivery may be preferred due to high risk of labor dystocia from a deflexed head [68].

Fetal hypothyroidism secondary to ATD drugs

Fetuses of mothers with GH on ATD can develop hypothyroidism and/or goiter due to overtreatment with ATDs [34]. Signs of hypothyroidism on FUS include fetal goiter, growth restriction, and delayed bone age [63]. ATD dose reduction or discontinuation should restore normal fetal thyroid function and decrease the size of the fetal goiter [56]. Rarely, intra-amniotic levothyroxine injections in conjunction with reduction of ATD dose may be indicated as combination therapy may lead to faster resolution of fetal goiter and recovery from hypothyroidism [67].

In the rare circumstance where the diagnosis remains unclear, cordocentesis remains the method of choice for confirmation of fetal thyroid status [1, 2, 57, 64]. Known as fetal blood sampling, cordocentesis involves US guided placement of a needle into the fetal circulation usually through direct placement into a free loop of umbilical cord or at the cord insertion site. Alternatively, TH concentrations in the amniotic fluid can be measured [58, 65]. While less hazardous, amniotic fluid hormone levels have not been validated as a reliable measure of fetal thyroid function [56].

Injection of levothyroxine into the umbilical vein should be restricted to cases of confirmed fetal hypothyroidism and progressive polyhydramnios in spite of repeated intra-amniotic injections [56, 69]. Overall risk of fetal complications associated with cordocentesis and intra-amniotic injection is low at 0.5% to 1% when performed at experienced centers [2, 57, 66]. The change in size of fetal goiter and extent of polyhydramnios help determine the response to treatment [64]. Repeat cordocentesis may be necessary to monitor therapy [70].

Fetal thyrotoxicosis

Isolated fetal hyperthyroidism in a euthyroid mother is treated with MMI 10-20 mg daily or larger doses if necessary after the first trimester with adjustment of the dose every few days based on fetal tachycardia and goiter size [34]. The lowest dose necessary to normalize the fetal heart rate (110–160 beats per minute) should be used [1]. Fetal assessment should then be performed every 1–2 weeks or as necessary with evaluation of fetal heart tones with hand-held doppler and US to assess growth, size of fetal thyroid gland, and amniotic fluid index. Care must be taken to prevent inducing fetal hypothyroidism due to excessive administration of ATD.

Neonatal management

The neonatology team or treating pediatrician should be alerted regarding the mother's diagnosis of thyroid disease before delivery [63]. Maternal use of ATDs during gestation, presence of TRAbs, and degree of control should be communicated directly. Progressive or complex thyroid illness during pregnancy warrants consideration of consultation with a pediatric endocrinologist prior to delivery [2].

Newborns of hyperthyroid mothers should be evaluated soon after birth. Neonates are at risk of hypothyroidism secondary to maternal ATD therapy, central hypothyroidism from untreated mothers via suppression of fetal TSH production that impairs the hypothalamic-pituitary-thyroid maturation [1, 71] and hyperthyroidism after the effect of maternal ATDs dissipates [33]. All newborns should be screened for thyroid dysfunction within 2 to 4 days after birth as early postnatal treatment reduces the risk of intellectual impairment [2].

TRAb can remain in the infant's circulation for up to four months after delivery leading to postnatal thyrotoxicosis in 1–5% of infants of mothers with GH [34]. The diagnosis may be delayed by 48–72 h due to the transplacental passage of ATD medication [59]. FT4 measurement at birth should be repeated between days 3 and 5 of life and continuously followed if elevated [40]. TRAb positive neonates without biochemical or clinical evidence of thyroid dysfunction should have weekly clinical and laboratory follow up until the TRAb test becomes negative [40].

Some hyperthyroid neonates are first diagnosed at birth. Signs of neonatal thyrotoxicosis include tachycardia, tachypnea, pulmonary arterial hypertension, systemic hypertension and heart failure. They may also be small for gestational age with accelerated bone maturation and craniosynostosis [34, 63]. The recommended treatment regimen for neonatal hyperthyroidism is MMZ 0.5–1 mg/day with addition of propranolol (2 mg/kg/d) if severe [2]. PTU is not recommended as a first line treatment due to the high frequency of hepatotoxicity, liver failure and death, particularly in children [72]. Follow up is necessary until the hyperthyroidism resolves which may take months.

In cases of non-transient hypothyroidism, the recommended starting dose of levothyroxine is 10–15 mcg/kg/day in term neonates. Therapy should be initiated within two weeks of life for optimal outcomes and the infant should be followed for the first three years of life [2]. Most children do well with treatment and higher initial thyroxine dosage combined with shorter time to normalization contribute to improved neurodevelopmental outcome [61].

Maternal post-partum management

GH mothers taking ATD at time of delivery should continue ATD after delivery even if breastfeeding. Those in remission are at risk for developing recurrent GH 4 to 12 months after delivery [73]. Elevated TRAb titers would favor relapse of GH. TSH and FT4 should be checked routinely the first year starting at 6 weeks after delivery.

GH in the postpartum period needs to be distinguished from postpartum thyrotoxicosis (PPT), a de novo auto-immune thyroid condition that occurs in approximately 5% of pregnancies in the first year postpartum [74]. PPT classically begins with a transient hyperthyroid phase followed by transient hypothyroidism before a return to euthyroidism. PPT does not require treatment with ATD. High TRAb titers would support relapse of GH. If the diagnosis remains unclear, 123-I RAIA uptake can help distinguish between GH and PPT in a non-breast-feeding woman [75]. If a woman is breastfeeding and a 123-I RAIA study must be done, the mother should discard the breast milk for 3–4 days [2].

Breastfeeding
Breastfeeding has been shown to be safe in mothers taking ATDs in appropriate doses. MMI and PTU both appear in breast milk in very small concentrations [76–78]. Studies of infants exposed to ATDs in breast milk in doses sufficient to control maternal GH had normal thyroid function and normal intellectual development [79, 80]. MMI is generally preferred in breastfeeding mothers because of hepatotoxicity associated with PTU. Experts recommend using the lowest effective doses possible with maximal doses of MMI 20 mg daily and PTU 300 mg daily [42, 81]. Doses should be split into 2 to 3 doses and administered after the mother has breastfed.

Conclusions
The goal in the care of women with GH is the delivery of a euthyroid healthy newborn to a healthy mother. Establishing the diagnosis of GH can be challenging for the physician. Physical exam, history, and occasionally TRAb levels, can help distinguish GH from GTT, the most common cause of hyperthyroidism in pregnancy. Maintaining euthyroidism throughout pregnancy is key to reducing the risk of maternal, fetal, and newborn complications. ATDs remain the cornerstone of treatment of GH in pregnancy, with the lowest doses needed to maintain TT4 at 1.5× the upper limit of the non-pregnant reference range or FT4I in the upper limit of the reference range. PTU is preferred in the first trimester. In women with mild GH controlled on low doses of ATD with mildly elevated TRAb levels, ATD may be stopped in the last 4–8 weeks of pregnancy. Limited course of β-adrenergic blockers may be used to control symptoms of GH. Surgery in the second trimester may be indicated for women unable to take ATD, uncontrolled on high doses of ATD, or with large goiters. Persistently elevated levels

of TRAb > 3× upper limit of normal is prognostic of fetal thyroid dysfunction and calls for close attention of the fetus and newborn. In the postpartum period, women are at risk for recurrence of GH symptoms and thyroid function tests should be evaluated at 6 weeks.

A multidisciplinary approach involving collaboration between the endocrinologist, maternal-fetal specialist, obstetrician, neonatologist, pediatric endocrinologist, and anesthesiologist is essential to the successful management of these complex patients. The key to a successful pregnancy begins with preconception counseling.

Abbreviations
ATDs: antithyroid drugs; cAMP: cyclic adenosine monophosphate; f: fetal; FT3: free triiodothyronine; FT4: free thyroxine; FT4I: FT4 index; FUS: fetal ultrasound; GH: Graves' Hyperthyroidism; GTT: gestational transient thyrotoxicosis; hCG: human chorionic gonadotropin; IUGR : intrauterine growth restriction; IVF: intravenous fluids; LT4: excessive levothyroxine; MMI: methimazole; NGT: nasogastric tube; PO: per oral; PR: per rectum; PTU: propylthiouracil; RAIA: 131-I radioactive iodine ablation; SGA: small for gestational age; TBG: thyroxine-binding globulin; TBI: TSH-binding inhibiting immunoglobulin; TBII: thyrotropin binding inhibitory immunoglobulin; TPO-Ab: Thyroid peroxidase antibody; TRAb: TSH Receptor Antibodies; TS: Thyroid Storm; TSH: Thyroid-stimulating hormone; TSI: Thyroid-stimulating immunoglobulin; TT3: total triiodothyronine; TT4: total thyroxine; ULN: upper limit of normal

Authors' contributions
CN and ES performed the literature review and drafted the manuscript. LB and JM provided guidance and edits. All authors read and approved the final manuscript.

Competing interests
The authors declare that they have no competing interests.

Author details
[1]Division of Endocrinology, Diabetes, & Metabolism, Department of Medicine, Keck School of Medicine, University of Southern California, 1540 Alcazar Street, CHP 204, Los Angeles, Ca 90033, USA. [2]Division of Maternal Fetal Medicine, Department of Obstetrics and Gynecology, Keck School of Medicine, University of Southern California, 2020 Zonal Avenue, IRD 220, Los Angeles, CA 90033, USA. [3]Division of Neonatology, Department of Pediatrics, LAC+USC Medical Center, Keck School of Medicine, University of Southern California, Los Angeles, Ca 90033, USA. [4]Division of Endocrinology, Diabetes & Metabolism, Department of Medicine and Obstetrics and Gynecology, Keck School of Medicine, University of Southern California, 1540 Alcazar Street CHP 204, Los Angeles, California 90033, USA.

References
1. Cooper DS, Laurberg P. Hyperthyroidism in pregnancy. Lancet Diabetes Endocrinol. 2013;1:238–49.
2. Alexander EK, Pearce EN, Brent GA, Brown RS, Chen H, Dosiou C, Grobman WA, Laurberg P, Lazarus JH, Mandel SJ, Peeters RP, Sullivan S. 2017 guidelines of the American Thyroid Association for the diagnosis and Management of Thyroid Disease during Pregnancy and the postpartum. Thyroid. 2017;27:315–89.
3. Zimmerman D. Fetal and neonatal hyperthyroidism. Thyroid. 1999;9:727–33.
4. Kautbally S, Alexopoulou O, Daumerie C, Jamar F, Mourad M, Maiter D. Greater efficacy of Total thyroidectomy versus radioiodine therapy on

hyperthyroidism and thyroid-stimulating immunoglobulin levels in patients with Graves' disease previously treated with Antithyroid drugs. Eur Thyroid J. 2012;1:122–8.

5. Laurberg P, Wallin G, Tallstedt L, Abraham-Nordling M, Lundell G, Torring O. TSH-receptor autoimmunity in Graves' disease after therapy with anti-thyroid drugs, surgery, or radioiodine: a 5-year prospective randomized study. Eur J Endocrinol. 2008;158:69–75.

6. Banige MEC, Biran V, Desfrere L, Champion V, Benachi A, Ville Y, Dommergues M, Jarrau PH, Mokhtari M, Boithias C, Brioude F, Mandelbrot L, Ceccaldi PF, Mitanchez D, Polak M, Luton D. Study of the factors leading to fetal and neonatal Dysthyroidism in children of patients with graves disease. Journal of endocrine. Society. 2017;1:751–61.

7. Laurberg P, Andersen SL. Therapy of endocrine disease: antithyroid drug use in early pregnancy and birth defects: time windows of relative safety and high risk? Eur J Endocrinol. 2014;171:R13–20.

8. Casey BM, Dashe JS, Wells CE, McIntire DD, Leveno KJ, Cunningham FG. Subclinical hyperthyroidism and pregnancy outcomes. Obstet Gynecol. 2006;107:337–41.

9. Goldman AM, Mestman JH. Transient non-autoimmune hyperthyroidism of early pregnancy. J Thyroid Res. 2011;2011:142413.

10. Niebyl JR. Clinical practice. Nausea and vomiting in pregnancy. N Engl J Med. 2010;363:1544–50.

11. Grun JP, Meuris S, De Nayer P, Glinoer D. The thyrotrophic role of human chorionic gonadotrophin (hCG) in the early stages of twin (versus single) pregnancies. Clin Endocrinol. 1997;46:719–25.

12. Lip GY, Beevers M, Churchill D, Shaffer LM, Beevers DG. Effect of atenolol on birth weight. Am J Cardiol. 1997;79:1436–8.

13. Nakhai-Pour HR, Rey E, Berard A. Antihypertensive medication use during pregnancy and the risk of major congenital malformations or small-for-gestational-age newborns. Birth Defects Res B Dev Reprod Toxicol. 2010;89:147–54.

14. Andersen SL, Olsen J, Carle A, Laurberg P. Hyperthyroidism incidence fluctuates widely in and around pregnancy and is at variance with some other autoimmune diseases: a Danish population-based study. J Clin Endocrinol Metab. 2015;100:1164–71.

15. Amino N, Tanizawa O, Mori H, Iwatani Y, Yamada T, Kurachi K, Kumahara Y, Miyai K. Aggravation of thyrotoxicosis in early pregnancy and after delivery in Graves' disease. J Clin Endocrinol Metab. 1982;55:108–12.

16. Weetman AP. Immunity, thyroid function and pregnancy: molecular mechanisms. Nat Rev Endocrinol. 2010;6:311–8.

17. Tagami T, Hagiwara H, Kimura T, Usui T, Shimatsu A, Naruse M. The incidence of gestational hyperthyroidism and postpartum thyroiditis in treated patients with Graves' disease. Thyroid. 2007;17:767–72.

18. Haddow JE, McClain MR, Lambert-Messerlian G, Palomaki GE, Canick JA, Cleary-Goldman J, Malone FD, Porter TF, Nyberg DA, Bernstein P, D'Alton ME, First, second trimester evaluation of risk for fetal aneuploidy research C. Variability in thyroid-stimulating hormone suppression by human chorionic [corrected] gonadotropin during early pregnancy. J Clin Endocrinol Metab. 2008;93:3341–7.

19. Roti E, Gardini E, Minelli R, Bianconi L, Flisi M. Thyroid function evaluation by different commercially available free thyroid hormone measurement kits in term pregnant women and their newborns. J Endocrinol Investig. 1991;14:1–9.

20. Berta E, Samson L, Lenkey A, Erdei A, Cseke B, Jenei K, Major T, Jakab A, Jenei Z, Paragh G, Nagy EV, Bodor M. Evaluation of the thyroid function of healthy pregnant women by five different hormone assays. Pharmazie. 2010;65:436–9.

21. Lee RH, Spencer CA, Mestman JH, Miller EA, Petrovic I, Braverman LE, Goodwin TM. Free T4 immunoassays are flawed during pregnancy. Am J Obstet Gynecol. 2009;200:260:e261–6.

22. Wilke TJ. Diagnostic value of three methods for assessing free thyroxine in pregnancy. Ann Clin Biochem. 1983;20(Pt 1):60–1.

23. Hesarghatta Shyamasunder A, Abraham P. Measuring TSH receptor antibody to influence treatment choices in Graves' disease. Clin Endocrinol. 2017;86:652–7.

24. Barbesino G, Tomer Y. Clinical review: Clinical utility of TSH receptor antibodies. J Clin Endocrinol Metab. 2013;98:2247–55.

25. Kahaly GJ. Bioassays for TSH receptor antibodies: quo Vadis? Eur Thyroid J. 2015;4:3–5.

26. Tozzoli R, Bagnasco M, Giavarina D, Bizzaro N. TSH receptor autoantibody immunoassay in patients with Graves' disease: improvement of diagnostic accuracy over different generations of methods. Systematic review and meta-analysis. Autoimmun Rev. 2012;12:107–13.

27. Davis LE, Lucas MJ, Hankins GD, Roark ML, Cunningham FG. Thyrotoxicosis complicating pregnancy. Am J Obstet Gynecol. 1989;160:63–70.

28. Mestman JH. Hyperthyroidism in pregnancy. Best Pract Res Clin Endocrinol Metab. 2004;18:267–88.

29. Laurberg P, Bournaud C, Karmisholt J, Orgiazzi J. Management of Graves' hyperthyroidism in pregnancy: focus on both maternal and foetal thyroid function, and caution against surgical thyroidectomy in pregnancy. Eur J Endocrinol. 2009;160:1–8.

30. Millar LK, Wing DA, Leung AS, Koonings PP, Montoro MN, Mestman JH. Low birth weight and preeclampsia in pregnancies complicated by hyperthyroidism. Obstet Gynecol. 1994;84:946–9.

31. Hamburger JI. Diagnosis and management of Graves' disease in pregnancy. Thyroid. 1992;2:219–24.

32. Abeillon-du Payrat J, Chikh K, Bossard N, Bretones P, Gaucherand P, Claris O, Charrie A, Raverot V, Orgiazzi J, Borson-Chazot F, Bournaud C. Predictive value of maternal second-generation thyroid-binding inhibitory immunoglobulin assay for neonatal autoimmune hyperthyroidism. Eur J Endocrinol. 2014;171:451–60.

33. Mestman JH. Hyperthyroidism in pregnancy. Curr Opin Endocrinol Diabetes Obes. 2012;19:394–401.

34. Patil-Sisodia K, Mestman JH. Graves hyperthyroidism and pregnancy: a clinical update. Endocr Pract. 2010;16:118–29.

35. Rubin PC. Current concepts: Beta-blockers in pregnancy. N Engl J Med. 1981;305:1323–6.

36. Laurberg P, Nygaard B, Glinoer D, Grussendorf M, Orgiazzi J. Guidelines for TSH-receptor antibody measurements in pregnancy: results of an evidence-based symposium organized by the European thyroid association. Eur J Endocrinol. 1998;139:584–6.

37. Mortimer RH, Tyack SA, Galligan JP, Perry-Keene DA, Tan YM. Graves' disease in pregnancy: TSH receptor binding inhibiting immunoglobulins and maternal and neonatal thyroid function. Clin Endocrinol. 1990;32:141–52.

38. Luton D, Le Gac I, Vuillard E, Castanet M, Guibourdenche J, Noel M, Toubert ME, Leger J, Boissinot C, Schlageter MH, Garel C, Tebeka B, Oury JF, Czernichow P, Polak M. Management of Graves' disease during pregnancy: the key role of fetal thyroid gland monitoring. J Clin Endocrinol Metab. 2005;90:6093–8.

39. Peleg D, Cada S, Peleg A, Ben-Ami M. The relationship between maternal serum thyroid-stimulating immunoglobulin and fetal and neonatal thyrotoxicosis. Obstet Gynecol. 2002;99:1040–3.

40. Besancon A, Beltrand J, Le Gac I, Luton D, Polak M. Management of neonates born to women with Graves' disease: a cohort study. Eur J Endocrinol. 2014;170:855–62.

41. Momotani N, Hisaoka T, Noh J, Ishikawa N, Ito K. Effects of iodine on thyroid status of fetus versus mother in treatment of Graves' disease complicated by pregnancy. J Clin Endocrinol Metab. 1992;75:738–44.

42. Mandel SJ, Cooper DS. The use of antithyroid drugs in pregnancy and lactation. J Clin Endocrinol Metab. 2001;86:2354–9.

43. Nakamura H, Miyauchi A, Miyawaki N, Imagawa J. Analysis of 754 cases of antithyroid drug-induced agranulocytosis over 30 years in Japan. J Clin Endocrinol Metab. 2013;98:4776–83.

44. Watanabe N, Narimatsu H, Noh JY, Yamaguchi T, Kobayashi K, Kami M, Kunii Y, Mukasa K, Ito K, Ito K. Antithyroid drug-induced hematopoietic damage: a retrospective cohort study of agranulocytosis and pancytopenia involving 50,385 patients with Graves' disease. J Clin Endocrinol Metab. 2012;97:E49–53.

45. Yoshihara A, Noh J, Yamaguchi T, Ohye H, Sato S, Sekiya K, Kosuga Y, Suzuki M, Matsumoto M, Kunii Y, Watanabe N, Mukasa K, Ito K, Ito K. Treatment of graves' disease with antithyroid drugs in the first trimester of pregnancy and the prevalence of congenital malformation. J Clin Endocrinol Metab. 2012;97:2396–403.

46. Cooper DS, Rivkees SA. Putting propylthiouracil in perspective. J Clin Endocrinol Metab. 2009;94:1881–2.

47. Andersen SL, Olsen J, Wu CS, Laurberg P. Birth defects after early pregnancy use of antithyroid drugs: a Danish nationwide study. J Clin Endocrinol Metab. 2013;98:4373–81.

48. Hoyert DL, Mathews TJ, Menacker F, Strobino DM, Guyer B. Annual summary of vital statistics: 2004. Pediatrics. 2006;117:168–83.

49. Andersen SL, Olsen J, Laurberg P. Antithyroid drug side effects in the population and in pregnancy. J Clin Endocrinol Metab. 2016;101:1606–14.

50. Clementi M, Di Gianantonio E, Cassina M, Leoncini E, Botto LD, Mastroiacovo P, Group SA-MS. Treatment of hyperthyroidism in pregnancy and birth defects. J Clin Endocrinol Metab. 2010;95:E337-41.

51. Andersen SL, Olsen J, Wu CS, Laurberg P. Severity of birth defects after propylthiouracil exposure in early pregnancy. Thyroid. 2014;24:1533-40.

52. Bahn RS, Burch HS, Cooper DS, Garber JR, Greenlee CM, Klein IL, Laurberg P, McDougall IR, Rivkees SA, Ross D, Sosa JA, Stan MN. The role of Propylthiouracil in the Management of Graves' disease in adults: report of a meeting jointly sponsored by the American Thyroid Association and the Food and Drug Administration. Thyroid. 2009;19:673-4.

53. Song R, Lin H, Chen Y, Zhang X, Feng W. Effects of methimazole and propylthiouracil exposure during pregnancy on the risk of neonatal congenital malformations: a meta-analysis. PLoS One. 2017;12:e0180108.

54. Gianetti E, Russo L, Orlandi F, Chiovato L, Giusti M, Benvenga S, Moleti M, Vermiglio F, Macchia PE, Vitale M, Regalbuto C, Centanni M, Martino E, Vitti P, Tonacchera M. Pregnancy outcome in women treated with methimazole or propylthiouracil during pregnancy. J Endocrinol Investig. 2015;38:977-85.

55. Patel J, Landers K, Li H, Mortimer RH, Richard K. Delivery of maternal thyroid hormones to the fetus. Trends Endocrinol Metab. 2011;22:164-70.

56. Polak M, Van Vliet G. Therapeutic approach of fetal thyroid disorders. Horm Res Paediatr. 2010;74:1-5.

57. Fisher DA. Fetal thyroid function: diagnosis and management of fetal thyroid disorders. Clin Obstet Gynecol. 1997;40:16-31.

58. Munoz JL, Kessler AA, Felig P, Curtis J, Evans MI. Sequential amniotic fluid thyroid hormone changes correlate with goiter shrinkage following in utero thyroxine therapy. Fetal Diagn Ther. 2016;39:222-7.

59. Polak M. Human fetal thyroid function. Endocr Dev. 2014;26:17-25.

60. Andersen SL, Olsen J, Laurberg P. Foetal programming by maternal thyroid disease. Clin Endocrinol. 2015;83:751-8.

61. Simpser T, Rapaport R. Update on some aspects of neonatal thyroid disease. J Clin Res Pediatr Endocrinol. 2010;2:95-9.

62. American College of O, Gynecologists. Practice bulletin no. 116: Management of intrapartum fetal heart rate tracings. Obstet Gynecol. 2010;116:1232-40.

63. King JR, Lachica R, Lee RH, Montoro M, Mestman J. Diagnosis and Management of Hyperthyroidism in pregnancy: a review. Obstet Gynecol Surv. 2016;71:675-85.

64. Gruner C, Kollert A, Wildt L, Dorr HG, Beinder E, Lang N. Intrauterine treatment of fetal goitrous hypothyroidism controlled by determination of thyroid-stimulating hormone in fetal serum. A case report and review of the literature. Fetal Diagn Ther. 2001;16:47-51.

65. American College of O, Gynecologists. Practice Bulletin No. 148: Thyroid disease in pregnancy. Obstet Gynecol. 2015;125:996-1005.

66. Nachum Z, Rakover Y, Weiner E, Shalev E. Graves' disease in pregnancy: prospective evaluation of a selective invasive treatment protocol. Am J Obstet Gynecol. 2003;189:159-65.

67. Bliddal S, Rasmussen AK, Sundberg K, Brocks V, Feldt-Rasmussen U. Antithyroid drug-induced fetal goitrous hypothyroidism. Nat Rev Endocrinol. 2011;7:396-406.

68. Aubry G, Pontvianne M, Chesnais M, Weingertner AS, Guerra F, Favre R. Prenatal diagnosis of fetal Goitrous hypothyroidism in a Euthyroid mother: a management challenge. J Ultrasound Med. 2017;36(11):2387-92.

69. Davidson KM, Richards DS, Schatz DA, Fisher DA. Successful in utero treatment of fetal goiter and hypothyroidism. N Engl J Med. 1991;324:543-6.

70. Srisupundit K, Sirichotiyakul S, Tongprasert F, Luewan S, Tongsong T. Fetal therapy in fetal thyrotoxicosis: a case report. Fetal Diagn Ther. 2008;23:114-6.

71. Kempers MJ, van Tijn DA, van Trotsenburg AS, de Vijlder JJ, Wiedijk BM, Vulsma T. Central congenital hypothyroidism due to gestational hyperthyroidism: detection where prevention failed. J Clin Endocrinol Metab. 2003;88:5851-7.

72. Rivkees SA, Mattison DR. Propylthiouracil (PTU) Hepatoxicity in children and recommendations for discontinuation of use. Int J Pediatr Endocrinol. 2009;2009:132041.

73. Rotondi M, Cappelli C, Pirali B, Pirola I, Magri F, Fonte R, Castellano M, Rosei EA, Chiovato L. The effect of pregnancy on subsequent relapse from Graves' disease after a successful course of antithyroid drug therapy. J Clin Endocrinol Metab. 2008;93:3985-8.

74. Stagnaro-Green A. Approach to the patient with postpartum thyroiditis. J Clin Endocrinol Metab. 2012;97:334-42.

75. Gorman CA. Radioiodine and pregnancy. Thyroid. 1999;9:721-6.

76. Kampmann JP, Johansen K, Hansen JM, Helweg J. Propylthiouracil in human milk. Revision of a dogma. Lancet. 1980;1:736-7.

77. Johansen K, Andersen AN, Kampmann JP, Molholm Hansen JM, Mortensen HB. Excretion of methimazole in human milk. Eur J Clin Pharmacol. 1982;23:339-41.

78. Cooper DS, Bode HH, Nath B, Saxe V, Maloof F, Ridgway EC. Methimazole pharmacology in man: studies using a newly developed radioimmunoassay for methimazole. J Clin Endocrinol Metab. 1984;58:473-9.

79. Cooper DS. Antithyroid drugs. N Engl J Med. 2005;352:905-17.

80. Eisenstein Z, Weiss M, Katz Y, Bank H. Intellectual capacity of subjects exposed to methimazole or propylthiouracil in utero. Eur J Pediatr. 1992;151:558-9.

81. Karras S, Tzotzas T, Kaltsas T, Krassas GE. Pharmacological treatment of hyperthyroidism during lactation: review of the literature and novel data. Pediatr Endocrinol Rev. 2010;8:25-33.

82. Lo JC, Rivkees SA, Chandra M, Gonzalez JR, Korelitz JJ, Kuzniewicz MW. Gestational thyrotoxicosis, antithyroid drug use and neonatal outcomes within an integrated healthcare delivery system. Thyroid. 2015;25:698-705.

83. Momotani N, Ito K, Hamada N, Ban Y, Nishikawa Y, Mimura T. Maternal hyperthyroidism and congenital malformation in the offspring. Clin Endocrinol. 1984;20:695-700.

84. Ishikawa N. The relationship between neonatal developmental dysplasia of the hip and maternal hyperthyroidism. J Pediatr Orthop. 2008;28:432-4.

85. Benvenga S, Amato A, Calvani M, Trimarchi F. Effects of carnitine on thyroid hormone action. Ann N Y Acad Sci. 2004;1033:158-67.

21

Liraglutide and Dulaglutide therapy in addition to SGLT-2 inhibitor and metformin treatment in Indian type 2 diabetics

S. Ghosal[1,3]* 🆔 and B. Sinha[2,3]

Abstract

Background: Therapy for Type 2 diabetes (T2D) has been transformed by the introduction of newer agents like Glucagon like Peptide Receptor Agonists (GLP-1RA) and Sodium-glucose linked transporter inhibitors (SGLT2i). However with co-initiation of SGLT2i and GLP-1RA in the DURATION 8 trial an improvement in HbA1c was noted but the beneficial effect was not equal to the sum of its parts. In view of this we proceeded to test the hypothesis that sequential addition of GLP-1RA therapy to metformin and SGLT-2i may be more beneficial.

Methods: A retrospective real world observational case note study conducted in two diabetes care centres in India analyzed the first 60 consecutive T2D patients who could afford this therapy and had not achieved their glycaemic target (HbA1c < 7%)on metformin and SGLT2i. All these patients were additionally treated with either Dulaglutide or Liraglutide and followed up for 13 weeks.

Results: Across the entire 13-week study period, both liraglutide and dulaglutide proved to be an excellent add on to metformin and SGLT-2 inhibitor. There was significant reduction in HbA1c and body weight. Liraglutide had an additional significant impact on systolic blood pressure reduction in contrast to the dulaglutide arm. Comparatively, liraglutide and dulaglutide achieved similar metabolic control. However, a larger proportion of patients achieved HbA1c below 7.0% in the liraglutide arm (63.3%) compared to the dulaglutide arm (30%) and this difference was statistically significant.

Conclusion: In this retrospective study in Indian type 2 diabetic patients poorly controlled with metformin and SGLT-2 inhibitor we found a meaningful impact of adding a GLP-1 RA on all metabolic parameters. There were additional advantages seen with liraglutide as far achieving target HbA1c of less than 7% and also on the quantum of weight loss and systolic blood pressure reduction.

Keywords: Diabetes, Liraglutide, Dulaglutide, SGLT-2i , HbA1c, Weight

Background

The combination of Glucagon like Peptide Receptor Agonists (GLP-1RA) with a Sodium-glucose linked transporter inhibitor (SGLT2i) addresses many of the pathophysiological defects seen in Type 2 Diabetes (T2D), according to certain researchers [1]. In the EDICT trial, using the strategy of treating T2D, using multiple agents addressing the pathophysiological defects of the disease (insulin resistance, beta-cell dysfunction and hyperglucagonaemia) was found to be superior to the traditional step wise approach to glycaemic control in terms of HbA1c reduction and reduction of hypoglycaemia [2]. There have also been robust positive outcomes from the recent cardiovascular outcome trials (CVOT) with SGLT2i (empagliflozin and canagliflozin) and GLP-1 RA(liraglutide and semaglutide), establishing cardiovascular benefits attributable to these agents [3–6]. Hence there is a good scientific rationale for using them in combination.

* Correspondence: ramdasghosal@gmail.com
[1]Nightingale Hospital, 11 Shakespeare Sarani, Kolkata, India
[3]Kolkata, India
Full list of author information is available at the end of the article

The recent DURATION 8 study, testing the above rationale, demonstrated an additive effect on weight and systolic blood pressure reduction but not HbA1c reduction when exenatide LAR, a GLP-1 RA and dapagliflozin, a SGLT2i were used in combination as a co-initiation strategy [7, 8]. However multiple observational studies suggested that GLP-1 RA and SGLT2i are additive from a metabolic perspective as well, when SGLT2i was added to GLP-1 RA (sequential initiation instead of co-initiation) [9, 10]. This is contrary to a real world scenario where usually injectable are added only when oral drugs fail. This differing data therefore poses a conundrum for the physician as to whether to combine these drugs together or not, particularly keeping in mind that these drugs are very expensive. In a resource poor setting such as India where patients pay 'out-of-pocket', injectable therapies are usually used as a third-line agent when oral therapy fails. Hence, data on this combination mimicking a real-life setting i.e. oral therapy followed by injectable would be useful in guiding physician choices for intensification options in Type 2 diabetes.

We therefore designed this study to look into the sequential additive benefit of GLP-1 RA therapy to preexisting SGLT2i and Metformin therapy as well as comparing Dulaglutide with Liraglutide, in combination with SGLT2i and Metformin. The aim of this study is to evaluate real-life data from clinical practice using this combination of drugs and assess how the results compare with the available data from randomized controlled trials.

Methods

A retrospective, real world observational study to evaluate the efficacy of triple-anti-hyperglycemic agent therapy namely metformin, sodium glucose co-transporter 2 Inhibitors (SGLT2i) and glucagon like peptide receptor agonists (GLP-1 RAs) for patients failing on a combination of full dose metformin 2000 mg/day and SGLT2i for at least 3 months, was conducted in the outpatient clinics associated with two hospitals in Kolkata, India, from May 2016 to August 2016. The baseline characteristics of the patients included for analysis are detailed in Table 1.

After clearance from the local ethics committee (Nightingale Hospital ethics committee), the case notes of the first 30 consecutive patients who had been commenced on Metformin plus SGLT2i plus Dulaglutide, in addition to the first 30 patients who had been commenced on Metformin plus SGLT2i plus Liraglutide were collated after signing patient consent form to use their data for publication purpose. The ethics committee decided that consent of the patients was not required as this was a completely retrospective study of case notes with no intervention required.

Furthermore when the patients' data was entered into the database the patient could only be identified by a number; so there was no chance of the patients' confidentiality being compromised.

After adequate counseling, patients *who could **afford** this expensive combination of medications for at least 3 months* were commenced on this therapy. The

Table 1 Baseline Characteristics of the Patients (N = 60)

Demographic profile.		Liraglutide, N = 30	Dulaglutide, N = 30	P value
Male, n (%)	28(46.7%)	13 (43.3%)	15 (50%)	0.605
Female, n (%)	32 (53.3%)	17 (56.7%)	15 (50%)	
Age(years), Mean ± SEM	47.75 ± 1.22	47.33 ± 1.91	48.17 ± 1.55	0.736
Height (centimeters), Mean ± SEM	161.53 ± 1.2	159.97 ± 1.52	163.10 ± 1.83	0.193
Body weight(Kg), Mean ± SEM	88.3 ± 1.68	89.43 ± 2.60	87.17 ± 2.16	0.506
Diabetes duration, (years), Mean ± SEM	6.07 ± 0.70	5.55 ± 0.94	6.59 ± 1.03	0.46
SBP(mmHg), Mean ± SEM	136.07 ± 1.84	137.83 ± 2.50	134.30 ± 2.71	0.342
DBP(mmHg), Mean ± SEM	82.1 ± 1.15	83.47 ± 1.58	80.73 ± 1.64	0.236
BMI(kg/m2), Mean ± SEM	34.99 ± 5.66	34.92 ± 0.86	32.84 ± 0.77	0.078
BMI – 25 -29.9	10 (16.67%)			
BMI - 30-34.9	30 (50%)			
BMI - 35-39.9	12 (20%)			
BMI - ≥40	8 (13.33%)			
FPG(mg/dL), Mean ± SEM	167.83 ± 7.04	160.13 ± 8.17	175.53 ± 11.45	0.278
HbA1c(%), Mean ± SEM	8.46 ± 0.17	8.49 ± 0.26	8.43 ± 0.21	0.847
On Metformin, n (%)	60 (100%)	30 (100%)	30 (100%)	1.00
On SGLT-2is, n (%)	60 (100%)	30 (100%)	30 (100%)	1.00

following inclusion and exclusion criteria decided by the two centres:

Inclusion criteria

Adult Type 2 diabetics with HbA1C ≥ 7.0% on
Metformin plus SGLT2i
Body mass index (BMI) ≥ 25 kg/m^2,
eGFR> 45 ml/min

Exclusion criteria

Type 1 Diabetes
Pregnancy
Deranged liver function tests
Any major organ system disease as determined by
physical examination, medical history and screening
blood tests
Recent insulin therapy
Recent anti obesity therapy
Recent treatment with any other oral anti diabetics
History of pancreatitis
Family history of Medullary Thyroid cancer or MEN 2

Patients received treatment as per routine standard of care. All anti hypertensives, anti hyperlipidaemics and anti platelet agents and other preexisting medications (not related to diabetes) were continued as per the patients' requirements. All patients' records with respect to age, gender, height, body weight, body mass index (BMI), duration of diabetes, glycosylated hemoglobin (HbA1c), fasting plasma glucose, blood pressure and adverse effects were collected from the case note database. Blood glucose was measured by hexokinase method and HbA1c was measured by high performance liquid chromatographic (HPLC) method (Bio-RAD D-10, Bio-RAD, Hercules, CA, USA).

All 30 patients had been maintained on Liraglutide in a dose of 1.2 mg per day and all 30 patients on dulaglutide 1.5 mg dose once-weekly during the 13 weeks of the study period. Both the arms were well matched as far as baseline characteristics were concerned. (Table 1).

All 60 patients received either of the SGLT-2 Inhibitors namely dapagliflozin 10 mg/day (n = 28), canagliflozin 100 mg/day (n = 20), empagliflozin 10 mg/day (n = 12), as per the treating physicians' decision. All patients were on Metformin 2000 mg per day. Other OADs had not been initiated.

Statistical methods

Descriptive statistical analysis were carried out with SAS (Statistical Analysis System) version 9.2 for windows, SAS Institute Inc. Cary, NC, USA and Statistical Package for Social Sciences (SPSS Complex Samples) Version 21.0 for windows, SPSS, Inc., Chicago, IL, USA, with Microsoft Word and Excel being used to generate graphs and tables. Results on continuous measurements are presented as Mean ± SEM and results on categorical measurements are presented in Number (%). Significance is assessed at a level of 5%.

The following assumptions were made of the data: 1) Cases of the samples should be independent, 2) The populations from which the samples are drawn have the same variance (or standard deviation) and 3) The samples are drawn from different populations are random.

Normality of data was tested by Anderson Darling test, Shapiro-Wilk, Kolmogorov-Smirnoff test and visually by QQ plot. Paired t-test was used to find the significance of study parameters within groups of patients measured on two occasions. Chi-square/ Fisher Exact test was used to find the significance of study parameters on categorical scale between two or more groups.

Results
Impact of adding either Dulaglutide or Liraglutide to metformin and SGLT2 inhibitors
Dulaglutide
Adding dulaglutide to the combination of metformin 2000 mg/day and aSGLT2i resulted in a significant reduction in fasting plasma glucose (– 41.87 ± 12.72 mg/dL; p = 0.003) and HbA1c at 3 months follow up (– 1.017 ± 0.22%; p << 0.001) [Table 2]. The reduction in glycemic parameters was accompanied by a significant impact on body weight (– 4.20 ± 0.47 kg; p << 0.001

Table 2 Change in study parameters during the follow-up period

Cohort	Dulaglutide, n = 30				Liraglutide, n = 30			
Parameter	Baseline Mean ± SEM	Follow-up Mean ± SEM	Change Mean ± SEM	P	Baseline Mean ± SEM	Follow-up Mean ± SEM	Change Mean ± SEM	P
Body weight (kg)	87.17 ± 2.16	82.97 ± 2.05	−4.20 ± 0.47	< 0.001	89.43 ± 2.60	83.60 ± 2.35	−5.83 ± 0.87	< 0.001
BMI (kg/m^2)	32.84 ± 0.77	31.312 ± 0 .68	−1.53 ± 0.21	< 0.001	34.92 ± 0.868	32.650 ± 0.77	−2.27 ± 0.33	< 0.001
SBP (mmHg)	134.30 ± 2.71	130.87 ± 2.49	−3.43 ± 2.97	0.258	137.83 ± 2.503	127.60 ± 2.07	−10.23 ± 2.36	< 0.001
DBP (mmHg)	80.73 ± 1.64	78.43 ± 0.914	− 2.30 ± 1.79	0.208	83.47 ± 1.587	80.67 ± 1.51	− 2.80 ± 1.85	0.141
FPG(mg/dl)	175.53 ± 11.45	133.67 ± 6.90	− 41.87 ± 12.72	0.003	160.13 ± 8.17	115.93 ± 5.69	− 44.20 ± 8.05	< 0.001
HbA1c (%)	8.43 ± 0.21	7.411 ± 0.15	−1.017 ± 0.22	< 0.001	8.49 ± 0.26	6.95 ± 0.21	− 1.547 ± 0.22	< 0.001

and BMI ($- 1.53 \pm 0.21\%$; $p < 0.001$) without an impact on blood pressure.

Liraglutide

As with dulaglutide, treatment with liraglutide in addition to Metformin and a SGLT2i resulted in a significant reduction in fasting plasma glucose ($- 44.20 \pm 8.05$ mg/dL; $p < 0.001$), HbA1c ($1.547 \pm 0.22\%$; $p < 0.001$), weight ($- 5.83 \pm 0.87$ kg; $p < 0.001$) and BMI ($2.27 \pm 0.33\&$; $p < 0.001$) at 3 months follow up [Table 2]. However in contrast to dulaglutide, liraglutide was associated with a significant reduction in systolic blood pressure ($- 10.23 \pm 2.36$ mm of Hg; $p < 0.001$) [Table 2].

Dulaglutide versus Liraglutide failing OHA regime

We analyzed the data to compare the effects of dulaglutide with liraglutide, when they were both added to existing therapy of Metformin and SGLT2i.

Glycemic parameters

There was a comparable reduction in FPG and HbA1c in both the arms. However, 63.3% of patients in the liraglutide achieved an HbA1c of $< 7.0\%$ compared to only 30% in the dulaglutide arm. This difference was statistically significant (0.019) [Table 3].

Weight

There was comparable weight loss in both the arms [Table 4]. A similar proportion of patients in both the arms experienced a weight loss between 5 and 10% (53.3% with dulaglutide vs. 50.0% with liraglutide). A highly significant weight loss of greater than 15% from baseline was seen in 6.7% patients in the liraglutide arm, but not in the dulaglutide arm [Fig. 1].

Blood pressure

There was similar reduction in systolic and diastolic blood pressure in both the arms [Table 4].

Dulaglutide vs. Liraglutide: Impact on the metabolic composite of HbA1creduction AND weight loss

The composite end point of HbA1creduction to below 7% and a greater than 5% of body weight loss was attained by 5 (16.7%) patients in the dulaglutide arm, while 20 (50%) patients on liraglutide arm reached this composite ($p = 0.75$). (Fig. 2).

Adverse events

No serious adverse event was reported during this 3 month follow up. There was no hypoglycaemia reported. The commonest adverse event was nausea in 14 (23%) patients, 6 (20%) in the dulaglutide group compared to 8 (26.6%) in the liraglutide group. One patient who was on liraglutide complained of 1 -2 episode of vomiting and diarrhoea, which responded to a week's treatment with a proton pump inhibitor and domperidone. There were no complaints of diarrhoea, vomiting or abdominal pain from the patients on dulaglutide. Two patients complained of genital irritation, which responded to topical anti mycotics. Both these patients were on dapagliflozin, with one of them taking dulaglutide and the other being on liraglutide. There were no dropouts from the cohort over the 3-month period of our study, which though surprising in the real world, was quite opportune.

Discussion

Recent publications of positive CV outcome trials with SGLT2i (empagliflozin and canagliflozin) and GLP1 RA (liraglutide and semaglutide) and the positive effects of treatment with these drugs utilizing the pathophysiological defects of T2D have caused a paradigm shift in the way the disease is treated [1–4]. Quite naturally, researchers have been interested to study the effects of co-initiating SGLT2i and GLP-1 RA. The DURATION 8 study was published recently showing a robust weight loss and reduction in systolic blood pressure in the dapagliflozin plus Exenatide arm [7]. Strangely, this benefit did not extend to HbA1c reduction [8]. Nauck et al. in their editorial accompanying the publication of DURATION 8 postulated that since the additive effect of the two molecules were "disappointing" when co initiated,

Table 3 Proportion of patients achieving HbA1c less than 7%

| | | | Follow-up A1c < 7% | | Total | p (2-sided) |
			No	Yes		
Cohort	Dulaglutide	Number of Patients	21	9	30	0.019
		%	70.0%	30.0%	100.0%	
	Liraglutide	Number of Patients	11	19	30	
		%	36.7%	63.3%	100.0%	
Total		Number of Patients	32	28	60	
		%	53.3%	46.7%	100.0%	

Table 4 Percentage Reduction in Study Variables

Study Variables	Liraglutide, N = 30	Dulaglutide, N = 30	p
Percent Change in Body weight Mean ± SEM	−5.83 ± 0.87	−4.2 ± 0.46	0.103
Percent Change in BMI, Mean ± SEM	−2.27 ± 0.33	1.53 ± 0.20	0.061
Percent Change in SBP, Mean ± SEM	−10.23 ± 2.36	−3.43 ± 2.98	0.079
Percent Change in DBP, Mean ± SEM	−2.8 ± 1.85	−2.3 ± 1.79	0.847
Percent Change in FPG, Mean ± SEM	−44.2 ± 8.05	−41.87 ± 12.72	0.877
Percent Change in HbA1c, Mean ± SEM	−1.55 ± 0.22	−1.02 ± 0.22	0.091

it would be prudent to test their effectiveness when started sequentially as would happen "probably in most clinical cases" [8].

A real-world observational data looked at the effect of sequential addition of canagliflozin after receiving GLP-1RA for 30 months [9]. This study documented a very modest HbA1c reduction. In another small retrospective study (n = 14) from the United Kingdom sequential addition of GLP-1RA followed by SGLT-2 inhibitor was analyzed [10]. On addition of a GLP1 RA, HbA1c came down by 8 mmol/mol (0.7%), with an associated 4.9 kg weight loss. After 20 weeks, a SGLT-2 inhibitor was added in sequence and followed up for 48 weeks. There was an additional significant reduction in HbA1calong with 5.47 kg weight loss.

However, the authors find in their clinical practice, injectables are tried or accepted by patients only after oral therapy has been exhausted, for obvious reasons. In the studies described above, SGLT2i (oral therapy) was added to preexisting injectable (GLP-1 RA) therapy or the drugs were co initiated, differing from a real world situation. In this real world study from India, we looked at the more realistic scenario of GLP-1 RA therapy being instituted when oral medicines have been suboptimal and this is the first data using this combination in this sequence.

Since it was a dual arm comparative study we could assess both the impact of adding a GLP-1 RA to a SGLT-2 inhibitor based regimen as well as compare the metabolic impact of liraglutide versus dulaglutide.

Both liraglutide as well as dulaglutide resulted in a significant reduction in fasting plasma glucose (− 41.87 ± 12.72 mg/dL with dulaglutide and − 44.20 ± 8.05 mg/dL with liraglutide), HbA1c (− 1.017 ± 0.22% with dulaglutide and − 1.547 ± 0.22%) as well as weight (− 4.20 ± 0.47 kg with dulaglutide and − 5.83 ± 0.87 kg with liraglutide) from baseline. Only liraglutide not dulaglutide had a significant impact on the reduction of systolic blood pressure (− 10.23 ± 2.36 mm of Hg). It should be noted here that all patients in this cohort had a reasonably well-controlled blood pressure at baseline and no antihypertensive medications were changed during the study.

This data would therefore suggest that as a first injectable, GLP-1 RA is a very effective option when it is used along with a SGLT-2 inhibitor on background metformin therapy in a sequential approach.

Our study also looked at the comparative effectiveness of liraglutide versus dulaglutide when added sequentially to a SGLT-2 inhibitor and metformin. There seems to be a trend favoring liraglutide in comparison to dulaglutide in reduction of fasting plasma glucose, HbA1c, weight and systolic blood pressure (statistically non significant)

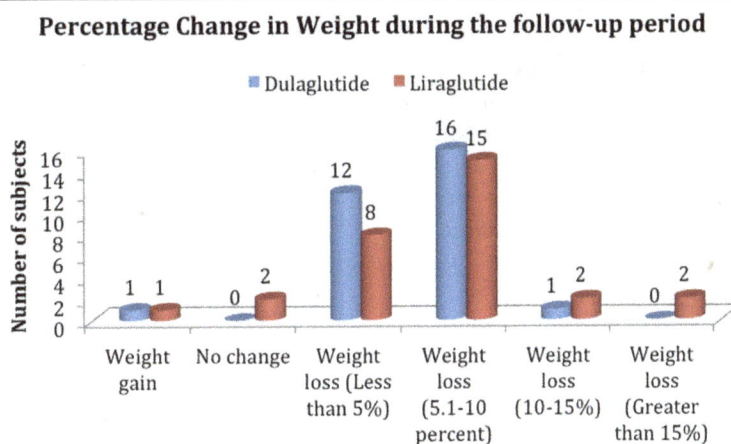

Fig. 1 Percentage Change in Weight during the follow-up period

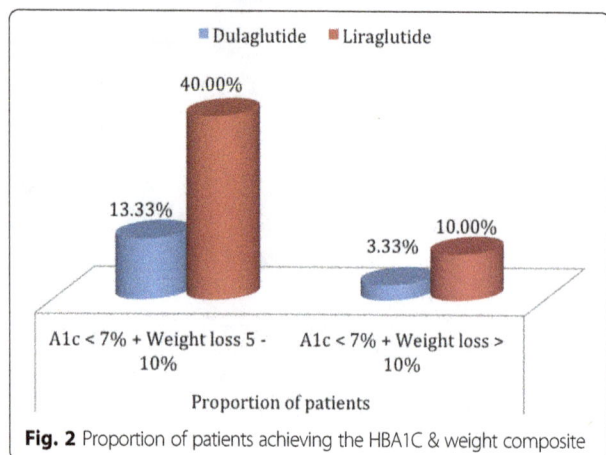

Fig. 2 Proportion of patients achieving the HBA1C & weight composite

(Table). However, there was a statistically significant difference favoring liraglutide (63.3% with liraglutide and 30% with dulaglutide) in the proportion of patients achieving HbA1c less than 7.0%.

The modern goal of therapy is to achieve target HbA1c without gaining weight. Larger proportion of patients achieved this end point on liraglutide. But this did not reach statistical significance probably due to the small number of patients.

In all the CV outcome trials there was very modest impact on weight that could not have contributed to the CV benefits. However, the LOOK-AHEAD trial provided us some insight that a weight loss of more than 10% from baseline has the potential to alter the CV risks substantially [11]. In our study this degree of weight loss was achieved in 13.4% in the liraglutide arm.

Off note, no serious adverse events were noted during the study and the combination of metformin, SGLT2i with GLP-1 RA, seems to be efficacious and also reasonably well tolerated. Off the 60 patients who had been commenced on this therapy, no dropouts were seen, indicating that this therapy would be quite well accepted if the patients were chosen and counseled properly.

There are several limitations in this study. Firstly it was open label and not controlled. Hence this data could not correct for numerous confounding factors that could have influenced the results. Secondly the small sample size could have influenced the quantum of metabolic impact. We are aware that this size was small also because only a small percentage of our patients could afford this very expensive therapy in our "pay from pocket" setting and were "chosen" based on their ability to afford this treatment. This would also be considered a major selection bias. But in spite of these limitations this data definitely points to the safety and efficacy of using GLP1RA on a background of metformin and SGLT2i in poorly controlled diabetes and this method of treatment could be further tested in larger trials.

Conclusion

In this retrospective study in Indian type 2 diabetic patients poorly controlled with metformin and SGLT-2 inhibitor we found a meaningful impact of adding a GLP-1 RA on all metabolic parameters. Both liraglutide and dulaglutide were effective in this regard. There were additional advantages seen with liraglutide as far achieving target HbA1c of less than 7% and also on the quantum of weight loss and systolic blood pressure reduction.

This study therefore provides a pilot and indeed generates a hypothesis supporting the sequential addition of a GLP-1 RA after metformin and SGLT-2 inhibitor, in the management of T2D, which needs to be tested in a more systematic manner on a larger population.

Abbreviations
BMI: Body mass index; CVOT: Cardiovascular outcome trials; GLP-1RA: Glucagon like Peptide Receptor Analogues; HbA1c: Glycosylated hemoglobin; HPLC: High performance liquid chromatography; OAD: Oral antidiabetic drugs; SGLT-2i: Sodium-glucose linked transporter inhibitor; T2D: Type 2 diabetes

Acknowledgements
The authors acknowledge the patients for agreeing to be a part of this study and Mr. Kingshuk Bhattacharya an independent bio-statistician for helping us analyze the data.

Funding
The study was self-funded. There was no external contribution for the same.

Authors' contributions
SG conceptualized the study design. BS prepared the protocol as well as the data needed to be captured. SG prepared an excel sheet for data capturing and prepared the patient consent form. SG presented the study protocol to Nightingale Hospital Ethics Committee. After ethics committee clearance both SG & BS started collecting data from their respective hospitals and data was entered into the excel sheet. The completed dataset was handed over to KB (biostatistician) who is also acknowledged in the manuscript. BS wrote the abstract, introduction, discussions and conclusion. The body of the manuscript was written by SG. Both authors read and approved the final manuscript.

Competing interests
The authors declare that they have no competing interests.

Author details
¹Nightingale Hospital, 11 Shakespeare Sarani, Kolkata, India. ²AMRI Hospitals, JC-16-17, Salt Lake City, Kolkata 700091, India. ³Kolkata, India.

References
1. DeFronzo RA. From the triumvirate to the ominous octet: a new paradigm for the treatment of type 2 diabetes mellitus. Diabetes. 2009;58(4):773–95.
2. Abdul-Ghani MA, Puckett C, Triplitt C, Maggs D, Adams J, Cersosimo E, DeFronzo RA. Initial combination therapy with metformin, pioglitazone and exenatide is more effective than sequential add-on therapy in subjects with new-onset diabetes. Results from the efficacy and durability of initial combination therapy for type 2 diabetes (EDICT): a randomized trial. Diabetes Obes Metab. 2015;17:268–75.
3. Zinman B, Wanner C, Lachin JM, Fitchett D, Bluhmki E, Hantel S, et al. Empagliflozin, cardiovascular outcomes, and mortality in type 2 diabetes. N Engl J Med. 2015;373:2117–28.

4. Marso SP, Daniels GH, Brown-Frandsen K, Kristensen P, Mann JFE, Nauck M, et al. Liraglutide and cardiovascular outcomes in type 2 diabetes. N Engl J Med. 2016;375:311–22.
5. Marso SP, Bain SC, Consoli A, Eliaschewitz FG, JoÅLdar E, Leiter LA, et al. Semaglutide and cardiovascular outcomes in patients with type 2 diabetes. N Engl J Med. 2016;375:1834–44.
6. Neal B, Perkovic V, Mahaffey KW, Zeeuw D, Fulcher G, Erondu N, et al. Canagliflozin and cardiovascular and renal events in type 2 diabetes. N Engl J Med. 2017;377:644–57.
7. Frías JP, Guja C, Hardy E, Ahmed A, Dong F, Öhman P, et al. Exenatide once weekly plus dapagliflozin once daily versus exenatide or dapagliflozin alone in patients with type 2diabetes inadequately controlled with metformin monotherapy (DURATION-8): a 28 week, multicentre, double-blind, phase 3, randomized controlled trial. Lancet Diabetes Endocrinol. 2016;4:1004–16.
8. Nauck AM, Meier J. GLP-1 receptor agonists and SGLT2 inhibitors: a couple at last? Lancet Diabetes Endocrinol. 2016;4(12):963–4.
9. Saroka RM, Kane MP, Busch RS, Watsky J, Hamilton RA. SGLT-2 inhibitor therapy added to GLP-1 agonist therapy in the management of type 2 diabetes. Endocr Pract. 2015;21:1315–22.
10. Curtis L, Humayun MA, Walker J, Hampton K, Partridge H. Addition of SGLT2 inhibitor to GLP-1 agonist therapy in people with type 2 diabetes and suboptimal glycaemic control. Practical. Diabetes. 2016;33(4):129–32.
11. Gregg EW, Jakicic JM, Blackburn G, Bloomquist P, Bray GA, Clark JM, et al. Look AHEAD Research group. Association of the magnitude of weight loss and changes in physical fitness with long-term cardiovascular disease outcomes in overweight or obese people with type 2 diabetes: a post-hoc analysis of the Look AHEAD randomised clinical trial. Lancet Diabetes Endocrinol. 2016;4(11):913–21.

22

Why do endocrine profiles in elite athletes differ between sports?

Peter H. Sönksen[1*], Richard I. G. Holt[1], Walailuck Böhning[1], Nishan Guha[1,3], David A. Cowan[4], Christiaan Bartlett[4] and Dankmar Böhning[2]

Abstract

Background: Endocrine profiles have been measured on blood samples obtained immediately post-competition from 693 elite athletes from 15 Olympic Sports competing at National or International level; four were subsequently excluded leaving 689 for the current analysis.

Methods: Body composition was measured by bioimpedance in a sub-set of 234 (146 men and 88 women) and from these data a regression model was constructed that enabled 'estimated' lean body mass and fat mass to be calculated on all athletes. One way ANOVA was used to assess the differences in body composition and endocrine profiles between the sports and binary logistical regression to ascertain the characteristic of a given sport compared to the others.

Results: The results confirmed many suppositions such as basketball players being tall, weightlifters short and cross-country skiers light. The hormone profiles were more surprising with remarkably low testosterone and free T3 (tri-iodothyronine) in male powerlifters and high oestradiol, SHBG (sex hormone binding globulin) and prolactin in male track and field athletes. Low testosterone concentrations were seen 25.4% of male elite competitors in 12 of the 15 sports and high testosterone concentrations in 4.8% of female elite athletes in 3 of the 8 sports tested. Interpretation of the results is more difficult; some of the differences between sports are at least partially due to differences in age of the athletes but the apparent differences between sports remain significant after adjusting for age. The prevalence of 'hyperandrogenism' (as defined by the IAAF (International Association of Athletics Federations) and IOC (International Olympic Committee)) amongst this cohort of 231 elite female athletes was the highest so far recorded and the very high prevalence of 'hypoandrogenism' in elite male athletes a new finding.

Conclusions: It is unclear whether the differences in hormone profiles between sports is a reason why they become elite athletes in that sport or is a consequence of the arduous processes involved. For components of body composition we know that most have a major genetic component and this may well be true for endocrine profiles.

Keywords: Elite-sport, Endocrine-profiles, Body-composition, BMI, Collagen biomarkers

Background

The first report on endocrine hormone profiles was in a group of 693 elite athletes across a range of Olympic Sports in 2014 [1]. In addition to statistically significant differences in profiles between men and women, there were considerable differences between athletes from various sports.

It has long been known that different sports attract athletes who differ in body composition; for example, marathon runners and cross-country skiers are thin and light while weightlifters and powerlifters are short and stocky and basketball players tall. Healy et al. also showed that on average elite female athletes had a lean body mass (LBM) that was 85% of the LBM of elite male athletes and proposed that the differences in strength and world records between men and women reflected this [1]. There is no clear indication why men and women develop bodies that show a fundamental difference in lean and fat mass but it is possible, if not likely,

---
* Correspondence: phsonksen@aol.com
[1]Human Development and Health Academic Unit, University of Southampton Faculty of Medicine, Southampton, UK
Full list of author information is available at the end of the article

that it is partly due to differences in hormonal profiles between the sexes [2].

There are very limited published data on endocrine profiles in sport, most being confined to a single sport. One unexpected finding of Healy et al. [1] was that 16.5% of male elite athletes had testosterone concentrations less than the lower limit of the laboratory reference range for 'normal' men and that 13.7% of elite female athletes had a testosterone concentration greater than the laboratory reference interval for 'normal' women including several with values within the reference range for men.

This paper examines these differences in endocrine profiles discovered by Healy et al. in more detail and attempts to interpret some of the findings.

Methods

Participants

The details of recruitment of the volunteer elite athletes as part of the GH-2000 study (A Methodology for the Detection of Doping with Growth Hormone & Related Substances. EU Contract Number: BMH4 CT950678) and the subsequent collection of data including analysis of blood samples have been published previously [3] as has the selection of the sub-set of these athletes in whom endocrine profiles were measured [1]. The participants in this study are those previously published. In brief, athletes were recruited on an 'opportunistic' basis from the 15 Olympic sports that were interested and prepared to co-operate with the GH-2000 research project whose aim was to develop a test to detect growth hormone misuse in professional athletes. Samples were collected within two hours of completion of their event. The project was funded mainly by the European Union and International Olympic Committee with further support from the industries and universities involved. Volunteers gave written consent to participation and this included a statement confirming that they had not misused any banned drug or anabolic agent and this was confirmed by finding no abnormal testosterone/LH ratios. Results of endocrine profiles were available in 694 of the original cohort of 813 elite athletes recruited for the original GH-2000 'Cross-Sectional' study [3]; they were those individuals with sufficient serum left for analysis of an endocrine profile after completion of the main study. Three participants were excluded as there was only 1 volunteer from each sport (women Powerlifting, Marathon and Canoeing) and one man was excluded as his thyroid profile showed him to be markedly hyperthyroid (high fT3 and suppressed TSH (thyroid stimulating hormone)) leaving 689 individuals for the current analysis.

Ethics approval

All volunteers gave written informed consent to participate in the original study including subsequent analysis and publication of the data. The study was approved by the Ethics Committee of West Lambeth Health Authority (as the committee covering the co-ordinating centre St Thomas' Hospital, London) and the appropriate local ethics committees of all participating partners.

Body composition

Demographic data included self-reported height, weight and age. Weight and body composition was measured on a sub-set of 234 (146 men and 88 women) at events where it was possible to use the Tanita TB7–305 bioimpedance analyser; this was only swimming, rowing and track and field. Since the measured body composition data were only available for three sports, estimated lean body mass (eLBM) and estimated fat mass (eFM) were calculated for everyone using regression equations (for each sex, using height and weight) derived from those in the three sports in whom body composition was measured; these data are shown in Fig. 1. Estimated fat mass was calculated by subtracting eLBM from total body weight. The large R^2 values and slope of almost unity indicate that the statistical models have a reasonable degree of validity.

$$\text{For men}: \text{ eLBM} = \text{-43.68} + 0.4598 \text{ weight} \\ +0.4285 \text{ height } \left(N = 146; R^2 = 85.6\%\right)$$

$$\text{For women}: \text{ eLBM} = \text{-22.68} + 0.5157 \text{ weight} \\ +0.2354 \text{ height}; R^2 = 86.1\% \left(N = 88\right)$$

Endocrine measurements

The endocrine profiles and the methods used are detailed in Healy et al. [1] and [3]. Serum growth hormone (GH), IGF-I (Insulin-like growth factor 1), pro-collagen type III N-terminal peptide (P-III-NP), carboxy-terminal cross-linked telopeptide of type I collagen (ICTP), carboxy-terminal propeptide of type I collagen (PICP) and osteocalcin were determined at the Sahlgrenska Hospital (Gothenburg, Sweden) and IGFBP-2 (IGF Binding Protein #2), IGFBP-3 (IGF Binding Protein #3) and acid-labile subunit (ALS) were measured at the Kolling Institute (Sydney, Australia). Serum luteinising hormone (LH), follicle-stimulating hormone (FSH), prolactin, thyroid-stimulating hormone (TSH), free tri-iodothyronine (fT3), free thyroxine (fT4), oestradiol, cortisol, testosterone and sex-hormone binding globulin (SHBG) were measured in the endocrine laboratory at St Thomas' Hospital (London, UK) using the Siemens Centaur and Immulite platforms. Many of the oestradiol concentrations (160/644 men and 64/234 women) were less than the laboratory Lower Limit of Quantification of 34 pmol/l and in the statistical analyses these were treated as missing data. The lower part of

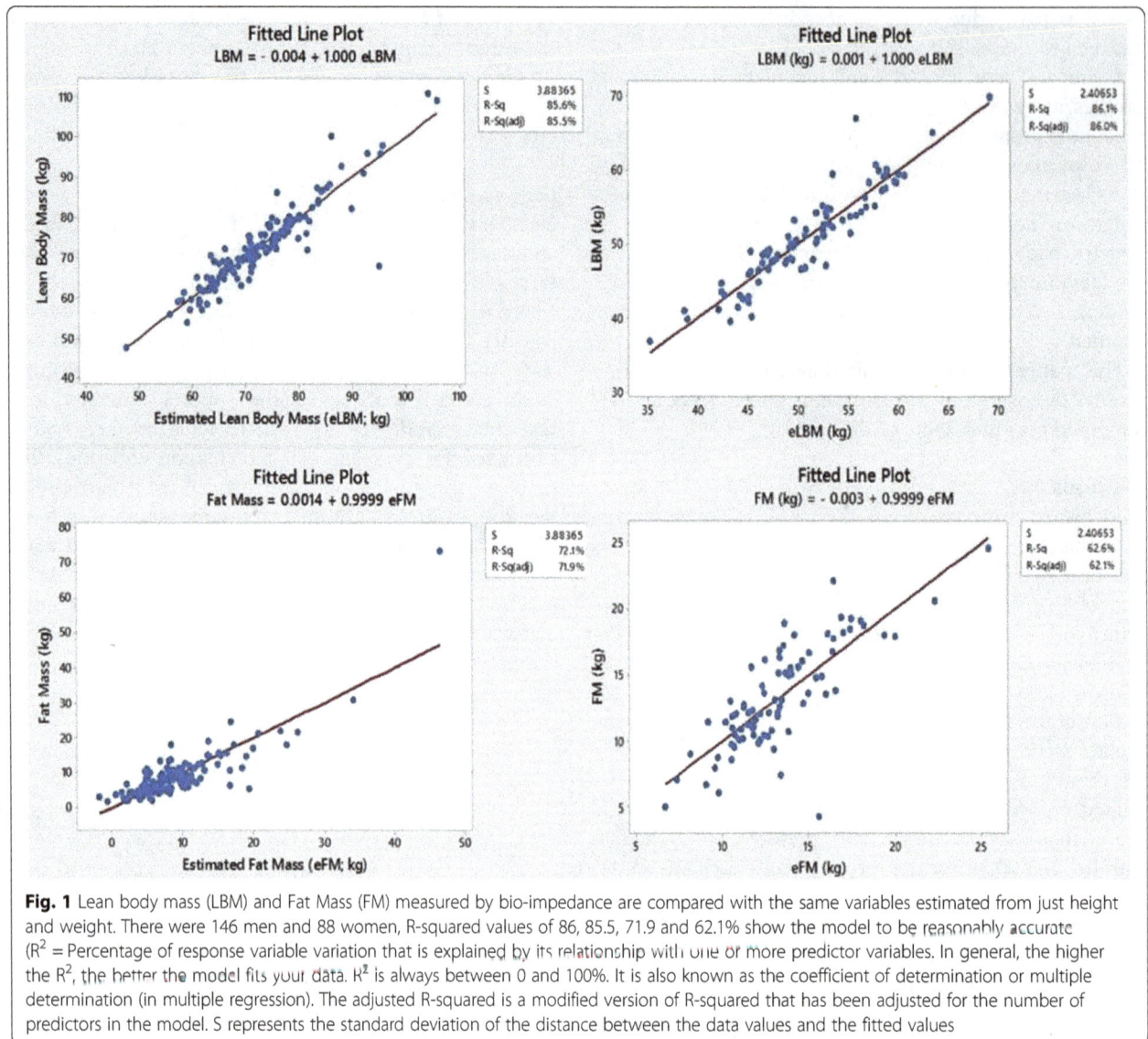

Fig. 1 Lean body mass (LBM) and Fat Mass (FM) measured by bio-impedance are compared with the same variables estimated from just height and weight. There were 146 men and 88 women, R-squared values of 86, 85.5, 71.9 and 62.1% show the model to be reasonably accurate (R^2 = Percentage of response variable variation that is explained by its relationship with one or more predictor variables. In general, the higher the R^2, the better the model fits your data. R^2 is always between 0 and 100%. It is also known as the coefficient of determination or multiple determination (in multiple regression). The adjusted R-squared is a modified version of R-squared that has been adjusted for the number of predictors in the model. S represents the standard deviation of the distance between the data values and the fitted values

the female range of testosterone was initially established with a radio-immunoassay (RIA) and then the RIA was correlated with the automated method. The automated assay had a between-assay imprecision of 20% at 1.5 nmol/l.

Statistical analysis

All analyses were performed using Minitab 17 with a significance level set at 0.05 unless stated to the contrary.

Comparison of concentration of a given hormone or marker between sports was by one-way analysis of variance. Comparison between the sport with the lowest mean value of a given endocrine variable and the results from other sports was performed using Dunnett's method (Minitab 17).

On occasions where a given variable was known to be age-dependent (e.g. growth hormone, IGF-I and the collagen biomarkers), multiple regression analysis with sport and age as independent variables, was used to examine their relative contributions to the observed differences. Outliers were included in the data for analysis and not treated separately; however, in these cases analysis was repeated after log-transformation of the data and no occasion did this affect the outcome.

Using Binary Logistic Regression the demographic data and endocrine profiles of a given sport was compared with that of the 'control' group created from all the other sports combined. This approach allowed the determination of the endocrine variables that were statistically characteristic in a given sporting group (either positively or negatively associated with that sport).

There are in all 390 comparisons so one would expect 20 to be positive by chance alone at the $p < 0.05$ level (in fact 21 men and 12 women), 4 at the $p < 0.01$ level (21 men and 7 women) and 1 at the level of $p < 0.001$

(39 men and 16 women)). Thus only variables with an association at the 1/100 (p < 0.01) or better were accepted as relevant.

Results

Using one-way analysis of variance the differences in means for each variable between sports and for men and women separately are illustrated in Figs. 2, 3, 4, 5, 6, 7, 8 and 9. Sports are represented by codes and the key to these is in the legend to each figure together with the number of volunteer elite athletes of each sex in each group.

Thus in Fig. 2, for men, weightlifters are older and shorter than in other sports while cross-country skiers are the youngest and lightest and basketball players the tallest. There are fewer volunteers and thus less data for women elite athletes but again basketball players are the

tallest, weightlifters the shortest and cross-country skiers the lightest. Swimmers of both sexes were both young and relatively tall.

Figure 3 compares eLBM, eFM and BMI between the sporting groups. Cross-country skiers were not only lightest but also had the lowest (estimated) lean body mass, fat mass and BMI for both men and women. The differences in BMI between the groups closely match the differences in (estimated) fat mass. Surprisingly both LBM and eLBM were relatively small in Powerlifters where mean fat mass (FM) and eFM were large partly due to one outlier with a measured FM of 74 kg. In women there was a similar pattern in eLBM, eFM and BMI between sports.

Figure 4 shows LH, FSH and Testosterone between sports and between sexes. The testosterone concentrations in the powerlifters are on average remarkably

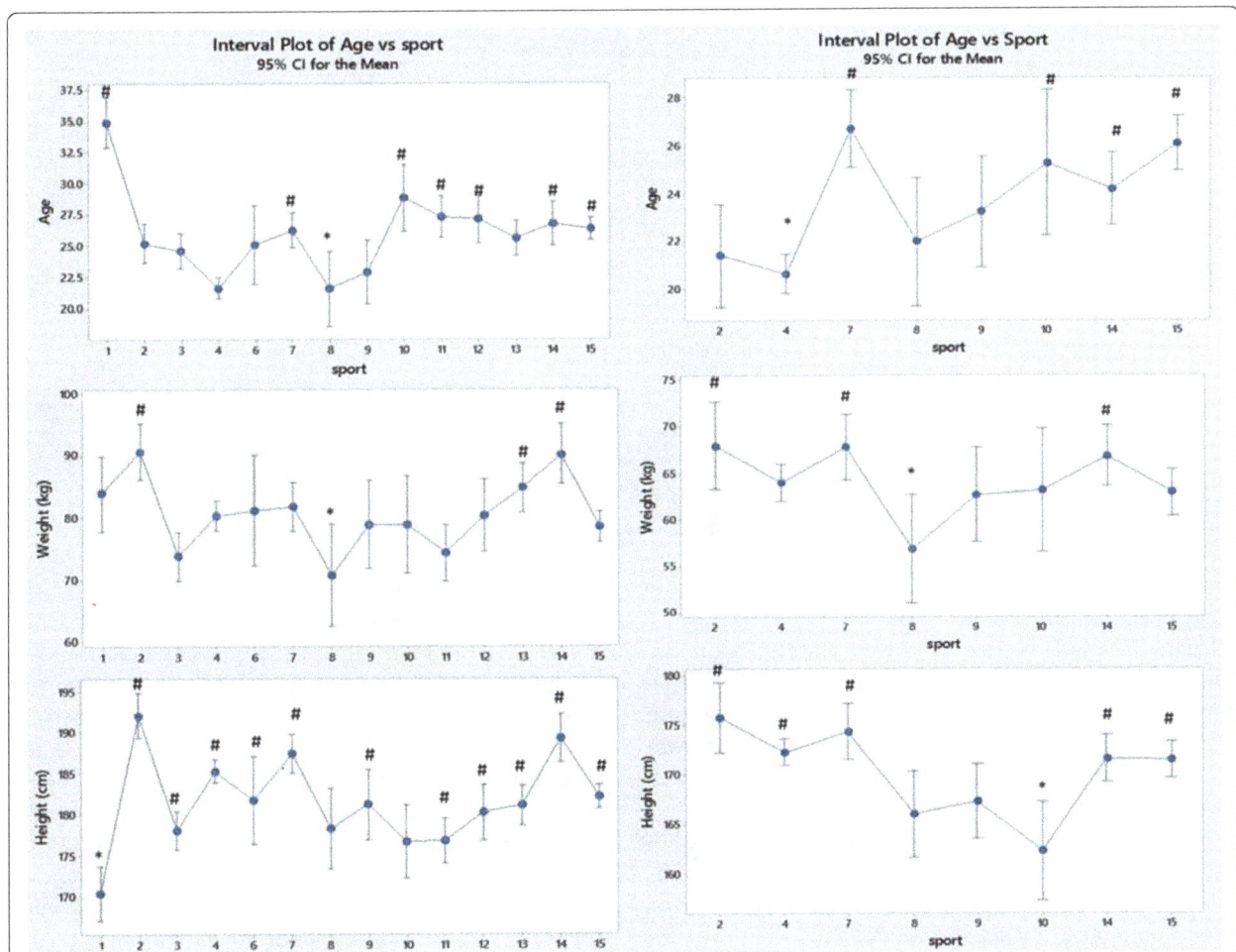

Fig. 2 The differences in mean age, weight and height between sports. For all the figures data from men are shown in the left panel and those from women are in the right panel. The lowest mean for each variable is marked with * and means that are significantly higher than this by one-way analysis of variance are marked with #. Each sport is represented by a numerical code and M = men and W = women: 1-Power Lifting (18 M and 1 W), 2-Basketball (27 M and 14 W), 3-Football (Soccer; 37 M), 4 Swimming (100 M and 91 W), 5-Marathon (1 W), 6-Canoeing (7 M and 1 W), 7-Rowing (36 M and 25 W), 8-Cross Country Skiing (8 m and 9 W), 9-Alpine Skiing (11 M and 12 W), 10-Weight Lifting (10 M and 7 W), 11-Judo (26 M), 12-Bandy (19 M), 13-Ice Hockey (38 M), 14 Handball (23 M and 29 W) and 15-Track and Field (95 M and 49 W)

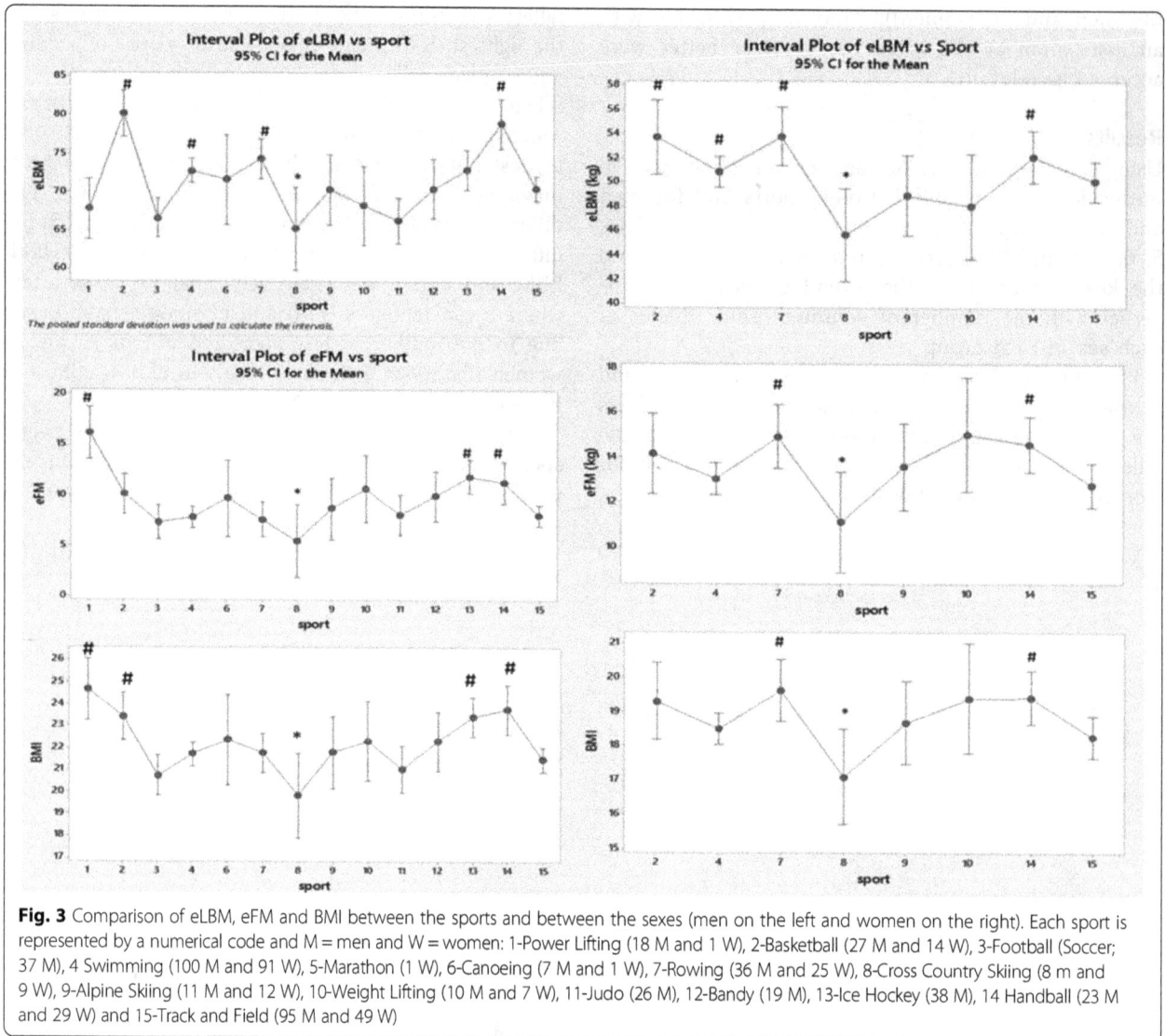

Fig. 3 Comparison of eLBM, eFM and BMI between the sports and between the sexes (men on the left and women on the right). Each sport is represented by a numerical code and M = men and W = women: 1-Power Lifting (18 M and 1 W), 2-Basketball (27 M and 14 W), 3-Football (Soccer; 37 M), 4 Swimming (100 M and 91 W), 5-Marathon (1 W), 6-Canoeing (7 M and 1 W), 7-Rowing (36 M and 25 W), 8-Cross Country Skiing (8 m and 9 W), 9-Alpine Skiing (11 M and 12 W), 10-Weight Lifting (10 M and 7 W), 11-Judo (26 M), 12-Bandy (19 M), 13-Ice Hockey (38 M), 14 Handball (23 M and 29 W) and 15-Track and Field (95 M and 49 W)

small and 8 of the remaining sports had significantly larger values.

Figure 5 shows oestradiol, SHBG and Prolactin between sports and between sexes. All three were high in men from track and field sports where prolactin was also high in women. The 'stress hormones' cortisol, growth hormone and prolactin [4] were all high in both men and women from track and field.

Figure 6 provides the thyroid function test results between sports in men and women. The most notable feature is the low free T3 in male powerlifters and weightlifters and track and field athletes while free T4 was low in male canoeists. In women, TSH was high in track and field and free T4 low in cross-country skiers while swimmers and track and field athletes had significantly raised values.

Figure 7 shows the results for three IGF binding-proteins between sports. IGFBP-2 was high in male

rowers and both men and women from track and field, while it was low in both alpine and cross-country skiing in men. IGFBP-3 was low in male powerlifters (but not weightlifters), canoers and rowers where it was also low in women. In both men and women the acid-labile subunit was low in basketball, weightlifting and track and field while it was relatively high in swimmers and rowers from both sexes.

Figure 8 shows the data on the bone marker osteocalcin and collagen markers ICTP and PICP. Most notably osteocalcin and ICTP are low in male powerlifters while osteocalcin was low in women from track and field.

Figure 9 shows data on growth hormone (GH) and the GH-sensitive markers IGF-I and P-III-NP. All three are relatively low in male powerlifters and weightlifters from both sexes. The GH-sensitive collagen marker P–III-NP and GH are relatively high in track and field in both sexes.

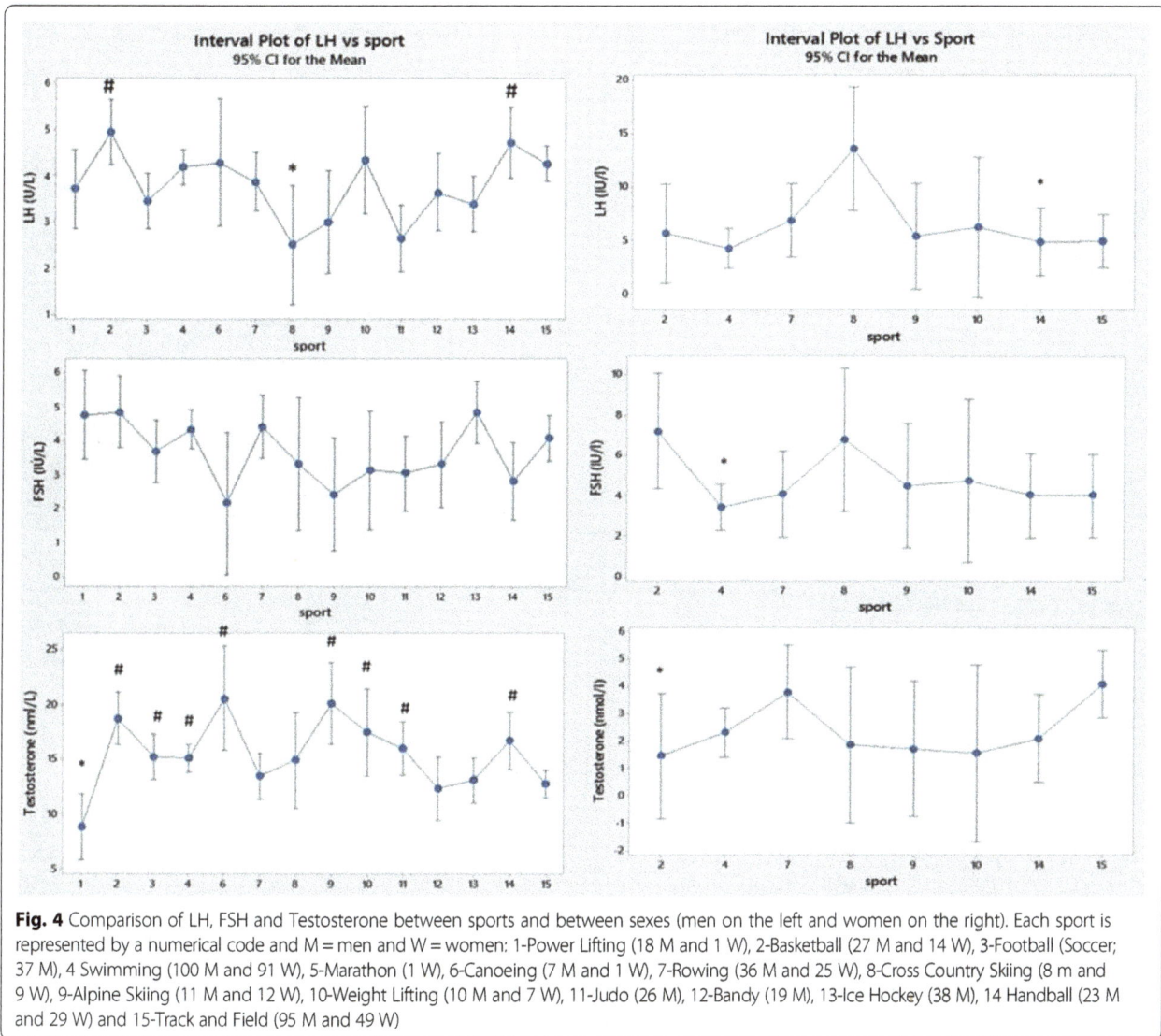

Fig. 4 Comparison of LH, FSH and Testosterone between sports and between sexes (men on the left and women on the right). Each sport is represented by a numerical code and M = men and W = women: 1-Power Lifting (18 M and 1 W), 2-Basketball (27 M and 14 W), 3-Football (Soccer; 37 M), 4 Swimming (100 M and 91 W), 5-Marathon (1 W), 6-Canoeing (7 M and 1 W), 7-Rowing (36 M and 25 W), 8-Cross Country Skiing (8 m and 9 W), 9-Alpine Skiing (11 M and 12 W), 10-Weight Lifting (10 M and 7 W), 11-Judo (26 M), 12-Bandy (19 M), 13-Ice Hockey (38 M), 14 Handball (23 M and 29 W) and 15-Track and Field (95 M and 49 W)

Figure 10 shows the individual testosterone levels in the different sports for male and female elite athletes. The horizontal line is set at 10 nmol/l which is the lower end of the reference range for non-elite men and the level set by the IAAF and IOC when setting up the 'hyperandrogenism' rule for female elite athletes [5, 6]. It shows a significant proportion of elite male athletes with a low concentration of testosterone (25.4%) and a smaller but significant proportion of women elite athletes with high values (4.8%).

Tables 1 and 2 contains the results of the binary logistic regression, showing which variables were significantly associated with a given sport either positively or negatively and the statistical level of this association and its direction (positive or negative). Thus, unsurprisingly basketball players were characteristically tall and powerlifters short.

Male powerlifters tended to be older while swimmers and cross-country skiers were younger than their colleagues in other sports. The data support the hypothesis that height was likely to be an advantage in basketball and may also be an advantage in rowing and handball but a disadvantage in powerlifting and football. Weight seemed a disadvantage in rowing but an advantage in ice-hockey. A higher testosterone was seen in basketball and alpine skiing while powerlifters had lower testosterone levels. BMI was not different in any group. LH was lower in alpine skiing and judo while FSH was lower in handball players. SHBG, like BMI and cortisol, showed no significant differences between sports. Oestradiol was lower in cross-country skiers and higher in track and field athletes. TSH was lower in rowers and track & field (athletes) and higher in ice hockey players. Free T3 was lower in powerlifters and track and field while it was higher in alpine skiers, bandy and ice hockey players. Free T4 was lower in canoeing and rowing.

IGFBP-2 was lower in basketball players and higher in rowers. IGFBP-3 was lower in rowers and judo players

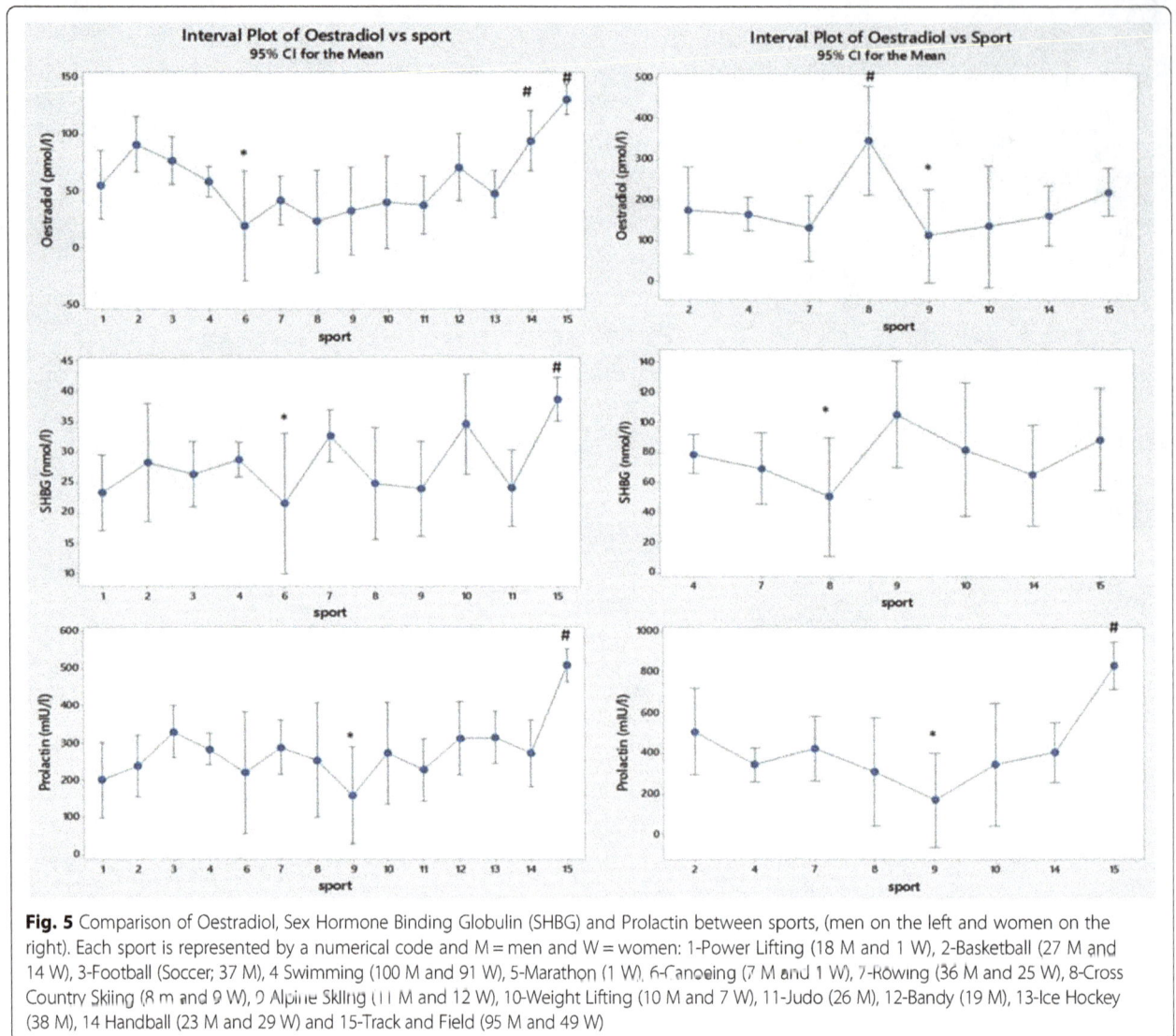

Fig. 5 Comparison of Oestradiol, Sex Hormone Binding Globulin (SHBG) and Prolactin between sports, (men on the left and women on the right). Each sport is represented by a numerical code and M = men and W = women: 1-Power Lifting (18 M and 1 W), 2-Basketball (27 M and 14 W), 3-Football (Soccer; 37 M), 4 Swimming (100 M and 91 W), 5-Marathon (1 W), 6-Canoeing (7 M and 1 W), 7-Rowing (36 M and 25 W), 8-Cross Country Skiing (8 m and 9 W), 9 Alpine Skiing (11 M and 12 W), 10-Weight Lifting (10 M and 7 W), 11-Judo (26 M), 12-Bandy (19 M), 13-Ice Hockey (38 M), 14 Handball (23 M and 29 W) and 15-Track and Field (95 M and 49 W)

and higher in ice-hockey and handball players. ALS showed a different pattern being lower in basketball, Ice hockey and track and field while higher in swimmers. IGF-I showed a weak positive association with rowers while GH was lower in football players and higher in track and field.

Osteocalcin was higher in weight-lifters, bandy and ice hockey players while PICP was characteristically lower in rowers and bandy players. The other collagen markers ICTP was lower in swimmers and handball players and P-III-NP was lower in ice-hockey players.

Estimated body composition showed lean body mass to be lower in power-lifters and in football and judo players. LBM was higher in basketball players, rowers and handball players. Fat mass was lower in rowers but relatively high in power-lifters and ice-hockey players.

In women, there are fewer athletes and fewer significant findings. Basketball players, swimmers and cross-country skiers were characteristically younger than other sports while as with men, cross-country skiers were lighter than other sports. Like men, rowers were taller while unlike with men but as might be expected weightlifters were shorter. Again BMI showed no discriminating tendency, neither did testosterone, LH, FSH, cortisol, fT3, IGFBP-2 or IGF-I.

SHBG was higher in alpine skiers while oestradiol was higher in cross-country skiers. Prolactin was lower in alpine skiers, TSH lower in rowers and fT4 lower in cross-country skiers. ALS was higher in swimmers while it was lower in alpine skiers and track and field athletes. Growth hormone was lower in handball players, osteocalcin lower in track and field athletes who characteristically had higher levels of PICP. Basketball players and swimmers had lower levels of ICTP while P-III-NP was higher basketball and handball players.

Estimated lean body mass was surprisingly lower in weight-lifters who had a higher estimated fat mass.

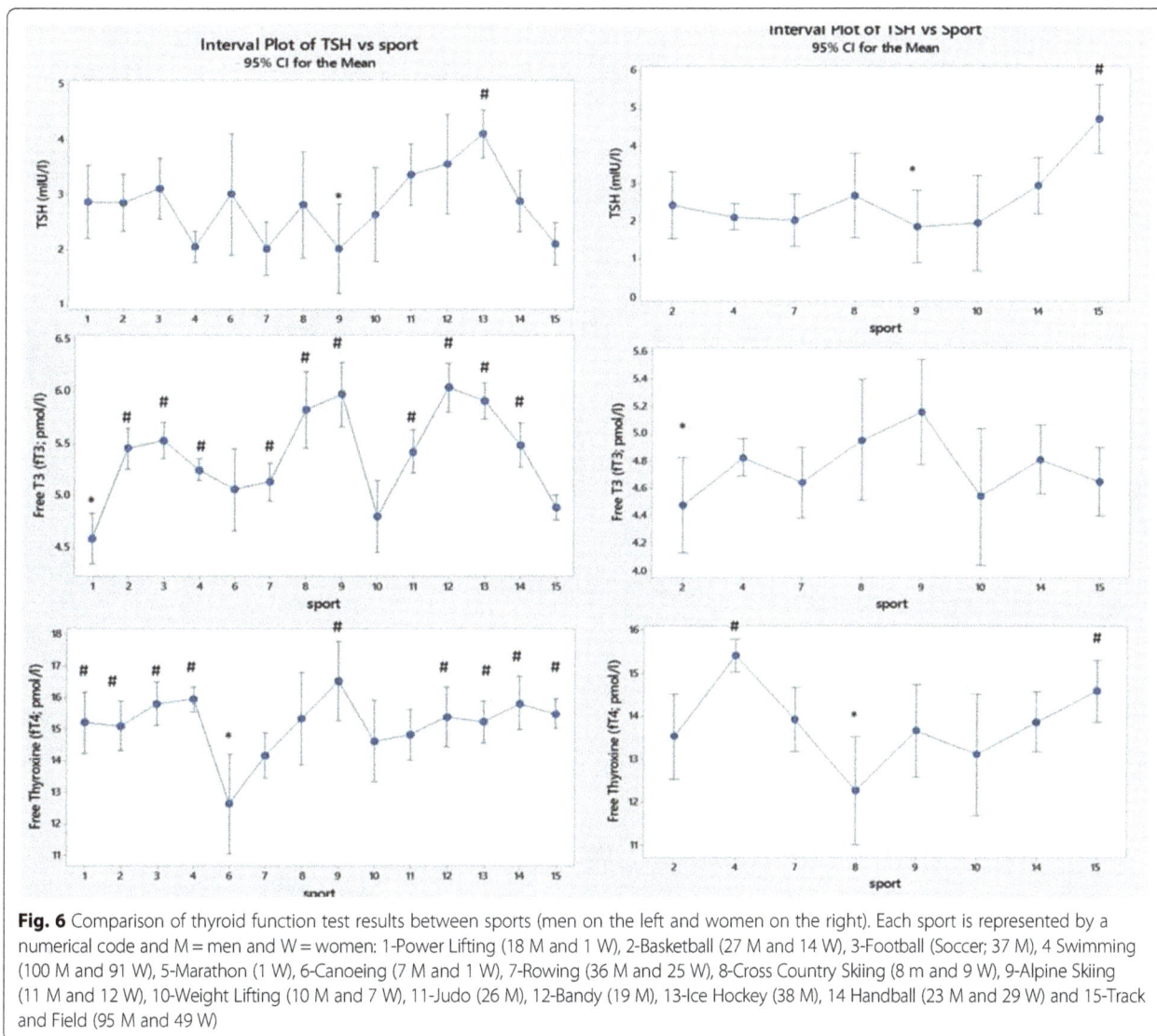

Fig. 6 Comparison of thyroid function test results between sports (men on the left and women on the right). Each sport is represented by a numerical code and M = men and W = women: 1-Power Lifting (18 M and 1 W), 2-Basketball (27 M and 14 W), 3-Football (Soccer; 37 M), 4 Swimming (100 M and 91 W), 5-Marathon (1 W), 6-Canoeing (7 M and 1 W), 7-Rowing (36 M and 25 W), 8-Cross Country Skiing (8 m and 9 W), 9-Alpine Skiing (11 M and 12 W), 10-Weight Lifting (10 M and 7 W), 11-Judo (26 M), 12-Bandy (19 M), 13-Ice Hockey (38 M), 14 Handball (23 M and 29 W) and 15-Track and Field (95 M and 49 W)

Discussion

This study has shown clear body composition and hormone concentration differences between athletes of different sporting disciplines of both sexes. These differences may contribute to the differences in *milieu interior* needed to excel in a given sport. We have used two complementary statistical methods to explore further the data. Firstly, analysis of variance has examined the magnitude of the differences between the body composition and endocrine profiles of the 15 Olympic sports that have been tested and is an extension of the analysis reported first in Healy et al. 2014 [1]. Secondly, in order to explore further the profile of body composition and hormone milieu for a given sport, we have used binary logistic regression to determine which of the measured variables appear 'characteristic' of a given sport. This has been done by comparing the profile of each sport against a pool of all the other sports and performed separately for men and women.

The results from the binary logistic regression may be compared with the differences in mean values of the variables shown in the figures. On most, but not all, occasions the results show a similar pattern; for example in men, there is a significantly higher age in powerlifters and weightlifters and younger age in swimmers and cross-country skiers. There are also several examples where there is little or no match. As might be expected female weight lifters were characteristically short but this was not the case with men.

For practical reasons it was only possible to measure body composition in 6 of the 15 sports in men and three in women. This was done at the time of data and blood sample collection post-event with a bioimpedance device of proven reliability and easy and fast to use in field studies such as this [7]. Bioimpedance analysis is to a degree dependent on hydration and ideally conditions of measurement should be standardised so far as hydration

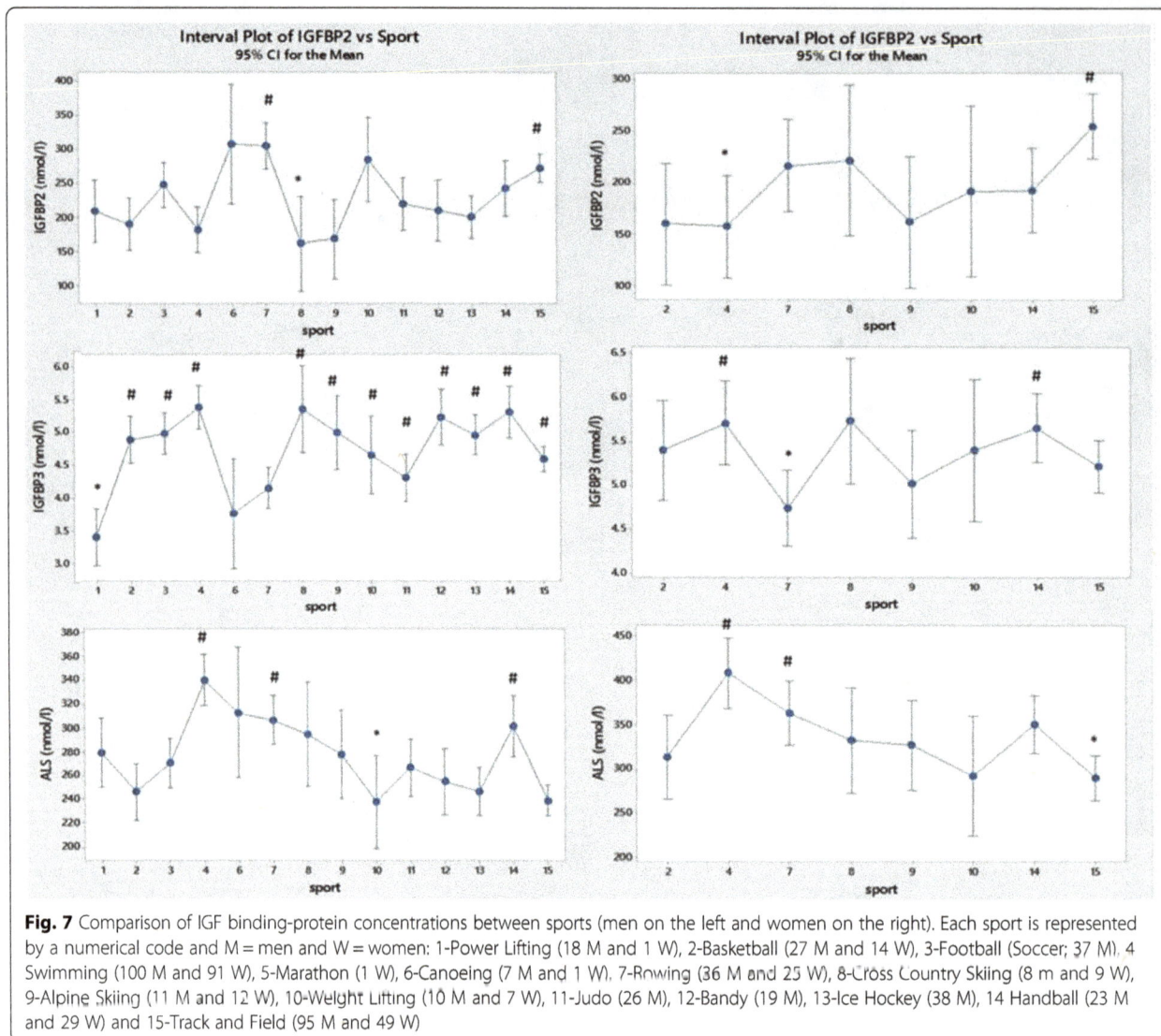

Fig. 7 Comparison of IGF binding-protein concentrations between sports (men on the left and women on the right). Each sport is represented by a numerical code and M = men and W = women: 1-Power Lifting (18 M and 1 W), 2-Basketball (27 M and 14 W), 3-Football (Soccer; 37 M), 4 Swimming (100 M and 91 W), 5-Marathon (1 W), 6-Canoeing (7 M and 1 W), 7-Rowing (36 M and 25 W), 8-Cross Country Skiing (8 m and 9 W), 9-Alpine Skiing (11 M and 12 W), 10-Weight Lifting (10 M and 7 W), 11-Judo (26 M), 12-Bandy (19 M), 13-Ice Hockey (38 M), 14 Handball (23 M and 29 W) and 15-Track and Field (95 M and 49 W)

is concerned; this was not possible in this study and the results should be interpreted with this knowledge. Likewise the extreme ranges of body composition seen are beyond those used in validation of the method. The key factors in determining body composition are height, weight and sex [8]. In order to examine the effects of body composition across the whole group of 15 sports we analysed the available measured data and established a regression model from which we calculated an 'estimated' lean body mass (eLBM) and by subtracting this from the measured mass (M), and estimated fat mass (eFM). From Fig. 1 it can be seen that although we are comparing the model with the data from which it was derived, there is a very good fit between this model and the measured data for LBM and a less good but reasonable fit for FM.

Most surprisingly eLBM was low (and eFM high) in male powerlifters and women weightlifters. This may be

true or possibly an artefact due to the bioimpedance method being unreliable in people with extreme variations in body composition. Apart from these observations body composition (in terms of muscle and fat) seemed little different between sports in women according to the logistic model although cross-country skiers (of both sexes) had the lowest eLBM, eFM and BMI by ANOVA. In men, basketball and handball players and rowers had the highest eLBM by both models. The differences in BMI between sports closely matched the differences in eFM in both sexes.

In both models testosterone concentrations were surprisingly low in powerlifters but not weightlifters, while large testosterone concentrations were a feature of basketball players and alpine skiers in the logistic model in men. There were no significant differences between sports in women for testosterone, LH or FSH. In the logistic model a low LH featured in male alpine skiers (where an association

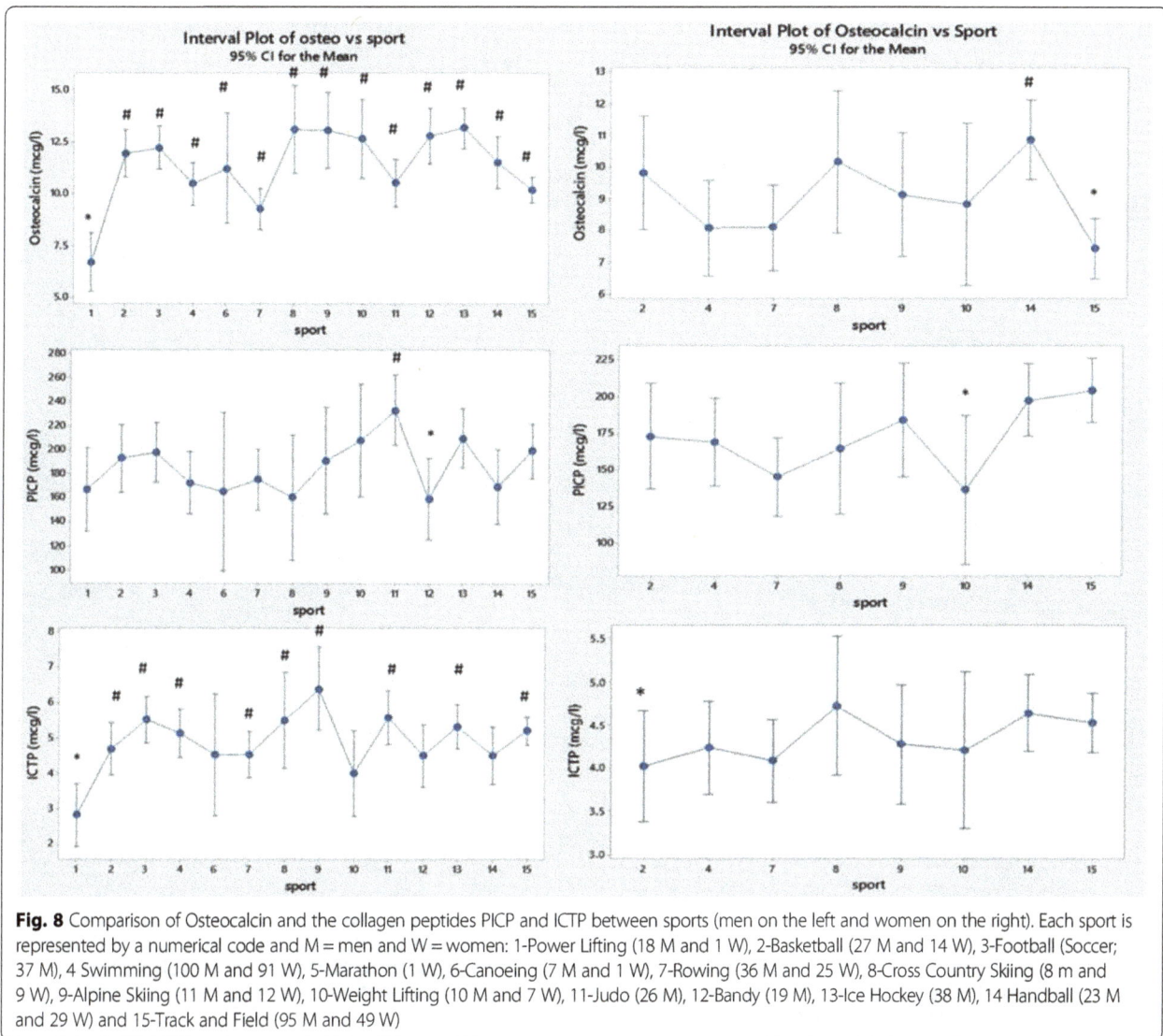

Fig. 8 Comparison of Osteocalcin and the collagen peptides PICP and ICTP between sports (men on the left and women on the right). Each sport is represented by a numerical code and M = men and W = women: 1-Power Lifting (18 M and 1 W), 2-Basketball (27 M and 14 W), 3-Football (Soccer; 37 M), 4 Swimming (100 M and 91 W), 5-Marathon (1 W), 6-Canoeing (7 M and 1 W), 7-Rowing (36 M and 25 W), 8-Cross Country Skiing (8 m and 9 W), 9-Alpine Skiing (11 M and 12 W), 10-Weight Lifting (10 M and 7 W), 11-Judo (26 M), 12-Bandy (19 M), 13-Ice Hockey (38 M), 14 Handball (23 M and 29 W) and 15-Track and Field (95 M and 49 W)

with a high testosterone was seen) and judo athletes while FSH was low in male handball players.

In men a low oestradiol was a feature of cross-country skiers in the logistic model while in contrast a high oestradiol was seen in women cross-country skiers. In men the highest average levels were in handball and track and field. In women a high SHBG was a feature of alpine skiers but SHBG did not feature in men. In both men and women a low prolactin characterised alpine skiers.

In the logistic model in both men and women, a low TSH was a distinguishing feature of rowers but mean values were equally low in swimmers, alpine skiers and track and field athletes while high values characterised male ice hockey players in the both models. Women from track and field had the highest mean TSH concentration but this was not a feature of the logistic model. Low average fT3 was seen in male power and weight-lifters and track and field athletes but was only important in power-

lifters in the logistic model where a high fT3 distinguished alpine skiers and bandy and ice-hockey players; fT3 appeared of little significance in women. In men fT4 was low in both models for canoeing and rowing while for women it was low in both models for cross-country skiers.

In men, in the logistic model IGF-BP2 is low in basketball players and high in rowers, similar to the mean values where in addition IGF-BP2 was low in both cross-country and alpine skiers. In women although there are a few significant differences by ANOVA between sports for IGF-BP2 and -BP3 there are no differences between sports by binary logistic regression. In the logistic model in men however, IGF-BP3 is low in rowing and judo and high in ice hockey and handball. These results differ considerably from the means where power lifting is the lowest and rowing and judo not noticeably low, nor ice hockey and handball noticeably high. In both men and women there are peaks in the mean

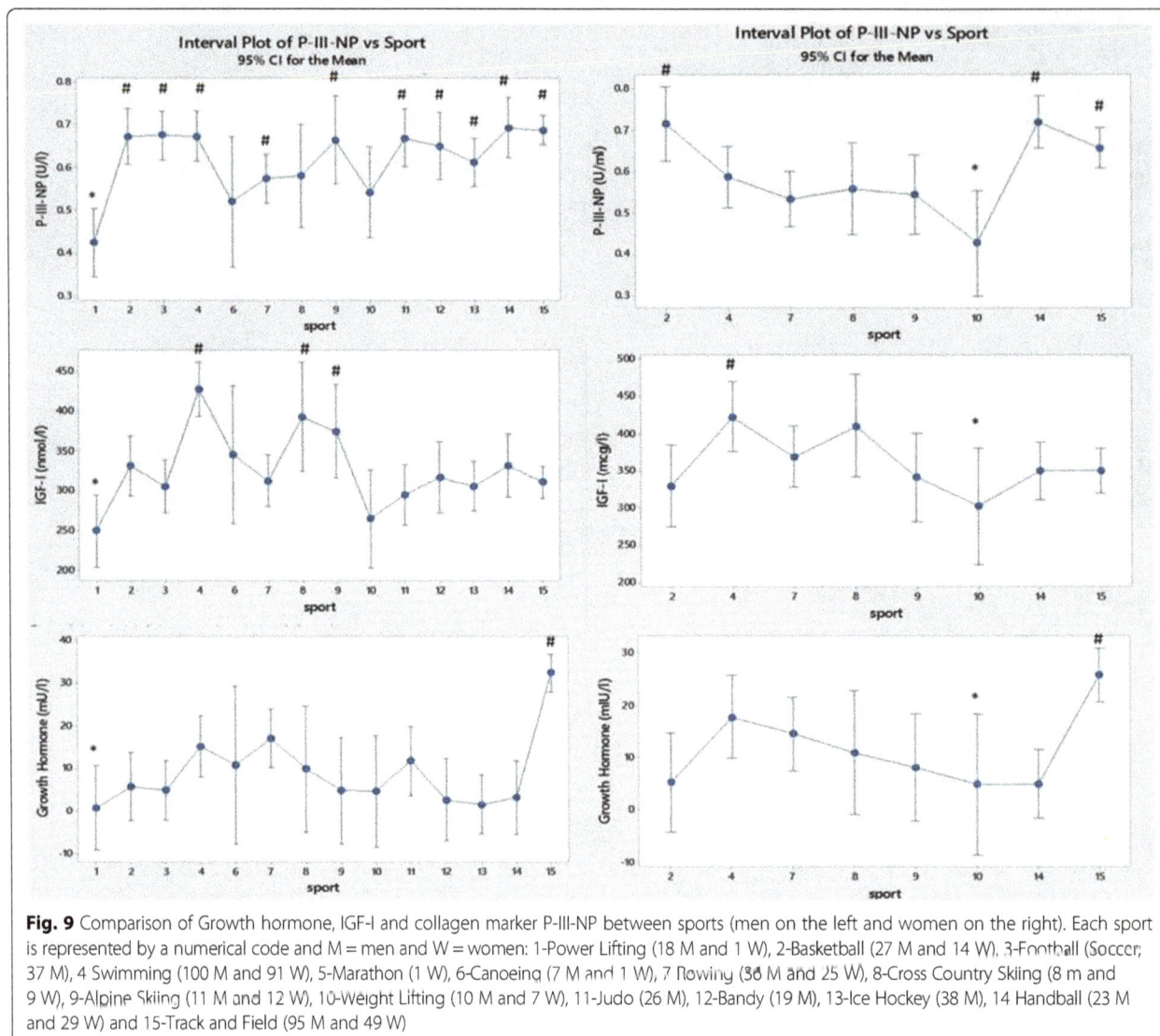

Fig. 9 Comparison of Growth hormone, IGF-I and collagen marker P-III-NP between sports (men on the left and women on the right). Each sport is represented by a numerical code and M = men and W = women: 1-Power Lifting (18 M and 1 W), 2-Basketball (27 M and 14 W), 3-Football (Soccer; 37 M), 4 Swimming (100 M and 91 W), 5-Marathon (1 W), 6-Canoeing (7 M and 1 W), 7 Rowing (36 M and 25 W), 8-Cross Country Skiing (8 m and 9 W), 9-Alpine Skiing (11 M and 12 W), 10-Weight Lifting (10 M and 7 W), 11-Judo (26 M), 12-Bandy (19 M), 13-Ice Hockey (38 M), 14 Handball (23 M and 29 W) and 15-Track and Field (95 M and 49 W)

concentrations of IGF-BP3 and ALS in swimming and handball, this concordance between the sexes is not seen in the logistic model where IGF-BP3 is high in handball but not in swimmers while ALS is high in swimmers but not in handball. In men the logistic model shows ALS to be low in basketball, ice-hockey and track and field which matches the lows in ANOVA but here there is also the lowest mean in weight-lifters. It is noticeable that although IGF-BP3 and ALS are both GH-sensitive their patterns between sports in both mean values and in the logistic model are not always similar. This is also true for the other known GH-sensitive endocrine markers where in many instances the logistic model bears little likeness to the mean values from ANOVA.

Osteocalcin mean concentration is very low in power-lifters but this does not appear of any significance in the logistic model where low values characterise track and field where mean values are substantially higher than in

power-lifters. In men weight-lifting, bandy and ice-hockey are characterised by high values that do not distinguish themselves in the ANOVA model. In women both models are in agreement over the low osteocalcin values in athletes from track and field. There is some discord between the models and the sexes for PICP, according to the logistic model a low value in men predicts rowers and bandy players while a high predicts track and field; by ANOVA although bandy players have a low mean PICP concentration there is no trough for rowers or peak for track and field. In women a high PICP is seen in track and field in both models.

One of the biggest discordances between models is for ICTP where low values are seen in the logistic model in men for swimming and handball but only in power-lifting by ANOVA while in women a low value strongly predicts basketball and swimming in the logistic model but there are no significant differences in ICTP concentrations

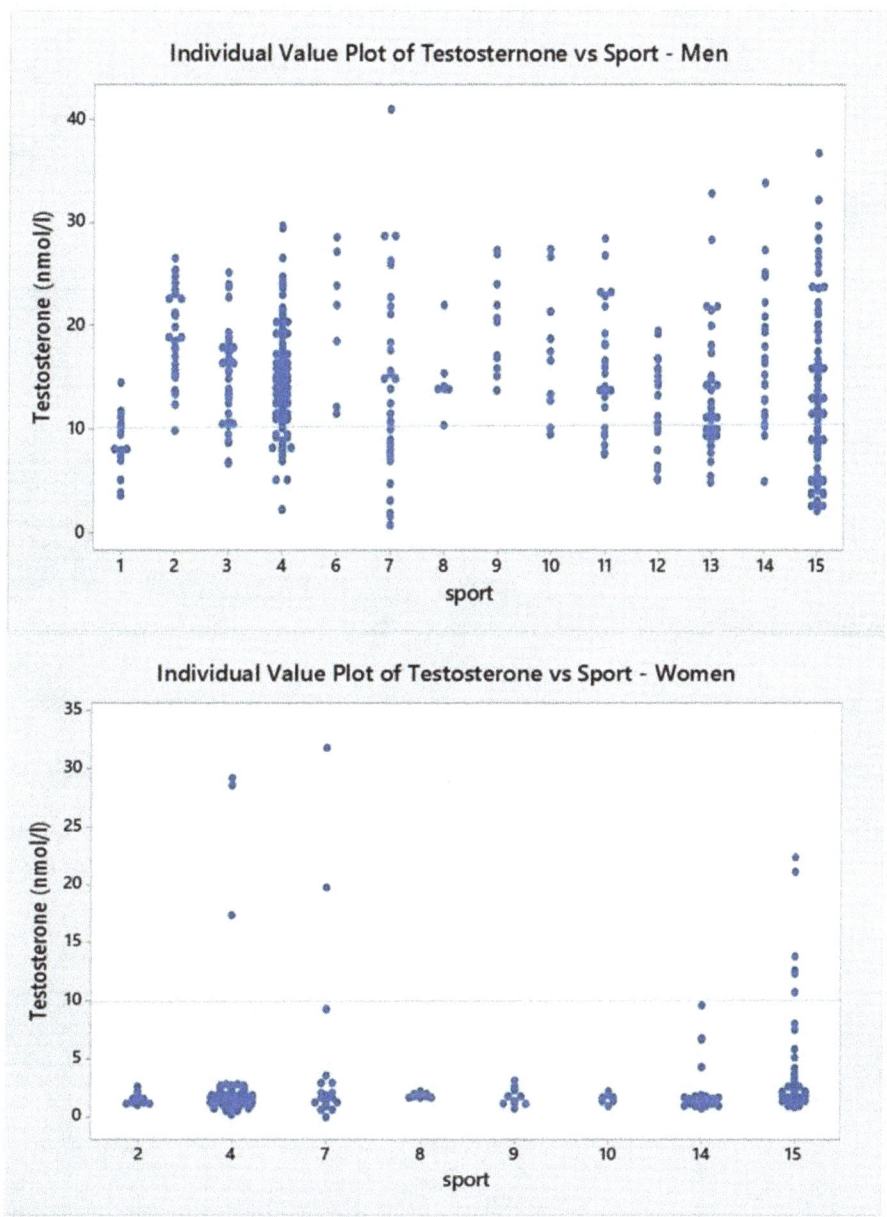

Fig. 10 Above –Serum testosterone in 445 elite male athletes. The horizontal line is at 10 nmol/l. There were 113 (25.4%) men with a testosterone value less than 10 nmol/l. Below - Serum testosterone in 231 elite female athletes. Horizontal line is at 10 nmol/l. There were 11 of 231 (4.8%) athletes with testosterone level above 10 nmol/l; 3 of 88 swimmers, 2 of 25 rowers and 6 of 48 track and field athletes. Each sport is represented by a numerical code and M = men and W = women: 1-Power Lifting (18 M and 1 W), 2-Basketball (27 M and 14 W), 3-Football (Soccer; 37 M), 4 Swimming (100 M and 91 W), 5-Marathon (1 W), 6-Canoeing (7 M and 1 W), 7-Rowing (36 M and 25 W), 8-Cross Country Skiing (8 m and 9 W), 9-Alpine Skiing (11 M and 12 W), 10-Weight Lifting (10 M and 7 W), 11-Judo (26 M), 12-Bandy (19 M), 13-Ice Hockey (38 M), 14 Handball (23 M and 29 W) and 15-Track and Field (95 M and 49 W)

between sports. There is no agreement between the models in men for P-III-NP where low values are observed in ice-hockey players (by logistic model) which is not reflected by ANOVA as the mean value is amongst the highest in ice hockey and a very low value seen in power-lifters. In women however, there is concordance between the models with high values in basketball and handball.

IGF-I levels are not associated with membership of any sporting group in women but high levels are associated with male rowers in the logistic model; rowers also have the highest mean level of IGF-I in both sexes. Low levels of growth hormone predict football in the logistic model in men and handball in women these results being discordant with the results from

Table 1 Significances of Logistic Regression of selective sports on body measurements (men)

Sport's Code	1	2	3	4	5	6	7	8	9	10	11	12	13	14	15
Sport	Power Lifting	Basketball	Football	Swimming	Marathon	Canoeing	Rowing	X-Skiing	Alpine	Weight Lifting	Judo	Bandy	Ice Hockey	Handball	Track & Field
Total Number	18	27	37	100	0	7	36	8	11	10	26	19	38	23	95
Number in Model	17	26	34	31		5	32	8	11	10	26	19	36	23	42
Age	**		*	***				**		*					
Weight							**	*			***			***	
Height	***	***	***				***							***	
BMI															
Testosterone	***	**				*			***		*				
LH									***		***			*	
FSH														***	
SHBG						*									
Estradiol								***							***
Cortisol								*							
Prolactin									***						*
TSH				*			***						**		***
fT3	**								***			***	***		***
fT4						**	***								*
IGF-BP2		**					***								
IGF-BP3			*				***				**		**	***	
ALS		***		**									***		**
IGF-I			*				**							*	
GH			***				*								***
Osteo										***		***	***		
PICP							***				*	***			
ICTP				**								*	*	**	
P-III-NP													***	*	
eLBM	**	**	***				***				**			***	
eFM	***						***						**	*	

* Inverse   * Direct
*<0.05
**<0.01
***<0.001

ANOVA where high values are seen in track and field in both men and women.

In power-lifting in men where mean GH levels are lowest is concordant with the low levels of GH-sensitive BP3, osteocalcin, ICTP, P-III-NP, and IGF-I. In each of these cases although the marker has a strong age-dependence and the power-lifters are the oldest, the differences between sports remains significant after adjusting for age (by regression analysis – data not shown).

Table 2 Significances of Logistic Regression of selective sports on body measurements (women)

Sport's Code	1	2	3	4	5	6	7	8	9	10	11	12	13	14	15
Sport	Power Lifting	Basketball	Football	Swimming	Marathon	Canoeing	Rowing	X-Skiing	Alpine	Weight Lifting	Judo	Bandy	Ice Hockey	Handball	Track & Field
Total Number	1	14	0	91	1	1	25	9	12	7	0	0	0	29	49
Number in Model	1	14		19			19	9	11	7				29	34
Age		***		***			*	**	*						
Weight								**							
Height		*					**			***					
BMI															
Testosterone							*								
LH															
FSH															
SHBG									**						
Estradiol							*	***							*
Cortisol				*			*								
Prolactin										***					
TSH							**								
fT3															
fT4								***							
IGF-BP2															
IGF-BP3															
ALS				**						**					***
IGF-I		*													
GH														***	
Osteo															***
PICP															***
ICTP		***		***											
P-III-NP		***												***	
eLBM		*		*			*			***					
eFM				*						***					

* Inverse   * Direct
*<0.05
**<0.01
***<0.001

In the first publication arising from this GH-2000 project the differences between marker levels between sports was attributed to differences in ages [3] but more detailed analysis has shown that although age plays an important part there are factors relating to the sport that prevail even when adjusting for age in all but two cases [1]. When allowing for age by regression analysis the differences between sports remain significant except for IGF-BP2 and BP3 in women [1].

It is difficult to compare these results with other published data as there are little comparable data available. Rickenlund et al. [9] examined endocrine profiles in a group of female university athletes and matched controls but this paper focussed on hyperandrogenicity and menstrual status and not differences between sports. In our case the 'hyperandrogenic' (as defined by IAAF and IOC as having testosterone above 10 nmol/l [5, 6]) women were in swimming, rowing as well as track and field sports; the overall prevalence was 11/231 (4.8%, Fig. 10). This is highly relevant to the comparison of our data and those of Bermon et al. [10] who reported limited endocrine profiles in 849 elite female track and field athletes taking part in the 2011 IAAF World Championship in Daegu (South Korea). They removed the data from 5 women 'suspected' of doping and 5 'later diagnosed with hyperandrogenic 46 XY disorder of sex development (DSD)' before analysis. They observed significant differences in testosterone, DHEAS and SHBG but not free testosterone between sports with 'Throwers, sprinters and to a lesser extent jumpers having higher levels of androgenic hormones than long distance runners'. This may be simply because long distance runners are prone to develop a form of functional hypogonadism and thus have low testosterone levels [11]. They calculated the prevalence of 'this type of medical condition' (hyperandrogenism) as 7.1 per 1000. The prevalence of 'hyperandrogenism' in our smaller group of randomly selected elite female athletes from 8 Olympic sports is nearly seven times greater. The high prevalence of hyperandrogenic disorders of sex development (46,XY DSD) in sport has been explained by genes for stature that occur on the Y-chromosome rather than the high testosterone levels [12], which in normal people have only a small influence on the development of lean body mass [2].

Looking at the converse and accepting the IOC and IAAF value of 10 nmol/l as being the lower limit of the 'normal' range for serum testosterone in men, 'hypoandrogenism' was present in 113 of 445 (25.4%) elite male athletes from 15 Olympic sports. Since these blood samples were taken within 2 h of completing their event in a National or International competition there can be no doubt that these were elite athletes competing at the highest level. The low testosterone may be related to the gruelling training that elite athletes have to maintain as it has been shown that exercise to exhaustion in young troops can lead to a state of 'functional hypogonadism' that resolves spontaneously with rest and a good night's sleep [13]. On the other hand it is possible that in some cases the low testosterone with normal LH and FSH may indicate the use of anabolic steroids that had been discontinued some time before the competition [14]. This example shows that simple correlations involving hormone levels and events does not necessarily indicate causation but may simply be a consequence of that event. Acute exercise itself has little effect on testosterone levels and so in the case of the data presented here, the timing of the blood sampling is unlikely to affect the number of low values [15]. There were no low values in basketball, canoeing, cross-country and alpine skiing and weight lifting but all other sports had a significant number of competing athletes with 'hypoandrogenism'. Low free testosterone levels (0.23 nmol/l) were found by Bermon and Garnier in 101 of 795 (12.7%) elite male track and field athletes in their sample from the World athletics championship in Daegu [10]; they did not report the data for total testosterone. Thus it is clear that a very low testosterone level does not prevent an elite male athlete from competing in top events. In addition Bermon and Garnier [16] found no correlation between serum testosterone and performance in either men or women.

Cardinale and Stone [17] demonstrated higher testosterone levels in female sprinters than volleyball players as well higher testosterone levels in male sprinters than soccer and handball players. They also showed that both male and female sprinters managed a higher 'countermovement jump (CMJ)' than the volleyball players. By correlating the results between these two groups they showed an apparent correlation between endogenous testosterone and performance. They did not consider that this was more likely a 'false correlation' as they were effectively drawing a line between two distinct groups and the use of correlation in this situation is inappropriate [18], they should have looked at the relationship between CMJ and testosterone levels by adjusting for sports discipline; this was a serious methodological limitation. More recently Eklund et al. [19] related serum androgen levels to performance in a group of female Olympic athletes. They found no differences in testosterone levels between sports and no correlation between serum testosterone and performance but were able to show weak correlations between some androgen precursors and performance. In a recent review Bermon reported that he was able to find a relationship between free testosterone levels and performance such that those with the highest free testosterone levels had between 1.8 and 4.5% advantage [20]; they found no relation between free testosterone and performance in the elite men. In the full paper [16] it is clear that they showed no relationship between endogenous testosterone concentration and performance in elite women athletes nor, unlike the men, any differences in free testosterone between sports. Thus neither group showed a significant correlation between serum total testosterone (the endocrine variable used in the 'hyperandrogenism' rule) and performance. They did claim to show a relationship between (estimated) free testosterone and performance in five out of 21 sub-groups but in nine of these sub-groups, those with the lower testosterone performed better.

Strengths and weaknesses
Our main strength is that we have examined comprehensive endocrine and anthropomorphic profiles in a large cohort of elite athletes of both sexes from a wide range of Olympic sports who were competing at national or international events. The blood samples were taken using a standardised protocol within two hours of completing their event, the serum separated promptly and stored at −80 °C until analysed. Analyses of serum samples were made by experts familiar with the methods and we have analysed the data extensively.

Our main weakness is that this was a supplementary study to the main GH-2000 project using remaining serum aliquots and consequently not all variables were measured on all athletes, thus the data set is incomplete. We did not know where volunteer athletes finished in their events and so we cannot match hormone profile to performance. We cannot exclude the possibility that any athlete was 'doping' although we consider that the fact that they volunteered to participate in a research study and signed a consent form that specifically excluded anyone who was currently or had previously used performance enhancing drugs made this unlikely together with the fact that there were no suspicious results to suggest this as a possibility. As the blood samples were taken within two hours of completing their event, they could have been taken at any time of day and thus they represent a random sample and may not be a true representative of the daily secretion. Likewise, the degree of hydration was not standardised although athletes had access to water and other drinks. This obligatory timing of sampling of the athletes was mandated by the agreement with the sporting authorities. It also meant that the state of hydration of each athlete at the time of body composition measurement was not standardised. The wide ranges of body composition in the volunteers is also outside the ranges of normal where the machines have been validated; measures of body composition must therefore be understood as measurements taken 'in the field'. Likewise, the estimated body composition data can only be considered approximate.

Conclusion
We have shown that, just as there are anthropomorphic differences between elite athletes from different events, there are also different hormonal profiles. We have not been able to elucidate whether this is the reason why athletes choose their events or whether this is a consequence of having trained and competed in their selected event over many years. There are clearly certain physical attributes that encourage individuals to pursue particular events (e.g. height and basketball) but also other events where they can modify their body to suit the event (e.g. weight control and cross-country skiing); it is possible that certain endocrine profiles favour success in a particular sport. We have shown that this is an area fertile for further research; an important 'next step' would be to examine endocrine profiles in relation to performance within events.

Abbreviations
ALS: Acid-labile subunit; ANOVA: Analysis of variance; DSD: Disorder of sex development; eFM: Estimated fat mass; eLBM: Estimated lean body mass; FM: Fat mass; FSH: Follicle stimulating hormone; fT3: Free tri-iodothyronine; fT4: Free thyroxine; GH: Growth hormone; GH-2000: GH-2000 A Methodology for the Detection of Doping with Growth Hormone & Related Substances. EU Contract Number: BMH4 CT950678 Official Contractual period: 1st January 1996-31st January 1999; IAAF: International Association of Athletics Federations; ICTP: Carboxy-terminal cross-linked telopeptide of type I collagen; IGFBP-3: IGF Binding protein #3; IGFBP-2: IGF binding protein #2; IGF-I: Insulin-like growth factor 1; IOC: International Olympic Committee; LBM: Lean body mass; LH: Luteinising hormone; M: Mass (weight); PICP: Carboxy-terminal propeptide of type I collagen; P-III-NP: Pro-collagen type III N-terminal peptide; SHBG: Sex hormone binding globulin; TSH: Thyroid stimulating hormone

Funding
There was no specific funding for this publication.

Authors' contributions
PHS analysed the data and wrote the first and subsequent drafts of the paper. DB and WB advised on and supervised statistical analyses of the data. All authors discussed and commented on the results during statistical analysis and drafting of the paper and subsequently read the first and subsequent drafts of the paper and made comments and suggestions as it went through several revisions. All authors read and approved the final manuscript.

Competing interests
The authors declare that they have no competing interests.

Author details
[1]Human Development and Health Academic Unit, University of Southampton Faculty of Medicine, Southampton, UK. [2]Southampton Statistical Sciences Research Institute, University of Southampton, Southampton, UK. [3]Nuffield Division of Clinical Laboratory Sciences, University of Oxford, Oxford, UK. [4]Department of Pharmacy and Forensic Science, Drug Control Centre, King's College London, London, UK.

References

1. Healy ML, Gibney J, Pentecost C, Wheeler MJ, Sonksen PH. Endocrine profiles in 693 elite athletes in the postcompetition setting. Clin Endocrinol. 2014;81:294–305.

2. Sonksen P. Determination and regulation of body composition in elite athletes. Br J Sports Med. 2016; https://doi.org/10.1136/bjsports-2016-096742.

3. Healy M-L, Dall R, Gibney J, Bassett E, Ehrnborg C, Pentecost C, et al. Toward the development of a test for growth hormone (GH) abuse: a study of extreme physiological ranges of GH-dependent markers in 813 elite athletes in the postcompetition setting4. J Clin Endocrinol Metab. 2005;90:641–9.

4. Ranabir S, Reetu K. Stress and hormones. Indian J Endocrinol Metab. 2011; 15:18–22. https://doi.org/10.4103/2230-8210.77573.

5. International Association of Athletics Federations. (IAAF). (2011). IAAF regulations governing eligibility of females with hyperandrogenism to compete in women's competitions. http://www.iaaf.org/about-iaaf/documents/medical.

6. IOC Regulations on Female Hyperandrogenism. 2012. http://www.olympic.org/Documents/Commissions_PDFfiles/Medical_commission/2012-06-22-IOC-Regulations-on-Female-Hyperandrogenism-eng.pdf. Accessed 17 Nov 2017.

7. Jebb SA, Cole TJ, Doman D, Murgatroyd PR, Prentice AM. Evaluation of the novel Tanita body-fat analyser to measure body composition by comparison with a four-compartment model. Br J Nutr. 2000;83(2):115-22. https://doi.org/10.1017/S0007114500000155.

8. Hume R. Prediction of lean body mass from height and weight. J Clin Pathol. 1966;19:389–91.

9. Rickenlund A, Carlstrom K, Ekblom B, Brismar TB, Von SB, Hirschberg AL. Hyperandrogenicity is an alternative mechanism underlying oligomenorrhea or amenorrhea in female athletes and may improve physical performance. Fertil Steril. 2003;79:947–55.

10. Bermon S, Garnier PY, Hirschberg AL, Robinson N, Giraud S, Nicoli R, et al. Serum androgen levels in elite female athletes1. J Clin Endocrinol Metab. 2014;99:jc20141391-.

11. Bennell KL, Brukner PD, Malcolm SA. Effect of altered reproductive function and lowered testosterone levels on bone density in male endurance athletes. Br.J. Sports Med. 1996;30:205–8.

12. Ferguson-Smith MA, Bavington LD. Natural selection for genetic variants in sport: the role of y chromosome genes in elite female athletes with 46,XY DSD1. Sport Med. 2014;44:1629–34.

13. Aakvaag A, Sand T, Opstad PK, Fonnum F. Hormonal changes in serum in young men during prolonged physical strain. Eur J Appl Physiol Occup Physiol. 1978;39:283–91.

14. Markku A, Matti, R. Reijo V. Response of serum hormones to androgen administration in pow... : Medicine & Science in Sports & Exercise. 1985;354–9. http://journals.lww.com/acsm-msse/Abstract/1985/06000/Response_of_serum_hormones_to_androgen..aspx. Accessed 20 Oct 2017.

15. Jensen J, Oftebro H, Breigan B, Johnsson A, Ohlin K, Meen HD, et al. Comparison of changes in testosterone concentrations after strength and endurance exercise in well trained men. Eur.J.Appl.Physiol Occup. Physiol. 1991;63:467–71.

16. Bermon S, Garnier P-Y. Serum androgen levels and their relation to performance in track and field: mass spectrometry results from 2127 observations in male and female elite athletes. Br J Sports Med. 2017. https://doi.org/10.1136/bjsports-2017-097792.

17. Cardinale M, Stone MH. Is testosterone influencing explosive performance? J Strength Cond Res. 2006;20:103–7.

18. Berndsen M, Spears R, Pligt J, McGarty C. Determinants of intergroup differentiation in the illusory correlation task. Br J Psychol. 1999;90:201–20. https://doi.org/10.1348/000712699161350.

19. Eklund E, Berglund B, Labrie F, Carlstrom K, Ekstrom L, Hirschberg AL. Serum androgen profile and physical performance in women Olympic athletes. Br J Sports Med. 2017. https://doi.org/10.1136/bjsports-2017-097582.

20. Bermon S. Androgens and athletic performance of elite female athletes. Curr Opin Endocrinol Diabetes Obes. 2017;24:246–51. https://doi.org/10.1097/MED.0000000000000335.

23

Growth hormone: isoforms, clinical aspects and assays interference

Júnia Ribeiro de Oliveira Longo Schweizer[1], Antônio Ribeiro-Oliveira Jr[1] and Martin Bidlingmaier[2]* ⓘ

Abstract

The measurement of circulating concentrations of growth hormone (GH) is an indispensable tool in the diagnosis of both GH deficiency and GH excess. GH is a heterogeneous protein composed of several molecular isoforms, but the physiological role of these different isoforms has not yet been fully understood. The 22KD GH (22 K-GH) is the main isoform in circulation, followed by 20KD GH (20 K-GH) and other rare isoforms. Studies have been performed to better understand the biological actions of the different isoforms as well as their importance in pathological conditions. Generally, the non-22 K- and 20 K-GH isoforms are secreted in parallel to 22 K-GH, and only very moderate changes in the ratio between isoforms have been described in some pituitary tumors or during exercise. Therefore, in a diagnostic approach, concentrations of 22 K-GH accurately reflect total GH secretion. On the other hand, the differential recognition of GH isoforms by different GH immunoassays used in clinical routine contributes to the known discrepancy in results from different GH assays. This makes the application of uniform decision limits problematic. Therefore, the worldwide efforts to standardize GH assays include the recommendation to use 22 K-GH specific GH assays calibrated against the pure 22 K-GH reference preparation 98/574. Adoption of this recommendation might lead to improvement in diagnosis and follow-up of pathological conditions, and facilitate the comparison of results from different laboratories.

Keywords: Growth hormone, Growth hormone isoform, Growth hormone molecule, 22 k growth hormone isoform, 20 k growth hormone isoform, Acromegaly, Growth hormone deficiency, Growth hormone assays, IRP 98/574

Background

The measurement of circulating concentrations of growth hormone (GH) is an indispensable tool in the diagnosis of both GH deficiency and GH excess. GH is a heterogeneous protein composed of several molecular isoforms, but the physiological role of the different isoforms has not yet been clarified. Owing to the fact that assays to specifically measure the different GH isoforms are not easily available, only a limited number of studies have investigated them under various clinical conditions. Most commercially available GH assays have not been fully characterized with respect to their cross-reactivity with the different isoforms. It must be assumed that most assays measure a mixture of isoforms with differences in affinity. This in part explains why despite some advances in design, practicability and sensitivity of the

assays, discrepancies between GH concentrations reported from different GH assays increased over the last decades [1–3]. This article reviews available information on the main GH isoforms as well as their impact on GH measurements in clinical practice.

GH molecule

Growth hormone belongs to a superfamily of cytokines, which includes interleukins, cytokines, as well as leukemic, neurotropic, and growth factors [4]. GH is a polypeptide hormone exhibiting molecular heterogeneity. It consists of a complex mixture of molecular isoforms and their multimers. In humans, the genetic locus that codes GH resides on chromosome 17q24.2 [4, 5], has 46.83 kilobases and contains five GH related genes. These multiple genes most likely arose from gene duplication. Each of these genes is composed of five exons and four introns: GH1 (or GH-N), GH2 (or GH-V), CS1, CS2 and CSL. While the GH1 is mainly expressed in somatotropes of the pituitary gland, the GH2 and CS (chorionic somatomammotropin also

* Correspondence: martin.bidlingmaier@med.uni-muenchen.de
[2]Endocrine Laboratory, Medizinische Klinik und Poliklinik IV, Klinikum der Universität München, Ziemssenstraße 1, 80336 Munich, Germany
Full list of author information is available at the end of the article

known as placental lactogen) are expressed exclusively by the placenta in females during pregnancy. The CSL (CS-like protein) is expressed at low levels and its function remains unclear [6].

Pituitary GH - isoforms and fragments
22 K-GH

The GH1 is expressed mainly in somatotrope cells of the pituitary gland. Expression in the immune system has been described, although there is no evidence that lymphocyte derived GH significantly contributes to circulating GH concentrations. The main product of this gene is a 191 amino acids single-chain protein stabilized by two disulphide bridges. The molecular weight is 22,129 Da [7]. This 22 K-GH molecule is the main GH isoform, representing more than 90% of total GH in circulation. Its tertiary structure is a 4-helical (Fig. 1) twisted bundle with unusual connectivity. The helices run up-up-down-down instead of the more usual up-down-up-down form. There are two binding-sites interacting with the GH receptor, namely site I and site II. Spectrums of posttranslational modifications of this isoform, including acetylation, phosphorylation, deamidation and glycosylation have been described, which can potentially modify GH actions [8, 9]. GH is best known from its growth promoting activity in children, but also has important biological activities in adults. These include lipolysis, glucose-, calcium- and phosphorous-metabolism as well as lactogenesis and immune function. The previous knowledge that some hormones and cleaved fragments have biological actions, like POMC (proopiomelanocortin), ACTH (adrenocorticotrophic hormone) and β-endorphin, as well as ANP (atrial natriuretic peptide) and BNP (brain natriuretic peptide), has led to the suspicion of GH isoforms existence and possible functions.

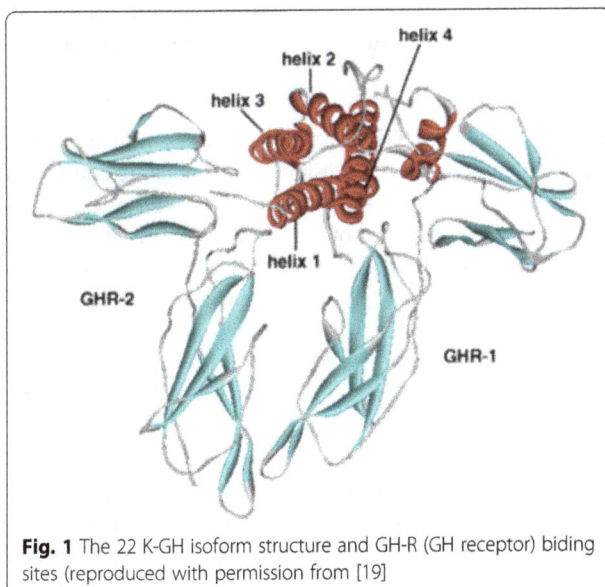

Fig. 1 The 22 K-GH isoform structure and GH-R (GH receptor) biding sites (reproduced with permission from [19]

20 K-GH

The second most abundant GH isoform is the 20 K-GH molecule. It is derived from GH-1 by alternative pre-messenger ribonucleic acid (pre mRNA) splicing of exon 3. The structure is similar to 22 K-GH except for a deletion of the internal residues 32–46 (Fig. 2). Therefore, 20 K-GH consists of 176 amino acids only. The molecular weight is 20,274 Da. This smaller GH isoform represents about 10% of total circulating GH. There is controversy in the literature regarding the biological function of 20 K-GH [10–13]. Most in vitro and animal studies report similar activities to promote growth and stimulate lipolysis, while some authors discussed reduced diabetogenic and anti-natriuretic activities [14–17]. The 20 K-GH isoform is more prone to dimerize, leading to slower clearance when compared to 22 K-GH. This potentially could lead to a change in the relative abundance of 20 K- and 22 K-GH isoforms in plasma over time following a secretory burst and possibly an extended action of the 20 K-GH isoform. Since the residues 32–46 missing in the 20 K-GH isoform overlap with the GH receptor binding site 1 (Figs. 1 and 2), the strength of interaction with the GH receptor could be different from the 22 K-GH [14]. However, there is compelling evidence that both 22 K- and 20 K-GH can activate Janus Kinase 2 (JAK2), signal transducers and activators of transcription 1, 3 and 5 (STATs 1/3/5), although the level of STAT 1/3/5 phosphorylation induced by 22 K-GH are higher than those of 20 K-GH [18].

GH fragments

As aforementioned, although the 22 K-GH is the main predicted protein product from the GH gene, posttranscriptional and posttranslational processing can lead to different GH isoforms. A number of such smaller fragments or isoforms has been described, but not all of them could be independently confirmed [10, 19]. It is important to realize that methodological differences in the experimental approach to identify these fragments as well as differences between species or matrices might explain the inconsistency of some findings. It has been reported that a single specific cleavage can generate two contiguous GH fragments of 5 K (fragment 1–43) and 17 K (fragment 44–191). These isoforms were synthesized and isolated from pituitary extract but have also been reported to occur in significant amounts in circulation. It has been suggested that 5 K-GH has similarity with the GH N-terminal region, has insulin-like activity and can be an in-vitro substrate of dipeptidyl peptidase [20]. Independently, a polypeptide of 17.5 K resulting from GH exon 3 skipping has been described in pituitary and circulation, representing 1 to 5% of GH transcripts. It reportedly exists mainly under pathological conditions. However, identity to the above mentioned 17 K-GH fragment 44–191 could not be demonstrated by the assay

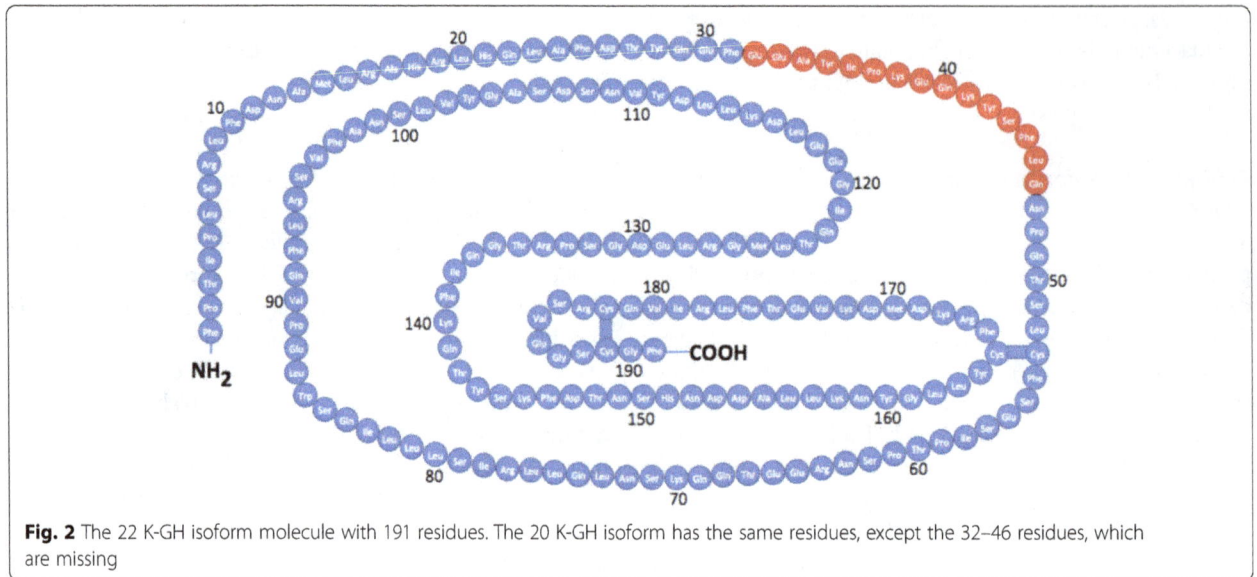

Fig. 2 The 22 K-GH isoform molecule with 191 residues. The 20 K-GH isoform has the same residues, except the 32–46 residues, which are missing

used [21]. Another synthetic peptide obtained by stop sense molecular inclusion in the GH gene sequence (fragment 53–134) was also discussed to correspond to 17 K-GH isoform. Other molecular variants including 12 K-GH, glycosylated GH, deamidated GH, and phosphorylated GH have also been described. However, more research is obviously needed to fully understand the nature of the smaller isoforms [7, 22–24].

At the other end of the molecular weight spectrum, larger forms of GH molecules can be found: 35 K-GH and 45 K-GH, as well as GH homo- and hetero-dimers and -oligomers have been found [10, 19]. It is still uncertain whether these isoforms could have the same biological actions potency of the 22 K-GH. They may act as either 22 K-GH agonists or antagonists, thus regulating biological functions of GH.

In addition to naturally occurring GH isoforms, additional isoforms and fragments have been synthesized. Currently, the GH receptor antagonist pegvisomant is the most relevant example of an artificial GH isoform. The amino acid sequence differs from that of naturally occurring 22 K-GH in only eight amino acids in binding site 1 (H18D, H21N, R167N, K168A, D171S, K172R, E174S, I179T), and one amino acid in binding site 2 (G120R). Also, pegylated residues were added to Lys residues in the 22KD-GH, producing a molecule with 42-46 K. These targeted mutations led to the generation of a GH molecule which can bind to one GH receptor molecule by very high affinity but does not correctly bind to the other molecule of the dimeric GH receptor. This prevents signal transduction, making the molecule a potent GH antagonist used to the treatment of acromegaly [25–27].

Among the smaller GH molecules, which have been synthesized is GH 30–54 [19]. It contains the segment GH32–46, which distinguishes the two main GH isoforms, i.e. the 22 K- and 20 K-GH. Its presence in biological fluid and the biological effects are not known. Another fragment, GH 108–129, may be originated from natural biosynthesis or GH fragmentation. It encompasses the helix 3 and site-II regions, the latter related to GH receptor interaction. Since mutations in this site could result in GH receptor binding interference and ultimately in growth disruption, this peptide could potentially serve as another GH antagonist and has been patented. A fragment 147–191 is obtained by enzymatic proteolysis and may be responsible for the generation of the fragment 177–191 (AOD9401). This late fragment is a short peptide, and one group has claimed it has GH like activity and the potential for treating obesity, due to its action on lipolysis [28, 29]. Interestingly, many of the fragments first were theoretically hypothesized, and then produced later on [30]. However, the significance of all these products for routine treatment remains unclear.

Placental GH

The placental GH (GH2 or GH-V) shares similarity with GH1 gene, except for 13 residues difference. It contains a consensus sequence for N-glycosylation at position 140, suggesting the existence of two GH2 isoforms: a glycosylated and a non-glycosylated form. The placental GH is a more basic protein, expressed exclusively in syncytiotrophoblast of the placenta. It is progressively released into the maternal circulation with peak concentrations reached in late pregnancy. Due to its high somatogenic activity, IGF-I concentrations in pregnant females tend to increase. In turn, these increasing IGF-I concentrations lead to an almost complete suppression of the pituitary GH-N secretion with advancing pregnancy. Although there is evidence of 20 K-GH isoform derived from placental GH, this gene is less prone of alternative splicing and does not represent the major origin of this isoform [31]. There is also evidence that placental derived 20 K-GH has lower diabetogenic and lactogenic activities when compared to the placental 22 K-GH [32]. Chorionic somatomammotropin (CS), the other important product of the GH gene family expressed in the placenta, has 85% structural homology with pituitary GH but does not have important somatogenic bioactivity. GH-V and CS will not be further discussed herein, as their importance are limited to the gestational period, which is not an objective of this article.

GH isoform secretion in healthy and disease
Physiology
22 K-GH is secreted from the pituitary gland under hypothalamic control. Secretion is classically stimulated by GHRH and inhibited by somatostatin. 22 K-GH secretory pulses occur every 2–3 h with great amplitude variance. The largest pulses usually occur at night, during slow wave sleep [33]. The 22 K-GH secretion pattern may differ between sexes, mainly due to estrogenic effect in females. Females usually have higher secretion rates, higher interpeak levels and more erratic secretion patterns of this isoform than males [34]. The 20 K-GH isoform has been reported to be higher in females than males, although the ratio of 20- to 22 K-GH usually does not differ between sexes [35, 36]. 22 K-GH secretion patterns also change with age. The 22 K-GH peaks are higher in puberty, and secretion rates decrease later in life by approximately 15% per decade. Other factors also affect GH secretion: Obesity is known to attenuate GH secretion whereas physical activity, stress and fasting are acute stimuli. In physiological state, the 20 K-GH and the 22 K-GH isoforms are secreted in a pulsatile manner, in a constant molar ratio and the peaks from both isoforms were coincident in healthy individuals, although much lower for 20 K-GH isoform [36].

Although there are other sites of GH clearance (e.g. the liver), the major portion of the metabolic clearance of monomeric GH occurs in the kidney. There is an efficient glomerular filtration and degradation in the proximal tubule. The urinary GH corresponds to only 1/10,000th of glomerular filtered GH. Some studies reported differences in clearance of isoforms, with a slower clearance for oligomeric GH and 20 K-GH compared to the main 22 k isoform. One study demonstrated an approximately 30% reduced clearance for 20 K-GH [37], although direct comparison of results from isoform specific assays might be difficult. There is little information about salivary GH, but in normal subjects it seems to be 1000-fold lower than serum GH. Since both, urinary and salivary GH are present in much smaller quantities than serum GH, methods to assess GH in these matrices are difficult and less standardized. Urinary GH has also been shown to be less stable than serum GH.

Thus, it is no surprise the main matrix to measure 22 K- and 20 K-GH, and also the main source of our knowledge about GH isoforms is serum.

Exercise
Exercise is a well-recognised condition that naturally stimulates GHRH and GH release in the circulation [38]. It can alter nocturnal GH secretion pattern by attenuating burst mass and amplitude, but increasing burst frequency. Therefore, the total nocturnal GH secretion is not altered [39]. Exercise can increase lactate acid, and there is a relation between GH secretion and blood lactate [39].

Some GH isoform studies measured various GH isoforms with distinct methods under different physical activity protocols. Wallace et al. [40] showed that all GH isoforms (22 K-, 20 K- and non-22 K-GH isoforms) increased during acute exercise. The 22 K-GH (polyclonal immunoradiometric assay) was the main GH isoform produced during physical activity and peaked at 30 min. The 20 K-GH (ELISA) and the non 22 K-GH measured by the 22 K-GH exclusion assay exhibited a somewhat greater increase during the post exercise period. This temporarily increased the relative abundance of the non-22 K-GH isoforms. The authors suggested that these isoforms might play a role in preventing post-training hypoglycemia, as the GH isoforms could have diabetogenic effects. Another study [41] found a moderate modulation of GH isoforms after acute exercise. As expected, concentrations of 22 K-GH (IFMA) and 20 K-GH (specific ELISA) isoforms increased, but – in contrast to the above mentioned study – the increase was greater for 22 K-GH. Accordingly, in this study the ratio 22 K-/20 K-GH was slightly increased for a short period after acute physical activity. After chronic resistance exercise, most studies did not find major alteration in different molecular weight GH isoforms [42]. However, in a study by Pierce et al. [43] it was shown that acute and chronic resistance exercise led to the appearance of similar amounts of disulphide-linked GH aggregates. The physiological significance of this alteration is unknown. Some studies used a very different analytical approach to study different molecular weight GH isoforms in physical activity. In these studies, GH isoforms were separated into categories greater than 60 K (> 60 K), 30-60 K and less than 30 K (< 30 K). In females, acute heavy resistance exercise led to an increase in 30-60 k and > 60 k, but not in the < 30 K molecular weight GH [44]. Before exercise, stronger women had greater total GH than the weaker ones, while the latter had higher smaller weight GH fractions (< 30 K). All GH isoforms increased after exercise in both, strong and weak untrained women, although the lower molecular weight variants were less responsive to greater amounts of exercise in stronger women [45]. The use of oral contraceptive (OC) in untrained women also seemed to influence the GH response during exercise when assessed by these assay methods, with higher abundance of high molecular weight GH in both resting and post exercise states in the OC group [46]. In contrast, other studies only confirmed that in the basal state all GH isoforms tend to be higher in females, but the 20 K–22 K-GH ratio was not different between sexes. In addition, oral contraceptive administration to postmenopausal women and testosterone administration to hypogonadal men also led to an increase in both 20 K- and 22 K-GH isoforms, but did not alter the 20-to-22 K-GH ratio [36]. The latter study used specific immunoassays to measure the 20 K- and 22 K-isoforms separately.

In summary, though the exercise induced increase in GH is known since a long time and has convincingly been demonstrated by several groups, any potential alterations in the relative abundance of the different isoforms have never been uniformly shown across studies. The use of different in-house research-type assay methodologies to measure concentrations of isoforms makes it very difficult directly comparing results from different studies. However, regardless of the assay methods used, the changes in isoform composition with exercise – if any - were small and of short duration.

Doping

Although evidence supporting performance enhancing effects in healthy trained subjects are lacking, it is known that GH is abused by some athletes [47]. For this reason, the World Anti-Doping Agency (WADA) classifies GH as a prohibited substance. Detection of GH doping, however, was considered I possible for a long time because recombinant GH is identical in its amino acid sequence and physicochemical properties to the main isoform of endogenous GH. The pulsatile secretion pattern of GH also makes it impossible to use high serum GH levels as evidence for exogenous GH administration. The improved understanding of the physiology of GH isoforms and their regulation by the administration of the other GH isoforms, however, has helped to develop a valid doping test. It has been shown that administration of the 20 K-GH isoform reduces secretion of the 22 K-GH isoform levels [48]. In turn, administration of exogenous recombinant 22 K-GH administration rapidly suppresses non-22 K- and 20 K-GH isoforms. Isoforms other than 22 K-GH remain low for approximately 24 h, coupled to a reduction in the 20 K-to-22 K-GH ratio [36, 49, 50]. This knowledge enabled the development of the so-called GH isoform test as one WADA's recommended anti-doping tests [51, 52]. Its advantage is the direct detection of the molecular changes induced by the administration of recombinant GH, although the short time window limits its use to the first 12-36 h after recombinant GH administration.

Pathological conditions
Acromegaly

In acromegaly, the rhythmicity of GH secretion seems to be preserved [34]. There were some studies evaluating the GH isoforms in acromegaly in the past decades, although the studies used different methods and measured different isoform fractions. Boguszewski et al. [53] evaluated the "non-22 K-GH isoform" in men with acromegaly before and 1 year after transsphenoidal surgery. The relative abundance of the non-22 K-GH isoform was increased in active acromegaly when compared to inactive acromegaly and healthy controls. Interestingly, the proportion of non-22 K-GH isoform in active acromegaly remained high after non-curative surgery, while patients with controlled acromegaly achieved a percentage of the non-22 K-GH isoform similar to healthy individuals. Tsushima et al. [54] for the first time studied the 20 K-GH isoform in acromegaly (by ELISA). They showed an increase of this isoform in active acromegaly, and also an increased 20- to 22 K-GH ratio in acromegaly compared to healthy controls. Another group [36] studied GH secretion pattern in acromegaly and healthy controls by measuring 20 K- and 22 K-GH every 20 min for 24 h. Although there was an increase in 20 K-GH isoform in patients with acromegaly, this isoform increased in parallel with 22 K-GH, keeping the 20- to 22 K-GH ratio very similar to the ratio seen in healthy controls. There is also conflicting data regarding GH isoforms after somatostatin analogue treatment in patients with acromegaly. Although Murakami et al. did not find a modification in the 20- to 22 K-GH ratio after acute octreotide treatment [55], Leung et al. [36] described a rapid reduction in both isoforms, but with a relative increased in the 20- to 22 K-GH isoform ratio. The authors speculate that this was caused by a shorter half-life and thus a faster decrease in the 22 K-GH isoform when compared to the 20 K-GH isoform. A more recent study [56] evaluated patients with acromegaly before and after 6 months of octreotide LAR treatment. The 20 K- and 22 K-GH were increased in patients with acromegaly when compared to healthy controls, but the 20- to 22 K-GH isoform proportion did not change. Furthermore, this study did not find alterations in the 20 K- to 22 K-GH ratio before and 6 months after initiation of octreotide treatment. A limitation of this study was that only 13% (3/23) of acromegaly patients were controlled after octreotide treatment, precluding final conclusions about potential changes in the 20 K- to 22 K-GH ratio related to octreotide therapy.

GH deficiency

GH deficiency obviously more likely is associated with very low GH concentrations. The very low concentrations provide a limitation to the study of GH isoforms, since the smaller, less abundant isoforms (eg. 20 K-GH) are even lower and commonly below the detection limit of most assays. Accordingly, there are only very few studies on GH isoform secretion in the GH deficiency field, and these studies also differ considerably in the analytical methods used. To overcome the problem, some of the studies used various stimulation test protocols to increase GH concentrations and make the isoforms accessible to existing analytical methods. Some studies reported no influence of age, pubertal stage and sex on the 20 K/22 K-GH ratio in normal and GH deficient children and adults. There was also no change in 24-h GH secretion pattern after arginine and hypoglycemia stimulation tests [17, 35, 36]. Another group studied normal children after a different stimulation test (GHRH). They found that both, the non-22 K-GH and 22 K-GH isoforms increased after GHRH administration, but no change in the ratio. After a second GHRH stimulus, patients who still responded with a GH peak secretion greater than 10 ng/mL had lower non-22 K-GH levels than non-responders. These data could suggest isoform related differences in the recovery of somatotrope function or differences in GH isoforms metabolic clearance, but also could be related to assay sensitivity [57]. Pagani et al. [41] studied 22 K- and 20 K-GH isoforms in GH deficient patients before and after several pharmacologic stimuli such as arginine, L-dopa or glucagon. They found a significant increase in both 22- and 20 K-GH isoforms, but describe a slight increase in the 22 K-/20 K-GH ratio. The 22 K-GH was the most abundant isoform even in a state of reduced GH secretion. As discussed above the use of different assays to assess GH isoforms could explain the difference in results. Furthermore, the groups studied different stimuli during dynamic tests.

Prader-Willi syndrome

Prader-Willi syndrome (PW) is a complex disorder associated to hypogonadism, behavioural and cognitive impairment, alongside with obesity and short stature. The GH secretion is abnormal, but the etiology is unknown. One study has evaluated GH isoforms in obese and non-obese, and GH deficient and non-GH deficient patients with PW submitted to GHRH plus arginine test [58]. There was no difference in the 22 K- and 20 K-GH isoform ratio at baseline between obese and non-obese patients. The stimulation test increased 22 K- and 20 K-GH isoforms in non-obese and non-GH deficient PW patients. The GH response for both isoforms was higher in non-obese PW patients and there was no difference in isoforms between GH deficient and non-GH deficient in these non-obese PW patients. The ratio of circulating levels of 22 K-to-20 K-GH did not alter during the test in all studied groups. This study shows that alteration in GH isoforms generation may not be implicated in etiology of GH

pattern alteration in PW [58]. Furthermore, this group compared GHRH plus arginine (GHRH+ARG) stimulation test with arginine (ARG) only in PW. Although both tests increased 20 K-GH peak, it was higher in GHRH+ARG than in ARG group. This study further confirmed absence of alterations in the 20/22 K-GH ratio in both stimulation tests [59].

Other conditions

Little data exist regarding GH isoforms in other conditions. One study showed that anorexia was associated with a higher abundance of the 20 K-GH isoform (20 K/20 K-GH + 22 K-GH), but there was no difference in hypothyroidism, hyperthyroidism and non-insulin dependent diabetes [35].

Impact of molecular heterogeneity on GH measurement in clinical routine

The study of GH isoforms in physiology and in pathologic states was only possible with the development of more sensitive, isoform specific assays. Historically, GH has been measured by a wide spectrum of different analytical methods ranging from bioassays to radio receptor assays, immunoassays and mass spectrometry approaches. For a long time, isoform specificity on most methods was unknown, and for many assays used in clinical routine it is still unknown. Cell based and radio receptor assays do not distinguish specifically between isoforms, while mass spectrometry assays today still lack sensitivity particularly to measure the less abundant isoforms. Mass spectrometry assays also not used in clinical routine. The most commonly used method to assess GH concentrations in clinical routine are antibody-based immunoassays. Theoretically, detailed investigation of the epitopes recognized by the antibodies used in these assays would allow characterization of each assays isoform specificity. In fact, most of the studies on regulation of GH isoforms reviewed above have used some well-characterized isoform specific immunoassays. However, for GH assays used in high throughput routine laboratories the extra effort to characterize the isoform specificity of the assays is rarely done. However, it is important to be aware that each of this routine GH immunoassay – depending on the antibodies used - will pick a different spectrum of total GH isoforms. Many factors potentially affecting comparability of GH immunoassay have been described. These include nature and composition of the assay calibrator, interference from the growth hormone binding protein (GHBP) and also matrix effects. However, the differential recognition of GH isoforms remains one of the key problems of assay comparability. It inherently leads to issues regarding the quantification of GH and contributes to the known discrepancies between GH concentrations in a given sample obtained from measurements by different assays.

Generally, older assays based on polyclonal antibodies commonly measured a broader isoform spectrum. The advent of monoclonal antibody assays brought more specificity to one or few of GH isoforms. It has been described that this increased specificity led to greater differences between the absolute concentrations reported from assays using different antibodies. Because of the recognition of only a certain spectrum of isoforms, the newer, monoclonal antibody based assays also have a tendency to report lower GH concentrations compared to older assays using polyclonal antisera. This is important to keep in mind when applying cut-offs from guidelines to the interpretation of GH data: If cut-offs were established by polyclonal assays, but in clinical routine today monoclonal antibody based assays are in use, the cut-offs might have to be adapted to reflect the lower GH concentrations reported by modern GH assays.

To facilitate the uniform adoption of cut-offs from guidelines continued efforts have been undertaken to harmonize results from different immunoassays for GH. General recommendations for performance characteristics of ideal GH assays have been published by scientific societies to guide physicians working in the field [1–3].

Isoform specificity for common assays

The existence of GH isoforms affects the comparability of GH assays in two ways: As described above, different assays recognize different isoforms. In addition to this, different reference preparations are in use to calibrate the GH assays – the older ones consisting of a mixture of pituitary GH isoforms, the newer ones – of recombinant origin – consisting of the 22 K-GH isoform only. In an immunoassay, the analyte concentration is determined by comparing the signal generated in the sample to a signal from samples with known amounts of the analyte. Consequently, the preparation used for GH assay standard curve has an important impact on GH measurement and results. In the past, the GH assays were done with pituitary extracts, and international reference preparations (IRP) were 66/217 and 80/505. Both contained a variety of GH isoforms and the exact amount of GH was unknown. The concentrations were arbitrarily assigned as 2.0 and 2.6 U/mg for IRP 66/217 and 80/505, respectively. Subsequently, new reference preparations were produced by recombinant technologies. These reference preparations consist of the 22 K-GH exclusively (IRP 88/624 and 98/574). Now it became possible to make GH assays traceable to a mass unit of the IRP 88/624 (micrograms per liter). For historic reasons, a conventional unit was also assigned (3.0 U/mg), though recent guidelines do no longer support the use of conventional units. Recently, the next generation of the recombinant international IRP has been introduced (98/574). Basically identical to 88/624, the new preparation is of high purity (> 96% 22 K-GH) and shows adequate stability, bioactivity and availability [2].

Table 1 lists a number of GH immunoassays commonly used in clinical routine. All these assays meanwhile are calibrated to the recombinant IRP 98/574. Though the use of a common calibrator has slightly improved assay agreement over the last years [60], there is still considerable disagreement between GH assay results, and the disagreement still has considerable impact on the diagnosis of GH related disorders [61]. For many of the assays information on isoform specificity of the antibodies is not available or incomplete. One of the assays with published characterization of the antibodies (IDS) does not cross-react with an artificial GH isoform: pegvisomant is a mutated GH molecule, which is used as a drug to treat GH excess (acromegaly) by blocking the GH receptor. Most other available GH assays cross-react with pegvisomant, leading to falsely high or low results depending on antibody specificity and assay design.

Data on clinical impact

The variability of GH secretion itself, the lack of a perfect correlation with other biochemical markers like IGF-I and other factors make the evaluation of disease amelioration and remission in GH related diseases challenging [62–65]. Problems with standardization or harmonization of GH assays add to the complexity and make the applicability of international guidelines difficult. Therefore, improvements in the assay agreement could help to permit comparability of published data and the clinical use of the information. For the clinician it is important to realize and understand the potential impact of assay problems on GH assay results to allow interpretation of local results in relation to published cut-offs and recommendations.

Acromegaly

There are increasing data regarding the use of criteria for GH in the diagnosis of acromegaly [66]. Recommendations about the cut-off for GH during OGTT (oral glucose tolerance test) changed over time, with more recent publications recommending a nadir of 0.4 ng/mL or 1 ng/mL to exclude acromegaly and evaluate remission. In 2000, the "Cortina criteria" recommended a random GH concentration below 0.4 ng/mL or a GH nadir during OGTT below 1 ng/mL, together with normal IGF-I for age and sex [67]. After a decade, another consensus statements for "controlled acromegaly" recommended different GH cut-off values together with normal IGF-I. The recommendation stated a random GH concentration below 1 ng/mL and a GH nadir below 0.4 ng/mL. The current Endocrine Society Clinical Practice Guideline [68] requests the lack of suppression of GH below 1 ng/mL (and elevated IGF-I for age and sex) for diagnosing acromegaly. The suggested therapeutic

Table 1 Characteristics of commonly used commercial assays for GH (according to manufacturers instructions/kit inserts available to the authors or according to published data). Calibration has changed for several assays in recent years, and the process is ongoing. To the best of the authors knowledge the assays listed here have uniformly adopted the latest recombinant standard for all countries. The list of assays is not complete. Additional hGH assays exist, including an unknown number of in-house assays. (modified from [3]

Manufacturer	Name	Assay principle	Calibration	Isoform-specificity	Measuring range	Recommended sample material	Comment
Siemens	Immulite 2000	Two-site Chemilumminescent immunometric assay	98/574	Not provided	0.05 to 40 ng/mL Analytical sensitivity: 0.01 ng/mL	Serum	ng/mL × 3.0 →mIU/L
Diasorin	Liaison hGH	Chemiluminescent sandwich immunoassay	98/574	Not provided	0.009–80 ng/mL	Serum	
Beckmann-Coulter	Access Ultrasensitive hGH	Automated immunometric assay, Chemiluminescence	98/574	See comment	0.002–35 ng/mL (μ/L)	Serum or plasma (heparin)	Cross reaction analysed with GH 8 ng/mL for 20 K-GH: – 2542%
IDS	iSYS hGH	Chemilumminescent assay	98/574	22kD GH: 100%	0.05–100 ng/mL	Serum or plasma (heparin or EDTA)	Do not cross react with substances in these concentrations: 20 K-GH (10 ng/mL); placental GH (200 ng/mL); HPL (10,000 ng/mL); prolactin (40.000 ng/mL); pegvisomant (50,000 ng/mL); biotin 300 nmol/L); GHBP: 140 ng/mL. ng/mL × 3.0=μIU/mL
DIASource	hGH IRMA	Immunometric assay enzyme amplified sensitivity	98/574	Not provided	1–120 ng/mL Sensitivity: ng/mL	Serum, plasma	Conversion factor: 1μIU = 0.33 ng
	hGH EASIA	Enzyme-Immunoassay	98/574	Not provided	0.45–98 ng/mL Sensitivity:0.17 ng/mL	Serum, plasma	Conversion factor: 1μIU = 0.33 ng
CisBio	hGH-RIACT	Immunoradiometric	98/574	Not provided	0.03–75 ng/mL	Serum	1 ng = 3μIU; do not cross react with prolactin and hPL. Cross reaction with 20kD GH is less than 5% for the concentration up to 3750 ng/mL (22kD GH proportional concentration above 24,000 ng/mL)

goal was a random GH below 1 ng/mL coupled to a normal age-adjusted IGF-I. In part, the differences in the published cut-offs are related to differences in the assays used, although most guidelines do not specify the assay used to generate the GH concentrations stated. Some authors have published convincing evidence that prevalence of acromegaly as well as percentages for remission largely depend on cut-off values used [60, 61, 64, 65, 69, 70]. More recent publications on studies using modern, more specific GH assays calibrated against the latest recombinant standard clearly indicated that the above mentioned cut.-off of 1 ng/mL is inappropriately high and should be adapted for modern assays. The use of the "traditional" cut-off of 1 ng/mL can contribute to a delayed diagnosis in patients with milder forms of acromegaly. Using such assays, in cases of mild acromegaly GH can be suppressed to concentrations significantly below 1 ng/mL [65]. Apart from the fact that different assays have different sensitivity and therefore, different limits of quantification, it must be kept in mind that different assays also do measure different - though for most assays unspecified or unknown – subgroups of GH isoforms. Although the 22 K-GH is the most abundant and biological active isoform, in borderline cases the degree of specificity of the assay for the 22 K-GH or other isoforms could significantly affect the classification of the patient [71]. It is important to keep this in mind when applying cut-offs from guideline in such cases in clinical practice. A better standardization of GH assays is of great importance to facilitate diagnosis and to avoid misdiagnosis and insufficient treatment. In a complex disease like acromegaly undesirable consequences for patients have to be avoided. Uncertainties in monitoring the success of the sophisticated and expensive treatment options also have significant economic impacts to the health system.

Obviously, in addition to analytical factors, biological variables must also be taken into account when interpreting GH concentrations measured during the biochemical workup of suspected acromegaly. As an example, it has been proposed to adjust GH cut-offs for OGTT for sex and BMI to increase sensitivity of the test in the detection of acromegaly [72, 73]. Furthermore, the presence of renal failure can make the exclusion of acromegaly challenging: In these patients, high baseline GH levels are observed due to GH resistance – including an increase in the 20KD GH isoform [74]. The reduction in GH levels following oral glucose load might also be compromised. Although the literature is scarce, a case report on the exclusion of acromegaly in a patient with renal failure suggested that diagnosis must be made following dialysis: Baseline GH levels were lower compared to the situation before dialysis, and GH suppression during OGTT was normal [74].

GH deficiency

Also in the diagnosis of GH deficiency biological variables like body mass index (BMI) can be important. Stimulation of GH by the insulin tolerance test might be affected only if BMI is greater than 35 kg/m^2, but response to GHRH + arginine test generally has to be evaluated with cut-offs adjusted to BMI. Some authors advocate reducing the cut-off when the glucagon test is used in overweight/obese adults [69, 75]. Age and the stimulus used should also be considered as factors interfering with test interpretation [76, 77]. However, besides these interfering biological factors, it is important to recognize that different GH assays can reveal different GH concentrations in the same sample. Therefore, cut-offs need to be adjusted in an assay specific manner. Lower cut-off values are expected with the current recommended IS 98/574 when compared with the IS 80/505 [78], reflecting differences in isoform composition of the calibrators. Wagner et al. [76] analyzed samples from several stimulation tests in short children with and without GHD by distinct GH assays and proposed different cut-off values depending on the GH assay used. Such assay specific data are required for each GH assay used to allow an unbiased interpretation of the stimulation test outcome (Table 2). Using "general" cut-offs frequently quoted in guidelines with no reference for a specific assay is associated with the risk of misinterpretation, potentially leading to over- or under treatment.

Conclusion

GH is a complex and heterogeneous mixture of molecular isoforms and not a single, homogenous molecule. Although 22 K-GH is the main isoform in circulation, there are other GH isoforms that can represent approximately 10–20% of GH under physiological conditions.

Table 2 Cut-off limits derived from the same cohort of short children with different GH assays (adapted from reference [76])

Assay	Cut off limit (ng/mL)
Immulite 2000 (Siemens)	7.77
AutoDELFIA (Perkin-Elmer)	7.44
iSYS (IDS)	7.09
Liaison (DIASorin)	6.25
RIA (in-house Tübingen)	5.28
DxI (Beckmann-Coulter)	5.15
ELISA (Mediagnost)	5.14
BC-IRMA (Beckmann-Coulter)	4.32

Usually, GH isoforms are secreted in parallel in response to various stimuli, with changes in 22 K-GH mirroring changes in all isoforms. Some studies have reported minor changes in the non-22 K/22 K-GH and 22 K/20 K-GH ratio under certain conditions, mostly with elevated abundance of the non-22 K isoforms. Such variation might be due to differences in the half-life of the isoforms, but might also be related to limitations in current assay methods to accurately quantify the various isoforms over a wide concentration range. More studies are needed to better understand why some diseases including pituitary adenomas might lead to changes in the isoform ratios, and to evaluate if changes in isoforms might be of clinical relevance. More importantly in clinical routine, the existence of GH isoforms represents one of the main reasons for discrepancies in GH concentrations measured by different common GH assays. Efforts to harmonize GH assays are under way but it remains important for the clinician to understand the potential impact of the specific GH assay used on the GH concentrations reported. Clinical decision limits and cut-off values not only must be adapted to biological variables, but also to the specific GH assay used by the local laboratory.

Funding
CNPq and FAPEMIG: AROJr, CAPES: JROLS.

Authors' contributions
The first author wrote the manuscript, and the second and third authors contributed in reviewing and editing the manuscript. All authors read and approved the final manuscript.

Competing interests
The authors declare that they have no competing interests.

Author details
[1]Endocrinology Laboratory of Federal University of Minas Gerais. Alfredo Balena, 190, Santa Efigênia, Belo Horizonte 30130-100, Brazil. [2]Endocrine Laboratory, Medizinische Klinik und Poliklinik IV, Klinikum der Universität München, Ziemssenstraße 1, 80336 Munich, Germany.

References

1. Clemmons DR. Consensus statement on the standardization and evaluation of growth hormone and insulin-like growth factor assays. Clin Chem. 2011;57:555–9.
2. Wieringa GE, Sturgeon CM, Trainer PJ. The harmonisation of growth hormone measurements: taking the next steps. Clin Chim Acta. 2014;432:68–71.
3. Bidlingmaier M, Freda PU. Measurement of human growth hormone by immunoassays: current status, unsolved problems and clinical consequences. Growth Hormon IGF Res. 2010;20:19–25.
4. Popii V, Baumann G. Laboratory measurement of growth hormone. Clin Chim Acta. 2004;350:1–16.
5. Chen EY, Liao YC, Smith DH, Barrera-Saldana HA, Gelinas RE, Seeburg PH. The human growth hormone locus: nucleotide sequence, biology, and evolution. Genomics. 1989;4:479–97.
6. Ho Y, Liebhaber SA, Cooke NE. Activation of the human GH gene cluster: roles for targeted chromatin modification. Trends Endocrinol Metab. 2004;15:40–5.
7. Lecomte CM, Renard A, Martial JA. A new natural hGH variant–17.5 kd–produced by alternative splicing. An additional consensus sequence which might play a role in branchpoint selection. Nucleic Acids Res. 1987;15:6331–48.
8. Lewis UJ, Singh RN, Bonewald LF, Seavey BK. Altered proteolytic cleavage of human growth hormone as a result of deamidation. J Biol Chem. 1981;256:11645–50.
9. Bustamante JJ, Gonzalez L, Carroll CA, Weintraub ST, Aguilar RM, Munoz J, Martinez AO, Haro LS. O-Glycosylated 24 kDa human growth hormone has a mucin-like biantennary disialylated tetrasaccharide attached at Thr-60. Proteomics. 2009;9:3474–88.
10. Baumann GP. Growth hormone isoforms. Growth Hormon IGF Res. 2009;19:333–40.
11. Wada M, Ikeda M, Takahashi Y, Asada N, Chang KT, Takahashi M, Honjo M. The full agonistic effect of recombinant 20 kDa human growth hormone (hGH) on CHO cells stably transfected with hGH receptor cDNA. Mol Cell Endocrinol. 1997;133:99–107.
12. Tsunekawa B, Wada M, Ikeda M, Uchida H, Naito N, Honjo M. The 20-kilodalton (kDa) human growth hormone (hGH) differs from the 22-kDa hGH in the effect on the human prolactin receptor. Endocrinology. 1999;140:3909–18.
13. Solomon G, Reicher S, Gussakovsky EE, Jomain JB, Gertler A. Large-scale preparation and in vitro characterization of biologically active human placental (20 and 22K) and pituitary (20K) growth hormones: placental growth hormones have no lactogenic activity in humans. Growth Hormon IGF Res. 2006;16:297–307.
14. Wada M, Uchida H, Ikeda M, Tsunekawa B, Naito N, Banba S, Tanaka E, Hashimoto Y, Honjo M. The 20-kilodalton (kDa) human growth hormone (hGH) differs from the 22-kDa hGH in the complex formation with cell surface hGH receptor and hGH-binding protein circulating in human plasma. Mol Endocrinol. 1998;12:146–56.
15. Ishikawa M, Tachibana T, Kamioka T, Horikawa R, Katsumata N, Tanaka T. Comparison of the somatogenic action of 20 kDa- and 22 kDa-human growth hormones in spontaneous dwarf rats. Growth Hormon IGF Res. 2000;10:199–206.
16. Satozawa N, Takezawa K, Miwa T, Takahashi S, Hayakawa M, Ooka H. Differences in the effects of 20 K- and 22 K-hGH on water retention in rats. Growth Hormon IGF Res. 2000;10:187–92.
17. Ishikawa M, Yokoya S, Tachibana K, Hasegawa Y, Yasuda T, Tokuhiro E, Hashimoto Y, Tanaka T. Serum levels of 20-kilodalton human growth hormone (GH) are parallel those of 22-kilodalton human GH in normal and short children. J Clin Endocrinol Metab. 1999;84:98–104.
18. Yao-Xia L, Jing-Yan C, Xia-Lian T, Ping C, Min Z. The 20kDa and 22kDa forms of human growth hormone (hGH) exhibit different intracellular signalling profiles and properties. Gen Comp Endocrinol. 2017;248:49–54.
19. De Palo EF, De Filippis V, Gatti R, Spinella P. Growth hormone isoforms and segments/fragments: molecular structure and laboratory measurement. Clin Chim Acta. 2006;364:67–76.
20. Such-Sanmartin G, Bosch J, Segura J, Wu M, Du H, Chen G, Wang S, Vila-Perello M, Andreu D, Gutierrez-Gallego R. Characterisation of the 5 kDa growth hormone isoform. Growth Factors. 2008;26:152–62.
21. Miletta MC, Lochmatter D, Pektovic V, Mullis PE. Isolated growth hormone deficiency type 2: from gene to therapy. Endocr Dev. 2012;23:109–20.
22. Hettiarachchi M, Watkinson A, Leung KC, Sinha YN, Ho KK, Kraegen EW. Human growth hormone fragment (hGH44-91) produces insulin resistance and hyperinsulinemia but is less potent than 22 kDa hGH in the rat. Endocrine. 1997;6:47–52.
23. Sinha YN, Jacobsen BP. Human growth hormone (hGH)-(44-191), a reportedly diabetogenic fragment of hGH, circulates in human blood: measurement by radioimmunoassay. J Clin Endocrinol Metab. 1994;78:1411–8.
24. Sinha YN, Jacobsen BP, Lewis UJ. Antibodies to newly recognized murine 13-18 KDa pituitary peptides crossreact with growth hormone and prolactin from several species, including man. Biochem Biophys Res Commun. 1989;163:386–93.
25. Pradhananga S, Wilkinson I, Ross RJ. Pegvisomant: structure and function. J Mol Endocrinol. 2002;29:11–4.
26. Kopchick JJ. Discovery and mechanism of action of pegvisomant. Eur J Endocrinol. 2003;148(Suppl 2):S21–5.
27. Kopchick JJ, Parkinson C, Stevens EC, Trainer PJ. Growth hormone receptor antagonists: discovery, development, and use in patients with acromegaly. Endocr Rev. 2002;23:623–46.
28. Ng FM, Jiang WJ, Gianello R, Pitt S, Roupas P. Molecular and cellular actions of a structural domain of human growth hormone (AOD9401) on lipid metabolism in Zucker fatty rats. J Mol Endocrinol. 2000;25:287–98.
29. Heffernan MA, Jiang WJ, Thorburn AW, Ng FM. Effects of oral administration of a synthetic fragment of human growth hormone on lipid metabolism. Am J Physiol Endocrinol Metab. 2000;279:E501–7.
30. Bustamante JJ, Grigorian AL, Munoz J, Aguilar RM, Trevino LR, Martinez AO, Haro LS. Human growth hormone: 45-kDa isoform with extraordinarily stable interchain disulfide links has attenuated receptor-binding and cell-proliferative activities. Growth Hormon IGF Res. 2010;20:298–304.
31. Boguszewski CL, Svensson PA, Jansson T, Clark R, Carlsson LM, Carlsson B. Cloning of two novel growth hormone transcripts expressed in human placenta. J Clin Endocrinol Metab. 1998;83:2878–85.
32. Vickers MH, Gilmour S, Gertler A, Breier BH, Tunny K, Waters MJ, Gluckman PD. 20-kDa placental hGH-V has diminished diabetogenic and lactogenic activities compared with 22-kDa hGH-N while retaining antilipogenic activity. Am J Physiol Endocrinol Metab. 2009;297:E629–37.
33. Surya S, Symons K, Rothman E, Barkan AL. Complex rhythmicity of growth hormone secretion in humans. Pituitary. 2006;9:121–5.
34. Ribeiro-Oliveira A Jr, Abrantes MM, Barkan AL. Complex rhythmicity and age dependence of growth hormone secretion are preserved in patients with acromegaly: further evidence for a present hypothalamic control of pituitary somatotropinomas. J Clin Endocrinol Metab. 2013;98:2959–66.
35. Tsushima T, Katoh Y, Miyachi Y, Chihara K, Teramoto A, Irie M, Hashimoto Y. Serum concentrations of 20K human growth hormone in normal adults and patients with various endocrine disorders. Study Group of 20K hGH. Endocr J. 2000;47(Suppl):S17–21.
36. Leung KC, Howe C, Gui LY, Trout G, Veldhuis JD, Ho KK. Physiological and pharmacological regulation of 20-kDa growth hormone. Am J Physiol Endocrinol Metab. 2002;283:E836–43.
37. Baumann G, Stolar MW, Buchanan TA. Slow metabolic clearance rate of the 20,000-Dalton variant of human growth hormone: implications for biological activity. Endocrinology. 1985;117:1309–13.
38. Nindl BC, Kraemer WJ, Marx JO, Tuckow AP, Hymer WC. Growth hormone molecular heterogeneity and exercise. Exerc Sport Sci Rev. 2003;31:161–6.
39. Tuckow AP, Rarick KR, Kraemer WJ, Marx JO, Hymer WC, Nindl BC. Nocturnal growth hormone secretory dynamics are altered after resistance exercise: deconvolution analysis of 12-hour immunofunctional and immunoreactive isoforms. Am J Physiol Regul Integr Comp Physiol. 2006;291:R1749–55.
40. Wallace JD, Cuneo RC, Bidlingmaier M, Lundberg PA, Carlsson L, Boguszewski CL, Hay J, Healy ML, Napoli R, Dall R, Rosen T, Strasburger CJ. The response of molecular isoforms of growth hormone to acute exercise in trained adult males. J Clin Endocrinol Metab. 2001;86:200–6.
41. Pagani S, Cappa M, Meazza C, Ubertini G, Travaglino P, Bozzola E, Bozzola M. Growth hormone isoforms release in response to physiological and pharmacological stimuli. J Endocrinol Investig. 2008;31:520–4.
42. Kraemer WJ, Nindl BC, Marx JO, Gotshalk LA, Bush JA, Welsch JR, Volek JS, Spiering BA, Maresh CM, Mastro AM, Hymer WC. Chronic resistance training in women potentiates growth hormone in vivo bioactivity: characterization of molecular mass variants. Am J Physiol Endocrinol Metab. 2006;291:E1177–87.
43. Pierce JR, Tuckow AP, Alemany JA, Rarick KR, Staab JS, Harman EA, Nindl BC. Effects of acute and chronic exercise on disulfide-linked growth hormone variants. Med Sci Sports Exerc. 2009;41:581–7.
44. Hymer WC, Kraemer WJ, Nindl BC, Marx JO, Benson DE, Welsch JR, Mazzetti SA, Volek JS, Deaver DR. Characteristics of circulating growth hormone in women after acute heavy resistance exercise. Am J Physiol Endocrinol Metab. 2001;281:E878–87.

45. Kraemer WJ, Rubin MR, Hakkinen K, Nindl BC, Marx JO, Volek JS, French DN, Gomez AL, Sharman MJ, Scheett T, Ratamess NA, Miles MP, Mastro A, VanHeest J, Maresh CM, Welsch JR, Hymer WC. Influence of muscle strength and total work on exercise-induced plasma growth hormone isoforms in women. J Sci Med Sport. 2003;6:295–306.

46. Kraemer WJ, Nindl BC, Volek JS, Marx JO, Gotshalk LA, Bush JA, Welsch JR, Vingren JL, Spiering BA, Fragala MS, Hatfield DL, Ho JY, Maresh CM, Mastro AM, Hymer WC. Influence of oral contraceptive use on growth hormone in vivo bioactivity following resistance exercise: responses of molecular mass variants. Growth Hormon IGF Res. 2008;18:238–44.

47. Nelson AE, Ho KK. Abuse of growth hormone by athletes. Nat Clin Pract Endocrinol Metab. 2007;3:198–9.

48. Hashimoto Y, Kamioka T, Hosaka M, Mabuchi K, Mizuchi A, Shimazaki Y, Tsunoo M, Tanaka T. Exogenous 20K growth hormone (GH) suppresses endogenous 22K GH secretion in normal men. J Clin Endocrinol Metab. 2000;85:601–6.

49. Wallace JD, Cuneo RC, Bidlingmaier M, Lundberg PA, Carlsson L, Boguszewski CL, Hay J, Boroujerdi M, Cittadini A, Dall R, Rosen T, Strasburger CJ. Changes in non-22-kilodalton (kDa) isoforms of growth hormone (GH) after administration of 22-kDa recombinant human GH in trained adult males. J Clin Endocrinol Metab. 2001;86:1731–7.

50. Keller A, Wu Z, Kratzsch J, Keller E, Blum WF, Kniess A, Preiss R, Teichert J, Strasburger CJ, Bidlingmaier M. Pharmacokinetics and pharmacodynamics of GH: dependence on route and dosage of administration. Eur J Endocrinol. 2007;156:647–53.

51. Baumann GP. Growth hormone doping in sports: a critical review of use and detection strategies. Endocr Rev. 2012;33:155–86.

52. Bidlingmaier M, Suhr J, Ernst A, Wu Z, Keller A, Strasburger CJ, Bergmann A. High-sensitivity chemiluminescence immunoassays for detection of growth hormone doping in sports. Clin Chem. 2009;55:445–53.

53. Boguszewski CL, Johannsson G, Bengtsson BA, Johansson A, Carlsson B, Carlsson LM. Circulating non-22-kilodalton growth hormone isoforms in acromegalic men before and after transsphenoidal surgery. J Clin Endocrinol Metab. 1997;82:1516–21.

54. Tsushima T, Katoh Y, Miyachi Y, Chihara K, Teramoto A, Irie M, Hashimoto Y. Serum concentration of 20K human growth hormone (20K hGH) measured by a specific enzyme-linked immunosorbent assay. Study group of 20K hGH. J Clin Endocrinol Metab. 1999;84:317–22.

55. Murakami Y, Shimizu T, Yamamoto M, Kato Y. Serum levels of 20 kilodalton human growth hormone (20K-hGH) in patients with acromegaly before and after treatment with octreotide and transsphenoidal surgery. Endocr J. 2004;51:343–8.

56. Lima GA, Wu Z, Silva CM, Barbosa FR, Dias JS, Schrank Y, Strasburger CJ, Gadelha MR. Growth hormone isoforms in acromegalic patients before and after treatment with octreotide LAR. Growth Hormon IGF Res. 2010;20:87–92.

57. Coya R, Algorta J, Boguszewski CL, Vela A, Carlsson LM, Aniel-Quiroga A, Busturia MA, Martul P. Circulating non-22 kDa growth hormone isoforms after a repeated GHRH stimulus in normal subjects. Growth Hormon IGF Res. 2005;15:123–9.

58. Rigamonti AE, Grugni G, Marazzi N, Bini S, Bidlingmaier M, Sartorio A. Unaltered ratio of circulating levels of growth hormone/GH isoforms in adults with Prader-Willi syndrome after GHRH plus arginine administration. Growth Hormon IGF Res. 2015;25:168–73.

59. Rigamonti AE, Crino A, Bocchini S, Convertino A, Bidlingmaier M, Haenelt M, Tamini S, Cella SG, Grugni G, Sartorio A. GHRH plus arginine and arginine administration evokes the same ratio of GH isoforms levels in young patients with Prader-Willi syndrome. Growth Horm IGF Res. 2017;

60. Katsumata N, Shimatsu A, Tachibana K, Hizuka N, Horikawa R, Yokoya S, Tatsumi KI, Mochizuki T, Anzo M, Tanaka T. Continuing efforts to standardize measured serum growth hormone values in Japan. Endocr J. 2016;63:933–6.

61. Kanakis GA, Chrisoulidou A, Bargiota A, Efstathiadou ZA, Papanastasiou L, Theodoropoulou A, Tigas SK, Vassiliadi DA, Tsagarakis S, Alevizaki M. The ongoing challenge of discrepant growth hormone and insulin-like growth factor I results in the evaluation of treated acromegalic patients: a systematic review and meta-analysis. Clin Endocrinol. 2016;85:681–8.

62. Casagrande A, Bronstein MD, Jallad RS, Moraes AB, Elias PC, Castro M, Czepielewski MA, Boschi A, Ribeiro-Oliveira A Jr, Schweizer JR, Vilar L, Nazato DM, Gadelha MR, Abucham J. All other investigators of the s. Long-term remission of acromegaly after octreotide withdrawal is an uncommon and frequently unsustainable event. Neuroendocrinology. 2017;104:273–9.

63. Ribeiro-Oliveira A Jr, Barkan A. The changing face of acromegaly--advances in diagnosis and treatment. Nat Rev Endocrinol. 2012;8:605–11.

64. Ribeiro-Oliveira A Jr, Faje A, Barkan A. Postglucose growth hormone nadir and insulin-like growth factor-1 in naive-active acromegalic patients: do these parameters always correlate? Arq Bras Endocrinol Metabol. 2011;55:494–7.

65. Ribeiro-Oliveira A Jr, Faje AT, Barkan AL. Limited utility of oral glucose tolerance test in biochemically active acromegaly. Eur J Endocrinol. 2011;164:17–22.

66. Abreu A, Tovar AP, Castellanos R, Valenzuela A, Giraldo CM, Pinedo AC, Guerrero DP, Barrera CA, Franco HI, Ribeiro-Oliveira A Jr, Vilar L, Jallad RS, Duarte FG, Gadelha M, Boguszewski CL, Abucham J, Naves LA, Musolino NR, de Faria ME, Rossato C, Bronstein MD. Challenges in the diagnosis and management of acromegaly: a focus on comorbidities. Pituitary. 2016;19:448–57.

67. Giustina A, Barkan A, Casanueva FF, Cavagnini F, Frohman L, Ho K, Veldhuis J, Wass J, Von Werder K, Melmed S. Criteria for cure of acromegaly: a consensus statement. J Clin Endocrinol Metab. 2000;85:526–9.

68. Katznelson L, Laws ER Jr, Melmed S, Molitch ME, Murad MH, Utz A, Wass JA, Endocrine S. Acromegaly: an endocrine society clinical practice guideline. J Clin Endocrinol Metab. 2014;99:3933–51.

69. Yuen KC, Tritos NA, Samson SL, Hoffman AR, Katznelson L. American Association of Clinical Endocrinologists and American College of endocrinology disease state clinical review: update on growth hormone stimulation testing and proposed revised cut-point for the glucagon stimulation test in the diagnosis of adult growth hormone deficiency. Endocr Pract. 2016;22:1235–44.

70. Freda PU, Nuruzzaman AT, Reyes CM, Sundeen RE, Post KD. Significance of "abnormal" nadir growth hormone levels after oral glucose in postoperative patients with acromegaly in remission with normal insulin-like growth factor-I levels. J Clin Endocrinol Metab. 2004;89:495–500.

71. Pokrajac A, Wark G, Ellis AR, Wear J, Wieringa GE, Trainer PJ. Variation in GH and IGF-I assays limits the applicability of international consensus criteria to local practice. Clin Endocrinol. 2007;67:65–70.

72. Endert E, van Rooden M, Fliers E, Prummel MF, Wiersinga WM. Establishment of reference values for endocrine tests--part V: acromegaly. Neth J Med. 2006;64:230–5.

73. Schilbach K, Strasburger CJ, Bidlingmaier M. Biochemical investigations in diagnosis and follow up of acromegaly. Pituitary. 2017;20:33–45.

74. Pena-Porta JM, Burgase-Estallo I, Nicolas-Sanchez F, Vicente-de Vera Floristan C. Chronic kidney disease and acromegaly: when appearances are deceptive. Nefrologia. 2014;34:800–2.

75. Feldt-Rasmussen U, Klose M. Adult Growth Hormone Deficiency Clinical Management. In: De Groot LJ, Chrousos G, Dungan K, Feingold KR, Grossman A, Hershman JM, Koch C, Korbonits M, Mc Lachlan R, New M, Purnell J, Rebar R, Singer F, Vinik A, editors. Endotext. South Dartmouth; 2000.

76. Wagner IV, Paetzold C, Gausche R, Vogel M, Koerner A, Thiery J, Arsene CG, Henrion A, Guettler B, Keller E, Kiess W, Pfaeffle R, Kratzsch J. Clinical evidence-based cutoff limits for GH stimulation tests in children with a backup of results with reference to mass spectrometry. Eur J Endocrinol. 2014;171:389–97.

77. Chinoy A, Murray PG. Diagnosis of growth hormone deficiency in the paediatric and transitional age. Best Pract Res Clin Endocrinol Metab. 2016;30:737–47.

78. Chaler EA, Ballerini G, Lazzati JM, Maceiras M, Frusti M, Bergada I, Rivarola MA, Belgorosky A, Ropelato G. Cut-off values of serum growth hormone (GH) in pharmacological stimulation tests (PhT) evaluated in short-statured children using a chemiluminescent immunometric assay (ICMA) calibrated with the international recombinant human GH standard 98/574. Clin Chem Lab Med. 2013;51:e95–7.

24

Characteristics of insulin-Naïve people with type 2 diabetes who successfully respond to insulin glargine U100 after 24 weeks of treatment

M. H. Cummings[1], D. Cao[2], I. Hadjiyianni[3], L. L. Ilag[2*] [ID] and M. H. Tan[4]

Abstract

Background: To identify baseline/clinical characteristics associated with clinically meaningful responses to insulin glargine 100 U/mL (IGlar) in insulin-naive people with type 2 diabetes mellitus (T2DM).

Methods: Individual participant data were pooled from 3 randomized trials to compare baseline characteristics and clinical outcomes associated with 24-week response to IGlar in combination with non-insulin antihyperglycemic agents in participants with T2DM. Responders were defined as achieving endpoint HbA1c target < 53 mmol/mol (< 7%) and/or ≥ 11 mmol/mol (≥ 1%) HbA1c reduction from baseline.

Results: Differences in baseline characteristics for responders versus nonresponders were higher HbA1c (99 vs 91 mmol/mol [9.1 vs 8.3%]; $P < 0.001$), higher fasting blood glucose (FBG; 10.4 vs 8.8 mmol/L [187 vs 159 mg/dL; $P < 0.001$), and fewer participants (94% vs 98%; $P = 0.006$) taking oral medications targeting postprandial blood glucose (BG). Most participants (80%) achieved one or both components of composite endpoint. 12-week response was a strong predictor of subsequent 24-week response (sensitivity, 85.9%; predictive positive value, 91.4%). At both 12 and 24 weeks, < 40% of responders and nonresponders reached target FBG ≤ 5.6 mmol/L (≤ 100 mg/dL). Responders at 24 weeks had higher incidence of hypoglycemia (total, 82.5% vs 70.4%; $P < 0.001$; nocturnal, 60.3% vs 50.5%; $P = 0.002$; documented symptomatic, 65.8% vs 55.6%; $P < 0.001$) than nonresponders.

Conclusions: Baseline characteristics associated with response were identified. The strong predictability of 12-week response suggests that the magnitude of early HbA1c reduction should be considered when assessing response to IGlar. More aggressive IGlar titration may be reasonable for nonresponders and responders who have not reached FBG and HbA1c targets, taking into account other BG timepoints.

Keywords: Type 2 diabetes, Insulin glargine, Insulin naïve, Responders, HbA1c composite endpoint, Baseline characteristics

* Correspondence: ilag_liza_l@lilly.com
[2]Eli Lilly and Company, Indianapolis, IN, USA
Full list of author information is available at the end of the article

Background

Dual or triple therapy with insulin (usually a basal insulin) in combination with metformin or other noninsulin antihyperglycemic medication is recommended for people with type 2 diabetes mellitus (T2DM) who do not attain glycemic target on noninsulin antihyperglycemic medications alone [1]. For people with newly diagnosed T2DM who are symptomatic and/or have highly elevated levels of glycated hemoglobin (HbA1c) ($\geq$ 86 mmol/mol [$\geq$ 10%]) and/or blood glucose (BG) ($\geq$ 16.7 mmol/L [$\geq$ 300 mg/dL]), basal-bolus insulin (preferred if symptomatic) or basal insulin plus a glucagon-like peptide-1 receptor agonist (GLP1-RA) should be considered for initial treatment [1]. Insulin glargine 100 units/mL (IGlar) was the first basal insulin analogue, which provided almost 24-h glycemic control with once-daily injection and lower risk for nocturnal hypoglycemia compared with human neutral protamine Hagedorn insulin, while having similar efficacy in terms of number of participants reaching HbA1c targets [2–6]. IGlar has since become a benchmark for the development of novel basal insulin analogues [7]. These newer marketed basal insulins, insulin degludec and insulin glargine 300 units/mL, are non-inferior to IGlar in terms of efficacy and in certain subpopulations may provide some advantages over IGlar, such as reduced nocturnal hypoglycemia, as shown in some insulin degludec 100 units/mL studies [8–10] and in insulin glargine 300 units/mL studies of participants already receiving high-dose basal insulin [11, 12]. IGlar, however, remains an important option for the management of T2DM.

In recent years, guidelines and position statements recommend that the choice of pharmacologic agents are to be guided by a patient-centered approach that considers factors like efficacy, hypoglycemia risk, and impact on weight. Even though this method allows for individualization of treatment based on several clinical and social factors, it has become increasingly challenging for healthcare providers to select from a plethora of antihyperglycemic classes and furthermore from different products within each class. Moreover, and specifically for basal insulin, recent literature emphasized the importance of proper titration before treatment intensification [13–15]. Anticipating treatment failures (e.g., minimal improvements, frequent and/or severe hypoglycemia) and establishing realistic expectations of treatment with individuals are important in clinical practice. To reach such decisions, it would be helpful to understand the characteristics of people with T2DM who do or do not respond to a common starter insulin, IGlar.

A few studies have investigated clinical characteristics of people with diabetes on IGlar achieving a target HbA1c of 53 mmol/mol (7%) [13–16]. These studies showed that only a few baseline characteristics were consistently associated with reaching target: lower HbA1c at baseline and shorter duration of diabetes [14, 16]. Furthermore, it was shown that as baseline HbA1c increased, so did mean reduction in HbA1c from baseline; however, progressively fewer participants achieved target HbA1c at study endpoint with every 1% increase in baseline HbA1c. Therefore, these studies were focused mainly on whether patients reached target or not, with no particular attention to patients who may have experienced clinically significant reductions in HbA1c (albeit short of reaching the HbA1c of 7%).

Recent analyses have shown that a composite HbA1c measured by a decrease from baseline in HbA1c of $\geq$ 11 mmol/mol ($\geq$ 1%) and/or achievement of HbA1c target < 53 mmol/mol (< 7%) identifies more patients with clinically meaningful responses to insulin therapy than attainment of target HbA1c alone [17, 18]. Indeed, it has been shown that a decrease in the HbA1c value of $\geq$11 mmol/mol ($\geq$1%) may confer clinical benefit, as demonstrated by the UK Prospective Diabetes Study: every 11 mmol/mol (1%) reduction in mean HbA1c level was associated with reductions of 21% for any diabetes-related endpoint, 21% for diabetes-related deaths, 14% for myocardial infarctions, and 37% for microvascular complications [19].

This current post hoc analysis was conducted using an integrated database of prospective clinical studies of once-daily IGlar treatment among insulin-naïve people with T2DM. The aims of this analysis were two-fold: 1) to identify factors/characteristics of responders to once-daily IGlar at 24 weeks, and 2) to assess the sensitivity and specificity of this composite HbA1c response measure at 12 weeks in predicting response at 24 weeks. Response was defined as a composite endpoint: achieving HbA1c < 53 mmol/mol (< 7%) and/or a $\geq$ 11 mmol/mol ($\geq$ 1%) reduction in HbA1c from baseline. This definition of response has been previously studied [17, 18], and therefore was selected for this analysis based on previous findings and its practical application in the real-world setting.

Methods

Integrated database

Individual participant data from 2 randomized clinical trials sponsored by Eli Lilly and Company [20, 21] and 1 randomized trial sponsored by Eli Lilly and Company and Boehringer Ingelheim [22] were used for meta-analyses. These studies were identified by an exhaustive search of Eli Lilly and Company's integrated clinical trial database based on the following inclusion criteria: 1) participants were insulin-naïve with T2DM, 2) a sufficient number of participants received IGlar (Basaglar®/Abasaglar®, Boehringer Ingelheim and Eli Lilly and Company, or Lantus®, Sanofi-Aventis) for at least 24 weeks, and 3) IGlar was the only insulin component in the antihyperglycemic treatment.

Buse et al. [20] compared the efficacy and safety of twice-daily (BID) insulin lispro mixture 75/25 and once-daily (QD) IGlar in a randomized, open-label, 24-week, non-inferiority trial conducted in 11 countries (Argentina, Australia, Brazil, Canada, Greece, Hungary, India, the Netherlands, Romania, Spain, and the United States). Eligible participants were insulin-naïve adults ≥ 18 years of age with T2DM and taking ≥ 2 oral antihyperglycemic medications (OAMs). Jain et al. [21] compared the efficacy and safety of 2 progressive insulin regimens, QD insulin glargine plus insulin lispro administered up to 3 times daily (TID) versus insulin lispro mixture 50/50 administered up to TID, in a randomized, open-label, 36-week, non-inferiority trial conducted in 9 countries (Australia, Canada, France, Greece, India, Republic of Korea, Mexico, Russian Federation, and Spain). Eligible participants were insulin-naïve adults ≥ 18 years of age with T2DM and taking ≥ 2 OAMs. Rosenstock et al. [22] compared the efficacy and safety of 2 IGlar products, LY IGlar versus Lantus®, in a phase 3, randomized, double-blind, 24-week, non-inferiority trial conducted in 11 countries (Czech Republic, France, Germany, Greece, Hungary, Italy, South Korea, Mexico, Poland, Spain, and the United States). Eligible participants were adults ≥ 18 years of age with T2DM who were either insulin-naïve or previously on Lantus® and taking ≥ 2 OAMs.

In each of these trials [20–22], postprandial glucose (PPG) was collected through 7-Point self-monitored blood glucose (SMBG) at weeks 0, 12, and 24 on 3 separate days in the 2-week period prior to each visit. Participants were also given a diary to record hypoglycemia events experienced throughout each study. For each hypoglycemia episode, the participant was asked to record the glucose value, if measured, and to describe the treatment, including if the participant was able to self-treat, and the outcome of the episode. At the onsite visit, the investigator reviewed the diary with the participant to verify and assess any need for treatment adjustment. Further study design details and key outcomes from each trial are summarized in Additional files 1 and 2, respectively.

Statistical analysis

Participants with non-missing HbA1c at 24 weeks were analyzed and classified into 2 responder cohorts (yes vs no) according to the composite HbA1c responder measure: HbA1c < 53 mmol/mol (< 7%) at 24 weeks or reduction in HbA1c from baseline to 24 weeks ≥ 11 mmol/mol (≥ 1%). Responders were the participants who either had HbA1c < 53 mmol/mol (< 7%) or had HbA1c reduction ≥ 11 mmol/mol (≥ 1%) at 24 weeks. Nonresponders did not meet either criterion. For the 3 SMBG profiles obtained at 0, 12, and 24 weeks, the average SMBG value was used for analysis. Missing data at week 24 was expected due to the self-monitoring nature of

SMBG and the attrition throughout the trials. Overall, about 60% of participants had non-missing PPG data at week 24. More specifically, among the 1485 patients who had non-missing HbA1c values at 24 weeks, 826 participants had non-missing glucose values post-breakfast and post-midday meal and 829 participants had non-missing post-dinner glucose at week 24. This was considered adequate for analysis with the majority of participants contributing data and a total sample size of > 800.

Heterogeneity across the studies was assessed by study-by-responder interaction. P values for interaction were nonsignificant for the majority of outcomes measured indicating that results in these trials were relatively homogeneous and therefore justified the integration of these data. In 2 of the 3 studies analysed [20, 22], responders had greater reductions in fasting blood glucose (FBG) than nonresponders, while in the 3rd study [21], the 2 cohorts had similar reductions in FBG, thereby resulting in a statistically significant ($P = 0.012$) study-by-responder interaction (Additional file 2). Baseline participant characteristics and clinical profiles at 24 weeks (HbA1c, FBG, PPG, insulin dose, and hypoglycemia categories [total hypoglycemia (BG ≤ 3.9 mmol/L [≤ 70 mg/dL] or signs/symptoms), documented symptomatic (BG ≤ 3.9 mmol/L [≤ 70 mg/dL] and signs/symptoms), nocturnal (between bedtime and waking), and severe (required 3rd party assistance) were compared between the responder cohorts. A 2-sided P value of < 0.05 was considered statistically significant, with P values based on the Pearson's Chi-square test for categorical variables and fixed effects meta-regression model for continuous variables. Results presented are model-adjusted mean and standard error (SE). Relationships between improvements in glycemic outcomes as continuous variables (FBG, daily mean PPG, and HbA1c) and baseline variables (HbA1c, FBG), between improvements in glycemic outcomes as continuous variables (FBG, daily mean PPG, and HbA1c) and insulin dose, and between hypoglycemic rate and insulin dose, were explored graphically using scatter plots as post hoc analyses.

Sensitivity, specificity, positive predictive value, and negative predictive value were evaluated to assess if early response at 12 weeks could predict subsequent response at 24 weeks to support current guidelines that recommend evaluation of therapeutic response to pharmacologic interventions at 12 weeks after initiating therapy.

All analyses were performed using SAS Version 9.2® or higher.

Results
Composite versus single HbA1c measure

The majority (80%) of participants achieved a meaningful clinical reduction in HbA1c at 24 weeks, as defined by the composite endpoint of attainment of target

HbA1c < 53 mmol/mol (< 7%) and/or a ≥ 11 mmol/mol (≥ 1%) decrease in HbA1c from baseline (Table 1). Of those participants who responded to treatment, 50% achieved both components of the composite HbA1c endpoint, while 43% only experienced a ≥ 11 mmol/mol (≥1%) decrease in HbA1c and 7% only reached target HbA1c < 53 mmol/mol (< 7%). The composite HbA1c endpoint identified 34% more responders than would have been found by the single HbA1c endpoint, achievement of target HbA1c < 53 mmol/mol (< 7%), commonly used in diabetes clinical studies.

Baseline characteristics of responders and nonresponders

The baseline characteristics of responders ($N = 1188$) and nonresponders ($N = 297$) at 24 weeks were generally similar; however, there were some notable differences (Table 2). More men than women (54 vs 46%; $P = 0.012$) responded to treatment. Responders also had higher baseline HbA1c levels (mean, 9.1 vs 8.3% [99 vs 91 mmol/mol]; $P < 0.001$), higher FBG levels (10.4 vs 8.8 mmol/L [187 vs 159 mg/dL; $P < 0.001$), and had fewer participants (94 vs 98%; $P = 0.006$) who used OAMs targeting PPG than nonresponders. Overall, both responders and nonresponders at 24 weeks had a baseline mean duration of T2DM of 10 years and were generally Caucasian (71 vs 58%), less than 65 years of age (75 vs 76%), and overweight or obese (mean body mass index [BMI] for both, 31 kg/m^2) at baseline.

Glycemic response and insulin dose

Early response at 12 weeks was a strong predictor of subsequent response at 24 weeks as shown by the high sensitivity (85.9%) and predictive positive value (91.4%) (Table 3). Responders at 24 weeks had significantly greater reductions from baseline in adjusted mean (SE) HbA1c (– 2.2% [0.04] vs – 0.8% [0.06]; – 24 [0.44] vs – 9 [0.66] mmol/mol; $P < 0.001$) than nonresponders (Table 4), as to be expected per the definition of response. Responders compared with nonresponders also had significantly greater reductions from baseline in both adjusted mean (SE) daily FBG (– 4.0 [0.09] vs – 3.3 [0.16] mmol/L; – 71 [1.6] vs –

Table 1 Number of responders and nonresponders to insulin glargine 100 Units/mL at 24 weeks by composite HbA1c endpoint

HbA1c < 7% (Yes/No)	≥1% reduction in HbA1c (Yes/No)	Responders (HbA1c < 7% or ≥ 1% reduction) n (%)	Nonresponders (HbA1c ≥ 7% and < 1% reduction) n (%)
Yes	Yes	595 (50)	–
Yes	No	88 (7)	–
No	Yes	505 (43)	–
No	No		297 (20)
Total (N = 1485)		1188 (80)	297 (20)

Abbreviation: HbA1c glycated hemoglobin

Table 2 Baseline characteristics of responders and nonresponders to insulin glargine 100 Units/mL at 24 weeks

	Responders at 24 weeks (HbA1c < 7% or ≥ 1% reduction) n = 1188	Nonresponders at 24 Weeks (HbA1c ≥ 7% and < 1% reduction) n = 297	P value
Age, years	57.8 (9.9)	57.2 (10.1)	0.323
Age group			0.833
< 65 years	893 (75.2)	225 (75.8)	
≥ 65 years	295 (24.8)	72 (24.2)	
Gender			0.012
Women	543 (45.7)	160 (53.9)	
Men	645 (54.3)	137 (46.1)	
Duration of T2DM, years	10.3 (6.6)	9.7 (6.5)	0.159
Weight, kg	87.5 (19.7)	85.8 (21.6)	0.201
BMI, kg/m^2	31.3 (5.70)	30.9 (5.70)	0.213
HbA1c, %	9.1 (1.2)	8.3 (0.9)	< 0.001
HbA1c, mmol/mol	99 (13)	91 (10)	< 0.001
FBG, mg/dL	186.7 (52.0)	158.5 (42.2)	< 0.001
≥ 1 OAMs Targeting PPG[a]	1111 (93.5)	290 (97.6)	0.006
SU, yes	1067 (89.8)	284 (95.6)	0.002
2 OAMs	790 (66.5)	194 (65.3)	0.701
MET/SU	614 (51.7)	167 (56.2)	–
3 OAMs	389 (32.7)	100 (33.7)	0.761
MET/SU/TZD	346 (29.1)	89 (30.0)	–
4 OAMs	7 (0.6)	3 (1.0)	0.429

Individual participant data were pooled from 3 randomized clinical trials [20–22] and are mean (SD) or n (%). Patients are those who were randomized to insulin glargine as the only insulin treatment and with no missing HbA1c values at 24 weeks. Two-sided *P* values were considered statistically significant if < 0.05 and were calculated by ANOVA model (response = subgroup) for continuous variables and by Pearson's Chi-square or Fisher's exact (for OAM data with less than 80% of cells with an expected value ≥5) test for categorical variables. *Abbreviations: AGI* alpha glucosidase inhibitor, *BMI* body mass index, *DPP-IV* dipeptidyl peptidase IV, *FBG* fasting blood glucose, *HbA1c* glycated hemoglobin, *MEG* meglitinides, *MET* metformin, *OAM* oral antihyperglycemic medication, *PPG* postprandial blood glucose, *SD* standard deviation, *SU* sulphonylurea, *T2DM* type 2 diabetes mellitus, *TZD* thiazolidinedione. [a]OAMs targeting postprandial glucose were SU, DPP-IV, AGI, and MEG

59 [2.8] mg/dL; $P < 0.001$) and daily PPG (– 4.1 [0.11] vs – 3.0 [0.18] mmol/L; – 73 [1.9] vs – 54 [3.3] mg/dL; $P < 0.001$) (Table 4). The difference between responders and nonresponders in change from baseline adjusted mean daily BG levels at 24 weeks was small at pre-breakfast and 3 AM, but more pronounced at other time points (Fig. 1). More responders than nonresponders (39% vs 34%) reached FBG target ≤ 5.6 mmol/L (≤ 100 mg/dL) at 24 weeks (Fig. 2). Responders were also more likely to reach PPG target ≤ 10.0 mmol/L (≤ 180 mg/dL) after breakfast (77% vs 69%), lunch (81% vs 66%), and evening meal (79% vs 71%) than nonresponders (Fig. 2). (Note: the PPG target was defined for this analysis and was not given to investigators during these trials.) The adjusted mean

Table 3 Prediction of insulin glargine 100 Units/mL response at 24 weeks based on early response at 12 weeks

		Responders at week 24	
		Yes	No
Responders at Week 12	Yes	91%	9%
	No	46%	54%
Predictive parameters			
Odds ratio = 12.7 (P < 0.001)			
Sensitivity = 85.9%			
Specificity = 67.7%			
Positive predictive value = 91.4%			
Negative predictive value = 54.5%			

Sensitivity is the percentage of subsequent responders (HbA1c <7% or ≥ 1% reduction) correctly identified (true-positive rate). Specificity is the percentage of subsequent nonresponders (HbA1c ≥7% and < 1% reduction) correctly identified (true-negative rate). Positive predictive value is the percentage of subsequent responders among early responders. Negative predictive value is the percentage of subsequent nonresponders among early nonresponders. *Abbreviation: HbA1c glycated hemoglobin*

(SE) daily IGlar dose was similar between responders and nonresponders at 24 weeks (45.2 [1.4] vs 42.2 [2.3] units/day; 0.49 [0.01] vs 0.47 [0.02] units/kg/day) (Table 4). From a post hoc graphical assessment (data not shown), inverse linear relationships were observed between improvements in glycemic measures (FBG, daily mean PPG, HbA1c) and baseline HbA1c or FBG which confirm the findings mentioned above. Plots of improvements in glycemic measures and insulin dose (data not shown) did not reveal an informative pattern.

Hypoglycemia

At 24 weeks, responders compared with nonresponders had a significantly higher incidence of total (82.5 vs 70.4%; P < 0.001), nocturnal (60.3 vs 50.5%; P = 0.002) and documented symptomatic (65.8 vs 55.6%; P < 0.001) hypoglycemia and significantly higher adjusted mean 1-year event rates of total (20.3 vs 14.7; P = 0.004) and documented symptomatic (9.7 vs 7.1; P = 0.022) hypoglycemia (Fig. 3). Nocturnal hypoglycemia adjusted mean 1-year event rates (5.4 vs 5.0; P = 0.608) and severe hypoglycemia incidence (12 [1.0%] vs 0; P = 0.082) and adjusted mean 1-year event rates (0 for both; P = 1.000) were similar between groups. From a post hoc graphical assessment (data not shown), no meaningful pattern between hypoglycemia rate and insulin dose was revealed.

Discussion

This analysis showed that the composite HbA1c response at 12 weeks was a strong predictor of maintaining at least the same HbA1c response (composite) at 24 weeks. Responders had higher HbA1c and FBG levels at baseline with fewer participants using OAMs targeting PPG than nonresponders. Responders compared

with nonresponders were also more likely to reach target FBG ≤ 5.6 mmol/L (≤ 100 mg/dL) and *hypothetical* target PPG ≤ 10.0 mmol/L (≤ 180 mg/dL) at 24 weeks with similar IGlar doses. Moreover, adjusted mean IGlar doses at 24 weeks for both groups were still below the limit for basal insulin titration (> 0.5 units/kg/day) recommended by the American Diabetes Association and European Association for the Study of Diabetes [1]. Despite the relatively high averages for IGlar dose and hypoglycemia incidence and yearly event rates at 24 weeks, hypoglycemia incidence and yearly event rates were lower in nonresponders than responders, and both groups had similar yearly event rates of nocturnal hypoglycemia. Given that hypoglycemia data were collected systematically, the chance for under-estimation of hypoglycemia incidence is expected to be small. The high incidence of hypoglycemia in both groups may be explained in part by the aggressive dose-titration protocols used in these trials (Additional file 1), and therefore inadequate titration is unlikely to have caused a lower incidence of hypoglycemia in nonresponders. The mean IGlar dose was close to 0.5 units/kg. Scatter plots of HbA1c versus dose and hypoglycemia yearly event rate versus dose at 24 weeks did not show an informative pattern to suggest a relationship between dose and improvement in glycemic control or lower hypoglycemia incidence. Some people with T2DM, however, may need greater than 0.5 units/kg/day of basal insulin in case of higher insulin resistance. The first-up-titrate-basal insulin approach is expected to be useful in some patients and should be considered on an individual basis. Early introduction of a medication for the control of PPG to reduce the risk of hypoglycemia, especially if using a GLP1-RA, could also benefit some individuals. For nonresponders to IGlar who have reached FBG target or whose up-titration of IGlar dose is limited by the frequency and/or severity of hypoglycemia, diabetes treatment should be intensified with PPG-lowering agents, such as prandial insulin or GLP1-RA.

Our findings are consistent with several post hoc analyses of trials assessing differences between responders and nonresponders to basal insulin treatment. Scheen et al. [13] evaluated the relative contributions of FBG and PPG to overall hyperglycemia in insulin-naive participants who either reached or did not reach target HbA1c < 53 mmol/mol (< 7%) with IGlar or insulin lispro mix 25 at 24 weeks in the DURABLE trial. Insulin doses were higher but hypoglycemia yearly event rates were lower in nonresponders compared with responders at study endpoint. Failure to reach target FBG ≤ 5.6 mmol/L (≤ 100 mg/dL) was the primary reason for not achieving target HbA1c in both insulin groups, suggesting the need to first up titrate basal insulin before intensifying therapy with PPG-lowering agents. Similarly, Khunti et al.

Table 4 Glycemic response and insulin dose in responders and nonresponders to insulin glargine 100 Units/mL at 24 weeks

	Responders (HbA1c < 7% or ≥ 1% reduction)	Nonresponders (HbA1c ≥ 7% and < 1% reduction)
HbA1c (mmol/mol), n	1188	297
Endpoint	74 (0.44)	89 (0.66)
CFB	− 24 (0.44)	− 9 (0.66)
CFB, LSM Diff (95% CI)	− 15 (− 16.40, − 13.88); $P < 0.001$	
HbA1c (%), n	1188	297
Endpoint	6.76 (0.04)	8.14 (0.06)
CFB	− 2.16 (0.04)	− 0.78 (0.06)
CFB, LSM Diff (95% CI)	− 1.38 (− 1.50, − 1.27); $P < 0.001$	
Dose (units/day), n	1187	297
Endpoint	45.21 (1.36)	42.16 (2.29)
LSM Diff (95% CI)	3.05 (− 1.24, 7.34); $P = 0.164$	
Dose (units/kg/day), n	1187	297
Endpoint	0.49 (0.01)	0.47 (0.02)
LSM Diff (95% CI)	0.02 (− 0.02, 0.07); $P = 0.272$	
Fasting blood glucose, n	692	143
Endpoint (mmol/L)	6.13 (0.09)	6.83 (0.16)
CFB	− 3.97 (0.09)	− 3.26 (0.16)
CFB, LSM Diff (95% CI)	− 0.71 (− 1.00, − 0.41); $P < 0.001$	
Endpoint (mg/dL)	110.39 (1.63)	123.10 (2.81)
CFB	− 71.48 (1.63)	− 58.77 (2.81)
CFB, LSM Diff (95% CI)	−12.71 (− 18.00, − 7.42); $P < 0.001$	
Daily mean SMBG, n	640	128
Endpoint (mmol/L)	7.30 (0.09)	8.20 (0.16)
CFB	− 3.85 (0.09)	− 2.95 (0.16)
CFB, LSM Diff (95% CI)	− 0.90 (− 1.20, − 0.60); $P < 0.001$	
Endpoint (mg/dL)	131.45 (1.62)	147.70 (2.83)
CFB	− 69.33 (1.62)	− 53.08 (2.83)
CFB, LSM Diff (95% CI)	− 16.25 (− 21.60, − 10.89); $P < 0.001$	
Daily mean premeal SMBG, n	678	142
Endpoint (mmol/L)	6.59 (0.08)	7.51 (0.14)
CFB	− 3.70 (0.08)	− 2.78 (0.14)
CFB, LSM Diff (95% CI)	− 0.92 (− 1.19, − 0.65); $P < 0.001$	
Endpoint (mg/dL)	118.75 (1.52)	135.30 (2.58)
CFB	− 66.64 (1.52)	− 50.09 (2.58)
CFB, LSM Diff (95% CI)	− 16.55 (− 21.40, − 11.69); $P < 0.001$	
Daily mean postprandial SMBG, n	677	139
Endpoint (mmol/L)	8.31 (0.11)	9.32 (0.18)
CFB	− 4.03 (0.11)	− 3.02 (0.18)
CFB, LSM Diff (95% CI)	− 1.01 (− 1.36, − 0.66); $P < 0.001$	
Endpoint (mg/dL)	149.70 (1.93)	167.91 (3.33)
CFB	− 72.70 (1.93)	− 54.49 (3.33)
CFB, LSM Diff (95% CI)	− 18.21 (− 24.50, − 11.93); $P < 0.001$	

Table 4 Glycemic response and insulin dose in responders and nonresponders to insulin glargine 100 Units/mL at 24 weeks (Continued)

	Responders (HbA1c < 7% or ≥ 1% reduction)	Nonresponders (HbA1c ≥ 7% and < 1% reduction)
Intrapatient between-day SMBG variability, n	673	137
Endpoint (mmol/L)	0.62 (0.03)	0.71 (0.05)
CFB	− 0.27 (0.03)	− 0.18 (0.05)
CFB, LSM Diff (95% CI)	− 0.08 (− 0.18, 0.01); P = 0.070	
Endpoint (mg/dL)	11.20 (0.52)	12.74 (0.89)
CFB	− 4.86 (0.52)	− 3.33 (0.89)
CFB, LSM Diff (95% CI)	− 1.53 (− 3.19, 0.13); P = 0.070	

Endpoints and CFB values are expressed as LSM (SE) unless otherwise stated. Pearson's Chi-square test was used for categorical variables and ANCOVA model (response = baseline of the response variable + responder + study + study-by-responder interaction + sulphonylurea use [yes/no]) for continuous variables. P values are based on fixed effects meta-regression with a 2-sided α-level of 0.05. Heterogeneity was assessed by study-by-responder interaction. P values for interaction were nonsignificant (≥ 0.05) for outcomes presented with the exception of fasting blood glucose (P = 0.012), indicating results in these trials were relatively homogeneous. All patients had HbA1c values at 24 weeks and received insulin glargine as the only insulin therapy. *Abbreviations*: *CFB* change from baseline, *CI* confidence interval, *Diff* difference, *HbA1c* glycated hemoglobin, *LSM* least squares mean, *SE* standard error, *SMBG* self-monitored blood glucose, *T2DM* type 2 diabetes mellitus

[14] found that the suboptimally controlled group (HbA1c ≥ 53 mmol/mol [7%]) treated with once-daily insulin detemir in the SOLVE trial had a relatively low risk of hypoglycemia and suboptimal FBG levels at 24 weeks, which according to the authors suggested that 'a more aggressive titration regimen could be implemented to improve glycemic control'. A Spanish cross-sectional study looking at people with T2DM on basal insulin also showed that approximately half of the participants had high FBG and HbA1c levels, and hence for those participants, further adjustments of basal insulin would be necessary [15]. Similar patterns of response to basal insulin were observed in a recent meta-analysis of participant-level

data from 3415 insulin-naïve participants treated with IGlar in 16 randomized, treat-to-target trials [23]. Participants who reached target HbA1c < 53 mmol/mol (< 7%) at 24 weeks were more likely to achieve target FBG ≤ 5.5 mmol/L (≤ 100 mg/dL), as well as had greater likelihood of reaching target FBG levels without hypoglycemia. Nevertheless, responders had more hypoglycemia events than participants with HbA1c levels of 53 mmol/mol (7%) to 64 mmol/mol (8%) or > 64 mmol/mol (8%). The higher HbA1c groups also had more weight gain and a slightly greater insulin dose at 24 weeks. Interestingly, more frequent hypoglycemia was associated with lower baseline C-peptide levels and was associated with

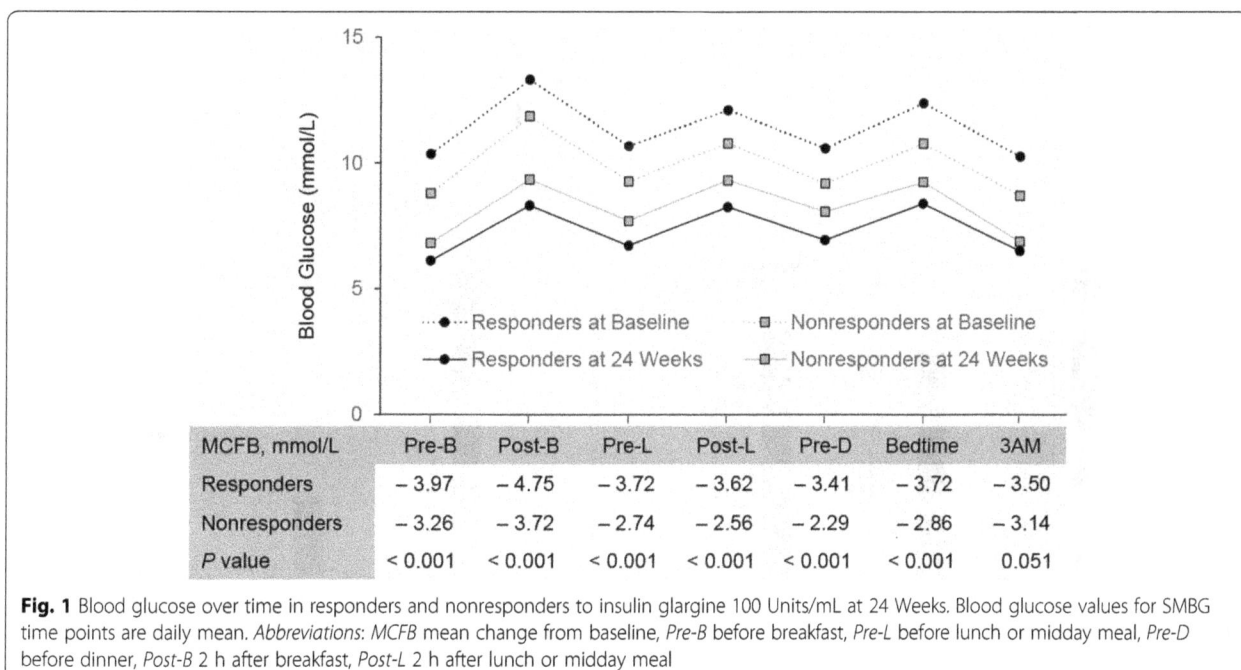

MCFB, mmol/L	Pre-B	Post-B	Pre-L	Post-L	Pre-D	Bedtime	3AM
Responders	− 3.97	− 4.75	− 3.72	− 3.62	− 3.41	− 3.72	− 3.50
Nonresponders	− 3.26	− 3.72	− 2.74	− 2.56	− 2.29	− 2.86	− 3.14
P value	< 0.001	< 0.001	< 0.001	< 0.001	< 0.001	< 0.001	0.051

Fig. 1 Blood glucose over time in responders and nonresponders to insulin glargine 100 Units/mL at 24 Weeks. Blood glucose values for SMBG time points are daily mean. *Abbreviations*: *MCFB* mean change from baseline, *Pre-B* before breakfast, *Pre-L* before lunch or midday meal, *Pre-D* before dinner, *Post-B* 2 h after breakfast, *Post-L* 2 h after lunch or midday meal

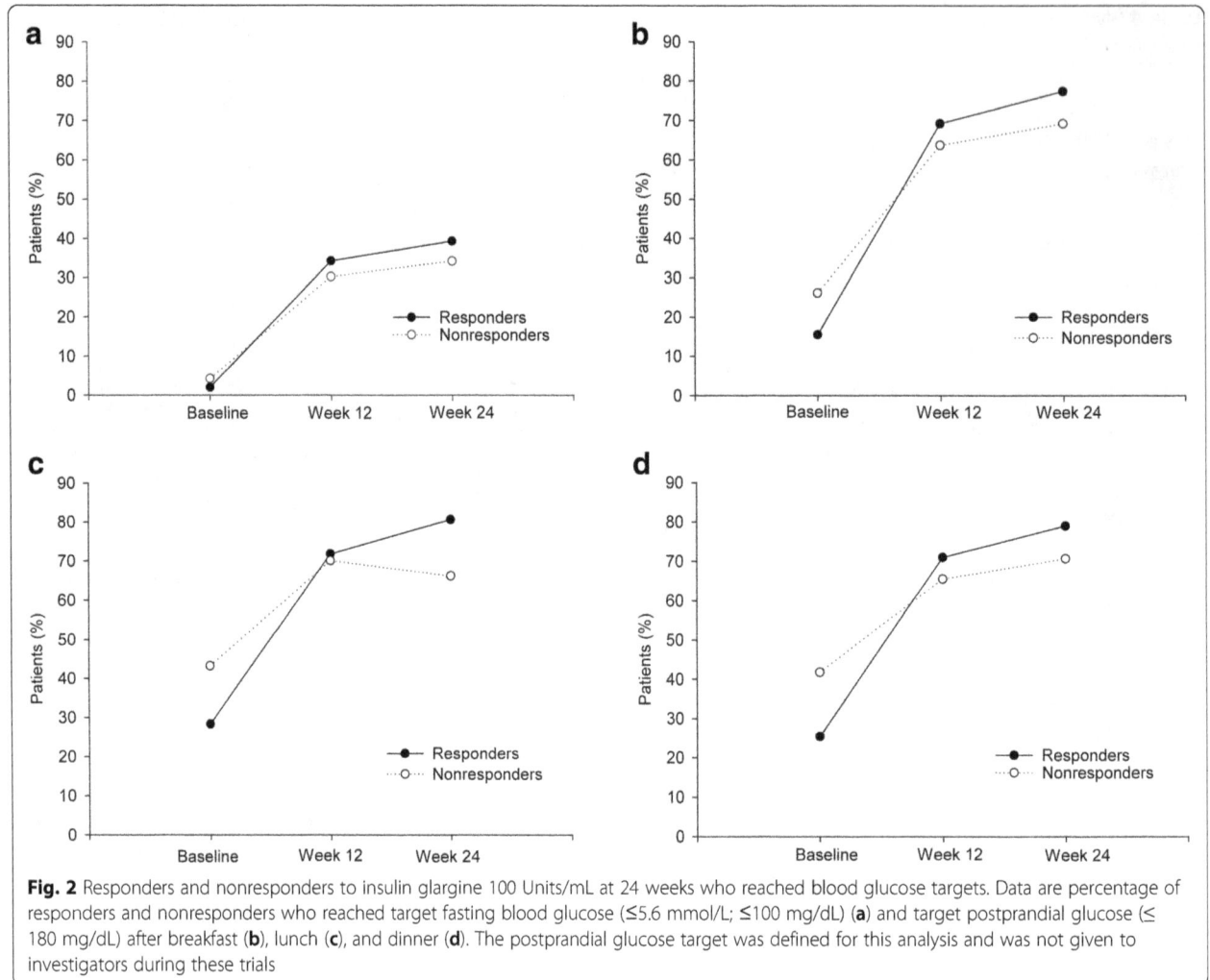

Fig. 2 Responders and nonresponders to insulin glargine 100 Units/mL at 24 weeks who reached blood glucose targets. Data are percentage of responders and nonresponders who reached target fasting blood glucose (≤5.6 mmol/L; ≤100 mg/dL) (**a**) and target postprandial glucose (≤ 180 mg/dL) after breakfast (**b**), lunch (**c**), and dinner (**d**). The postprandial glucose target was defined for this analysis and was not given to investigators during these trials

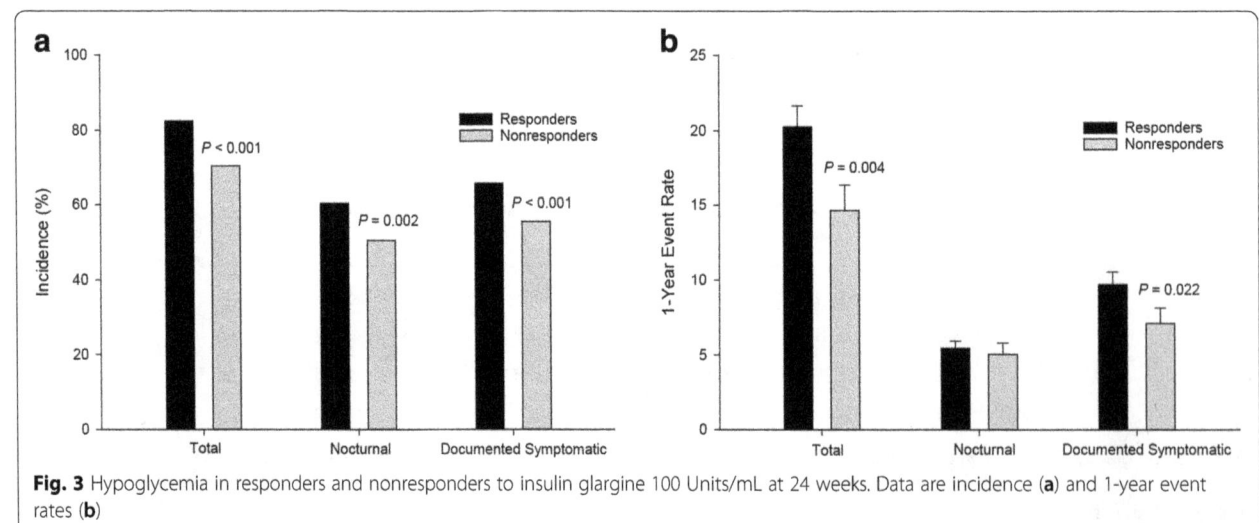

Fig. 3 Hypoglycemia in responders and nonresponders to insulin glargine 100 Units/mL at 24 weeks. Data are incidence (**a**) and 1-year event rates (**b**)

more weight gain at 24 weeks in all HbA1c groups. The authors concluded that people initiating therapy with IGlar are a heterogeneous group in terms of glycemic response and hypoglycemia risk. Our analysis focused on glycemic response, and therefore did not include weight changes from baseline. Baseline C-peptide values were not available to assess.

Studies analyzing the predictability of early response to IGlar for subsequent longer-term response are limited. The high predictive values of 12-week response for subsequent treatment success at 24 weeks in our meta-analysis are consistent with results of a pooled analysis of participant-level data by Fu et al. [17] using the same composite HbA1c endpoint to measure response to IGlar and to OAMs in 3 randomized clinical trials. The high predictive values of 12-week response in both analyses support current guidelines that recommend clinicians evaluate therapeutic responses to pharmacologic interventions 12 weeks after initiating therapy [1].

Participants with higher baseline HbA1c levels have been shown to be less likely to achieve target HbA1c < 53 mmol/mol (< 7%) with basal insulin therapy in randomized clinical trials [13, 16] and in observational studies [14]. Other baseline factors associated with not achieving this HbA1c target include longer duration of diabetes [14, 16], use of a sulphonylurea [16], number of OAMs and longer duration of OAM treatment [14], and higher BMI [14]. When achievement of HbA1c < 53 mmol/mol (< 7%) was further analysed by reaching target FBG < 7.2 mmol/L (< 130 mg/dL) in an observational cross-sectional study of 9899 participants with T2DM [15], only 18% of the study population achieved both HbA1c and FBG targets. Of the participants who did not reach HbA1c target (75% of the total population), those who reached target FBG (24%) were older, had a longer duration of diabetes, and had lower mean values for HbA1c, BMI, diastolic blood pressure, and low-density lipoprotein cholesterol at baseline than those who did not reach target FBG (51%).

Limitations of this meta-analysis are in part due to its post hoc design, and therefore a cause and effect relationship cannot be established. Additionally, data are from randomized clinical trials, thereby results may not reflect what would be seen in a real-world setting, where more aggressive titration of basal insulin is possible and the addition of prandial insulin or a GLP1-RA is an option. Additionally, a lesser reduction in HbA1c (e.g., 8.7 mmol/mol [0.8%] vs 11 mmol/mol [1%]) despite not reaching target HbA1c < 53 mmol/mol [< 7%] could be considered clinically significant. Reasons for not increasing IGlar dose to reach HbA1c goal, particularly for participants without hypoglycemia, were not assessed in these trials, and insulin resistance was not measured. Treatment algorithms and noninsulin treatment options have also changed since these studies were conducted, and therefore results of our analysis may not fully reflect today's clinical practice.

Conclusions

As would be expected, more participants with clinically meaningful reductions in HbA1c were identified in this analysis by expanding the definition of response to include a ≥ 11 mmol/mol (≥ 1%) reduction in HbA1c from baseline. Baseline HbA1c and FBG were also statistically higher in responders than nonresponders, although there was not a significant clinical difference to warrant a cut-off for basal insulin administration. At both 12 and 24 weeks, the majority of responders and nonresponders had not reached target FBG, suggesting that more aggressive insulin titration was still possible in responders who had not yet reached FBG and HbA1c goals, assuming hyper- or hypoglycemia at other self-monitoring BG time points were not the driving factors. These findings, coupled with the high predictability of 12-week response for subsequent longer-term response, suggest that the composite HbA1c endpoint is superior to the single HbA1c measure. Clinicians should consider the magnitude of reduction in HbA1c at 12 weeks in addition to achievement of target HbA1c to better recognize the potential for success with this effective starter basal insulin, especially for people with more advanced T2DM and/or higher HbA1c levels, which may require larger insulin doses to obtain glycemic control possibly related to higher insulin resistance. Moreover, sequentially targeting FBG and PPG levels could identify nonresponders to IGlar who could become responders with additional therapy beyond basal insulin. This approach could be encouraging to people with T2DM who are clinically benefiting early from IGlar therapy to continue treatment to get closer to desired goal. A better understanding of concerns of clinicians and/or people with T2DM and reasons for not up titrating or intensifying IGlar therapy is needed and is currently being assessed in a large observational study [24–26]. Studies evaluating the value of adding basal-only versus basal-bolus insulin or GLP1-RA treatment in people with T2DM not adequately controlled on current noninsulin combination therapies are needed to inform clinicians' treatment selection.

Our findings confirm the clinical utility of IGlar as a safe and effective starter basal insulin and offer insights about addressing an individual's response to treatment as early as 12 weeks. Timely adjustments to basal insulin therapy could help keep people with T2DM on track to benefit from better glycemic control.

Abbreviations

BG: Blood glucose; BMI: Body mass index; FBG: Fasting blood glucose; GLP1-RA: Glucagon-like peptide-1 receptor agonist; HbA1c: Glycated hemoglobin; IGlar: Insulin glargine 100 units/mL; OAM: Oral antihyperglycemic medication; PPG: Postprandial blood glucose; SE: Standard error; SMBG: Self-monitored blood glucose; T2DM: Type 2 diabetes mellitus; UK: United Kingdom

Acknowledgements

The authors would like to thank both Robyn Pollom and Tim Costigan for their reviews and valuable suggestions at the start of this project. We also thank Karen M. Paulsrud, RPh of Eli Lilly and Company for assistance with the preparation of this manuscript.

Funding

This research was funded by Eli Lilly and Company and Boehringer-Ingelheim. Eli Lilly and Company participated in data collection. Both Eli Lilly and Company and Boehringer-Ingelheim participated in the study design, data collection, data review, data analysis, and manuscript preparation and publication decisions.

Authors' contributions

MHC interpreted data and drafted the manuscript. DC participated in the design of the study, performed statistical analysis, and drafted the manuscript. IH and LLI participated in the design of the study, interpreted data, and drafted the manuscript. MHT interpreted data and drafted the manuscript. All authors read and approved the final manuscript.

Competing interests

MHC has participated in Abasaglar speaker events for which he received honorarium from Eli Lilly and Company and Boehringer-Ingelheim. LLI, DC, and IH are employees of and hold stock in Eli Lilly and Company. MHT is a retiree of Eli Lilly and Company. This study was previously published in part as two abstracts, the first at the American Diabetes Association's 76th Annual Scientific Sessions in New Orleans, LA, USA in June 2016 and the second at Diabetes UK Professional Conference, Manchester, UK in March 2017.

Author details

[1]Queen Alexandra Hospital, Portsmouth, UK. [2]Eli Lilly and Company, Indianapolis, IN, USA. [3]Lilly Deutschland GmbH, Bad Homburg, Germany. [4]University of Michigan, Ann Arbor, MI, USA.

References

1. Inzucchi SE, Bergenstal RM, Buse JB, Diamant M, Ferrannini E, Nauck M, et al. Management of hyperglycemia in type 2 diabetes, 2015: a patient-centered approach: update to a position statement of the American Diabetes Association and the European Association for the Study of diabetes. Diabetes Care. 2015;38:140–9.
2. Lantus® [prescribing information]. 2015. http://products.sanofi.us/lantus/lantus.html. Accessed 19 Apr 2017.
3. Abasaglar® [summary of product characteristics]. 2015. http://www.ema.europa.eu/ema/index.jsp?curl=pages/medicines/human/medicines/002835/human_med_001790.jsp&mid=WC0b01ac058001d124. Accessed 19 Apr 2017.
4. Riddle MC, Rosenstock J, Gerich J, on behalf of the Insulin Glargine 4002 Study Investigators. The treat-to-target trial: randomized addition of glargine or human NPH insulin to oral therapy of type 2 diabetic patients. Diabetes Care. 2003;26:3080–6.
5. Standl E, Owen DR. New long-acting basal insulins: does benefit outweigh cost? Diabetes Care. 2016;39(Suppl 2):S172–9.
6. Yki-Jarvinen H, Kauppinen-Makelin R, Tiikkainen M, Vahatalo M, Virtamo H, Nikkila K, et al. Insulin glargine or NPH combined with metformin in type 2 diabetes: the LANMET study. Diabetologia. 2006;49:442–51.
7. Hilgenfeld R, Seipke G, Berchtold H, Owens DR. The evolution of insulin glargine and its continuing contribution to diabetes care. Drugs. 2014;74:911–27.
8. Garber AJ, King AB, Del Prato S, Sreenan S, Balci MK, Munoz-Torres M, et al. Insulin degludec, an ultra-longacting basal insulin, versus insulin glargine in basal-bolus treatment with mealtime insulin aspart in type 2 diabetes (BEGIN Basal-Bolus Type 2): a phase 3, randomised, open-label, treat-to-target non-inferiority trial. Lancet. 2012;379:1498–507.
9. Zinman B, Philis-Tsimikas A, Cariou B, Handelsman Y, Rodbard HW, Johansen T, et al. Insulin degludec versus insulin glargine in insulin-naive patients with type 2 diabetes: a 1-year, randomized, treat-to-target trial (BEGIN once long). Diabetes Care. 2012;35:2464–71.
10. Wysham C, Bhargava A, Chaykin LB, de la Rosa R, Handelsman Y, Troelsen LN, et al. SWITCH 2: reduced risk of hypoglycaemia with insulin degludec vs insulin glargine U100 in a type 2 diabetes population on basal insulin: a randomised, double-blind, crossover trial. Oral presentation #82 presented at the European Association for the Study of Diabetes 52nd Annual Meeting 2016; Munich Germany. http://www.easdvirtualmeeting.org/resources/switch-2-reduced-risk-of-hypoglycaemia-with-insulin-degludec-vs-insulin-glargine-u100-in-a-type-2-diabetes-population-on-basal-insulin-a-randomised-double-blind-crossover-trial-86c59ec3-9ff2-42d3-aee3-203a79532b0f. Accessed 19 Apr 2017.
11. Riddle MC, Bolli GB, Ziemen M, Muehlen-Bartmer I, Bizet F, Home PD, et al. New insulin glargine 300 units/mL versus glargine 100 units/mL in people with type 2 diabetes using basal and mealtime insulin: glucose control and hypoglycemia in a 6-month randomized controlled trial (EDITION 1). Diabetes Care. 2014;37:2755–62.
12. Yki-Jarvinen H, Bergenstal R, Ziemen M, Wardecki M, Muehlen-Bartmer I, Boelle E, et al. New insulin glargine 300 units/mL versus glargine 100 units/mL in people with type 2 diabetes using oral agents and basal insulin: glucose control and hypoglycemia in a 6-month randomized controlled trial (EDITION 2). Diabetes Care. 2014;37:3235–43.
13. Scheen AJ, Schmitt H, Jiang HH, Ivanyi T. Factors associated with reaching or not reaching target HbA1c after initiation of basal or premixed insulin in patients with type 2 diabetes. Diabetes Metab. 2017;43:69–78.
14. Khunti K, Damci T, Husemoen LL, Babu V, Liebl A. Exploring the characteristics of suboptimally controlled patients after 24weeks of basal insulin treatment: an individualized approach to intensification. Diabetes Res Clin Pract. 2017;123:209–17.
15. Mata-Cases M, Mauricio D, Franch-Nadal J. Clinical characteristics of type 2 diabetic patients on basal insulin therapy with adequate fasting glucose control who do not achieve HbA1c targets. J Diabetes. 2017;9:34–44.
16. Riddle MC, Vlajnic A, Zhou R, Rosenstock J. Baseline HbA1c predicts attainment of 7.0% HbA1c target with structured titration of insulin glargine in type 2 diabetes: a patient-level analysis of 12 studies. Diabetes Obes Metab. 2013;15:819–25.
17. Fu H, Cao D, Boye KS, Curtis B, Schuster DL, Kendall DM, et al. Early glycemic response predicts achievement of subsequent treatment targets in the treatment of type 2 diabetes: a post hoc analysis. Diabetes Ther. 2015;6:317–28.
18. Conget I, Kirkman MS, Cao D, Wong M, Reviriego J, Kendall DM. Identifying insulin treatment responders with a composite measure: beyond Hba1c < 7% in patients with type 2 diabetes. CMRO. 2018;34(2):329–36.
19. Stratton IM, Adler AI, Neil HA, Matthews DR, Manley SE, Cull CA, et al. Association of glycaemia with macrovascular and microvascular complications of type 2 diabetes (UKPDS 35): prospective observational study. BMJ. 2000;321:405–12.
20. Buse JB, Wolffenbuttel BH, Herman WH, Shemonsky NK, Jiang HH, Fahrbach JL, et al. DURAbility of basal versus lispro mix 75/25 insulin efficacy (DURABLE) trial 24-week results: safety and efficacy of insulin lispro mix 75/25 versus insulin glargine added to oral antihyperglycemic drugs in patients with type 2 diabetes. Diabetes Care. 2009;32:1007–13.
21. Jain SM, Mao X, Escalante-Pulido M, Vorokhobina N, Lopez I, Ilag LL. Prandial-basal insulin regimens plus oral antihyperglycemic agents to improve mealtime glycaemia: initiate and progressively advance insulin therapy in type 2 diabetes. Diabetes Obes Metab. 2010;12:967–75.
22. Rosenstock J, Hollander P, Bhargava A, Ilag LL, Pollom RK, Zielonka JS, et al. Similar efficacy and safety of LY2963016 insulin glargine and insulin glargine (Lantus(R)) in patients with type 2 diabetes who were insulin-naive or previously treated with insulin glargine: a randomized, double-blind controlled trial (the ELEMENT 2 study). Diabetes Obes Metab. 2015;17:734–41.
23. Frier BM, Landgraf W, Zhang M, Bolli GB, Owens DR, Home PD. Association of hypoglycaemia with insulin titration and body weight in people with T2DM commencing insulin glargine 100 U/mL and achieving different HbA1c levels. ePoster #732 presented at the 53rd Annual Meeting of the European Association for the Study of Diabetes 2017; Lisbon, Portugal. https://www.easd.org/virtualmeeting/home.html#!resources/association-of-hypoglycaemia-with-insulin-titration-and-body-weight-in-people-with-type-2-diabetes-commencing-insulin-glargine-100-u-ml-and-achieving-different-hba-sub-1c-sub-levels-bd82eba4-0b0e-458b-a5c2-f0cd93b11832. Accessed 28 Sep 2017.

24. Polinski JM, Curtis BH, Seeger JD, Choudhry NK, Zagar A, Shrank WH. Rationale and design of the multinational observational study assessing insulin use: the MOSAIc study. BMC Endocr Disord. 2012; https://doi.org/10.1186/1472-6823-12-20.

25. Polinski JM, Kim SC, Jiang D, Hassoun A, Shrank WH, Cos X, et al. Geographic patterns in patient demographics and insulin use in 18 countries, a global perspective from the multinational observational study assessing insulin use: understanding the challenges associated with progression of therapy (MOSAIc). BMC Endocr Disord. 2015; https://doi.org/10.1186/s12902-015-0044-z.

26. Linetzky B, Jiang D, Funnell MM, Curtis BH, Polonsky WH. Exploring the role of the patient-physician relationship on insulin adherence and clinical outcomes in type 2 diabetes: insights from the MOSAIc study. J Diabetes. 2016; https://doi.org/10.1111/1753-0407.12443.

Published abstracts

1. Ilag LL, Cao D, Cummings M, Hadjiyianni I, Pollom RK, Costigan TM, Tan M. Characteristics of patients with type 2 diabetes (T2D) who successfully achieved A1c <7%. Diabetes. 2016;65(Suppl. 1) A568[2244-PUB]

2. Cummings M, Cao D, Hadjiyianni I, Ilag LL, Hassan SW, Tahbaz A, et al. Characteristics of patients with type 2 diabetes treated with insulin glargine U-100 who successfully achieved HbA1c <53 mmol/mol (<7%) or reduction in HbA1c of ≥11 mmol/mol (≥1%). Diabet Med. 2017;34(Suppl. s1):190.

3. Cummings M, Cao D, Hadjiyianni I, Ilag LL, Hassan SW, Tahbaz A, Tan MH. Characteristics of patients with type 2 diabetes (T2D) treated with insulin glargine U-100 who successfully achieved HbA1c <53 mmol/mol (<7%) or reduction in HbA1c of ≥11 mmol/mol (≥1%). Associazione Medici Diabetologi - XXI Congresso Nazionale. 2017.

4. Cummings M, Cao D, Hadjiyianni I, Ilag LL, Hassan SW, Tahbaz A, Tan MH. Characteristics of patients with type 2 diabetes (T2D) treated with insulin glargine who successfully achieved HbA1c <53 mmol/mol (<7%) or reduction in HbA1c of ≥11 mmol/mol (≥1%). Societe Francophone du Diabete - 43rd Congres Annuel 2017.

25

How is neighborhood social disorganization associated with diabetes outcomes? A multilevel investigation of glycemic control and self-reported use of acute or emergency health care services

Sarah D. Kowitt[1,2]*, Katrina E. Donahue[2,3], Edwin B. Fisher[1], Madeline Mitchell[3] and Laura A. Young[4]

Abstract

Background: Diabetes management is influenced by a number of factors beyond the individual-level. This study examined how neighborhood social disorganization (i.e., neighborhoods characterized by high economic disadvantage, residential instability, and ethnic heterogeneity), is associated with diabetes-related outcomes.

Methods: We used a multilevel modeling approach to investigate the associations between census-tract neighborhood social disorganization, A1c, and self-reported use of acute or emergency health care services for a sample of 424 adults with type 2 diabetes.

Results: Individuals living in neighborhoods with high social disorganization had higher A1c values than individuals living in neighborhoods with medium social disorganization (B = 0.39, $p = 0.01$). Individuals living in neighborhoods with high economic disadvantage had higher self-reported use of acute or emergency health care services than individuals living in neighborhoods with medium economic disadvantage (B = 0.60, $p = 0.02$).

Conclusions: High neighborhood social disorganization was associated with higher A1c values and high neighborhood economic disadvantage was associated with greater self-reported use of acute or emergency health care services. Controlling for individual level variables diminished this effect for A1c, but not acute or emergency health care use. Comprehensive approaches to diabetes management should include attention to neighborhood context. Failure to do so may help explain the continuing disproportionate diabetes burden in many neighborhoods despite decades of attention to individual-level clinical care and education.

Keywords: Health policy, Neighborhood, Environmental influences, Poverty, Emergency services, Social determinants, Psychosocial influences, Type 2 diabetes

* Correspondence: kowitt@email.unc.edu
[1]Peers for Progress and Department of Health Behavior, Gillings School of Global Public Health, University of North Carolina at Chapel Hill, Rosenau Hall, CB #7440, Chapel Hill, NC 27599-7440, USA
[2]Department of Family Medicine, University of North Carolina at Chapel Hill, Chapel Hill, NC 27599, USA
Full list of author information is available at the end of the article

Background

Diabetes is the seventh leading cause of death and associated with significant health complications [1]. Compared to individuals without diabetes, people with diabetes and particularly those with poor diabetes management, as evidenced through elevated glycemic control (A1c) are at greater risk for heart attack, stroke, kidney failure, and premature mortality [1]. Moreover, an estimated one in seven health care dollars is attributed to diabetes—resulting in a $327 billion total estimated cost [2]. For these reasons, diabetes management poses a significant problem that needs to be addressed, particularly for individuals in the Southeastern U.S. who experience greater rates of diabetes than the general population (colloquially called the "diabetes belt") [3].

Moving beyond the "self" in "diabetes self-management," research has shown that diabetes management is influenced by a number of ecological factors beyond the individual and that interventions focused solely on the individual are often insufficient to improve glycemic control over the long-term [4]. There is growing empirical evidence that even after controlling for individual level socioeconomic status (SES) and race/ethnicity, aspects of the neighborhood are associated with health status [5] and glycemic control [6] among individuals with diabetes, as well as risk of developing diabetes [7–10]. While most of the evidence to date has been observational, in one of the only randomized studies of neighborhood poverty, researchers found that individuals randomized to live in low poverty neighborhoods were less likely to develop diabetes than individuals randomized to live in high poverty neighborhoods [8]. In addition to the growing body of empirical evidence, researchers have also conceptualized *how* neighborhood characteristics are associated with health outcomes.

Social disorganization theory suggests that in addition to neighborhood disadvantage—a well-documented predictor of poor health status [11]—other features of neighborhoods, such as residential instability and ethnic heterogeneity (i.e., an index of neighborhood diversity) influence health outcomes [12]. Specifically, this theory posits that neighborhoods with social disorganization (i.e., neighborhoods characterized by high economic disadvantage, residential instability, and ethnic heterogeneity) have lower social control and collective efficacy and higher violence and crime. While this theory has mostly been applied to violence or substance use [12], researchers have hypothesized that neighborhood social disorganization (NSD) may also affect physical health outcomes [13] through its influence on: 1) health-related behaviors by constraining diffusion of health information and reducing social control over deviant health-related behavior; 2) access to services and amenities by affecting residents' ability to lobby for provision of services and use of such services (e.g., health care services) that are

directly related to health; and 3) psychosocial processes by influencing levels of affective support, stress, self-esteem and mutual respect—all of which are associated with immune response and overall health [14]. In a study of cardiometabolic risk factors among African Americans, for example, a composite measure of NSD was associated with presence of metabolic syndrome in women (defined as having 3 of 5 of the following risk factors: elevated serum triglycerides, fasting plasma glucose, blood pressure, waist circumference, and decreased high density lipoprotein cholesterol), even after adjusting for age, health behaviors, income, education, and family size [15].

While researchers have often examined economic disadvantage and residential instability as metrics of neighborhood functioning, the concept of ethnic heterogeneity is specific to social disorganization theory. Ethnic heterogeneity is hypothesized to affect health outcomes because it can contribute to lack of communication between neighborhoods, hinder social ties, and increase social isolation, leading to less social control and reduced neighborhood collective efficacy [12]. Indeed, a number of researchers have found increasing ethnic heterogeneity to be associated with increased rates of dating violence victimization [16], increased rates of assault, juvenile violence, or violent crime [17–20], and weakened perceptions of collective efficacy [21]. Even in the study described above examining cardiometabolic risk factors among African Americans, the composite measure of NSD included dimensions assessing ethnic heterogeneity [15]. However, other research suggests that associations between increasing ethnic heterogeneity and worse health outcomes may be misleading due to methodological artifacts or other confounding variables [22, 23]. Many arguments can also be made for the benefits of neighborhood racial and ethnic diversity, such as increased cultural sensitivity among residents, decreased racial and ethnic prejudice, broadened social networks, and increased social growth [24]. Given that social disorganization theory was first developed in 1969, it is possible that ethnic heterogeneity may no longer be relevant for health or social processes and further research is needed.

Despite the growing body of evidence examining associations between neighborhood characteristics and health outcomes among individuals with diabetes, few studies have used behavioral health theories to examine associations, which can help guide selection of appropriate variables for analyses and can also facilitate comparisons of results across studies. Moreover, no studies to our knowledge have examined NSD and its association with diabetes-related outcomes. Therefore, in the current study, we use social disorganization theory to examine how NSD may be associated with two diabetes outcomes: A1c and self-reported use of emergency and acute health care services. We chose A1c as an outcome given its importance as a marker of glycemic control and diabetes management [1]. In addition, we chose use of acute or emergency health care services given its impact on health care expenditures [2] and because few studies have examined how neighborhood characteristics may be associated with use of acute or emergency health care services among individuals with type 2 diabetes. Based on prior research [5–10, 25], we hypothesized that NSD would be associated with both A1c and self-reported use of emergency and acute health care services.

Methods

Data source

For this study, we used baseline data from a larger parent study investigating the impacts on patient-centered outcomes of three different approaches to self-monitoring of blood glucose among 450 adults with non-insulin dependent type 2 diabetes living in North Carolina [26, 27]. Patients from primary care practices within the central North Carolina area were recruited to take part in the parent study. Participants were aged 30 or over with an A1c between 6.5 and 9.5% within the 6 months preceding screening. All measurements were collected as part of the larger parent study. For the present study, we used baseline data from all participants. Baseline data were collected betwen January 2014 and June 2014. The University of North Carolina at Chapel Hill Institutional Review Board approved the parent study, as well as the present study.

Measures

A1c

To assess A1c, we collected blood at the time of the patient's baseline visit and measured total glycated hemoglobin using a published formula by the processing laboratory.

Self-reported use of acute or emergency health care services

To assess use of acute or emergency health care services, we asked participants "in the last year, how many times have you" 1) "gone to an urgent care clinic?" 2) "been seen in the Emergency Room?" 3) "been hospitalized overnight?" and 4) "had someone call EMS for you?". We summed responses to create a count of how many visits a participant made to the emergency room, urgent care, hospital, or ambulatory care in the previous year.

NSD

Of the 450 participants, we were able to geocode 436 addresses into 200 census tracts; the remaining 14 addresses were PO boxes, which we excluded for this study. We then downloaded 2013 American Community Survey census tract data and merged these with the individual-level dataset. Based on previous research [13, 28], we used seven census indicators to represent the three components of NSD. These census indicators were used to assess *neighborhood economic disadvantage* (i.e., the proportion of female-headed families, the proportion of individuals in poverty, the proportion of households receiving public assistance, and the proportion of unemployed individuals) [13, 28], *neighborhood residential instability* (i.e., the proportion of renter-occupied homes vs. owner-occupied and the proportion of residents who had lived in the neighborhood for less than 5 years) [28], and *neighborhood ethnic heterogeneity* (i.e., calculated as the sum of the squared proportions of each racial / ethnic group in the neighborhood subtracted from one) [29].

We analyzed NSD in two ways. First, in line with previous research [15], we averaged these seven indicators to create a score that ranged from 0 to 1 with higher values indicating greater NSD (Cronbach's alpha = 0.76). We then created tertiles of NSD with neighborhoods with low NSD defined as one standard deviation below the mean and neighborhoods and high NSD defined as one standard deviation above the mean—as has been done in previous research [28, 30–32]. Second, we examined these seven indicators separately as variables representing neighborhood economic disadvantage, neighborhood residential instability, and neighborhood ethnic heterogeneity, as has also been done previously [28]. Similar to the first approach, we averaged respective indicators and created tertiles with low defined as one standard deviation below the mean and high defined as one standard deviation above the mean.

Psychosocial and clinical variables

Psychosocial and clinical variables included: years with diabetes, diabetes distress, diabetes empowerment, self-care, and number of comorbidities. We measured *years with diabetes* by asking participants how long ago they were diagnosed with diabetes (in years). We measured *diabetes distress* with 20 items form the Problem Areas in Diabetes (PAID) scale, which assesses diabetes-specific emotional distress, including guilt, anger, depressed mood, worry, and fear [33]. Each item has five possible answers ranging from 0 (representing "no problem") to 4 ("a serious problem") [33]. We added the scores and multiplied by 1.25 to generate a total score between 0 and 100, with higher values indicating more distress [33]. We measured *diabetes empowerment* with eight items from Diabetes Empowerment Scale-Short Form (DES-SF), which assesses one's confidence in managing, coping, and making positive choices about diabetes care [34]. Each item has 5 response options (1 = strongly disagree to 5 = strongly agree), which we averaged for a scale ranging from 1 to 5, with higher values indicating higher diabetes empowerment [34]. We measured *self-care* with items from the Summary of Diabetes Self-Care Activities, which is a brief self-report questionnaire of general diet, specific diet, exercise, blood-glucose testing, foot care, and smoking [35]. For the purposes of this study, we only included self-care items for general diet, specific diet, exercise, blood-glucose testing, and footcare [35]. For each item, response options range from 0 to 7, indicating the frequency with which activities had been performed over the previous week (e.g., participating in at least 30 min of physical activities). We created a total mean score by averaging all items [35]. We measured *comorbidities* by asking participants to self-report other conditions, including chronic back pain, heart disease, high blood pressure, lung disease, stroke, high cholesterol, kidney disease, liver disease, anemia or other blood disease, cancer, depression / anxiety, arthritis, autoimmune disease, and stomach or bowel disease. We created a total score by summing the number of comorbidities; higher values indicate more comorbidities.

Demographic variables
Demographic variables included education (categorized as completed some high school, high school graduate, some college, college degree, or graduate degree), age, sex, ethnicity (Latino vs. not Latino), and race (options for American Indian or Alaska Native, Asian, Black or African American, Native Hawaiian or Pacific Islander, White, Other, and Mixed). Given the limited number of participants not identifying as Black or White, we collapsed race into the following categories: Black, White, and Other.

Data analysis
We collected data from January 2014 to June 2014 and conducted data analysis between September 2015 and February 2016. We used SAS version 9.3 survey procedures (SAS Inc., Cary, NC, USA) for descriptive statistics and multilevel modeling (Proc Mixed and Proc Glimmix). Of the 450 participants with baseline data, we dropped data for 14 participants (3.1%) who could not be geocoded and 12 participants (3%) who were missing data on any of the other variables examined, resulting in an analytic sample of 424 participants. We set critical α = .05 and used 2-tailed statistical tests.

Multilevel models
We applied two-level random intercept models to assess the associations between neighborhood characteristics and individual-level diabetes management outcomes [36].

Before constructing the multilevel models, we examined descriptive statistics and unadjusted associations between NSD and each outcome. Then we constructed the multilevel models in steps of increasing complexity. First, we constructed a null model to quantify the between and within-tract variance of the outcomes, or in

other words to estimate the intraclass correlation (ICC). This model was not presented in the tables. Next, we constructed a multilevel random intercept model (Model 1), with individual-level demographic predictors modeled as fixed effects, to examine the influence of individual-level characteristics on our outcomes. Third, we entered individual level demographic, psychosocial, and clinical variables into the model (Model 2) as fixed effects to determine the influence of psychosocial and clinical factors on our outcomes. Finally, we added neighborhood-level contextual factors in two ways: NSD modeld as three separate variables (Model 3) and NSD modeled as a composite variable (Model4). To model A1c, we used a linear multilevel modeling approach. For use of acute or emergency health care services (i.e., counts data), we used a series of Poisson models to account for the non-normal distribution of the data [37].

Finally, to determine if the individual-level variables mediated or confounded the relationship between NSD and our outcomes, we examined whether there was a significant relationship between NSD and our outcomes with and without individual-level variables in the model. We also ran sensitivity analyses to see if effects varied when individual-level factors were entered into the model as random effects (rather than fixed effects) and used Akaike Information Criteria and Bayesian Information Criterion values to determine which model had the best fit (smaller values indicate better fit).

In the results, regression coefficients ("B") and 95% confidence intervals (CIs) are presented. Within each model, the referent group was chosen as the group with the largest number of participants.

Results
Descriptive statistics
On average participants were 60.5 years old and majority White (63.9%) (Table 1). Most participants had completed some college (36.3%), had a college degree (20.8%), or had a graduate degree (13.4%). Mean A1c was 7.5 and, on average, participants reported using 1 acute or emergency health care service in the previous year (mean: 1.2, SD: 2.3). Participants also reported having between 3 and 4 comorbidities, on average (mean: 3.4, SD: 1.9). While most participants lived in neighborhoods with medium NSD (70.8%), an appreciable minority lived in neighborhoods with high NSD (12.5%), defined as one standard deviation above the mean.

Simple, unadjusted effects of neighborhood disadvantage
A1c
In an unadjusted model (Table 2), there were no associations between A1c and neighborhood economic disadvantage, neighborhood residential instability, or neighborhood ethnic heterogeneity, that is, the individual scales that comprised NSD. However, turning to the composite

Table 1 Participant characteristics, $n = 424$

Characteristic	N (%) or mean (SD)
Age, mean (SD)	60.5 (11.5)
Sex	
Female	224 (52.8)
Male	200 (47.2)
Educational level	
Some HS	24 (5.7)
HS grad or GED	101 (23.9)
Some college	154 (36.3)
College degree	88 (20.8)
Grad degree	57 (13.4)
Race	
White	271 (63.9)
Black	138 (32.6)
Other	15 (3.5)
Latino	
No	417 (98.4)
Yes	7 (1.7)
Duration of diabetes, mean (SD)	8.2 (7.6)
Diabetes empowerment, mean (SD)	4.3 (0.5)
Diabetes self-care, mean (SD)	3.4 (1.4)
Diabetes distress, mean (SD)	10.5 (12.8)
Comorbidities, mean (SD)	3.4 (1.9)
Self-reported use of acute or emergency health care services, mean (SD)	1.2 (2.3)
A1c, mean (SD)	7.5 (1.1)
Neighborhood economic disadvantage[a]	
Low	52 (12.3)
Medium	314 (74.1)
High	58 (13.7)
Neighborhood residential instability[a]	
Low	61 (14.4)
Medium	288 (67.9)
High	75 (17.7)
Neighborhood ethnic heterogeneity[a]	
Low	79 (18.6)
Medium	265 (62.5)
High	80 (18.9)
NSD[a]	
Low	71 (16.8)
Medium	300 (70.8)
High	53 (12.5)

NSD refers to neighborhood social disorganization
[a] For all of the neighborhood variables, low was defined as one standard deviation below the mean, and high was defined as one standard deviation above the mean

measure of NSD, individuals living in neighborhoods with high NSD had higher A1c values than individuals living in neighborhoods with medium NSD (B = 0.47, $p = 0.003$), whereas individuals living in neighborhoods with low NSD had similar A1c values compared to individuals living in neighborhoods with medium NSD (B = 0.17, $p = 0.21$).

Use of acute or emergency health care services

Turning to self-reported use of acute or emergency health care services (Table 2), individuals living in neighborhoods with high neighborhood economic disadvantage reported greater use of acute or emergency health care services (B = 0.49, $p = 0.04$) than individuals living in neighborhoods with medium economic disadvantage, while the individual measures of neighborhood residential instability and neighborhood ethnic heterogeneity were not significantly related to utilization. There were no associations with the composite measure of NSD.

Multilevel models examining A1c

Table 3 provides information from the four different models regarding individual and neighborhood-level predictors of A1c. In the null model, 3.3% of the total variability in A1c was due to variation between neighborhoods, while the remainder of the variation in A1c was due to variation within neighborhoods, that is, individual variation.

Model 1

We observed no significant relationships between A1c and demographic characteristics (i.e., race, age sex, educational level).

Model 2

Several psychosocial and clinical variables, including greater years with diabetes (B = 0.04, $p < 0.001$), greater diabetes distress (B = 0.02, $p < 0.001$), and greater diabetes empowerment (B = 0.24, $p = 0.03$) were significantly associated with higher A1c values, while greater self-care (B = − 0.10, $p = 0.02$) and comorbidities (B = − 0.07, $p = 0.03$) were associated with lower A1c values.

Model 3

There were no associations between A1c and neighborhood economic disadvantage, neighborhood residential instability, or neighborhood ethnic heterogeneity, that is, the individual scales that comprised NSD. Greater years with diabetes (B = 0.04, $p < 0.001$), greater diabetes distress (B = 0.02, $p < 0.001$), and greater diabetes empowerment (B = 0.25, $p = 0.02$) were all still associated with higher A1c values, while greater self-care (B = − 0.10, $p = 0.02$) and greater comorbidities (B = − 0.06, $p = 0.04$) were still associated with lower A1c values.

Table 2 Unadjusted effects of neighborhood variables on outcomes, $n = 424$

Variable	A1c[a]		Self-reported use of acute or emergency health care services[a]	
	Regression Coefficient B (95% CI)	p-value	Regression Coefficient B (95% CI)	p-value
Neighborhood economic disadvantage				
Low	0.26 (−0.06, 0.58)	0.11	−0.55 (−1.09, −0.01)	0.05
Medium	REF		REF	
High	0.23 (−0.08, 0.54)	0.15	0.49* (0.03, 0.95)	0.04
Neighborhood residential instability				
Low	0.07 (−0.23, 0.38)	0.63	−0.42 (−0.94, 0.09)	0.11
Medium	REF		REF	
High	0.19 (−0.09, 0.47)	0.18	−0.22 (−0.69, 0.24)	0.33
Neighborhood ethnic heterogeneity				
Low	−0.002 (−0.28, 0.27)	0.98	−0.27 (−0.74, 0.20)	0.25
Medium	REF		REF	
High	0.16 (−0.12, 0.43)	0.26	0.02 (−0.43, 0.46)	0.94
NSD (composite measure)				
Low	0.17 (−0.10, 0.45)	0.21	−0.25 (−0.72, 0.22)	0.29
Medium	REF		REF	
High	0.47** (0.16, 0.78)	0.003	0.04 (−0.44, 0.53)	0.86

NSD refers to neighborhood social disorganization

* $p < 0.05$

** $p < 0.01$

[a]Model adjusts for clustering of observations within census tract, but does not adjust for any individual-level demographic, psychosocial, or clinical variables. Each neighborhood variable was analyzed separately

Model 4

As hypothesized, individuals who lived in neighborhoods with high NSD (the composite measure) had higher A1c values (B = 0.39, $p = 0.01$), when compared to individuals who lived in neighborhoods with medium NSD. There was no difference in A1c values, however, for individuals living in neighborhoods with low NSD, compared to individuals living in neighborhoods with medium NSD (B = 0.09, $p = 0.52$). Greater years with diabetes (B = 0.04, $p < 0.001$), greater diabetes distress (B = 0.02, $p = 0.001$), and greater diabetes empowerment (B = 0.24, $p = 0.03$) were all still associated with higher A1c values, while greater self-care (B = −0.10, $p = 0.01$) and greater comorbidities (B = −0.06, $p = 0.04$) were still associated with lower A1c values.

Comparisons to unadjusted effects

The role of the composite measure of NSD was reduced somewhat by the inclusion of other variables in the models. Compared to the unadjusted effects in Table 2, the regression coefficient comparing high and medium NSD declined in magnitude (from B = 0.47 to B = 0.39) and level of significance (from $p = 0.003$ to p = 0.01).

Multilevel models examining self-reported use of acute or emergency health care services

For acute or emergency use of health care services, we used a series of Poisson models to model the non-normal data. In Poisson regression, there is no estimate of ICC [37]. As a result, we compared the magnitude of clustering by comparing an empty fixed model with a fixed intercept and no clustering of the data to a random intercept null model with clustering specified [37]. Results indicated that the model that incorporated clustering had lower Akaike Information Criteria and Bayesian Information Criterion values, suggesting better fit. Table 4 provides information from the four different models regarding individual and neighborhood-level predictors of acute or emergency health care utilization.

Model 1

We observed no significant relationships between self-reported use of acute or emergency health care services and some demographic characteristics (i.e., race, age sex, educational level), however, increasing age was negatively associated with self-reported use of acute or emergency health care service (B = −0.03, $p < 0.001$). In addition, individuals with a high school degree reported greater use of acute or emergency health care services (B = 0.33, $p = 0.02$), compared to individuals with some college.

Model 2

Turning to psychosocial and clinical variables, greater co-morbidities (B = 0.23, $p < 0.001$) was associated with greater self-reported use of acute or emergency health care

Table 3 Effects of neighborhood variables and correlates on A1c, $n = 424$

Variable[a]	Model 1		Model 2		Model 3		Model 4	
	Regression Coefficient B (95% CI)	p-value	Regression Coefficient B (95% CI)	p-value	Regression Coefficient B (95% CI)	p-value	Regression Coefficient B (95% CI)	p-value
Intercept	7.55 (7.48, 7.66)	< 0.001	7.55 (7.45, 7.65)	< 0.001	7.55 (7.45, 7.65)	< 0.001	7.55 (7.45, 7.64)	< 0.001
Sex								
Female	REF		REF		REF		REF	
Male	0.01 (−0.20, 0.22)	0.91	0.02 (−0.18, 0.22)	0.84	0.02 (−0.19, 0.22)	0.87	0.01 (−0.19, 0.22)	0.90
Age	−0.01 (−0.01, 0.00)	0.28	0.00 (−0.01, 0.01)	0.53	0.00 (−0.01, 0.01)	0.48	0.00 (−0.01, 0.01)	0.48
Race								
White	REF		REF		REF		REF	
Black	0.02 (−0.21, 0.25)	0.86	−0.03 (−0.26, 0.19)	0.77	−0.06 (−0.30, 0.18)	0.61	−0.07 (−0.30, 0.16)	0.54
Other	0.39 (−0.17, 0.96)	0.17	0.34 (−0.2, 0.88)	0.22	0.26 (−0.29, 0.81)	0.36	0.25 (−0.30, 0.79)	0.37
Educational level								
Some HS	0.16 (−0.31, 0.62)	0.51	0.03 (−0.42, 0.48)	0.91	0.05 (−0.41, 0.51)	0.83	0.05 (−0.40, 0.50)	0.84
HS grad	−0.05 (−0.32, 0.22)	0.73	−0.01 (−0.27, 0.25)	0.96	−0.01 (−0.28, 0.25)	0.93	−0.01 (−0.26, 0.25)	0.97
Some college	REF		REF		REF		REF	
College grad	0.14 (−0.14, 0.42)	0.34	0.10 (−0.17, 0.37)	0.45	0.09 (−0.18, 0.37)	0.49	0.13 (−0.14, 0.4)	0.34
Grad	−0.02 (−0.35, 0.31)	0.90	−0.05 (−0.36, 0.27)	0.77	−0.06 (−0.38, 0.26)	0.71	−0.03 (−0.34, 0.29)	0.87
Years with diabetes	–	–	0.04*** (0.02, 0.05)	< 0.001	0.04*** (0.02, 0.05)	< 0.001	0.04*** (0.02, 0.05)	< 0.001
Diabetes distress	–	–	0.02*** (0.01, 0.03)	< 0.001	0.02*** (0.01, 0.03)	< 0.001	0.02*** (0.01, 0.03)	< 0.001
Diabetes empowerment	–	–	0.24* (0.03, 0.45)	0.03	0.25* (0.04, 0.46)	0.02	0.24* (0.03, 0.45)	0.03
Self-reported use of acute or emergency health care services	–	–	−0.01 (−0.06, 0.03)	0.61	−0.01 (−0.06, 0.04)	0.65	−0.01 (−0.06, 0.03)	0.60
Self-care	–	–	−0.10* (−0.18, −0.02)	0.02	−0.10* (−0.18, −0.02)	0.02	−0.10* (−0.18, −0.02)	0.01
Comorbidities	–		−0.07* (−0.13, −0.01)	0.03	−0.06* (−0.12, 0.00)	0.04	−0.06* (−0.12, 0.00)	0.04
Neighborhood economic disadvantage								
Low	–	–	–	–	0.20 (−0.14, 0.54)	0.25	–	–
Medium	–	–	–	–	REF	–	–	–
High	–	–	–	–	0.11 (−0.21, 0.42)	0.51	–	–
Neighborhood residential instability								
Low	–	–	–	–	0.01 (−0.31, 0.33)	0.95	–	–
Medium	–	–	–	–	REF		–	–
High	–	–	–	–	0.18 (−0.10, 0.46)	0.21	–	–
Neighborhood ethnic heterogeneity								
Low	–	–	–	–	−0.03 (−0.3, 0.25)	0.84	–	–
Medium	–	–	–	–	REF		–	–
High	–	–	–	–	0.01 (−0.26, 0.28)	0.94	–	–
NSD (composite measure)								
Low	–	–	–	–	–	–	0.09 (−0.18, 0.36)	0.52
Medium	–	–	–	–	–	–	REF	
High	–	–	–	–	–	–	0.39* (0.08, 0.69)	0.01

Model 1 - Individual demographic variables. Model 2 - Individual demographic, psychosocial, and clinical variables. Model 3 - Individual demographic, psychosocial, and clinical variables and separate NSD measures. Model 4 - Individual demographic, psychosocial, and clinical variables and composite NSD measure

NSD refers to neighborhood social disorganization

* $p < 0.05$

*** $p < 0.001$

[a]In all models, variables were grand mean centered to increase interpretability

Table 4 Effects of neighborhood variables and correlates on self-reported use of acute or emergency health care services, $n = 424$

Variable[a]	Model 1		Model 2		Model 3		Model 4	
	Regression Coefficient	p-value	Regression Coefficient	p-value	Regression Coefficient	p-value	Regression Coefficient	p-value
	B (95% CI)		B (95% CI)		B (95% CI)		B (95% CI)	
Intercept	−0.31 (−0.53, −0.10)	0.003	−0.34 (−0.53, −0.14)	0.001	−0.33 (−0.53, −0.14)	0.001	−0.34 (−0.54, −0.14)	0.001
Sex								
Female	REF		REF		REF		REF	
Male	−0.07 (−0.15, 0.15)	0.52	0.12 (−0.11, 0.35)	0.30	0.12 (−0.11, 0.35)	0.32	0.12 (−0.11, 0.35)	0.32
Age	−0.03*** (−0.02, −0.02)	< 0.001	−0.04*** (−0.05, −0.02)	< 0.001	−0.03*** (−0.05, −0.02)	< 0.001	−0.04*** (−0.05, −0.02)	< 0.001
Race								
White	REF		REF		REF		REF	
Black	0.01 (−0.27, 0.26)	0.91	0.1 (−0.16, 0.37)	0.45	0.05 (−0.22, 0.32)	0.71	0.1 (−0.17, 0.36)	0.48
Other	−0.21 (−0.31, 0.44)	0.52	−0.26 (−0.94, 0.41)	0.44	−0.31 (−1.00, 0.37)	0.37	−0.27 (−0.95, 0.4)	0.43
Educational level								
Some HS	0.03 (−0.41, 0.53)	0.91	−0.13 (−0.65, 0.39)	0.63	−0.19 (−0.71, 0.33)	0.47	−0.13 (−0.65, 0.39)	0.63
HS grad	0.33* (−0.27, 0.59)	0.02	0.16 (−0.12, 0.44)	0.27	0.13 (−0.16, 0.41)	0.38	0.16 (−0.12, 0.44)	0.27
Some college	REF		REF		REF		REF	
College grad	−0.20 (−0.13, 0.12)	0.22	−0.24 (−0.58, 0.09)	0.16	−0.25 (−0.59, 0.08)	0.14	−0.24 (−0.58, 0.1)	0.16
Grad	−0.04 (−0.34, 0.34)	0.84	−0.15 (−0.53, 0.23)	0.43	−0.12 (−0.50, 0.26)	0.52	−0.15 (−0.53, 0.23)	0.43
Years with diabetes	–	–	0.00 (−0.02, 0.02)	0.91	0.00 (−0.02, 0.02)	0.92	0.00 (−0.02, 0.02)	0.91
Diabetes distress	–	–	0.00 (−0.01, 0.01)	0.33	0.01 (0.00, 0.02)	0.26	0.00 (−0.01, 0.01)	0.34
Diabetes empowerment	–	–	0.06 (−0.18, 0.3)	0.60	0.07 (−0.17, 0.31)	0.58	0.06 (−0.18, 0.3)	0.61
A1c	–	–	−0.05 (−0.17, 0.07)	0.42	−0.05 (−0.17, 0.07)	0.38	−0.05 (−0.17, 0.07)	0.41
Self-care	–	–	−0.06 (−0.15, 0.04)	0.23	−0.05 (−0.15, 0.04)	0.25	−0.06 (−0.15, 0.03)	0.21
Comorbidities	–		0.23*** (0.17, 0.3)	< 0.001	0.23*** (0.17, 0.29)	< 0.001	0.23*** (0.17, 0.3)	< 0.001
Neighborhood economic disadvantage								
Low	–	–	–	–	−0.34 (−0.92, 0.25)	0.26	–	–
Medium	–	–	–	–	REF		–	–
High	–	–	–	–	0.60* (0.10, 1.09)	0.02	–	–
Neighborhood residential instability								
Low	–	–	–	–	0.01 (−0.55, 0.57)	0.97	–	–
Medium	–	–	–	–	REF		–	–
High	–	–	–	–	−0.39 (−0.87, 0.09)	0.11	–	–
Neighborhood ethnic heterogeneity								
Low	–	–	–	–	−0.08 (−0.55, 0.39)	0.74	–	–
Medium	–	–	–	–	REF		–	–
High	–	–	–	–	−0.08 (−0.51, 0.36)	0.73	–	–
NSD (composite measure)								
Low	–	–	–	–	–	–	−0.04 (−0.50, 0.42)	0.87
Medium	–	–	–	–	–	–	REF	
High	–	–	–	–	–	–	0.08 (−0.40, 0.56)	0.75

Model 1 - Individual demographic variables. Model 2 - Individual demographic, psychosocial, and clinical variables. Model 3 - Individual demographic, psychosocial, and clinical variables and separate NSD measures. Model 4 - Individual demographic, psychosocial, and clinical variables and composite NSD measure

NSD refers to neighborhood social disorganization

* $p < 0.05$

** $p < 0.01$

*** $p < 0.001$

[a] In all models, variables were grand mean centered to increase interpretability

services. Age was still negatively associated with self-reported use of acute or emergency health care services (B = – 0.04, $p < 0.001$).

Model 3
In the disaggregated evaluation of NSD indicators (Model 3), individuals who lived in neighborhoods with high economic disadvantage reported using acute or emergency health care services more than individuals who lived in neighborhoods with medium economic disadvantage (B = 0.60, $p = 0.02$). Age was still negatively associated with self-reported use of acute or emergency health care services (B = – 0.03, $p < 0.001$). In addition, greater comorbidities was still associated with greater self-reported use of acute or emergency health care services (B = 0.23, $p < 0.001$).

Model 4
Turning finally to the composite measure of NSD, it showed no association with self-reported use of acute or emergency health. Age was still negatively associated with self-reported use of acute or emergency health care services (B = – 0.04, $p < 0.001$). In addition, greater comorbidities was still associated with greater self-reported use of acute or emergency health care services (B = 0.23, $p < 0.001$).

Comparisons to unadjusted effects
The role of neighborhood economic disadvantage in explaining acute/emergency utilization was not significantly altered by the inclusion of other variables in the models. Compared to the unadjusted model in Table 2, the regression coefficient comparing high and medium neighborhood economic disadvantage was of similar magnitude (from B = 0.49 to B = 0.60) and level of significance (from $p = 0.04$ to $p = 0.02$).

Model diagnostics
As a sensitivity analysis, we also entered in select individual-level variables as random effects into the models. However, when entered, the respective models for each outcome failed to converge, thereby indicating that this may not be an appropriate way to model the data. Additionally, we compared the Akaike Information Criteria and Bayesian Information Criterion values from the different models for A1c and use of acute or emergency health care services. These indicators suggested that the models with the composite and individual NSD variables respectively (Model 4 for A1c and Model 3 for acute or emergency health care service use) demonstrated the best fit (smallest Akaike Information Criteria and Bayesian Information Criterion values).

Discussion
In this study among individuals with type 2 diabetes, we found individuals living in neighborhoods with high NSD (a composite of economic, residential, and racial / ethnic diversity indicators) had greater A1c values than individuals living in neighborhoods with medium NSD and that individuals living in neighborhoods with high economic disadvantage had higher self-reported use of acute or emergency health care services than individuals living in neighborhoods with medium economic disadvantage. Controlling for individual level variables diminished this effect for A1c, but not for acute or emergency care.

When considered in light of previous research showing associations between neighborhood factors and diabetes outcomes [5–10, 25], our findings suggest that comprehensive approaches to diabetes management need to include attention to neighborhood context [8, 38]. Failure to do so may help explain the continuing disproportionate diabetes burden in many neighborhoods despite decades of attention to individual-level clinical care and education. While randomized controlled trials changing neighborhood disadvantage are almost nonexistent [8], there are innovative ways to encourage social interaction in neighborhoods (increasing vegetation and common spaces [39], designing homes with porches or stoops [40]), and encourage self-care behaviors, such as physical activity, through improvements to infrastructure like lighting or sidewalks [41]. However, care must be taken to design such interventions in culturally appropriate and sensitive ways by engaging community members and securing buy-in from neighborhood residents [42].

In addition, we found that *both* neighborhood and individual-level factors contributed to outcomes of individuals with type 2 diabetes (rather than one or the other). Some of the effects of the individual-level variables on diabetes outcomes ran counter to our expectation, e.g., that greater numbers of comorbidities was associated with lower A1c values, that increasing diabetes empowerment was associated with higher A1c values, and that increasing age was associated with greater self-reported use of acute or emergency health care services. Regarding the first unexpected finding, it is possible that individuals with more comorbidities had more reason to seek care from their physician and thus received more care. It is also important to note that this association was weak (p-values ranging from 0.03 to 0.04). Regarding the later unexpected finding, it should be noted that some research suggests that younger adults with diabetes may have worse glycemic control than older adults, may be less likely to take medication prescribed for diabetes, and may be less likely to visit health care professionals for services like blood pressure and cholesterol checks [43, 44].

For the most part, these findings—of both individual and neighborhood level variables being important for health—suggest that targeting factors at individual and larger ecological levels will remain important. Failing to acknowledge human agency downplays the important role that individuals and practitioners may play in making important lifestyle and behavioral changes. At the same time, relying too heavily on only individual-level change neglects the powerful role that environments and context have in influencing individuals' decisions and behaviors.

Multilevel level interventions, which target behavioral change at more than one ecological level [45], will remain important tools in improving health and reducing health disparities. Yet, most public health interventions are targeted at intrapersonal and interpersonal levels [46]. This is likely due to a number of reasons, including but not limited to: lack of training or resources for health professionals seeking to implement institutional, community, or policy-level programs; lack of theories or training in theories for creating interventions to change upper ecological levels; fewer metrics to evaluate changes at upper ecological levels; and added financial and logistical difficulty in trying to address upper ecological determinants. Transdisciplinary approaches, in which theories and methods are integrated across disciplines, may be particularly beneficial in disseminating lessons learned for future research on neighborhoods and health [47].

Recommendations for future research
Based on the results of the present study, we identified three recommendations for future research. First, while we found that broad aspects of neighborhood disorganization encompassing economic, racial / ethnic diversity, and residential indicators were associated with A1c, which aligns with previous research finding NSD to be associated with metabolic syndrome among African American women [15], we found non-significant effects of neighborhood residential instability or ethnic heterogeneity on either A1c or self-reported use of acute or emergency health care services. It is possible that these constructs may not have been as important for our sample, which was composed of mostly older adults in the Southeastern U.S. Future research examining associations between NSD and diabetes outcomes in other settings and among other populations may be helpful, as well as critical investigation of ethnic heterogeneity as a construct.

Second, mediation analysis with these and other variables may be an important, underutilized tool for future research. Brown et al. has theorized that socioeconomic position (both at the neighborhood level and at the level of the individual relative to his or her position in the neighborhood) influences health through proximal mediators that include: health behaviors (e.g., diet/medication adherence, exercise), availability of and access to health care resources, and processes of care (i.e., technical and interpersonal care provided to patients within the health care setting) [48]. However, studies examining variables that mediate associations between neighborhoods and

health are few and far between. For instance, in a systematic review examining associations between neighborhood characteristics and health outcomes among individuals with diabetes in the U.S., only 4 of the 38 identified studies conducted mediation analysis (Kowitt SD, Bhushan N, Fisher EB. Taking the "self" out of "self management": a systematic review of the effects of neighborhood and community characteristics on diabetes outcomes in the United States, in preparation). Structural equation modeling and longitudinal studies will surely advance understanding of how neighborhoods affect health outcomes and which variables may act as mediators, confounders, or controls.

Finally, this is a novel study illustrating associations between neighborhood disadvantage and self-reported use of emergency or acute health care services among individuals with diabetes. This points to the importance of these factors in efforts to decrease avoidable emergency and acute or hospital care, a major priority of "bending the curve" through health care reform in the US as well as internationally. This study also builds upon other observations of the importance of neighborhood factors in avoidable care [49–51] In the present study, neighborhood disadvantage was evaluated at the level of the census tract. In contrast, some of the work of Brenner and colleagues in Camden New Jersey has explored hot spots defined at more micro levels, such as buildings and neighborhood blocks. Other researchers have proposed the idea of "spatial polygamy," which refers to the idea that individuals are exposed to multiple contexts that interact to affect health (not just neighborhoods) [52]. Future research will address these various determinants and contexts, and importantly, will need to identify levels of influence that may be actionable at the level of individual or community interventions and policies.

Limitations
We acknowledge several limitations. Most notably, our study design was cross-sectional, which limits our ability to infer causality. Second, while we included individual-level control variables (demographic, psychosocial, and clinical), we did not have a measure of individual-level income or insurance, which may have accounted for the observed effects especially of neighborhood economic disadvantage. While we included a measure of education, which has been used as a proxy of income in previous studies, further research controlling for income *and* examining interactions between neighborhood income and individual income will be important. Third, data came from a convenience sample of individuals in central North Carolina; findings may not generalize to other populations or settings. Fourth, level 1 residuals for one of our outcomes (A1c) appeared to be mostly normally distributed but there was evidence of a slight violation of normality, which could have biased results (e.g.,

biased fixed effects, standard errors, or variance components).

Fifth, our measure of use of acute and emergency health care services was self-reported and therefore subject to a number of potential biases, including information / recall bias. Some individuals may have incorrectly recalled how many times they had used a specific acute or emergency health care service. Additionally, the four items used to assess self-reported use of acute or emergency health care services were not mutually exclusive. A participant that reported "yes" to being seen in the ER may have also reported "yes" to having EMS being called and this would have been counted as two visits. Moreover, the questions used to ascertain acute or emergency care visits were not disease specific and could have been related to factors beyond diabetes. However, it is important to note that previous research has found self-reported hospitalization and emergency department visits to have high concordance with medical chart data and claims databases [53]. Supporting the validity of our measure, we also found that increasing number of comorbidities was associated with increased self-reported use of acute or emergency health care services. In addition, when we dichotomized the measure of use of acute / emergency health care services as 1 = any reported encounter or 0 = no reported encounter, both diabetes distress and high NSD were still associated with use ($p < 0.05$; data not shown).

Finally, while we cannot determine the temporality of observed associations (i.e., whether individuals who use emergency health care services were more likely to choose to live in more disadvantaged neighborhoods, or whether some aspect of neighborhood disadvantage caused people use more emergency health care services), our findings suggest that future research should explore this association. Our study is strengthened by our use of multilevel modeling techniques to control for any clustering within census-tracts and our inclusion of both demographic, psychosocial, and clinical variables in our models.

Conclusions
Neighborhood and other ecological factors contributing to diabetes outcomes are poorly understood, yet growing research highlights the influence of neighborhoods and communities on management of diabetes as well as other chronic diseases. This research offers an in-depth exploration of how broad aspects of NSD are related to glycemic control and how economic disadvantage in particular is associated with avoidable use of acute and emergency health care.

Abbreviations
A1c: Glycemic control; CI: Confidence interval; DES-SF: Diabetes Empowerment Scale-Short Form; ICC: Intraclass correlation; NSD: Neighborhood social disorganization; PAID: Problem Areas in Diabetes scale; SES: Socioeconomic status

Funding
Research reported in this publication was partially funded through a Patient-Centered Outcomes Research Institute (PCORI) Award (CE-12-11-4980). The views in this article are solely the responsibility of the authors and do not necessarily represent the views of the Patient-Centered Outcomes Research Institute (PCORI), its Board of Governors or Methodology Committee. Research reported in this publication was also partially funded by a University of North Carolina at Chapel Hill Graduate School Summer Research Fellowship.

Authors' contributions
SK and EF designed the study. MM, KD, and LY were responsible for acquiring the data. SK was responsible for data analysis. SK drafted the manuscript. All authors provided critical revision of the manuscript. KD and LY obtained funding for the parent study. SK obtained funding for the present study's analysis. All authors take full responsibility for the work as a whole, including the study design, access to data, and the decision to submit and publish the manuscript. All authors read and approved the final manuscript

Competing interests
The authors declare that they have no competing interests.

Author details
[1]Peers for Progress and Department of Health Behavior, Gillings School of Global Public Health, University of North Carolina at Chapel Hill, Rosenau Hall, CB #7440, Chapel Hill, NC 27599-7440, USA. [2]Department of Family Medicine, University of North Carolina at Chapel Hill, Chapel Hill, NC 27599, USA. [3]Cecil G. Sheps Center for Health Services Research, University of North Carolina at Chapel Hill, Chapel Hill, NC 27599, USA. [4]Division of Endocrinology & Metabolism, School of Medicine, University of North Carolina at Chapel Hill, Chapel Hill, NC 27599, USA.

References
1. Centers for Disease Control and Prevention. National diabetes statistics report: estimates of diabetes and its burden in the United States, 2014. Atlanta: US Department of Health and Human Services, Centers for Disease Control and Prevention; 2014.
2. American Diabetes Association. Economic costs of diabetes in the U.S. in 2017. Diabetes Care. 2018;41(5):917–28.
3. Barker LE, Kirtland KA, Gregg EW, Geiss LS, Thompson TJ. Geographic distribution of diagnosed diabetes in the U.S.: a diabetes belt. Am J Prev Med. 2011;40(4):434–9.
4. Fisher EB, Brownson CA, O'Toole ML, Shelty G, Anwuri W, Glasgow RE. Ecological approaches to self-management: the case of diabetes. Am J Public Health. 2005;95(9):1523.
5. Gary-Webb TL, Baptiste-Roberts K, Pham L, Wesche-Thobaben J, Patricio J, Pi-Sunyer FX, et al. Neighborhood socioeconomic status, depression, and health status in the look AHEAD (action for health in diabetes) study. BMC Public Health. 2011;11:349.
6. Smalls BL, Gregory CM, Zoller JS, Egede LE. Direct and indirect effects of neighborhood factors and self-care on glycemic control in adults with type 2 diabetes. J Diabetes Complicat. 2015;29(2):186–91.
7. Mezuk B, Chaikiat A, Li X, Sundquist J, Kendler KS, Sundquist K. Depression, neighborhood deprivation and risk of type 2 diabetes. Health Place. 2013;23:63–9.
8. Ludwig J, Sanbonmatsu L, Gennetian L, Adam E, Duncan GJ, Katz LF, et al. Neighborhoods, obesity, and diabetes--a randomized social experiment. N Engl J Med. 2011;365(16):1509–19.
9. Auchincloss AH, Diez Roux AV, Mujahid MS, Shen M, Bertoni AG, Carnethon MR. Neighborhood resources for physical activity and healthy foods and incidence of type 2 diabetes mellitus: the multi-ethnic study of atherosclerosis. Arch Intern Med. 2009;169(18):1698–704.
10. Schootman M, Andresen EM, Wolinsky FD, Malmstrom TK, Miller JP, Yan Y, et al. The effect of adverse housing and neighborhood conditions on the development of diabetes mellitus among middle-aged African Americans. Am J Epidemiol. 2007;166(4):379–87.
11. Diez Roux AV, Mair C. Neighborhoods and health. Ann N Y Acad Sci. 2010;1186:125–45.
12. Browning CR. The span of collective efficacy: extending social disorganization theory to partner violence. J Marriage Fam. 2002;64(4):833–50.
13. Browning CR, Cagney KA. Neighborhood structural disadvantage, collective efficacy, and self-rated physical health in an urban setting. J Health Soc Behav. 2002;43(4):383–99.

14. Kawachi I, Berkman LF. Social Cohesion, Social Capital, and Health. In: Berkman LF, Kawachi I, Glymour M, editors. Social epidemiology. Second ed. New York: Oxford University Press; 2014.

15. Clark CR, Ommerborn MJ, Hickson DA, Grooms KN, Sims M, Taylor HA, et al. Neighborhood disadvantage, neighborhood safety and cardiometabolic risk factors in African Americans: biosocial associations in the Jackson heart study. PLoS One. 2013;8(5):e63254.

16. Foshee VA, Chang LY, McNaughton Reyes HL, Chen MS, Ennett ST. The synergy of family and neighborhood on rural dating violence victimization. Am J Prev Med. 2015;49(3):483–91.

17. Goodson A, Bouffard LA. The rural/urban divide: examining different types of assault through a social disorganization lens. J Interpers Violence. 2017:1–24. https://doi.org/10.1177/0886260517711179. [Epub ahead of print].

18. Bouffard LA, Muftić LR. The" rural mystique": social disorganization and violence beyond urban communities. West Criminol Rev. 2006;7(3):56.

19. Petee TA, Kowalski GS. Modeling rural violent crime rates: a test of social disorganization theory. Sociol Focus. 1993;26(1):87–9.

20. Osgood DW, Chambers JM. Social disorganization outside the metropolis: an analysis of rural youth violence. Criminology. 2000;38(1):81–116.

21. Browning CR, Dirlam J, Boettner B. From heterogeneity to concentration: Latino immigrant neighborhoods and collective efficacy perceptions in Los Angeles and Chicago. Soc Forces. 2016;95(2):779–807.

22. Abascal M, Baldassarri D. Love thy neighbor? Ethnoracial diversity and trust reexamined. Am J Sociol. 2015;121(3):722–82.

23. Laurence J, Bentley L. Does ethnic diversity have a negative effect on attitudes towards the community? A longitudinal analysis of the causal claims within the ethnic diversity and social cohesion debate. Eur Sociol Rev. 2015;32(1):54–67.

24. Turner MA, Rawlings L. Promoting neighborhood diversity: benefits, barriers, and strategies Washington DC: the Urban Institute; 2009 [June 13, 2018]. Available from: https://www.urban.org/sites/default/files/publication/30631/411955-Promoting-Neighborhood-Diversity-Benefits-Barriers-and-Strategies.PDF.

25. Karter AJ, Parker MM, Moffet HH, Ahmed AT, Ferrara A, Liu JY, et al. Missed appointments and poor glycemic control: an opportunity to identify high-risk diabetic patients. Med Care. 2004;42(2):110–5.

26. Young LA, Buse JB, Weaver MA, Vu MB, Mitchell CM, Blakeney T, et al. Glucose self-monitoring in non-insulin-treated patients with type 2 diabetes in primary care settings: a randomized trial. JAMA Intern Med. 2017;177(7):920–9.

27. Young LA, Buse JB, Weaver MA, Vu MB, Reese A, Mitchell CM, et al. Three approaches to glucose monitoring in non-insulin treated diabetes: a pragmatic randomized clinical trial protocol. BMC Health Serv Res. 2017;17(1):369.

28. Beyers JM, Bates JE, Pettit GS, Dodge KA. Neighborhood structure, parenting processes, and the development of youths' externalizing behaviors: a multilevel analysis. Am J Community Psychol. 2003;31(1–2):35–53.

29. Blau PM. Inequality and heterogeneity: a primitive theory of social structure. New York: Free Press; 1977.

30. Chang LY, Foshee VA, Reyes HL, Ennett ST, Halpern CT. Direct and indirect effects of neighborhood characteristics on the perpetration of dating violence across adolescence. J Youth Adolesc. 2015;44(3):727–44.

31. Reyes H, Foshee VA, Tharp AT, Ennett ST, Bauer DJ. Substance Use and Physical dating violence: the role of contextual moderators. Am J Prev Med. 2015;49(3):467–75.

32. Molnar BE, Cerda M, Roberts AL, Buka SL. Effects of neighborhood resources on aggressive and delinquent behaviors among urban youths. Am J Public Health. 2008;98(6):1086–93.

33. Welch GW, Jacobson AM, Polonsky WH. The problem areas in diabetes scale: an evaluation of its clinical utility. Diabetes Care. 1997;20(5):760–6.

34. Anderson RM, Fitzgerald JT, Gruppen LD, Funnell MM, Oh MS. The diabetes empowerment scale-short form (DES-SF). Diabetes Care. 2003;26(5):1641–2.

35. Toobert DJ, Hampson SE, Glasgow RE. The summary of diabetes self-care activities measure: results from 7 studies and a revised scale. Diabetes Care. 2000;23(7):943–50.

36. Snijders T, Bosker R. Multilevel analysis: an introduction to basic and advanced multilevel modeling. Thousand Oaks: Sage; 1999.

37. Aiken LS, Mistler SA, Coxe S, West SG. Analyzing count variables in individuals and groups: single level and multilevel models. Group Process Intergroup Relat. 2015;18(3):290–314.

38. Walker RJ, Smalls BL, Campbell JA, Strom Williams JL, Egede LE. Impact of social determinants of health on outcomes for type 2 diabetes: a systematic review. Endocrine. 2014;47(1):29–48.

39. Kweon B-S, Sullivan WC, Wiley AR. Green common spaces and the social integration of Inner-City older adults. Environ Behav. 1998;30(6):832–58.

40. Brown SC, Mason CA, Lombard JL, Martinez F, Plater-Zyberk E, Spokane AR, et al. The relationship of built environment to perceived social support and psychological distress in Hispanic elders: the role of "eyes on the street". J Gerontol B Psychol Sci Soc Sci. 2009;64(2):234–46.

41. Hajna S, Ross NA, Joseph L, Harper S, Dasgupta K. Neighbourhood walkability and daily steps in adults with type 2 diabetes. PLoS One. 2016;11(3):e0151544.

42. Dubowitz T, Ncube C, Leuschner K, Tharp-Gilliam S. A natural experiment opportunity in two low-income urban food desert communities: research design, community engagement methods, and baseline results. Health Educ Behav. 2015;42(1 Suppl):87s–96s.

43. Shamshirgaran SM, Mamaghanian A, Aliasgarzadeh A, Aiminisani N, Iranparvar-Alamdari M, Ataie J. Age differences in diabetes-related complications and glycemic control. BMC Endocr Disord. 2017;17:25.

44. Villarroel MA, Vahratian A, Ward BW. Health care utilization among U.S. adults with diagnosed diabetes, 2013. NCHS Data Brief. 2015;(183):1–8. https://www.cdc.gov/nchs/data/databriefs/db183.pdf.

45. Sallis JF, Owen N, Fisher EB. Ecological models of health behavior. Health behavior and health education: theory, research, and practice, vol. 4; 2008. p. 465–86.

46. Golden SD, Earp JA. Social ecological approaches to individuals and their contexts: twenty years of health education & behavior health promotion interventions. Health Educ Behav. 2012;39(3):364–72.

47. Wallerstein NB, Yen IH, Syme SL. Integration of social epidemiology and community-engaged interventions to improve health equity. Am J Public Health. 2011;101(5):822.

48. Brown AF, Ettner SL, Piette J, Weinberger M, Gregg E, Shapiro MF, et al. Socioeconomic position and health among persons with diabetes mellitus: a conceptual framework and review of the literature. Epidemiol Rev. 2004;26:63–77.

49. Burton J, Eggleston B, Brenner J, Truchil A, Zulkiewicz BA, Lewis MA. Community-based health education programs designed to improve clinical measures are unlikely to reduce short-term costs or utilization without additional features targeting these outcomes. Popul Health Manag. 2017;20(2):93–8.

50. Gross K, Brenner JC, Truchil A, Post EM, Riley AH. Building a citywide, all-payer, hospital claims database to improve health care delivery in a low-income, urban community. Popul Health Manag. 2013;16(Suppl 1):S20–5.

51. Kaufman S, Ali N, DeFiglio V, Craig K, Brenner J. Early efforts to target and enroll high-risk diabetic patients into urban community-based programs. Health Promot Pract. 2014;15(2 Suppl):62s–70s.

52. Matthews SA, Yang TC. Spatial polygamy and contextual exposures (SPACEs): promoting activity space approaches in research on place and health. Am Behav Sci. 2013;57(8):1057–81.

53. Dendukuri N, McCusker J, Bellavance F, Cardin S, Verdon J, Karp I, et al. Comparing the validity of different sources of information on emergency department visits: a latent class analysis. Med Care. 2005;43(3):266–75.

26

The association of depression and diabetes across methods, measures, and study contexts

Jaimie C. Hunter[1,2*], Brenda M. DeVellis[2], Joanne M. Jordan[3], M. Sue Kirkman[4], Laura A. Linnan[2], Christine Rini[5,6,7] and Edwin B. Fisher[2]

Abstract

Background: Empirical research has revealed a positive relationship between type 2 diabetes mellitus and depression, but questions remain regarding timing of depression measurement, types of instruments used to measure depression, and whether "depression" is defined as clinical depression or depressive symptoms. The present study sought to establish the robustness of the depression-diabetes relationship across depression definition, severity of depressive symptoms, recent depression, and lifetime depression in a nationally representative dataset and a large rural dataset.

Methods: The present examination, conducted between 2014 and 2015, used two large secondary datasets: the National Health and Nutrition Examination Survey (NHANES) from 2007 to 2008 ($n = 3072$) and the Arthritis, Coping, and Emotion Study (ACES) from 2002 to 2006 ($n = 2300$). Depressive symptoms in NHANES were measured using the Patient Health Questionnaire 9-item survey (PHQ-9). ACES used the Center for Epidemiologic Studies—Depression Scale (CES-D) to measure depressive symptoms and the Composite International Diagnostic Interview (CIDI) to measure diagnosable depression. Diabetes was modelled as the dichotomous outcome variable (presence vs. absence of diabetes). Logistic regression was used for all analyses, most of which were cross-sectional. Analyses controlled for age, ethnicity, sex, education, and body mass index, and NHANES analyses used sample weights to account for the complex survey design. Additional analyses using NHANES data focused on the addition of health behavior variables and inflammation to the model.

Results: *NHANES.* Every one-point increase in depressive symptoms was associated with a 5% increase in odds of having diabetes [OR: 1.05 (CI: 1.03, 1.07)]. These findings persisted after controlling for health behaviors and inflammation. *ACES.* For every one-point increase in depressive symptom score, odds of having diabetes increased by 2% [OR: 1.02 (CI: 1.01, 1.03)]. Recent (past 12 months) depression [OR: 1.49, (CI: 1.03, 2.13)] and lifetime depression [OR: 1.40 (CI: 1.09, 1.81)] were also significantly associated with having diabetes.

Conclusions: This study provides evidence for the robustness of the relationship between depression or depressive symptoms and diabetes and demonstrates that depression occurring over the lifetime can be associated with diabetes just as robustly as that which occurs more proximal to the time of study measurement.

Keywords: Depression, Diabetes, Psychosocial, Mental health

* Correspondence: jchunter@wakehealth.edu
[1]Department of Social Sciences and Health Policy, Division of Public Health Sciences, Wake Forest University School of Medicine, Medical Center Boulevard, Winston-Salem, NC 27157, USA
[2]Department of Health Behavior, Gillings School of Global Public Health, The University of North Carolina at Chapel Hill, Chapel Hill, NC, USA
Full list of author information is available at the end of the article

Background

Depression is devastating to productivity, relationships, and overall well-being and, in the United States (US), remains second only to back pain as a leading cause of disability [1]. Despite having an estimated lifetime prevalence of 20% in adults [2], it frequently goes undiagnosed and untreated, owing in part to a dramatic shortage of mental health care providers [3]. Untreated depression is associated with greater quantity and severity of physical and mental health comorbidities [4]. For instance, depression is frequently comorbid with sleep problems, [5] anxiety, [6] and cardiovascular disease [7]. Depression is often associated with risky health behaviors, such as poor diet, sedentariness, and smoking, which, in turn, increase risk for chronic diseases like obesity and diabetes [8].

Diabetes mellitus, a frequent comorbidity, impacts 26 million Americans. Approximately 95% of cases are type 2 [9]. The prevalence of diabetes has increased rapidly, fueled by a worldwide increase in obesity, population aging, and longer life expectancies [10]. Altering behavioral risk factors like unhealthy diet and sedentariness reduces diabetes risk [11, 12]. Innovative prevention efforts are needed, and, therefore, interest in psychosocial approaches to preventing diabetes has grown in recent years [13–15]. As one example, peer support programs, in which trained helpers offer guidance and support for people at risk for a health condition, have proven invaluable in encouraging individuals to follow recommended health behaviors. Improved health behaviors, in turn, reduce risk for diabetes and other chronic diseases [16, 17].

People with depression are more likely to have diabetes than those in the general population [18]. The reverse is also true; depression prevalence among individuals living with diabetes is estimated to range from 9% to 35% [19, 20]. Bidirectional pathways drive this comorbidity. Researchers using a decade of data from the Nurses' Health Study found a 17% increase in diabetes risk for individuals with depression and a 29% increase in depression risk for those with diabetes [21]. Another study showed a 43% increase in depression risk over six years for participants with baseline diabetes and a 102% increase in risk for diabetes among those with depression at baseline [22].

Knowing whether timing of depression diagnosis (recent versus at any point over the lifetime) matters in association with diabetes risk would prove informative for preventive interventions. The goal of the present study was therefore to explore the robustness of the relationship between depressive symptoms and diabetes status across varied samples, measures, and contexts. Analyses for this study were based on two distinct samples: a large, nationally representative sample (the National Health and Nutrition Examination Survey [NHANES]) [23] and a population sample addressing arthritis and other chronic diseases among rural communities in North Carolina (the Arthritis, Coping, and Emotion Study [ACES]), part of a larger study of osteoarthritis in the region known as the Johnston County Osteoarthritis Project (JoCo OA) [24]. Researchers hypothesized a robust, positive relationship between depression and diabetes status.

Methods

Study samples

The present investigation, conducted between 2014 and 2016, was a secondary analysis of data from two independent studies: NHANES and ACES. NHANES is a continuing series of independent studies of chronic disease risk factors among non-institutionalized civilians in the United States. Conducted in person, the study draws data from interviews and laboratory measures. The de-identified data are freely available from the National Center for Health Statistics [23]. Because the ACES study enrolled only individuals 45 years of age and older, the present NHANES analyses were restricted to adults in this age range.

ACES data were collected between 2002 and 2006 from a subset of individuals who participated in JoCo OA, a longitudinal, epidemiological study of knee and hip osteoarthritis in rural North Carolina (NC) [24]. Using in-person, in-depth interviews, ACES investigators collected data to identify psychosocial, behavioral, and disease-related factors that mitigate or exacerbate psychiatric comorbidity with physical illness in older adults. ACES included self-reported psychosocial data and collected participants' weight and height. Inclusion criteria were being Caucasian or African American, living in Johnston County, being a civilian, and being at least 45 years of age. The first wave of data, collected from 2001 to 2006, was used in the present study.

Measures

Depression

NHANES included the nine item Patient Health Questionnaire (PHQ-9) [25, 26]. Items assess the frequency of depressive symptoms as categorized in the fourth edition of the *Diagnostic and Statistical Manual for Mental Disorders* (DSM-IV) (e.g., "little interest or pleasure in doing things"), and responses are made on the following scale: not at all (0), several days (1), more than half the days (2), and nearly every day (3). Responses were summed to create a score with a possible range of 0 to 27; higher scores indicate higher levels of depressive symptoms. The PHQ-9 has been validated in individuals living with diabetes [27].

ACES included the Composite International Diagnostic Interview (CIDI), [28] which can identify probable cases of depression that occurred over the lifetime and over the previous 12 months using an algorithm based on third edition of the *Diagnostic and Statistical Manual for Mental Disorders, Revised* (DSM-III-R) criteria. The study also assessed depressive symptoms using the Center for Epidemiologic Studies–Depression (CES-D) scale [29]. The CES-D contains 20 items (e.g., "I was bothered by things that usually don't bother me"), and participants rated how often they were true: rarely or none of the time (0); some or a little of the time (1); occasionally or a moderate amount of time (2); or most or all of the time (3). The CES-D responses were summed to create a score of 0 to 60, with higher scores indicating higher levels of depressive symptoms. Reverse coding was used where appropriate.

Diabetes

Type 2 diabetes was a dichotomous outcome variable in both studies. The 2007–2008 NHANES study followed standards outlined by the Centers for Disease Control and Prevention (CDC): a respondent was classified as having diabetes if he or she had a fasting plasma glucose (FPG) level of at least 126 or a glycated hemoglobin (HbA$_1$c) level of at least 6.5, or if he or she reported having a doctor's diagnosis of diabetes [9]. For ACES, diabetes was defined using a dichotomous, self-reported item indicating that a doctor had "ever told" the respondent that he or she has diabetes or high blood sugar. Recent studies examining the veracity of self-reported diabetes status as compared to health insurance administrative records and measured diabetes indices revealed very strong correlations between the measures [30, 31].

Covariates

Both studies controlled for sex (female = 1, male = 0); ethnicity (Caucasians = 0, African Americans = 1, NHANES Latino = 2, NHANES Other = 3); age; body mass index (BMI); and education (high school or less = 1, more than high school education = 0). Income data were not collected in the ACES study because investigators felt they were too sensitive.

Statistical analysis

Analyses were conducted using SAS version 9.3 software (SAS Institute, Cary, NC). Descriptive statistics were used to examine the distribution of all variables. Univariate analyses of quantitative (continuous) variables proceeded using PROC MEANS and PROC UNIVARIATE to determine range, skewness and kurtosis, and statistical mean and standard deviation. PROC FREQ was used to provide a descriptive examination of each categorical variable. It was unnecessary to transform any variable to facilitate inclusion in subsequent multivariate analyses; all continuous variables met criteria for

normalcy according to these tests. Bivariate analyses (Wald chi-square tests) were conducted to determine the degree to which each predictor was related to diabetes status.

In multivariate analyses, categorical variables with more than two levels (e.g., "ethnicity" in NHANES) were entered into the model as ordinal variables. SAS PROC LOGISTIC (for ACES data) and PROC SURVEYLOGISTIC (for NHANES data, given the complex survey design) were used for logistic regression analysis. For the NHANES data, the logistic regression models were adjusted for the complex sampling design by using Mobile Examination Center (MEC) weights. Odds ratios and 95% Wald confidence limits were reported. Multivariate analyses statistically controlled for age, ethnicity, sex, education level, and body mass index.

Further analyses were conducted using the NHANES data, which included health behavior variables associated with diabetes that were not included in the ACES dataset, to gain a more robust understanding of the way health behaviors contributed to the relationship between depression and diabetes. These analyses allowed for evaluation of the association of depressive symptoms with diabetes after controlling for health behavior variables, which included: smoking (never = 0, former = 1, current = 2), sedentary behavior (self-reported lack of any physical activity; active = 0, sedentary = 1), and self-rated healthiness of diet (poor/fair = 1, good/very good/excellent = 0). This model also controlled for inflammation (C-reactive protein from laboratory blood draw, measured quantitatively).

The Institutional Review Board at the University of North Carolina at Chapel Hill reviewed the protocol for the present study and exempted it, as it involved only secondary analysis of de-identified data. Participants in each of the constituent studies provided informed consent at the time of data collection, and each parent study received approval and oversight from its respective ethics board.

Results

Sample characteristics

Descriptive statistics for the 3072 NHANES participants and the 2300 ACES participants are presented in Table 1. In both datasets, approximately one in five respondents had diabetes and 12–13% met the scale's requirements for significant depressive symptomatology. The lifetime prevalence or "history" of depression in ACES was nearly 23%, whereas the prevalence of "recent" (12-month) depression was 8%. The ACES sample was slightly older, was more likely to be female, and had fewer Caucasians than the NHANES sample. The NHANES sample had more than twice as many respondents having pursued education beyond high school. The mean body mass

Table 1 Description and comparison of NHANES and ACES samples

Characteristic	NHANES ($n = 3072$)	ACES ($n = 2300$)
Percent with diabetes	19.2%	20.7%
Percent with depression or mean depressive symptoms score	PHQ-9: 3.2 out of 27, SE[a] = 0.2	CES-D: 8.1 out of 60, SD[b] = 9.1 Recent (12 months): 8.1% Lifetime: 22.9%
Mean age	59.5 years, SE = 0.3	65.1 years, SD = 10.5
Ethnicity	African American: 10.0% Latino: 8.7% Caucasian: 76.2% Other: 5.1%	African American: 33.8% Caucasian: 66.2%
Sex: Female	53.6%	68.1%
Education: High school or less	47.3%	75.0%
Mean body mass index	29.0, SE = 0.2	29.8, SD = 6.8

[a]SD = Standard Error
[b]SE = Standard Deviation

indexes of both samples were comparable at 29 kg/m^2. For the PHQ-9 (NHANES depressive symptoms measure), the raw Cronbach's alpha was 0.85 in the present data, and raw alpha for the CES-D (ACES depressive symptoms measure) was 0.91 for the present data. Thus, the items in the scales were cohesive.

Bivariate models

In NHANES, without adjusting for covariates, every 1-point increase in PHQ-9 score above the mean was associated with a 5% increase in odds of having diabetes [OR: 1.05 (95% CL: 1.03, 1.07)] (Table 2). In general, being older, being African American or Latino, having a high school education or less, and high BMI were each

independently associated with increased diabetes risk over their respective comparison groups.

For the ACES data, before adjusting for covariates, depressive symptoms were independently associated with diabetes status such that a 1-point increase in CES-D score was associated with a 2% increase in likelihood of having diabetes [OR: 1.02 (1.01, 1.03)]. There was a 58% increase in diabetes risk for recent depression [OR: 1.58 (1.13, 2.20)] and 35% for lifetime depression [OR: 1.35 (1.07, 1.70)]. Being African American, having a high BMI, and having a high school education or less each increased the odds of diabetes. Age was not significantly associated with odds of having diabetes [OR: 1.00 (0.99, 1.01)], but it was included in the multivariate model for its theoretical and clinical importance.

Table 2 Odds ratios and confidence intervals indicating bivariate associations with diabetes status

Variable name	NHANES $n = 3072$		ACES $n = 2300$	
	OR[a]	95% CI[b]	OR	95% CI
Depressive symptoms	**1.05**	**1.03, 1.07**	**1.02**	**1.01, 1.03**
Depression, recent	–	–	**1.58**	**1.13, 2.20**
Depression, lifetime	–	–	**1.35**	**1.07, 1.70**
Age (in years)	**1.03**	**1.02, 1.04**	1.00	0.99, 1.01
Ethnicity (reference: Caucasian)				
African American	**2.46**	**1.86, 3.26**	**1.63**	**1.32, 2.00**
Latino	**1.76**	**1.29, 2.39**	–	–
Other	1.14	0.56, 2.32	–	–
Sex: Female (reference: male)	0.84	0.69, 1.02	1.23	0.99, 1.53
Education (reference: more than high school)	**2.02**	**1.66, 2.46**	**1.65**	**1.30, 2.09**
Body mass index (in kg/m^2)	**1.12**	**1.09, 1.15**	**1.07**	**1.06, 1.09**

Boldface indicates statistical significance ($p < 0.05$)
[a]OR = Odds Ratio
[b]CI = 95% Wald Confidence Interval

Multivariate models
NHANES

As shown in Table 3, the relationship between depressive symptoms and diabetes status seen in the bivariate model persisted after adjusting for sex, ethnicity, age, education, and BMI [OR: 1.05 (1.03, 1.07)]. Because depressive symptoms were measured continuously, the odds ratio indicates that the odds of having diabetes increased by 5% for every 1-point increase in PHQ-9 score above the mean.

Odds ratios were significant for all covariates except the "other" level of ethnicity, indicating protective effects for being female, being Caucasian, being younger (closer to age 40), and having at least some postsecondary education. For every year of age over the mean, the odds of having diabetes increased by 5% [OR: 1.05 (CI: 1.04, 1.06)]. The odds of diabetes were 2.4 times as high for African Americans and 1.8 times as high for Latinos as for Caucasians. The odds of diabetes in women were about one-third lower than those for men [OR: 0.66 (CI: 0.51, 0.85)]. Having a high school diploma or less was associated with a 68% increase in odds for diabetes compared to those who have at least some post-secondary education [OR: 1.68 (CI: 1.29, 2.17)]. Every 1 kg/m^2 increase in BMI over the mean was associated with a 13% higher odds of having diabetes [OR: 1.13 (CI: 1.10, 1.16)].

NHANES plus behavioral variables and inflammation

The relationship between depressive symptoms and diabetes status persisted even after the addition to the multivariate model of the three health behavior variables (smoking, diet, and sedentary behavior) and inflammation. For every 1-point increase in PHQ-9 score over the mean, odds of diabetes rose by 4% [OR: 1.04 (CI: 1.02, 1.06)] (Table 3). Former smoking, current smoking, inflammation, and self-reported unhealthy diet were not significantly associated with diabetes status in the multivariate model. Being sedentary, however, was associated with a 58% increase in odds of having diabetes as compared to having at least some physical activity [OR: 1.58 (CI: 1.23, 2.03)].

Aces

As shown in Table 4, self-reported diabetes was associated with CES-D depressive symptoms score [OR: 1.02 (CI: 1.01, 1.03)] and CIDI report of recent [OR: 1.49 (CI: 1.03, 2.13)] and lifetime [OR: 1.40 (CI: 1.09, 1.81)] depression after adjusting for covariates. Being older, having African American ethnicity, having a high school diploma or less, and having higher BMI were associated with increased odds of diabetes, while female gender was not significant in any model.

Discussion

This study demonstrated a consistent and robust relationship between depression and diabetes. These findings were substantial and significant across instruments used to measure depression (PHQ-9, CIDI, CES-D), timing of depression (recent versus lifetime exposure), classification of the "depression" variable (diagnosable depression versus depressive symptomatology), and

Table 3 ORs and CIs for the multivariate and full NHANES models ($n = 3072$)

Variable name	Main Model		Main model + health behaviors + inflammation	
	OR[a]	95% CI[b]	OR	95% CI
Depressive symptoms (PHQ-9 score)	**1.05**	**1.03, 1.07**	**1.04**	**1.02, 1.06**
Age (in years)	**1.05**	**1.04, 1.06**	**1.05**	**1.04, 1.06**
Ethnicity (reference: Caucasian)				
African American	**2.45**	**1.85, 3.25**	**2.51**	**1.91, 3.30**
Latino	**1.78**	**1.32, 2.40**	**1.77**	**1.34, 2.33**
Other	1.79	0.95, 3.37	1.89	0.96, 3.70
Sex: Female (reference: male)	**0.66**	**0.51, 0.85**	**0.64**	**0.49, 0.85**
Education (reference: more than high school)	**1.68**	**1.29, 2.17**	**1.52**	**1.19, 1.94**
Body mass index (in kg/m^2)	**1.13**	**1.10, 1.16**	**1.12**	**1.09, 1.16**
Smoking (reference: Never)				
Current	–	–	0.98	0.71, 1.36
Former	–	–	1.04	0.67, 1.61
Diet (reference: good/very good/excellent)	–	–	1.07	0.70, 1.63
Sedentariness (reference: active)	–	–	**1.58**	**1.23, 2.03**
C-reactive protein (in mg/L)	–	–	0.99	0.91, 1.07

Boldface indicates statistical significance ($p < 0.05$)
[a]OR = Odds Ratio
[b]CI = 95% Wald Confidence Interval

Table 4 ORs and CIs for the multivariate model in ACES (n = 2300)

Variable name	CES-D		Recent Depression		Lifetime Depression	
	OR[a]	95% CI[b]	OR	95% CI	OR	95% CI
Depression indicator	**1.02**	**1.01, 1.03**	**1.49**	**1.03, 2.13**	**1.40**	**1.09, 1.81**
Age (in years)	**1.02**	**1.01, 1.03**	**1.02**	**1.01, 1.03**	**1.02**	**1.01, 1.03**
African American ethnicity (reference: Caucasian)	**1.31**	**1.05, 1.63**	**1.34**	**1.08, 1.68**	**1.38**	**1.11, 1.73**
Sex: Female (reference: male)	1.02	0.81, 1.29	1.04	0.82, 1.30	1.01	0.80, 1.27
Education (reference: more than high school)	**1.35**	**1.05, 1.73**	**1.40**	**1.09, 1.79**	**1.43**	**1.12, 1.83**
Body mass index (in kg/m²)	**1.07**	**1.06, 1.09**	**1.07**	**1.06, 1.09**	**1.07**	**1.06, 1.09**

Boldface indicates statistical significance (p < 0.05)
[a]OR = Odds Ratio
[b]CI = 95% Wald Confidence Interval

study context (nationally representative versus representative of a specific rural county). The relationship between depression and diabetes persisted after controlling for the effects of body mass index and demographic characteristics on diabetes status and, for NHANES, remained robust even with the addition of three health behavior variables and a measure of inflammation.

The present findings add to empirical knowledge the observation that lifetime history of depression is associated with increased diabetes risk. Most previous studies of the relationship between depression and diabetes have used measures of depressive symptoms taken at the time of the baseline interview or within the previous year [22, 32, 33]. Having any history of experiencing depression was associated with significantly increased odds of having diabetes when compared to those who never had depression. The odds of diabetes diagnosis were sizeable for all measures of depression, and they remained robust across depression diagnosed proximally or over the lifetime and for both the nationally representative sample and the smaller rural study sample. Additional research is warranted to gain a better understanding of the relative importance of depression compared to other variables in the etiology of diabetes; some mechanisms, such as inflammation, [34] may impact both diabetes and depression. The findings here imply mental health, and specifically depression, should be considered when designing interventions.

Treatment studies suggest a causal association between diabetes and depression, although the direction of causality may be complex. When depression is treated in people with diagnosed diabetes, hemoglobin A_1c (HbA$_1$c), a biomarker for glucose control, decreases moderately [35]. The elevated risk for diabetes associated with depression remains even when other recognized diabetes risk factors are considered, including risk conferred by some antidepressants [32], poor diet, [36, 37] family history, [37] inflammation, [33] and sedentary lifestyle [36, 38].

Limitations

As with many studies of depression and diabetes, this study uses mostly cross-sectional data, precluding inferences of causality. It remains unclear whether depression produces diabetes, is produced by it, or co-evolves with it. However, history of depression could hint at depression's contribution to diabetes risk based on a retrospective-prospective study design [39]. Participants were asked to reflect retrospectively on symptoms they have experienced over the course of their lives, and these reflections were used by the CIDI computerized adaptive test to judge whether the symptoms were sufficient for a diagnosis of depression [28]. Then, lifetime depression status was used as a predictor of diabetes, providing some evidence for the claim that the two conditions are causally related.

There are other limitations to the present work. Researchers were unable to exclude individuals with type 1 diabetes from either analysis. For ACES, diabetes status was dichotomous and entirely self-reported, and no data were collected to indicate the type of diabetes a participant had. Also, it is no longer safe to assume that all diabetes that occurs during or before adolescence is Type 1, given the rise of Type 2 diabetes among teenagers [9]. However, it is estimated that only 5% of all diabetes cases are Type 1 [9]. Another limitation is that both datasets relied heavily on self-reported data for depression rather than clinical interviews or formal diagnoses, although the reliability and validity of instruments used is well-established [25–27, 29]. Self-report data are vulnerable to recall bias and other threats to validity. Finally, these analyses did not control for conditions that are frequently associated with depression and may also be associated with diabetes, such as anxiety and sleep disorders [5, 6].

Although generality cannot be proven, the present findings add substantially to previous evidence that the relationships between depression and diabetes are robust across methods and populations. The data analyzed were derived from large, community-based samples. The

NHANES random sample purports to be representative of the United States population when properly weighted, so results using these data should be generalizable to individuals outside of those studied directly. The ACES dataset was a biracial, older-aged sample from a rural North Carolina county and therefore may be less generalizable than NHANES. Nevertheless, taken together, the findings from national and local data are informative.

Conclusions

The strength of the relationship between lifetime experience of depression and diabetes risk suggests that interventions designed to lessen the burden of diabetes should focus on depression that occurs at any time over a person's lifespan rather than only that which is detected immediately at the time of diabetes diagnosis or treatment. Much of the ongoing research in this field is biomedical, yet a multilevel public health model is needed to move this research forward by considering the myriad factors that contribute to each health outcome. This wider-lens model would also allow researchers and clinicians to include social determinants like education, which in the present analyses had a strong relationship with diabetes even after controlling for depression, in interventions.

The results from the present analyses demand the reconstruction of the current biomedical model to be more inclusive of psychosocial factors associated with disease. This model can then be used to develop interventions that will treat both body and mind. For example, several randomized controlled trials are underway in which researchers are using cognitive behavioral therapy to relieve depression among people living with diabetes, with the ultimate goal of managing their diabetes more effectively [40, 41].

Amidst the burgeoning literature addressing relationships among depression and other mental health indicators on the one hand, and diabetes and other physical health conditions on the other, the present findings add evidence of the robustness of the depression-diabetes connection across several populations as well as sampling, measurement, and analytic approaches. They also add the novel finding that a reported history of depressive symptoms is predictive of later diabetes. In addition to reinforcing the general interest in these issues, the present findings add evidence for the importance of depression as an indicator for both prevention and treatment of diabetes.

Abbreviations
ACES: Arthritis, Coping, and Emotion Study; CDC: Centers for Disease Control and Prevention; CES-D: Center for Epidemiologic Studies Depression inventory; CIDI: Composite International Diagnostic Interview; DSM-III-R: Third edition of *Diagnostic and Statistical Manual for Mental Disorders*, Revised; DSM-IV: Fourth edition of *Diagnostic and Statistical Manual for Mental Disorders*; FPG: Fasting plasma glucose; HbA1c: Glycated hemoglobin (hemoglobin A1c); JoCo OA: Johnston County Osteoarthritis Study; MEC: NHANES Mobile Examination Center; NC: North Carolina; NHANES: National Health And Nutrition Examination Survey; PHQ-9: 9-Item Patient Health Questionnaire; US: United States of America.

Acknowledgements
At the time the study took place, Jaimie Hunter was a doctoral student in the Department of Health Behavior at the University of North Carolina at Chapel Hill. The present manuscript is derived from her dissertation work, which is published here: https://goo.gl/9EQDVv. Analyses have been rerun, and the text has been completely rewritten.
The authors wish to thank the United States National Center for Health Statistics for building and maintaining national data on important health issues. Data from the National Health and Nutrition Examination Survey (NHANES) are freely available on the Centers for Disease Control and Prevention website: https://www.cdc.gov/nchs/nhanes/.
We also wish to acknowledge and thank Dr. Chris Wiesen at the UNC Odum Institute for providing statistical assistance.

Funding
The Johnston County Osteoarthritis Project was supported in part by the Centers for Disease Control and Prevention / Association of Schools of Public Health (cooperative agreements S043, S1734, and S3486), the National Institute of Arthritis and Musculoskeletal and Skin Diseases Multipurpose Arthritis and Musculoskeletal Disease Center (grant 5-P60-AR30701), and the National Institute of Arthritis and Musculoskeletal and Skin Diseases Multidisciplinary Clinical Research Center (grant 5-P60-AR49465–03). The Arthritis, Coping and Emotions Study was supported by the National Institute of Mental Health (grant R01MH64034, Co-PIs Brenda DeVellis and Joanne Jordan).

Authors' contributions
JCH conceptualized the study and conducted the analysis as part of her dissertation project at the University of North Carolina at Chapel Hill. All authors contributed substantially to study concept, design, and interpretation of results. All authors contributed to the composition of this manuscript. EBF, JMJ, CR, LAL, and MSK served on the dissertation committee for JCH and thus were present with the study from conceptualization to completion. EBF served as the chair of the dissertation committee. BMD provided subject area expertise and guided the theoretical underpinnings of the study. All authors read and approved the final manuscript.

Competing interests
The authors declare that they have no competing interests.

Author details
[1]Department of Social Sciences and Health Policy, Division of Public Health Sciences, Wake Forest University School of Medicine, Medical Center Boulevard, Winston-Salem, NC 27157, USA. [2]Department of Health Behavior, Gillings School of Global Public Health, The University of North Carolina at Chapel Hill, Chapel Hill, NC, USA. [3]Division of Rheumatology, Allergy, and Immunology, Thurston Arthritis Research Center, University of North Carolina School of Medicine, Chapel Hill, NC, USA. [4]Diabetes Care Center Clinical Trials Unit, Division of Endocrinology and Metabolism, University of North Carolina School of Medicine, Chapel Hill, NC, USA. [5]Cancer Prevention and Control, John Theurer Cancer Center, Hackensack University Medical Center, Hackensack, NJ, USA. [6]Department of Biomedical Research, Hackensack University Medical Center, Hackensack, NJ, USA. [7]Department of Oncology, Georgetown University School of Medicine, Washington DC, USA.

References
1. Murray CJ, et al. The state of US health, 1990–2010: burden of diseases, injuries, and risk factors. JAMA. 2013;310(6):591–608.
2. Kessler RC, et al. Age differences in the prevalence and co-morbidity of DSM-IV major depressive episodes: results from the WHO world mental health survey initiative. Depress Anxiety. 2010;27(4):351–64.
3. WHO. Psychiatrists and nurses working in mental health sector (per 100,000) population, 2011. 2011; Available from: http://www.who.int/gho/mental_health/human_resources/psychiatrists_nurses/en/. Accessed 21 Dec 2017.
4. Ghio L, et al. Duration of untreated depression influences clinical outcomes and disability. J Affect Disord. 2015;175:224–8.
5. Zhang P, et al. Combined effects of sleep quality and depression on quality of life in patients with type 2 diabetes. BMC Fam Pract. 2016;17:–40. https://doi.org/10.1186/s12875-016-0435-x.

6. Tiller JW. Depression and anxiety. Med J Aust. 2013;199(6 Suppl):S28–31.
7. Joynt KE, Whellan DJ, O'Connor CM. Depression and cardiovascular disease: mechanisms of interaction. Biol Psychiatry. 2003;54(3):248–61.
8. Holt RI, de Groot M, Golden SH. Diabetes and depression. Curr Diab Rep. 2014;14(6):491. https://doi.org/10.1007/s11892-014-0491-3.
9. Centers for Disease Control and Prevention. National diabetes fact sheet: national estimates and general information on diabetes and prediabetes in the United States, 2011. Atlanta: Department of Health and Human Services, Centers for Disease Control and Prevention; 2011.
10. Ogden CL, et al. Prevalence of obesity in the United States, 2009–2010. NCHS Data Brief. 2012(82):1–8.
11. Knowler WC, et al. Reduction in the incidence of type 2 diabetes with lifestyle intervention or metformin. N Engl J Med. 2002;346(6):393–403.
12. Tuomilehto J, Schwarz PE. Preventing diabetes: early versus late preventive interventions. Diabetes Care. 2016;39(Suppl 2):S115–20. https://doi.org/10.2337/dcS15-3000.
13. Liburd LC, et al. Intervening on the social determinants of cardiovascular disease and diabetes. Am J Prev Med. 2005;29(5 Suppl 1):18–24.
14. Olson MM, et al. The biopsychosocial milieu of type 2 diabetes: an exploratory study of the impact of social relationships on a chronic inflammatory disease. Int J Psychiatry Med. 2010;40(3):289–305.
15. Peyrot M, McMurry JF Jr, Kruger DF. A biopsychosocial model of glycemic control in diabetes: stress, coping and regimen adherence. J Health Soc Behav. 1999;40(2):141–58.
16. Fisher EB, et al. Key features of peer support in chronic disease prevention and management. Health Aff (Millwood). 2015;34(9):1523–30. https://doi.org/10.1377/hlthaff.2015.0365.
17. Fisher EB, et al. Peer support in health care and prevention: cultural, organizational, and dissemination issues. Annu Rev Public Health. 2014;35: 363–83. https://doi.org/10.1146/annurev-publhealth-032013-182450. Epub 2014 Jan 2
18. Mezuk B, et al. Is ignorance bliss? Depression, antidepressants, and the diagnosis of Prediabetes and type 2 diabetes. Health Psychol. 2013; 32(3):254–63.
19. Ferreira MC, et al. Clinical variables associated with depression in patients with type 2 diabetes. Rev Assoc Med Bras. 2015;61(4):336–40.
20. Li C, et al. Prevalence and correlates of undiagnosed depression among U.S. adults with diabetes: the behavioral risk factor surveillance system, 2006. Diabetes Res Clin Pract, 2009. 83(2):268–79.
21. Pan A, et al. Bidirectional association between depression and type 2 diabetes mellitus in women. Arch Intern Med. 2010;170(21):1884–91.
22. Chen PC, et al. Population-based cohort analyses of the bidirectional relationship between type 2 diabetes and depression. Diabetes Care. 2013; 36(2):376–82.
23. CDC and NCHS, National Health and Nutrition Examination Survey Data, C.f. D.C.a.P. U.S. Department of Health and Human Services, Editor. 2007: Hyattsville, MD.
24. Jordan JM, et al. Prevalence of knee symptoms and radiographic and symptomatic knee osteoarthritis in African Americans and Caucasians: the Johnston County osteoarthritis project. J Rheumatol. 2007;34(1):172–80.
25. Kroenke K, Spitzer RL. The PHQ-9: a new depression and diagnostic severity measure. Psych Annals. 2002;32:509–21.
26. Kroenke K, Spitzer RL, William JB. The PHQ-9: validity of a brief depression severity measure. J Gen Intern Med. 2001;16:1606–13.
27. van Steenbergen-Weijenburg KM, et al. Validation of the PHQ-9 as a screening instrument for depression in diabetes patients in specialized outpatient clinics. BMC Health Serv Res. 2010;10:235.
28. Robins LN, et al. The composite international diagnostic interview. An epidemiologic instrument suitable for use in conjunction with different diagnostic systems and in different cultures. Arch Gen Psychiatry. 1988; 45(12):1069–77.
29. Radloff L. The CES–D scale: a self-report depression scale for research in the general population. Appl Psychol Meas. 1977;3:385–401.
30. Fortin M, et al. Self-reported versus health administrative data: implications for assessing chronic illness burden in populations. A cross-sectional study. CMAJ Open. 2017;5(3):E729–33. https://doi.org/10.9778/cmajo.20170029.
31. White K, et al. Diabetes risk, diagnosis, and control: do psychosocial factors predict hemoglobin A1c defined outcomes or accuracy of self-reports? Ethn Dis. 2014;24(1):19–27.
32. Atlantis E, et al. Diabetes incidence associated with depression and antidepressants in the Melbourne longitudinal studies on healthy ageing (MELSHA). Int J Geriatr Psychiatry. 2010;25(7):688–96.
33. Golden SH, et al. Examining a bidirectional association between depressive symptoms and diabetes. JAMA. 2008;299(23):2751–9.
34. Stuart MJ, Baune BT. Depression and type 2 diabetes: inflammatory mechanisms of a psychoneuroendocrine co-morbidity. Neurosci Biobehav Rev. 2012;36(1):658–76.
35. Echeverry D, et al. Effect of pharmacological treatment of depression on A1C and quality of life in low-income Hispanics and African Americans with diabetes: a randomized, double-blind, placebo-controlled trial. Diabetes Care. 2009;32(12):2156–60.
36. Carnethon MR, et al. Longitudinal association between depressive symptoms and incident type 2 diabetes mellitus in older adults: the cardiovascular health study. Arch Intern Med. 2007;167(8):802–7.
37. Mezuk B, et al. The influence of educational attainment on depression and risk of type 2 diabetes. Am J Public Health. 2008;98(8):1480–5.
38. Mezuk B, et al. Depression and type 2 diabetes over the lifespan: a meta-analysis. Diabetes Care. 2008;31(12):2383–90.
39. Kumar R. Research methodology: a step-by-step guide for beginners. London: Sage; 2011.
40. De Groot M, et al. Program ACTIVE II: design and methods for a multi-center community-based depression treatment for rural and urban adults with type 2 diabetes. J Diabetes Res Ther. 2015;1(2) [Epub ahead of print].
41. Hermanns N, et al. The effect of a diabetes-specific cognitive behavioral treatment program (DIAMOS) for patients with diabetes and subclinical depression: results of a randomized controlled trial. Diabetes Care. 2015;38:551–60.

Permissions

All chapters in this book were first published in CDE, by BioMed Central; hereby published with permission under the Creative Commons Attribution License or equivalent. Every chapter published in this book has been scrutinized by our experts. Their significance has been extensively debated. The topics covered herein carry significant findings which will fuel the growth of the discipline. They may even be implemented as practical applications or may be referred to as a beginning point for another development.

The contributors of this book come from diverse backgrounds, making this book a truly international effort. This book will bring forth new frontiers with its revolutionizing research information and detailed analysis of the nascent developments around the world.

We would like to thank all the contributing authors for lending their expertise to make the book truly unique. They have played a crucial role in the development of this book. Without their invaluable contributions this book wouldn't have been possible. They have made vital efforts to compile up to date information on the varied aspects of this subject to make this book a valuable addition to the collection of many professionals and students.

This book was conceptualized with the vision of imparting up-to-date information and advanced data in this field. To ensure the same, a matchless editorial board was set up. Every individual on the board went through rigorous rounds of assessment to prove their worth. After which they invested a large part of their time researching and compiling the most relevant data for our readers.

The editorial board has been involved in producing this book since its inception. They have spent rigorous hours researching and exploring the diverse topics which have resulted in the successful publishing of this book. They have passed on their knowledge of decades through this book. To expedite this challenging task, the publisher supported the team at every step. A small team of assistant editors was also appointed to further simplify the editing procedure and attain best results for the readers.

Apart from the editorial board, the designing team has also invested a significant amount of their time in understanding the subject and creating the most relevant covers. They scrutinized every image to scout for the most suitable representation of the subject and create an appropriate cover for the book.

The publishing team has been an ardent support to the editorial, designing and production team. Their endless efforts to recruit the best for this project, has resulted in the accomplishment of this book. They are a veteran in the field of academics and their pool of knowledge is as vast as their experience in printing. Their expertise and guidance has proved useful at every step. Their uncompromising quality standards have made this book an exceptional effort. Their encouragement from time to time has been an inspiration for everyone.

The publisher and the editorial board hope that this book will prove to be a valuable piece of knowledge for researchers, students, practitioners and scholars across the globe.

List of Contributors

Alex J. Graveling
JJR Macleod Centre for Diabetes and Endocrinology, Aberdeen Royal Infirmary, Foresterhill, Aberdeen AB25 2ZP, UK

Brian M. Frier
The Queen's Medical Research Institute, The University of Edinburgh, Edinburgh EH16 4TJ, UK

Priscila Novaes and Ana Beatriz Diniz Grisolia
Department of Ophthalmology and Visual Sciences, Kellogg Eye Center, University of Michigan Medical School, Ann Arbor, MI 48105, USA

Terry J. Smith
Department of Ophthalmology and Visual Sciences, Kellogg Eye Center, University of Michigan Medical School, Ann Arbor, MI 48105, USA
Division of Metabolism, Endocrinology, and Diabetes, Department of Internal Medicine, University of Michigan Medical School, Ann Arbor, MI 48105, USA
Department of Ophthalmology and Visual Sciences, Brehm Tower, Room 7112, 1000 Wall Street, Ann Arbor, MI 48105, USA

Ann-Marie Svensson and MirNabi Pirouzi Fard
Center of Registers in Region Västra Götaland, Göteborg, Sweden

Vincent Lak and Björn Eliasson
Department of Medicine, Sahlgrenska University Hospital, University of Gothenburg, S-413 45 Göteborg, Sweden

Balaji Bhavadharini, Manni Mohanraj Mahalakshmi, Ranjit Mohan Anjana, Kumar Maheswari, Mohan Deepa, Ranjit Unnikrishnan, Harish Ranjani and Viswanathan Mohan
Madras Diabetes Research Foundation, 4, Conran Smith Road, Gopalapuram, Chennai 600 086, India

Ram Uma
Seethapathy Clinic and Hospital, Chennai, India

Sonak D Pastakia
College of Pharmacy, Purdue University, West Lafayette, IN, USA

Arivudainambi Kayal, Lyudmil Ninov, Belma Malanda and Anne Belton
International Diabetes Federation, Brussels, Belgium

Alexander Faje
Neuroendocrine Unit, Massachusetts General Hospital and Harvard Medical School, 55 Fruit Street, Boston, MA 02114, USA

Sima Saberi
Ann Arbor Endocrinology and Diabetes, PC, Ypsilanti, Michigan, USA

Nazanene H. Esfandiari and Meng H. Tan
Division of Metabolism, Endocrinology and Diabetes, University of Michigan, Lobby C, 24 Frank Lloyd Wright Drive, Ann Arbor, MI 48106, USA

Mark P. MacEachern
Taubman Health Sciences Library, University of Michigan, Ann Arbor, Michigan, USA

Roma Y. Gianchandani
Frank Lloyd Wright Drive, Ann Arbor, MI 48106, USA
University of Michigan Health System, Ann Arbor, MI, USA

Timothy W. Bodnar
Ann Arbor Endocrinology and Diabetes Associates P.C., Ypsilanti, MI, USA

Jennifer J. Iyengar and Preethi V. Patil
University of Michigan Health System, Ann Arbor, MI, USA

Marcio W Lauria and Antonio Ribeiro-Oliveira Jr
Department of Internal Medicine (Endocrinology section and Transplantation unit), Federal University of Minas Gerais, Rua Alfredo Balena, 190, 30130-100 Belo Horizonte, MG, Brazil

Huan Wang and Peter T. Donnan
Dundee Epidemiology and Biostatistics Unit, Population Health Sciences, University of Dundee, The Mackenzie Building, Kirsty Semple Way, Dundee DD2 4BF, UK

Callum J. Leese
University of Edinburgh, Faculty of Medicine, Edinburgh, UK

Edward Duncan
NMAHP Research Unit, University of Stirling, Stirling, UK

David Fitzpatrick
NMAHP Research Unit, University of Stirling, Stirling, UK
Scottish Ambulance Service, National Headquarters, Edinburgh, UK

Brian M. Frier
BHF Centre for Cardiovascular Science, The Queen's Medical Research Institute, University of Edinburgh, Edinburgh, UK

Graham P. Leese
School of Medicine, Ninewells Hospital and Medical School, Dundee, UK

Saroj Khatiwada
Department of Pharmacy, Central Institute of Science and Technology (CIST) College, Pokhara University, Kathmandu, Nepal

Santosh Kumar Sah
Department of Biochemistry, Universal College of Medical Sciences, Bhairahawa, Nepal.

Rajendra KC
Department of Medical Laboratory Technology, Modern Technical College, Satdobato, Lalitpur, Nepal

Nirmal Baral and Madhab Lamsal
Department of Biochemistry, B P Koirala Institute of Health Sciences, Dharan, Nepal

William H. Herman
Diabetes Prevention Program Coordinating Center, The Biostatistics Center, George Washington University, 16110 Executive Blvd., Suite 750, Rockville, MD 20852, USA

Brijesh K. Singh and Paul M. Yen
Laboratory of Hormonal Regulation, Cardiovascular and Metabolic Disorders Program, Duke-NUS Graduate Medical School, 8 College Road, Singapore 169857, Singapore

Alberto Hayek
Scripps Whittier Diabetes Institute, La Jolla, CA 92037, USA

Charles C. King
Pediatric Diabetes Research Center, University of California, San Diego, La Jolla, CA 92093, USA

Giovanni Veronesi
Department of Clinical and Experimental Medicine, Research Centre in Epidemiology and Preventive Medicine, University of Insubria, Varese, Italy

Carmine S. Poerio and Antonio C. Bossi
Metabolic Diseases and Diabetes Unit, A.O. Ospedale Treviglio-Caravaggio, P.le Ospedale, 1 – 24047 Treviglio, BG, Italy

Alessandra Braus and Lavinia Gilberti
Pharmacy Unit, A.O. Ospedale Treviglio-Caravaggio, Treviglio, BG, Italy

Maurizio Destro
Medical Science Department, A.O. Ospedale Treviglio-Caravaggio, Treviglio, BG, Italy

Giovanni Meroni
Hospital Health Management Direction, A.O. Ospedale Treviglio-Caravaggio, Treviglio, BG, Italy

Estella M. Davis
Creighton University School of Pharmacy and Health Professions, Omaha, NE, USA

Shrikant Tamhane and Hossein Gharib
Mayo Clinic College of Medicine, Rochester, MN 55905, USA
Division of Endocrinology, Diabetes, Metabolism, and Nutrition, Mayo Clinic, 200 First Street SW, Rochester, MN 55905, USA

Viral N. Shah
Barbara Davis Center for Diabetes, University of Colorado Denver, 1775 Aurora Court, A140, Aurora, CO 80045, USA
School of Medicine, University of Colorado Denver, Aurora, CO, USA

Satish K. Garg
Barbara Davis Center for Diabetes, University of Colorado Denver, 1775 Aurora Court, A140, Aurora, CO 80045, USA
School of Medicine, University of Colorado Denver, Aurora, CO, USA
Diabetes Technology and Therapeutics, New Rochelle, USA

Anjali R. Shah
Departments of Ophthalmology and Visual Sciences, University of Michigan Medical Schoo, W.K. Kellogg Eye Center, 1000 Wall St, Ann Arbor, MI 48105, USA

Thomas W. Gardner
Departments of Ophthalmology and Visual Sciences, University of Michigan Medical Schoo, W.K. Kellogg Eye Center, 1000 Wall St, Ann Arbor, MI 48105, USA
Molecular and Integrative Physiology, University of Michigan Medical School, W.K. Kellogg Eye Center, 1000 Wall St, Ann Arbor, MI 48105, USA

Palak Choksi, Andrew Kraftson, Nicole Miller, Katherine Zurales and Catherine Van Poznak
Department of Internal Medicine, University of Michigan, 24 Frank Lloyd Wright Dr, Ann Arbor, MI 48106, USA

Amy Rothberg
Department of Internal Medicine, University of Michigan, 24 Frank Lloyd Wright Dr, Ann Arbor, MI 48106, USA
Department of Nutritional Sciences, University of Michigan, Ann Arbor, USA

Charles Burant
Department of Internal Medicine, University of Michigan, 24 Frank Lloyd Wright Dr, Ann Arbor, MI 48106, USA
Molecular and Integrative Physiology, University of Michigan, Ann Arbor, USA
Department of Nutritional Sciences, University of Michigan, Ann Arbor, USA

Mark Peterson
Department of Physical Medicine and Rehabilitation, University of Michigan, Ann Arbor, USA

Martin Eichholz
Kelton Communications, Culver City, CA, USA

Andrea H. Alexander, Patrick Hlavacek, Bruce Parsons and Alesia Sadosky
Pfizer Inc., 235 East 42nd Street, New York, NY 10017, USA

Joseph C. Cappelleri
Pfizer Inc., Groton, CT, USA

Michael M. Tuchman
Palm Beach Neurological Center, Palm Beach Gardens, FL, USA

Caroline T. Nguyen
Division of Endocrinology, Diabetes, and Metabolism, Department of Medicine, Keck School of Medicine, University of Southern California, 1540 Alcazar Street, CHP 204, Los Angeles, Ca 90033, USA

Elizabeth B. Sasso
Division of Maternal Fetal Medicine, Department of Obstetrics and Gynecology, Keck School of Medicine, University of Southern California, 2020 Zonal Avenue, IRD 220, Los Angeles, CA 90033, USA

Lorayne Barton
Division of Neonatology, Department of Pediatrics, LAC+USC Medical Center, Keck School of Medicine, University of Southern California, Los Angeles, Ca 90033, USA

Jorge H. Mestman
Division of Endocrinology, Diabetes and Metabolism, Department of Medicine and Obstetrics and Gynecology, Keck School of Medicine, University of Southern California, 1540 Alcazar Street CHP 204, Los Angeles, California 90033, USA

S. Ghosal
Nightingale Hospital, 11 Shakespeare Sarani, Kolkata, India
Kolkata, India

B. Sinha
AMRI Hospitals, JC-16-17, Salt Lake City, Kolkata 700091, India
Kolkata, India

Peter H. Sönksen, Richard I. G. Holt and Walailuck Böhning
Human Development and Health Academic Unit, University of Southampton Faculty of Medicine, Southampton, UK

Nishan Guha
Human Development and Health Academic Unit, University of Southampton Faculty of Medicine, Southampton, UK
Nuffield Division of Clinical Laboratory Sciences, University of Oxford, Oxford, UK

Dankmar Böhning
Southampton Statistical Sciences Research Institute, University of Southampton, Southampton, UK
Nuffield Division of Clinical Laboratory Sciences, University of Oxford, Oxford, UK

David A. Cowan and Christiaan Bartlett
Department of Pharmacy and Forensic Science, Drug Control Centre, King's College London, London, UK

Júnia Ribeiro de Oliveira Longo Schweizer and Antônio Ribeiro-Oliveira Jr
Endocrinology Laboratory of Federal University of Minas Gerais. Alfredo Balena, 190, Santa Efigênia, Belo Horizonte 30130-100, Brazil

Martin Bidlingmaier
Endocrine Laboratory, Medizinische Klinik und Poliklinik IV, Klinikum der Universität München, Ziemssenstraße 1, 80336 Munich, Germany

M. H. Cummings
Queen Alexandra Hospital, Portsmouth, UK

D. Cao and L. L. Ilag
Eli Lilly and Company, Indianapolis, IN, USA

I. Hadjiyianni
Lilly Deutschland GmbH, Bad Homburg, Germany

M. H. Tan
University of Michigan, Ann Arbor, MI, USA

Edwin B. Fisher
Peers for Progress and Department of Health Behavior, Gillings School of Global Public Health, University of North Carolina at Chapel Hill, Rosenau Hall, CB #7440, Chapel Hill, NC 27599-7440, USA

Sarah D. Kowitt
Peers for Progress and Department of Health Behavior, Gillings School of Global Public Health, University of North Carolina at Chapel Hill, Rosenau Hall, CB #7440, Chapel Hill, NC 27599-7440, USA
Department of Family Medicine, University of North Carolina at Chapel Hill, Chapel Hill, NC 27599, USA

Katrina E. Donahue
Department of Family Medicine, University of North Carolina at Chapel Hill, Chapel Hill, NC 27599, USA
Cecil G. Sheps Center for Health Services Research, University of North Carolina at Chapel Hill, Chapel Hill, NC 27599, USA

Madeline Mitchell
Cecil G. Sheps Center for Health Services Research, University of North Carolina at Chapel Hill, Chapel Hill, NC 27599, USA

Laura A. Young
Division of Endocrinology and Metabolism, School of Medicine, University of North Carolina at Chapel Hill, Chapel Hill, NC 27599, USA

Jaimie C. Hunter
Department of Social Sciences and Health Policy, Division of Public Health Sciences, Wake Forest University School of Medicine, Medical Center Boulevard, Winston-Salem, NC 27157, USA
Department of Health Behavior, Gillings School of Global Public Health, The University of North Carolina at Chapel Hill, Chapel Hill, NC, USA

Brenda M. DeVellis, Laura A. Linnan and Edwin B. Fisher
Department of Health Behavior, Gillings School of Global Public Health, The University of North Carolina at Chapel Hill, Chapel Hill, NC, USA

Joanne M. Jordan
Division of Rheumatology, Allergy, and Immunology, Thurston Arthritis Research Center, University of North Carolina School of Medicine, Chapel Hill, NC, USA

M. Sue Kirkman
Diabetes Care Center Clinical Trials Unit, Division of Endocrinology and Metabolism, University of North Carolina School of Medicine, Chapel Hill, NC, USA

Christine Rini
Cancer Prevention and Control, John Theurer Cancer Center, Hackensack University Medical Center, Hackensack, NJ, USA
Department of Biomedical Research, Hackensack University Medical Center, Hackensack, NJ, USA
Department of Oncology, Georgetown University School of Medicine, Washington DC, USA

Index

www.ingramcontent.com/pod-product-compliance
Lightning Source LLC
Chambersburg PA
CBHW080250230326

41458CB00097B/4197